MEDICAL MICROBIOLOGY

SECOND EDITION

CEDRIC MIMS
BSc, MD, FRCPath
Emeritus Professor
Department of Microbiology
Guy's Hospital Medical School
London, UK

JOHN PLAYFAIR
MB, Bchir, PhD, DSc
Emeritus Professor
Department of Immunology
University College and Middlesex
School of Medicine
London, UK

IVAN ROITT
MA DSc (Oxon), Hon FRCP (Lond), FRCPath FRS
Emeritus Professor of Immunology
Director of Institute of
Biomedical Science
University College London
Medical School
London, UK

DEREK WAKELIN
BSc, PhD, DSc, FRCPath
Professor,
School of Biological Sciences
University of Nottingham
Nottingham, UK

ROSAMUND WILLIAMS
PhD, FRCPath
Division of Emerging and other
Communicable Diseases,
Surveillance and Control
World Health Organization
Geneva, Switzerland

Mosby
London Philadelphia St Louis Sydney Tokyo

Editor	**Louise Crowe**
Project Manager	**Leslie Sinoway**
Design	**Pete Wilder**
Layout	**Rob Curran**
Cover Design	**Greg Smith**
Illustration Manager	**Danny Pyne**
Cover Illustration	**Mark Willey**
Illustrators	**Mike Saiz**
	Rob Dean
	Paul Bernson
	Debra Woodward
Production	**Gudrun Hughes**
Index	**Janine Ross**

MOSBY

© Mosby Publishers Limited 1998

M is a registered trademark of Harcourt Publishers Limited

The rights of C Mims, J Playfair, I Roitt, D Wakelin and R Williams to be identified as the authors of this work have been asserted by them in accordance with the Copyright, Designs and Patents Act, 1988.

First edition published by Mosby-Year Book Europe Ltd, 1993
This edition published 1998
  Reprinted 1999
  Reprinted 2000
  Reprinted 2001
ISBN 0 7234 2781 X

British Library Cataloguing in Publication Data
A catalogue record for this book is available from the British Library.

Library of Congress Cataloging-in-Publication data applied for.

Printed by Grafos S.A. Arte sobre papel, Barcelona, Spain

Preface

Medical Microbiology Second Edition maintains the innovative approach of the first edition in concentrating on the conflict between host and parasite. To address today's curricula, we have retained a systems-based treatment of microbiology, putting infectious diseases into clinically relevant sections and emphasizing their biologic context. Details about each microorganism are conveniently collected into an Appendix, together with updated information about relevant microbiologic methods and techniques.

A major improvement in this edition has been to focus the immunology directly onto the role of the immune system in infectious disease, both in contributing to defense against infection and in bringing about immunopathologic changes. New sections have been added to cover aspects of the molecular biology and genetics of pathogenic bacteria relating to disease mechanisms.

Case studies have been incorporated into the text, to focus attention on clinical relevance. Summaries of the key points in each chapter are a useful review tool and questions challenge the student's understanding of the subject.

The layout and illustration of the book have been extensively revised to improve readability and access to information. We are confident that this second edition of *Medical Microbiology* builds successfully on the excellent reputation of the first edition. It continues to offer the reader an informative and exciting insight into the means by which microorganisms cause disease and the ways in which these infectious diseases can be treated and controlled.

CM, JHLP, IMR, DW, RW
1998

Acknowledgements

We wish to express our appreciation of the generosity of many collegues throughout the world who supplied illustrative material, particularly W Edmund Farrar, Martin J Wood, John A Innes, Hugh Tubbs, James S Bingham, Ralph Muller, John R Baker and Dilip K Banerjee. We would like to thank the library of The Wellcome Institute for the History of Medicine for providing portrait photographs for the historical profiles. We are also grateful to David Jarvis for his invaluable help in compiling the Appendix, and Professor John Oxford for his advice on the cover illustration.

CM, JHLP, IMR, DW, RW
1998

Contributors

Roy M Anderson FRS
Linacre Professor and Head of Department
Director of Wellcome Trust Centre for
Epidemiology of Infectious Disease
Department of Zoology
University of Oxford
Oxford, UK

Timothy R Hirst BSc, DPhil
Professor of Microbiology
Department of Pathology and Microbiology
University of Bristol
Bristol, UK

Gillian Urwin MSc, MB, BS, MRCPath
Consultant Microbiologist
Department of Microbiology
Essex Rivers Healthcare NHS Trust
Colchester, UK

Mark Zuckerman BSc (Hons), MSc,
MRCP, MRCPath
Consultant Virologist and Honorary Senior
Registrar
Dulwich Public Health Laboratory and
Medical Microbiology
King's College School of Medicine and Dentistry
London, UK

Contents

diagnostic principles of clinical manifestations section 3

clinical manifestations and diagnosis of infections by body system section 4

control

appendix

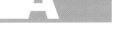

1

the adversaries

Introduction

The conventional distinction between 'microbes' and 'parasites' is essentially arbitrary
Microbiology is sometimes defined as the biology of microscopic organisms, its subject being the 'microbes'. Traditionally, clinical microbiology has been concerned with those organisms responsible for the major infectious diseases of humans and whose size makes them invisible to the naked eye. It is not surprising that the range of organisms included has reflected those diseases that have been (or continue to be) of greatest importance in those countries where the scientific and clinical discipline of microbiology developed, notably Europe and the USA. The term 'microbes' has usually been applied in a restricted fashion, primarily to viruses, bacteria and related organisms. Fungi and protozoans ('parasites') have sometimes been included as relatively minor contributors, but in general they have been treated as the subjects of other disciplines (mycology and parasitology).

Although there can be no argument that viruses and bacteria are the most numerous and most important pathogens, the conventional distinction between these as 'microbes' and the other infectious agents we know loosely as 'parasites' is essentially arbitrary, not least because the criterion of microscopic visibility cannot be applied rigidly *(Fig. 1.1)*. Perhaps we should remember that the first 'microbe' to be associated with a specific clinical condition was a parasitic worm – the nematode *Trichinella spiralis* – whose larval stages are just visible to the naked eye (though microscopy is needed for certain identification). *T. spiralis* was first identified in 1835 and causally related to the disease trichinellosis in the 1860s.

A New Approach to Microbiology

Many microbiology texts deal with infectious organisms as agents of disease in isolation – isolated both from other infectious organisms and from the biologic context in which they live and in which disease is caused. It is certainly convenient to list and deal with organisms group by group, to summarize the diseases they cause, and to review the forms of control available, but this approach produces a static picture of what is a dynamic relationship between the organism and its host.

Host response is the outcome of the complex interplay between host and parasite
Host response can be discussed in terms of pathologic signs and symptoms and in terms of immune control, but it is better treated as the outcome of the complex interplay between two organisms – host and parasite; without this dimension a distorted view of infectious disease results. It simply is not true that microbe + host = disease, and clinicians are well aware of this. Insights into understanding the reasons why this is not the case and the events that may make it the case are as important as the identification of infectious organisms and a knowledge of the ways in which they can be controlled.

We therefore believe that it is time to reconsider our approaches to microbiology, both in terms of the organisms that might usefully be considered within a textbook and also in terms of the contexts in which they and the diseases they cause, are discussed. There are many reasons for having reached this conclusion, the most important being:
- A comprehensive understanding now exists of the biologic bases of infection, of disease, of host–pathogen interactions, and of the epidemiology of infectious disease. It is important for students to be aware of this understanding so that they can grasp the connections between infection and disease within both individuals and communities and be able to use this knowledge in novel and changing clinical situations.
- It is now realized that the host's response to infection is a coordinated and subtle interplay involving the mechanisms of both innate and acquired resistance, and that these mechanisms are expressed regardless of the nature and identity of the pathogen involved. Our present understanding of the ways these mechanisms are stimulated and the ways in which they act is very sophisticated. We can now see that infection is a conflict between two organisms, with the outcome (resistance or disease) being critically dependent upon molecular interactions. Again, it is essential to understand the basis of this host–pathogen interplay if the processes of disease and disease control are to be interpreted correctly.

Opportunistic and tropical infections are increasingly common in developed countries
In addition, two other factors have helped to mould our concept of microbiology and our opinion that a broader view is needed to provide a firm basis for clinical and scientific practise:
- There is an increasing prevalence of a wide variety of opportunistic infections in patients who are immunosuppressed. Immunosuppressive therapies are now more common, as are diseases in which the immune system is compromised, notably, of course, AIDS.

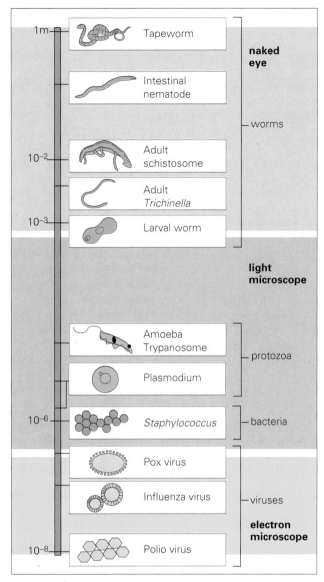

Fig. 1.1 Relative sizes of the organisms covered in this book.

- In the West, there has been a renewed interest in tropical medicine over recent years. Clinicians now see many tourists who have been exposed to the quite different spectrum of infectious agents found in tropical countries. There is also greater public concern over the health problems of the developing world *(Fig. 1.2)*.

The approach adopted in this book

The factors outlined above point towards the need for a text with a dual function:
- Firstly, it should provide a more inclusive treatment of the organisms responsible for infectious disease.
- Secondly, the purely clinical/laboratory approach to microbiology should be replaced with an approach that will stress the biologic context in which clinical/laboratory studies are to be undertaken.

The approach we have adopted in this book is to look at microbiology from the viewpoint of the conflicts inherent in all host–pathogen relationships. We first describe the adversaries, the infectious organisms on the one hand, and the innate and adaptive defense mechanisms of the host on the other. The outcome of the conflicts between the two is then amplified and discussed system by system. Rather than taking each organism or each disease manifestation in turn, we look at the major environments available for infectious organisms in the human body such as the respiratory system, the gut, the urinary tract, the blood and the central nervous system. The organisms that invade and establish in each of these are examined in terms of the pathologic responses they provoke. Finally, we look at how the conflicts we have described can be controlled or eliminated, both at the level of the individual patient and at the level of the community. We hope that such an approach will provide the reader with a dynamic view of host–pathogen interactions and allow them to develop a more creative understanding of infection and disease.

The Varieties of Microbes

Prokaryotes and eukaryotes

A number of important and distinctive biologic characteristics must be taken into account when considering any organism in relation to infectious disease. One of these is the way in which the organism is constructed, particularly the way in which genetic material and cellular components are organized.

All organisms other than viruses are made up of cells

Viruses are not cells – they do have genetic material (DNA or RNA) but lack cell membranes, cytoplasm and the machinery for synthesizing macromolecules, depending instead upon host cells for this process. Conventional viruses have their genetic material packed in capsules. Some organisms related to viruses are even simpler in their organization. The agents which cause diseases such as Creutzfeldt–Jakob disease, kuru, scrapie and BSE appear to lack nucleic acid and consist only of proteinaceous infectious particles.

All other organisms have a cellular organization, with bodies of single cells (most 'microbes') or of many cells. Each cell has genetic material (DNA) and cytoplasm with synthetic machinery, and is bounded by a cell membrane.

Bacteria are prokaryotes, all other organisms are eukaryotes

There are many differences between these two major divisions (prokaryotes and eukaryotes) of cellular organisms *(Fig. 1.3)*. One of the most striking is the absence of a distinct nucleus in prokaryotes. Their DNA, in the form of a single circular chromosome, is not contained in a nuclear membrane; additional DNA is carried in small plasmids. Transcription and translation from the genetic information can be carried out simultaneously. In eukaryotes, DNA is carried on several chromosomes contained within a nucleus and separated from

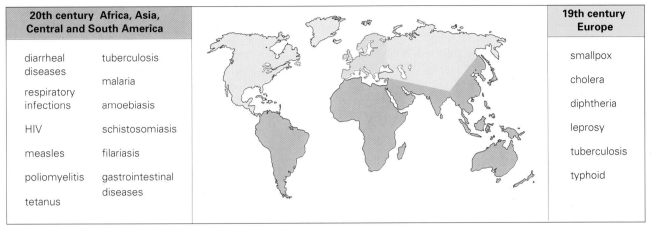

20th century Africa, Asia, Central and South America		19th century Europe
diarrheal diseases	tuberculosis	smallpox
respiratory infections	malaria	cholera
	amoebiasis	diphtheria
HIV	schistosomiasis	leprosy
measles	filariasis	tuberculosis
poliomyelitis	gastrointestinal diseases	typhoid
tetanus		

Fig. 1.2 Infectious diseases that were responsible for major mortality and morbidity in 19th century Europe, when the foundations of modern microbiology were laid down, and those which are of major importance in the 20th century.

the cytoplasm by a nuclear membrane. Transcription of DNA requires the formation of messenger RNA (mRNA) and movement of mRNA out of the nucleus into the cytoplasm before translation can take place on ribosomes. Whereas the cytoplasm of eukaryotes is rich in membrane-bound organelles (mitochondria, endoplasmic reticulum, Golgi apparatus, lysosomes), these do not occur in prokaryotes.

Gram-negative bacteria have an outer lipopolysaccharide-rich layer

Another important difference between prokaryotes and the majority of eukaryotes is that the cell membrane (plasma membrane) of prokaryotes is covered by a thick protective cell wall. In Gram-positive bacteria, this wall, made of peptidoglycan, forms the external surface of the cell, while in Gram-negative bacteria there is an additional outer layer rich in lipopolysaccharides. These layers play an important role in protecting the cell against the immune system and chemotherapeutic agents, and in stimulating certain pathologic responses. They also confer antigenicity.

Micro- and macroparasites
Microparasites replicate within the host

Identification of 'microbes' purely in terms of size and visibility distracts attention from other important characteristics. Organisms traditionally regarded as microbes are certainly small, but more significantly they can all replicate within the host. A single microbe can theoretically multiply to produce a very large number of progeny, thereby causing an overwhelming infection. Other organisms, although microscopic in size, do not have this ability: one infectious stage matures into one reproducing stage and the resulting progeny leave the host to continue the cycle. In both clinical and epidemiologic terms there is therefore an important distinction between microparasites, which replicate within the host (viruses, bacteria, protozoa, fungi), and macroparasites

(worms, arthropods), for which the level of infection is determined by the numbers of organisms that enter the body. Of course the boundary between micro- and macroparasites is not always clear. The progeny of some macroparasites do remain within the host and infections can lead to the

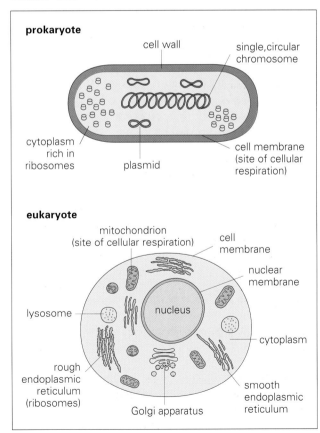

Fig. 1.3 Prokaryote and eukaryote cells. The major features of cellular organization are shown diagrammatically.

build-up of overwhelming numbers. The roundworms *Trichinella, Strongyloides stercoralis* and some filarial nematodes, and *Sarcoptes scabiei* (the itch mite) are examples of this type of parasite. Nevertheless, for most practical purposes, the division based on ability to replicate is helpful and informative.

Organisms that are small enough can live inside cells

Absolute size has other biologically significant implications for the host–pathogen relationship, which cut across the divisions between micro- and macroparasites. Perhaps the most important of these is the relative size of a pathogen and its host's cells. Organisms that are small enough can live inside cells and by doing so establish a biologic relationship with the host that is quite different from that of extracellular organism—one that influences both disease and control.

Living Inside or Outside Cells

The basis of all host–pathogen relationships is the exploitation by one organism (the pathogen) of the environment provided by another (the host). The nature and degree of exploitation varies from relationship to relationship, but the pathogen's primary requirement is a supply of metabolic materials from the host, whether provided in the form of nutrients or (as in the case of viruses) in the form of nuclear synthetic machinery. The reliance of viruses upon host synthetic machinery requires an obligatory intracellular habit; viruses must live within host cells. Some other groups of pathogens (*Chlamydia, Rickettsia*) also live only within cells, but in the remaining groups of pathogens different species have adopted either the intracellular or the extracellular habit, or, in a few cases, both. Intracellular organisms take their metabolic requirements directly from the pool of nutrients available in the cell itself, while extracellular organisms take theirs from the nutrients present in tissue fluids, or, occasionally, by feeding directly on host cells (e.g. *Entamoeba histolytica*, the organism associated with amebic dysentery). Macroparasites are almost always extracellular (though *Trichinella* is intracellular) and many feed by ingesting and digesting host cells, although others can take up nutrients directly from tissue fluids or intestinal contents.

Pathogens within cells are protected from many of the host's defense mechanisms

As will be discussed in greater detail in Chapter 2, the intracellular pathogens pose problems for the host that are quite different from those posed by extracellular organisms. Pathogens that live within cells are largely protected against many of the host's defense mechanisms while they remain there, particularly against the action of specific antibodies. Control of these infections depends therefore on the activities of short-range mediators or of cytotoxic agents, although a consequence of the latter may be the destruction of both the pathogen and the host cell, leading to tissue damage. This problem, of targeting activity against the pathogen when it lives within a vulnerable cell, also arises when using drugs or antibiotics as it is difficult to achieve selective action against the pathogen while leaving the host cell intact. Even more problematic is the fact that many intracellular pathogens live inside the very cells responsible for the host's immune and inflammatory mechanisms and therefore depress the host's defensive abilities. For example, a variety of viral, bacterial and protozoal pathogens live inside macrophages, and several viruses (including HIV) are specific for lymphocytes.

Intracellular life has many advantages for the pathogen. It provides access to the host's nutrient supply and its genetic machinery and allows escape from host surveillance and antimicrobial defenses. However, no organism can be wholly intracellular at all times: if it is to replicate successfully, transmission must occur between the host's cells and this inevitably involves some exposure to the extracellular environment. As far as the host is concerned, this extracellular phase in the development of the pathogen provides an opportunity to control infection through defense mechanisms such as phagocytosis, antibody and complement. However, transmission between cells can involve destruction of the initially infected cell and so contribute to tissue damage and general host pathology.

Living outside cells provides opportunities for growth, reproduction and dissemination

Extracellular pathogens can grow and reproduce freely, and may move extensively within the tissues of the body. However, they also face constraints on their survival and development. The most important is continuous exposure to components of the host's defense mechanisms, particularly antibody, complement and phagocytic cells.

The characteristics of extracellular organisms lead to pathologic consequences that are quite different from those associated with intracellular species. These are seen most dramatically with the macroparasites, whose sheer physical size, reproductive capacity and mobility can result in extensive destruction of host tissues. Many extracellular pathogens, including bacteria and viruses, have the ability to spread rapidly through extracellular fluids or to move rapidly over surfaces resulting in a widespread infection within a relatively short time. The rapid colonization of the entire mucosal surface of the small bowel by *Vibrio cholerae* is a good example. Successful host defense against extracellular parasites requires mechanisms that differ from those used in defense against intracellular parasites. The variety of locations and tissues occupied by extracellular parasites also poses problems for the host in ensuring effective deployment of defense mechanisms. These are most acute when macroparasites are concerned because their size often renders them insusceptible to defense mechanisms that can be used against smaller organisms.

- Our approach is to provide a comprehensive account of the organisms that cause infectious disease in humans, from the viruses to the worms, and to cover the biologic bases of infection, disease, host–pathogen interactions, disease control and epidemiology.
- The diseases caused by microbial pathogens will be placed in the context of the conflict that exists between them and the innate and adaptive defenses of their hosts.
- Infections will be described and discussed in terms of the major body systems, treating these as environments in which microbes can establish themselves, flourish and give rise to pathologic changes.

1. What are the major groups of pathogenic organisms that cause disease in humans?
2. List the key differences between prokaryotes and eukaryotes.
3. What are the important differences between micro- and macroparasites?
4. List three advantages that organisms gain by living within cells.

Further Reading

Mims CA, Dimmock NJ, Nash A *et al. Mims' Pathogenesis of Infectious Disease,* 4th edition. London: Academic Press, 1995.

The Host–Parasite Response

Introduction

Approaching medical microbiology solely in terms of the identification and treatment of disease-causing pathogens can convey the mistaken impression that pathogens form discrete and readily defined categories quite distinct from related, but non-pathogenic, organisms. In fact, pathogenesis is not the inevitable consequence of host–microbe associations. Many factors influence the outcome of a particular association and organisms may be pathogenic in one situation, but harmless in another. To understand the microbiologic basis of infectious disease, host–microbe associations need to be placed firmly in the context of other interspecies association, such as commensalism or mutualism, where the outcome for the host does not normally involve any damage or disadvantage.

Symbiotic Association

All living animals are used as habitats by other organisms; none is exempt from such invasion – even protozoans have their own flora and fauna. Animal evolution, with the development of larger, more complex and better regulated bodies, has increased the number and variety of habitats for other organisms to colonize. The most complex and best regulated bodies, those of warm-blooded birds and mammals (including humans), provide the most nutritious, favorable and diverse environments, and these groups of animals are the most heavily colonized.

Commensalism, mutualism and parasitism are categories of symbiotic association

All associations in which one species lives in or on the body of another can be grouped under a single description –

'symbiosis' (literally 'living together'). This term has no overtones of benefit or harm, but includes a wide diversity of associations. Attempts have been made to categorize types of association very specifically, but these have failed because all associations form part of a continuum *(Fig. 2.1)*. Three broad categories – commensalism, mutualism and parasitism – can be identified based on the relative benefit obtained by each partner. None of these categories of association is restricted to any particular taxonomic group. Indeed some organisms fit into each category depending upon the circumstances in which they live *(Fig. 2.2)*.

Commensalism

In commensalism one species of organism uses the body of a larger species

At its simplest, a commensal association is one in which one species of organism uses the body of a larger species as its

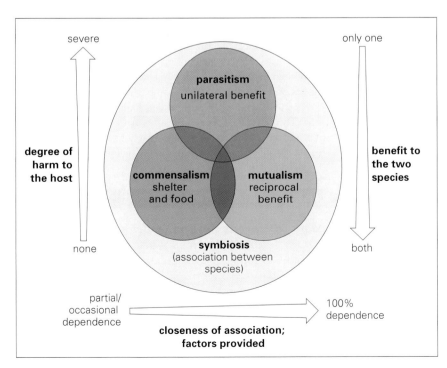

Fig. 2.1 The relationships between symbiotic associations. Most species are independent of other species or rely on them only temporarily for food (e.g. predators and their prey). Some species form closer associations termed 'symbioses' and there are three major categories – commensalism, parasitism and mutualism – though each merges with the other and no definition separates one absolutely from the others.

commensalism – large intestine of man

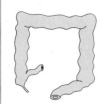

Bacteroides spp.

Host provides total environment – surface, temperature, pH, nutrition, anaerobic. Bacteria ferment digested food; host may use some fermentation products. Present in large numbers (10^{10}/g) but usually harmless; may become pathogenic if tissues damaged (surgery), if gut changes (antibiotics) or immunity reduced

parasitism – large intestine of man

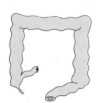

Entamoeba histolytica

Host provides total environment (as above). Protozoan feeds on intestinal mucosa, causes formation of ulcers and dysentery, but can live as harmless commensal, feeding on digested food material

mutualism – rumen of cattle

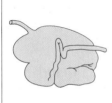

Bacteroides spp.

Host provides total environment (as above). Bacteria decompose cellulose or starch from host food, reduce to volatile fatty acids and gases. Host takes up acids across rumen wall, providing major energy sources.

Fig. 2.2 Examples of commensalism, parasitism and mutualism. The first two examples show how difficult it is to categorize any organism as entirely harmless, entirely harmful or entirely beneficial.

physical environment and may make use of that environment to acquire nutrients.

Like all animals, humans support an extensive commensal microbial flora on the skin, in the mouth and in the alimentary tract. The majority of these microbes are bacteria and their relationship with the host may be highly specialized, with specific attachment mechanisms and precise environmental requirements. Normally such microbes are harmless, but they can become harmful if their environmental conditions change in some way (e.g. *Bacteroides, Escherichia coli, Staphylococcus aureus*). Conversely, commensal microbes can benefit the host:

- By preventing colonization by more pathogenic species (e.g. the intestinal flora).
- By producing metabolites that are used by the host (e.g. the bacteria and protozoa in the ruminant stomach).

It follows that the normal definition of commensalism is merely one of convenience as the association can merge into either mutualism or parasitism.

Mutualism
Mutualistic relationships confer reciprocal benefits on the two organisms involved

Frequently the relationship is obligatory for at least one member, and may be for both. Good examples are the bacteria and protozoa living in the stomachs of domestic ruminants, which play an essential role in the digestion and utilization of cellulose, receiving in return both the environment and the nutrition essential for their survival. The dividing line between commensalism and mutualism can be hard to draw. For example, in humans good health and resistance to colonization by pathogens can depend upon the integrity of the normal commensal enteric bacteria (see Chapter 3), many of which are highly specialized for life in the human intestine, but there is certainly no strict mutual dependence in this relationship.

Parasitism
In parasitism the symbiotic relationship benefits only the parasite

Classic definitions of parasitism state that the relationship is not only one-sided in its benefits to the parasite, but is also positively harmful to the host. Certainly parasites do benefit from the association, being provided with their physicochemical environment, food, respiratory and other metabolic needs, and often the signals that regulate their development. Equally, many parasites are harmful to their hosts, but to some extent this is a view colored by human and veterinary clinical medicine, and by the results of laboratory experimentation. In fact many 'parasites' establish quite innocuous associations with their natural hosts and are not at all pathogenic under normal circumstances (e.g. when their natural host is in good health); the rabies virus for example coexists with many wild mammals but can cause fatal disease in humans. This state of 'balanced pathogenicity' is sometimes explained as the outcome of selective pressures acting upon a relationship over a long period of evolutionary time. 'Balanced pathogenicity' may simply reflect selection of an increased level of genetically determined resistance in the host population. Alternatively, it may be the evolutionary norm and 'unbalanced pathogenicity' simply the consequence of organisms becoming established in 'unnatural' (i.e. new) hosts. So, like the other categories of symbiosis, parasitism is impossible to define exclusively except in the context of clearcut and highly pathogenic organisms. The belief that 'harmfulness' is a necessary characteristic of a parasite is difficult to sustain in any broader view and the reasons for this are discussed in more detail below.

The Characteristics of Parasitism

Many different groups of organisms are parasitic and all animals are parasitized

Parasitism as a way of life has been adopted by many different groups of organisms. Some, such as viruses, are exclusively parasitic (see below), but the majority include both parasitic and free-living representatives. Parasites occur in all animals, from the simplest to the most complex, and are an almost inevitable accompaniment of organized animal existence. We can see, then, that parasitism has been an evolutionary success; as a way of life it must confer very considerable advantages.

Parasitism has metabolic, nutritional and reproductive advantages

The most obvious advantage of parasitism is metabolic. The parasite is provided with a variety of metabolic requirements by the host, at no energy cost to itself, so it can devote a large proportion of its own resources to replication or reproduction. This one-sided metabolic relationship shows a broad spectrum of dependence, both within and between the various groups of parasites. Some parasites are totally dependent upon the host, while others are only partly dependent.

Unlike non-viral parasites viruses are completely dependent upon the host for all their metabolic needs

At one extreme of the 'parasite dependency' spectrum are the viruses. They possess the genetic information required for production of new viruses, but none of the cellular machinery necessary to transcribe or translate this information, to assemble new virus particles or to produce the energy for these processes. The host provides not only the basic building blocks for the production of new viruses, but also the synthetic machinery and the energy required *(Fig. 2.3)*. Retroviruses go one stage further in dependence, inserting their own genetic information into the host's DNA in order to parasitize the transcription process. Viruses therefore represent the ultimate parasitic condition and are qualitatively different from all other parasites in the nature of their relationship with the host.

The basis for the fundamental difference between viruses and other parasites is the difference between virus organization and the cellular organization of prokaryotic and eukaryotic parasites. Non-viral parasites have their own cellular machinery and multi-enzyme systems for independent metabolic activity and macromolecular synthesis (see Chapter 1). The degree of reliance on the host for nutritional requirements varies considerably and follows no consistent phylogenetic pattern, nor does it follow that smaller parasites tend to be more dependent – some of the largest parasites, the tapeworms, are wholly reliant upon the host's digestive machinery to provide their nutritional needs. All, of course, receive nutrition from the host, but whereas some use macromolecular material (proteins, polysaccharides) of host origin and digest it using their own enzyme systems, others rely on the host for the process of digestion as well, being able to take up only low molecular weight materials (amino acids, monosaccharides). Nutritional dependence may also include host provision of growth factors that the parasite is unable to synthesize itself. All internal parasites rely upon the host's respiratory and transport systems to provide oxygen, although some respire anaerobically in either a facultative or obligate manner.

Parasite development can be controlled by the host

The very considerable advantage that parasitism confers in reproductive terms places a premium upon the coordination of parasite development with the availability of suitable hosts.

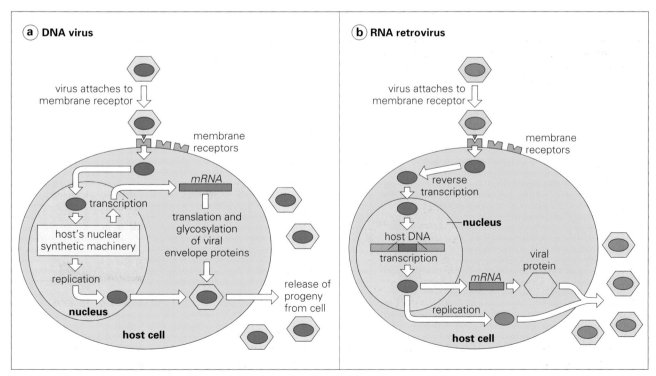

Fig. 2.3 How DNA and RNA viruses invade and infect cells. (a) DNA viruses such as the herpesviruses have their own DNA, and use only the host's cellular machinery to make more DNA and more virus protein and glycoprotein. These are then reassembled into new virus particles before they are released from the cell. (b) RNA retroviruses (e.g. HIV) first make viral DNA, using their reverse transcriptase, insert this DNA into the host's genetic material so that viral RNA can be transcribed, and then translate some of the RNA into virus protein. The viral protein and RNA are then reassembled into new particles and released.

Indeed, one of the characteristic features of parasites is that their development may be controlled partly or completely by the host; the parasite has lost the ability to initiate or to regulate its own development. At its simplest, host control is limited to providing the cell surface molecules necessary for parasite attachment and internalization. Many parasites, from viruses to protozoa, rely on the recognition of such molecular signals for their entry into host cells, and this process provides the trigger for their replicative or reproductive cycles.

Other parasites, primarily the eukaryotes, require more comprehensive and sophisticated signals, often a complex of signals, to initiate and regulate their entire developmental cycle. The complexity of the signal required for development is one of the factors determining the specificity of the host–parasite relationship. Where the availability of one of the signals means that parasite development can occur in only one species, host specificity is high. Where many host species are capable of providing the necessary signals for a parasite, specificity is low.

Disadvantages of parasitism

The most obvious disadvantage of parasitism has its basis in the control of parasite development by the host. No development is possible without a suitable host, and many parasites will die if no host becomes available. For this reason, several adaptations have evolved to promote prolonged survival in the outside world and so maximize the chances of successful host contact (e.g. virus particles, bacterial spores, protozoan cysts and worm eggs). The prolific replication of parasites is another device to achieve the same end. Nevertheless, where parasites fail to make contact with a host, their powers of survival are necessarily limited. Adaptation to host signals can therefore have a reproductive cost (i.e. the loss of many potential parasites).

The Evolution of Parasitism

As such a wide range of organisms is parasitic and every group of animals is subject to invasion by parasites, the development of parasitism as a way of life must have occurred at an early stage in evolution and at frequent intervals thereafter. How this occurred is not fully understood and it may well have been different in different groups of organisms. In many, parasitism most probably arose as a consequence of accidental contacts between organism and host. Of many such contacts some would have resulted in prolonged survival, and under favorable nutritional circumstances prolonged survival would have been associated with enhanced replication, giving the organism a selective advantage within the environment.

Bacterial parasites evolved through accidental contact

In the case of bacteria, it is easy to see how accidental contact in environments rich in free-living bacteria could lead to successful colonization of the gastrointestinal tract and external orifices. Initially the organisms concerned would have had to be facultative parasites, capable of life both within or outside host organisms (many pathogenic bacteria still have this property, e.g. *Legionella*, *Vibrio*), but selective

pressures would have forced others into obligatory parasitism. Such events are of course speculative, but are supported by the close relationship of enteric bacteria such as *E. coli* with free-living photosynthetic purple bacteria.

Many bacteria and related parasites of humans and other mammals may have originated via the route of accidental contact, but it is clear that others have become adapted to these hosts after initially becoming parasitic in other species. Blood-feeding arthropods provide an example of the most obvious route for this, as their parasites have ready access to the tissues of the animals on which the arthropods feed.

Many bacterial parasites have evolved to live inside host cells

Bacteria that became parasitic by accidental contact would have lived outside host cells at first and would not have had the advantages of being intracellular. The evolution of the intracellular habit required further modifications to allow survival within host cells, but could easily have been initiated by passive phagocytic uptake. Subsequent survival of the microbe would depend upon the possession of surface or metabolic properties that prevented digestion and destruction by the host cell. The success of intracellular life can be measured not only by the large number of bacteria that have adopted this habit, but also by the extent to which some organisms have integrated their biology with that of the host cell. The endpoint of such integration is perhaps to be seen in the evolution of the eukaryote mitochondrion, which is widely considered to be the product of symbiotically associated heterotrophic purple bacteria *(Fig. 2.4)*.

The pathway of virus evolution is uncertain

Clearly, parasitism by bacteria, which are undoubtedly ancient organisms (they can be traced back 3–5 billion years in the fossil record), depended upon the evolution of higher organisms to act as hosts. Whether the same is true of viruses is open to question, and depends upon whether viruses are considered primarily or secondarily simple. If viruses evolved from cellular ancestors by a process of secondary simplification then parasitism must have evolved long after the evolution of prokaryotes and eukaryotes. If viruses are primitively non-cellular then it is possible that they became parasitic at a very early stage in the evolution of cellular life, at some point when, because of environmental change, independent existence became impossible. A third alternative is that viruses were never anything other than fragments of the nuclear material of other organisms and have in effect always been parasitic. Modern viruses may, in fact, have arisen by all three pathways.

Eukaryote parasites have evolved through accidental contact

The evolution of parasitism by eukaryotes is likely to have arisen much as it may have done in prokaryotes (i.e. through accidental contact and via blood-feeding arthropods, *(Fig. 2.5)*. Examples can be found among both protozoan and worm parasites to support this view:

- There are protozoa such as the free-living ameba *Naegleria*, which can opportunistically invade the human body and cause severe and sometimes fatal disease.

- There are several species of nematode worms that can live either as parasites or as free-living organisms, *Strongyloides stercoralis* being the most important in humans.
- It is likely that trypanosomes (the protozoans responsible for sleeping sickness) were primarily adapted as parasites of blood-feeding flies and only secondarily become established as parasites of mammals.

Parasite adaptations to overcome host inflammatory and immune responses

We can view the evolution of parasitism and the adaptations necessary for life within another animal as being exactly analogous to the adaptations necessary for life within any other specialized habitat: the environment in which parasites live is merely one of the many to which organisms have become adapted in evolution (comparable with life in soil, freshwater, salt water, decaying material and so on). Such a viewpoint has some fruitful consequences, but it is always necessary to remember that in one major respect parasitism is quite different from any other specialist mode of life. This difference is that the environment in which a parasite lives, the body of the host, is not passive; on the contrary it is capable of an active response to the presence of the parasite.

The attractiveness of animal bodies as environments for parasites means that hosts are under continual pressures from infection and these pressures are increased when hosts live:

- Close together.
- In insanitary conditions.
- In climates that favor the survival of parasite stages in the external world.

Pressure of infection has been a major influence in evolution

Pressure of infection has been a major selective influence in evolution, and there is little doubt that it has been largely responsible for the development of the sophisticated inflammatory and immune responses of humans and other mammals. In evolutionary terms all infection has its costs to the host because it diverts valuable resources from the activities of survival and reproduction; there has therefore

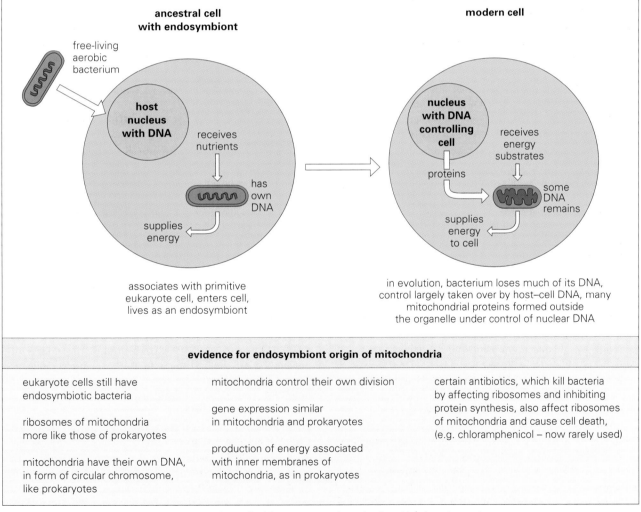

Fig. 2.4 The evolution of mitochondria. Many lines of evidence suggest that mitochondria of modern eukaryote cells evolved from bacteria that established symbiotic (mutualistic) relationships with ancestral cells.

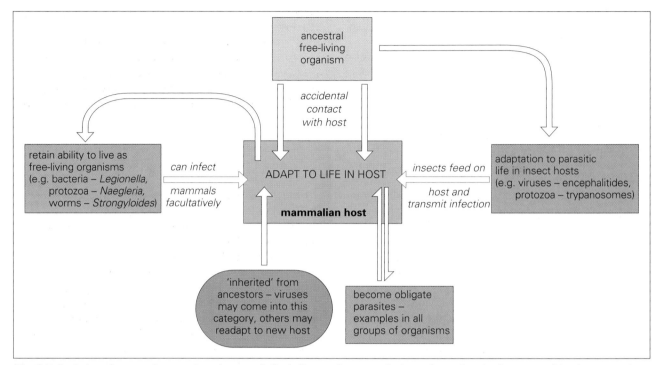

Fig. 2.5 Evolution of present day parasites of mammals (including humans). Most have probably come from free-living ancestral organisms or readapted to mammals after becoming parasites in other vertebrates. Some have been transmitted from blood-feeding insects and other arthropods, adapting to parasitize the mammal as well. Some viruses at least may have been inherited in a genetic sense (i.e. entering the host with inherited DNA).

been pressure to develop means of overcoming infection whether or not it causes disease. Of course, this is not the focus of clinical microbiology, which legitimately places emphasis on the costs of infection in terms of frank disease, but it should be remembered because it explains more fully the nature of the continuing battle between host and parasite – the former attempting to contain or destroy, the latter attempting to evade or suppress – and why the emergence of new, and the return of old, infectious diseases are a constant threat.

Parasites are therefore faced not only with the problems of surviving within the environment they experience initially, but of surviving in that environment as it changes in ways that are likely to be deleterious to them. The inflammatory and immune responses that follow the establishment of infection are the most important means by which the host can control infections by those organisms able to penetrate its natural barriers and survive within its body. These responses represent formidable obstacles to the continued survival of parasites, forcing them to evolve strategies to cope with harmful changes in their environment. The successful parasite is therefore one that can cope with, or evade, the host's response in one of the ways shown in *Figure 2.6*.

All of these adaptations are known to exist within different groups of parasites and they are well documented in the case of some of the major human pathogens. Indeed they are often the very reason why such organisms are major pathogens. Nevertheless, transmission and survival of many parasites depends upon the existence of particularly susceptible host individuals (e.g. children) to provide a continuing reservoir of infective stages.

Changes in parasites create new problems for hosts

From what has been said above, it can be appreciated that there is no such thing as a static host–parasite relationship, and that concepts of unchanging 'pathogenicity' or 'harmlessness' cannot be justified. Each relationship is an 'arms race', changes in one member being countered by changes in the other. Quite subtle changes in either can completely change the balance of the relationship, towards greater or lesser pathogenicity for example.

Perhaps the most important contemporary illustration of this situation is the dramatic and explosive appearance of HIV infections. Although there is still debate, one view is that this group of viruses was originally restricted to non-human primates, but that changes in the virus have permitted extensive infections in humans. Of a different nature, but relevant to the general theme, is the acquisition of drug resistance in bacteria and protozoa *(Fig. 2.7)*. Although the underlying genetic and metabolic changes do not by themselves influence pathogenicity, the expression of such changes in the face of intense and selective chemotherapy certainly does so.

Host adaptations to overcome changes in parasites

Changes in the host can also alter the balance of a host–parasite relationship. A particularly dramatic example is the intense selection for resistant genotypes in rabbit populations exposed to the myxomatosis virus, which took place concurrently with selection for reduced pathogenicity in the virus itself (see Chapter 7). There are no exactly equivalent examples in humans, but in evolutionary time there have been

EVASION STRATEGIES	
strategy	**example**
elicit minimal response	herpes simplex virus – survives in host cells for long periods in a latent stage – no pathology
evading effects of response	mycobacteria – survive unharmed in granulomatous response designed to localize and destroy infection
depress host's response	HIV – destroys T cells malaria – depresses immune responsiveness
antigenic change	viruses, spirochetes, trypanosomes – all change target antigens so host response is ineffective
rapid replication	viruses, bacteria, protozoa – producing acute infections before recovery and immunity
survival in weakly responsive individuals	genetic heterogeneity in host population means some individuals respond weakly or not at all, allowing organism to reproduce freely; examples in all groups

Fig. 2.6 Evasion strategies of parasites.

major selective influences on populations prompting changes to permit survival in the face of life-threatening infections. A good example is the selective pressure exerted by falciparum malaria, which has been responsible for the persistence of many alleles associated with hemoglobinopathies (e.g. sickle cell hemoglobin): although these abnormalities are detrimental to a varying degree, they persist because they are associated with resistance to infection.

Social and behavioral changes can be as important as genetic changes in altering host–parasite relations

Social and behavioral changes can alter host–parasite relations both positively and negatively (*Fig. 2.8*). Although many bacterial infections of the intestine have declined in importance with changes in human life style, there are other contemporary microbiological problems in the developed world whose onset can be traced directly to sociologic, environmental and even medical change (*Fig. 2.8*). A particularly good example is disease arising from domestication of pets (e.g. toxoplasmosis) because it illustrates that human freedom from some infections arises primarily because of lack of contact with the organisms and not from any innate resistance to the establishment of the infection itself. Diseases arising from contact with infected animals or animal products (zoonotic infections) constitute a constant threat that can be realized by behavioral or environmental changes that alter established patterns of human–animal contact.

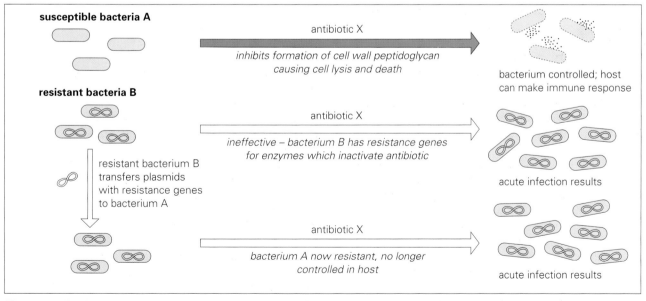

Fig. 2.7 Antibiotic resistance in bacteria. The activity of many antibiotics can be blocked by bacterial enzymes coded for by genes located on cytoplasmic DNA in plasmids. The ability of bacteria to transfer plasmids between individual organisms means that strains or species previously susceptible to an antibiotic can acquire the ability to produce such enzymes and so gain antibiotic resistance directly from resistant organisms. These newly resistant forms are then differentially selected under antibiotic treatment, the susceptible individuals being deleted from the population.

SOCIAL AND BEHAVIORAL CHANGES AND INFECTIOUS DISEASES		
	the causes	**the results**
living	altered environments (e.g. air conditioning)	water used in cooling systems provides suitable growth conditions for *Legionella* bacteria spread in aerosols
food	changes in food production and food handling practises	intensive husbandry under antibiotic protection leads to drug-resistant bacteria in animal products deep-freeze storage, fast-food production and inadequate cooking allows bacteria and toxins to enter body (e.g. *Listeria, Salmonella*)
medicine	routine use of antibiotics in medicine	emergence of antibiotic-resistant bacteria as hazards to hospitalized patients (e.g. multiply-resistant *Staphylococcus aureus*)
	routine use of immunosuppressive therapy	development of opportunistic infections in patients with reduced resistance (e.g. *Pseudomonas, Candida, Pneumocystis*)
sex	altered sexual habits	promiscuity increases transmission of sexually transmitted diseases (e.g. gonorrhea, genital herpes, AIDS)
water	breakdown of filtration systems overuse of limited water supplies	transmission of animal infections through contaminants leading to diarrheal and other infections (e.g. cryptosporidiosis, giardiasis, leptospirosis)
pets	increase in ownership of pets, particularly exotic species	transmission of animal infections through contamination (e.g. *Chlamydia, Salmonella, Toxoplasma, Toxocara*)
travel	increased frequency of journeys to tropical and subtropical countries	exposure to organisms and vectors not found in country of origin (e.g. malaria, viral encephalitides)

Fig. 2.8 Life style changes and infectious diseases.

- Clinical microbiology concentrates upon the identification and treatment of the major infectious diseases, primarily those caused by viruses and bacteria.
- Changes in medical practise, in human behavior, in international relationships and, not least, in infectious organisms, create a situation in which a wider spectrum of infectious organisms needs to be considered and a wider view of host–parasite relationships developed.
- It is as important to understand the causes of infection, resistance and pathology as it is to be able to identify organisms and prescribe appropriate treatment.
- Such understanding must be based upon the biologic context of host–parasite relationships and the dynamic conflict between two species, of which frank disease is merely one possible outcome.

1. What are the three major categories of symbiotic relationships?
2. What is a facultative parasite? Give an example.
3. List four strategies adopted by parasites to maximize their survival in hosts.
4. List four social and behavioral changes that have increased the prevalence of human infectious diseases.

Introduction

Infectious diseases are caused by organisms belonging to a very wide range of different groups – viruses, bacteria, protozoa, helminths (worms) and arthropods. Each has its own system of classification, making it possible to identify and categorize the organisms concerned. Correct identification is an essential requirement for accurate diagnosis and effective treatment. Viruses differ from all other organsims in the lack of metabolic machinery, so that they can only reproduce within host cells. Their genomic information is carried in RNA or DNA and may become incorporated into host DNA. Some viruses are associated with development of tumors. Bacteria are prokaryotes, their DNA lacks introns and is not contained within a distinct nucleus. Their cellular organization shows many differences from that of eukaryotes (all other cellular organisms). Bacterial cell walls play an important part in the biology and host–parasite relationships of these pathogens. Much is known of bacterial molecular genetics in particular of the genes that determine virulence and antibiotic resistance, and which can be transferred between individual bacteria. The human body contains very large numbers of overgrowth of pathogenic species. When immunity is suppressed, when the body is subject to trauma, or when the normal flora is depleted by antibiotic treatment, some of these organisms can be pathogenic. Protozoa, helminths and arthropods are of greatest importance in tropical regions, but occur in temperate countries as well. Their frequency often reflects standards of public and individual hygiene. Some species are important opportunistic pathogens in individuals whose immune competence is depressed.

Systems of Classification

The binomial system is used for eukaryote and some prokaryote organisms. The fundamental units of this system are the 'species' (similar, interbreeding organisms), which in turn are grouped into a 'genus' (closely related but non-interbreeding species). Each organism is identified by two names, indicating the 'genus' and the 'species', respectively. For example, *Homo sapiens* and *Escherichia coli*. Related genera are grouped into progressively broader and more inclusive categories.

Classification of bacteria and viruses

A basic difficulty in classifying prokaryotes and viruses is the concept of 'species'. Classification of bacteria uses a mixture of easily determined practical characteristics, based on size, shape, color, staining properties, respiration and reproduction, and a more sophisticated analysis of immunologic and biochemical criteria. The former characteristics can be used to divide the organisms into conventional taxonomic groupings, as shown for the Gram-positive bacteria in *Figure 3.1* (see Chapter 14).

Correct identification of bacteria below the species level is often vital to differentiate pathogenic and non-pathogenic forms

Correct treatment is possible after correct identification. For some bacteria the important subspecies groups are identified on the basis of their immunologic properties.

staining	shape	respiration	shape/reproduction	genus	species
Gram-positive	cocci	aerobic	clusters	*Staphylococcus*	*S. aureus*
			chains/pairs	*Streptococcus*	*S. faecalis*
		anaerobic		*Peptococcus*	*P. magnus*
	bacilli	aerobic	sporing	*Bacillus*	*B. anthracis*
			non-sporing	*Listeria*	*L. monocytogenes*
		anaerobic	sporing	*Clostridium*	*C. tetani*
			non-sporing	*Propionibacterium*	*P. acnes*

Fig. 3.1 How the characteristics of bacteria can be used in classification, taking Gram-positive bacteria as an example.

Cell wall, flagellar and capsule antigens are used in tests with specific antisera to define serogroups and serotypes (e.g. in salmonellae, streptococci, shigellae, *E. coli*). In others, biochemical characteristics are used to define other subspecies groupings (biotypes, strains, groups). For example, certain strains of *Staphylococcus aureus* release a β-hemolysin (causing red blood cells to lyse). Production of other toxins is also important in differentiating between groups, as in *E. coli*. Bacteria can also be classified below species level by their susceptibility to particular bacteriophage viruses. Phage typing is used, for example, in differentiating between isolates of *Staph. aureus*, *Vibrio cholerae* and *Salmonella typhi*.

Direct genetic approaches can also be used in identification and classification. These include:

- Measuring total genome size (the molecular weight of the DNA present).
- Determining the amount of the bases guanine and cytosine in the DNA.
- Using specific probes to identify particular sequences of DNA in the genome.

Classification of viruses departs even further from the binomial system

Families and, sometimes, genera are used, but not species. Groupings are based on characteristics such as the type of nucleic acid present (DNA or RNA), the symmetry of the virus particle (icosahedral, helical or complex), the presence or absence of an external envelope, as shown for the DNA viruses in *Fig. 3.2*. The equivalents of subspecies categories are also used, and indeed are more easily determined than species could be, given the peculiar biologic characteristics of viruses. These categories include factors such as serotypes, strains, variants and isolates and are determined primarily by serologic reactivity of virus material. The influenza virus, for example, can be considered as the equivalent of a genus containing three types (A, B, C). Identification can be carried out using the stable nucleoprotein antigen, which differs between the three types. The neuraminidase and hemagglutinin antigens are not stable and show variation within types. Characterization of these antigens in an isolate enables the particular variant to be identified (see Chapter 17). A further example is seen in adenoviruses, for which the various antigens associated with a component of the capsid can be used to define groups, types and finer subdivisions.

Classification assists diagnosis and the understanding of pathogenicity

Prompt identification of organisms is necessary clinically so that diagnoses can be made and appropriate treatments advised. To understand host–parasite interactions, however, not only should the identity of an organism be known, but as much as possible of its general biology; useful predictions can then be made about the consequences of infection. For these reasons we have included outline classifications of the important pathogens, accompanied by brief accounts of their structure (gross and microscopic), modes of life, molecular biology, biochemistry, replication and reproduction, in the Appendix. Here we will emphasize those aspects of the cellular and molecular biology of the major groups of parasites that determine their interactions with the host, and therefore the outcome of infection.

The Viruses

Viruses differ from all other infectious organisms in their structure and biology, particularly in their reproduction.

Viruses infect every form of life

Although viruses carry conventional genetic information in their DNA or RNA, they lack the synthetic machinery necessary for this information to be processed into new virus material. A virus by itself is metabolically inert – it can replicate only after infection of a host cell, when it can parasitize the host's ability to transcribe and/or translate genetic information.

Viruses range from very small (poliovirus at 30 nm) to quite large (vaccinia virus at 400 nm is as big as small bacteria). Their organization varies considerably between the different groups, but there are some general characteristics common to all:

- The genetic material, in the form of single-stranded (ss) or double-stranded (ds), linear or circular RNA or DNA, is contained within a capsule or capsid, made up of a number of individual protein molecules (capsomeres).

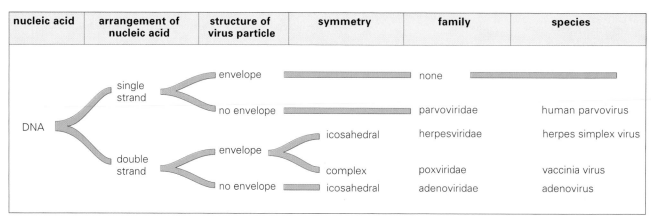

nucleic acid	arrangement of nucleic acid	structure of virus particle	symmetry	family	species
DNA	single strand	envelope		none	
		no envelope		parvoviridae	human parvovirus
	double strand	envelope	icosahedral	herpesviridae	herpes simplex virus
			complex	poxviridae	vaccinia virus
		no envelope	icosahedral	adenoviridae	adenovirus

Fig. 3.2 How the characteristics of viruses can be used in classification, taking DNA viruses as an example.

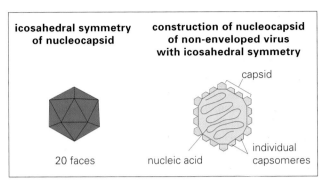

Fig. 3.3 Symmetry and construction of the viral nucleocapsid.

- The complete unit of nucleic acid and capsid is called the 'nucleocapsid', and often has a distinctive symmetry depending upon the ways in which the individual capsomeres are assembled *(Fig. 3.3)*. Symmetry can be icosahedral, helical or complex.
- In many cases the entire 'virus particle' or 'virion' consists only of a nucleocapsid. In others the virion consists of the nucleocapsid surrounded by an outer envelope or membrane *(Fig. 3.4)*. This is generally a lipid bilayer of host cell origin, into which virus proteins and glycoproteins are inserted.

The outer surface of the virus particle is the part that first makes contact with the membrane of the host cell

The structure and properties of the outer surface of the virus particle are therefore of vital importance in understanding the process of infection. In general, naked (envelope-free) viruses are resistant and survive well in the outside world; they may also be bile-resistant allowing infection through the alimentary canal. Enveloped viruses are more susceptible to environmental factors such as drying, gastric acidity and bile. These differences in susceptibility influence the ways in which these viruses can be transmitted.

Infection of host cells

The stages involved in infection of host cells are summarized in *Fig. 3.5* (see also *Fig. 2.3*).

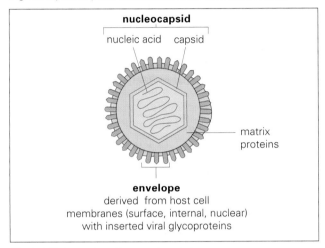

Fig. 3.4 Construction of an enveloped virus.

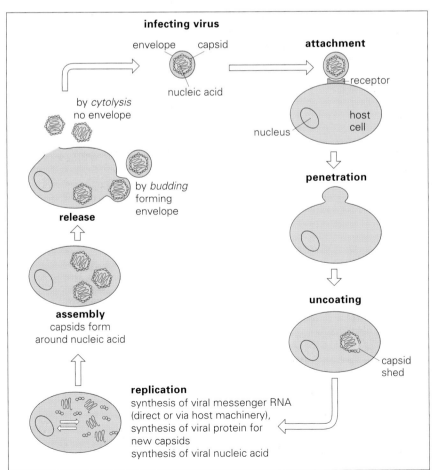

Fig. 3.5 Stages in the infection of a host's cell and replication of a virus. Several thousand virus particles may be formed from each cell.

Virus particles enter the body of the host in many ways

The commonest forms of virus transmission (*Fig. 3.6*; see Chapter 8) are:

- Via inhaled droplets (rhinovirus).
- In food and water (hepatitis A).
- Direct transfer from other infected hosts (HIV).
- Bites of vector arthropods (yellow fever).

Viruses show host specificity, which is initally based upon an ability to attach to the host cell

Like all pathogens, viruses usually infect only one or a restricted range of host species. The initial basis of specificity is the ability of the virus particle to attach to the host cell.

The process of attachment to, or adsorption by, a host cell depends first upon the operation of general intermolecular forces, then upon more specific interactions between the molecules of the nucleocapsid (in naked viruses) or the virus membrane (in enveloped viruses) and the molecules of the host cell membrane. In many cases there is a specific interaction with a particular host molecule, which therefore acts as a receptor. Influenza virus, for example, attaches by its hemagglutinin to a glycoprotein (sialic acid) found on cells of mucous membranes and on red blood cells; other examples are given in *Figure 3.7*. Attachment to the receptor is followed by entry into the host cell.

Once in the host's cytoplasm the virus is no longer infective

After fusion of viral and host membranes, or uptake into a phagosome, the virus particle is carried into the cytoplasm across the plasma membrane. At this stage, the envelope and/or the capsid are shed and the viral nucleic acids released. The virus is now no longer infective: this 'eclipse phase' persists until new complete virus particles reform after replication. The way in which replication occurs is determined by the nature of the nucleic acid concerned.

Replication
Viruses must first synthesize messenger RNA (mRNA)

Viruses contain either DNA or RNA, never both. The nucleic acids are present as single or double strands in a linear (DNA or RNA) or circular (DNA) form. The total genetic information (genome) of the virus may be carried on a single molecule of nucleic acid or on several molecules. With this diversity it is not surprising that the process of replication in the host cell is also diverse. In viruses containing DNA, mRNA can be formed using the host's own RNA polymerase to transcribe directly from the viral DNA. The RNA of viruses cannot be transcribed in this way, as host polymerases do not work from RNA. If transcription is necessary, the virus must provide its own polymerases. These may be carried in the nucleocapsid or may be synthesized after infection.

RNA viruses produce mRNA by several different routes

In dsRNA viruses, one strand is first transcribed by viral polymerase into mRNA (*Fig. 3.8*). In ssRNA viruses there are three distinct routes to the formation of mRNA:

- Where the single strand has the positive sense configuration (i.e. has the same base sequence as that required for translation) it can be used directly as mRNA.
- Where the strand has the negative sense configuration it must first be transcribed, using viral polymerase, into a positive sense strand, which can then act as mRNA.
- Retroviruses follow a completely different route. Their positive sense ssRNA is first made into a negative sense ssDNA, using the viral reverse transcriptase enzyme carried in the nucleocapsid and dsDNA is then formed, which enters the nucleus and becomes integrated into the host genome. This integrated viral DNA is then transcribed by host polymerase into mRNA.

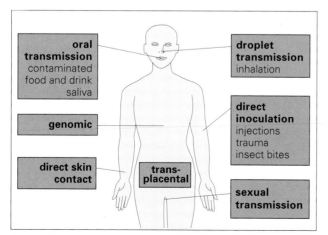

Fig. 3.6 Routes by which viruses enter the body.

CELL MEMBRANE RECEPTORS FOR VIRUSES	
virus	**receptor molecule**
influenza	sialic acid on glycoproteins, including the glycophorin A molecule
rabies	acetylcholine receptor
HIV	CD4 molecule on T cells
Epstein–Barr	C3d receptor on B cells
vaccinia	epidermal growth factor receptor
reovirus type 3	β-adrenergic hormone receptor
encephalomyocarditis	glycophorin A molecule
rhinovirus	intercellular adhesion molecule-1

Fig. 3.7 Molecules used by viruses in attaching to host cells.

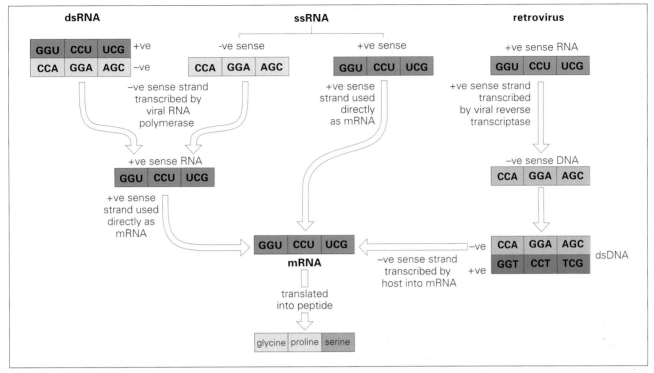

Fig. 3.8 Ways in which genomic RNA of RNA viruses can be transcribed into messenger RNA (mRNA) before translation into proteins. (+ve, positive sense; –ve, negative sense; ds, double stranded; ss, single stranded.)

Viral mRNA is then translated in the host cytoplasm to produce viral proteins

Once viral mRNA has been formed, it is translated using host ribosomes to synthesize viral proteins *(Fig. 3.9)*. Viral mRNA, which is usually 'monocistronic' (i.e. has a single coding region) can displace host mRNA from ribosomes so that viral products are synthesized preferentially. In the early phase, the proteins produced (enzymes, regulatory molecules) are those that will allow subsequent replication of viral nucleic acids; in the later phase, the proteins necessary for capsid formation are produced.

In viruses where the genome is a single nucleic acid molecule, translation produces a large multifunctional protein, a polyprotein, which is then cleaved enzymatically to produce a number of distinct proteins. In viruses where the genome is distributed over a number of molecules, several mRNAs are produced, each being translated into separate proteins. After translation the proteins may be glycosylated, again using host enzymes.

Viruses must also replicate their nucleic acid

In addition to producing molecules for the formation of new capsids, the virus must replicate its nucleic acid to provide genetic material for packaging into these capsids. In positive sense, ssRNA viruses such as poliovirus, a polymerase translated from viral mRNA produces negative sense RNA from the positive sense template, which is then repeatedly transcribed into more positive strands. Further cycles of transcription then occur, resulting in the production of very large numbers of positive strands, which are packaged into new particles using structural proteins translated earlier from mRNA *(Fig. 3.10)*.

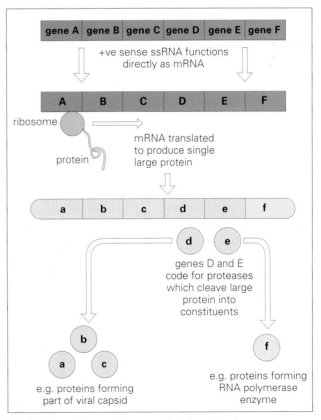

Fig. 3.9 Translation and cleavage of viral proteins from messenger RNA (mRNA). (+ve, positive sense; ss, single stranded.)

In negative sense ssRNA viruses (e.g. rabies virus) transcription by viral polymerase produces positive sense RNA strands from which new negative sense RNA is produced *(Fig. 3.10)*. In the rabies virus this replication occurs in the host cell cytoplasm, but in others (e.g. measles and influenza virus) replication takes place within the nucleus, large numbers of negative sense RNA molecules being transcribed for new particles.

Nucleic acid replication follows a similar pattern in dsRNA viruses (e.g. rotavirus) in that positive sense RNA strands are produced. These then act as templates in a subviral particle for the synthesis of new negative sense strands to restore the ds condition.

Replication of viral DNA occurs in the host nucleus, except for poxviruses where it takes place in the cytoplasm

Viral DNA may become complexed with host histones to produce stable structures. With herpes viruses, mRNA translated in the cytoplasm produces a DNA polymerase that is necessary for the synthesis of new viral DNA; adenoviruses use both viral and host enzymes for this purpose. With retroviruses, synthesis of new viral RNA occurs in the nucleus, host RNA polymerase transcribing from the viral DNA that has become integrated into the host genome *(Fig. 3.8)*. Hepatitis B virus, a dsDNA virus, is unique in using a ssRNA intermediate transcribed from its DNA, in order to synthesize new DNA.

The final stage of replication is assembly and release of new virus particles

Assembly of virus particles involves the association of replicated nucleic acid with newly synthesized capsomeres to form a new nucleocapsid. This may take place in the cytoplasm or in the nucleus of the host cell. Enveloped viruses go through a further stage before release. Envelope proteins and glycoproteins, translated from viral mRNA, are inserted into areas of the host cell membrane (usually the plasma membrane). The progeny nucleocapsids associate specifically with the membrane in these areas, via the glycoproteins, and bud through it *(Fig. 3.11)*. The new virus acquires the host cell membrane plus viral molecules as an outer envelope (see Chapter 17). Viral enzymes (e.g. the neuraminidase of influenza virus) may assist in this process. Host enzymes (e.g. cellular proteases) may cleave the initial large envelope proteins, a process that is necessary if the progeny viruses are to be fully infectious. In herpesviruses, acquisition of a membrane occurs as the nucleocapsids bud from the inner nuclear membrane. Release of enveloped viruses can occur without causing cell death so that infected cells continue to shed virus particles for long periods.

Insertion of viral molecules into the host cell membrane results in the host cell becoming antigenically different. Expression of viral antigens in this way is a major factor in the development of antiviral immune responses.

Outcome of viral infection
Viral infections may cause cell lysis or be persistent or latent

In 'lytic' infections, the virus goes through a cycle of replication, producing many new virus particles. Release of these particles is associated with lysis (i.e. destruction of the cell). This is the typical consequence of infection with polio- or influenza virus. With other infections, such as hepatitis B, the

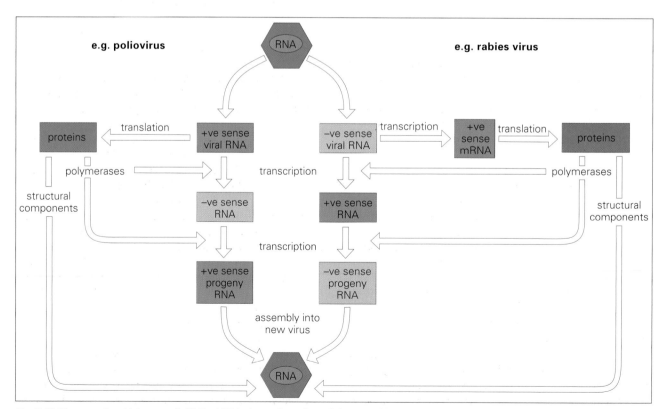

Fig. 3.10 The ways in which genomic RNA of RNA viruses is replicated. (+ve, positive sense; –ve, negative sense; mRNA, messenger RNA.)

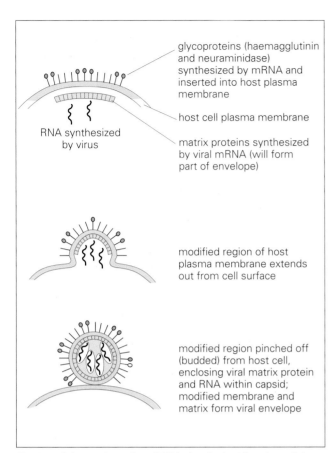

glycoproteins (haemagglutinin and neuraminidase) synthesized by mRNA and inserted into host plasma membrane

host cell plasma membrane

matrix proteins synthesized by viral mRNA (will form part of envelope)

RNA synthesized by virus

modified region of host plasma membrane extends out from cell surface

modified region pinched off (budded) from host cell, enclosing viral matrix protein and RNA within capsid; modified membrane and matrix form viral envelope

Fig. 3.11 Release of enveloped RNA virus by budding through host cell membrane. Influenza A virus is shown in this example.

cell may remain alive and continue to release virus particles at a slow rate. These 'persistent' infections are of great epidemiologic importance, as the infected person may act as a symptomless carrier of the virus, providing a continuing source of infection (see Chapter 11). In both lytic and persistent infections the virus undergoes replication. However, in latent infections the virus remains quiescent and the genetic material of the virus may:

- Exist in the host cell cytoplasm (herpesvirus).
- Be incorporated into the genome (retroviruses).

Replication does not take place until some signal triggers a release from latency. The stimuli that result in release are not fully understood in all cases. In herpes simplex infection stress can activate the virus, resulting in an active infection seen as cold sores. With HIV, antigenic stimulation of infected cells may provide the signal that leads to activation.

Some viruses can 'transform' the host cell into a tumor or cancer cell

Lytic, persistent and latent infections involve essentially normal host cells, although cellular metabolic and regulatory processes can be severely disrupted. Some viruses, however, can 'transform' the host cell, malignant transformation being the change of a differentiated host cell into a tumor or cancer

cell (see Chapter 12). Transformed cells show changes in morphology, behavior and biochemistry. Controlled growth patterns and contact inhibition are lost, so that cells continue to divide and form random aggregations. They become invasive and can form tumors if injected into animals. However, not all transformed cells give rise to harmful tumors *in vivo*. Warts, for example, are benign growths caused by one group of papovaviruses.

Cancer-inducing viruses are found in several different groups of virus and include both DNA and RNA viruses (see Chapter 12). Although the end results of transformation may be similar, the mechanisms involved differ between different viruses. However, all involve interference with the normal regulation of division and response to external growth-promoting and growth-inhibiting factors. These changes come about after viral nucleic acid is incorporated into the host genome. In one of the best-analysed cases, that of the Rous sarcoma virus (a retrovirus that causes cancer in chickens), transformation arises from the introduction into the host genome of a viral 'oncogene', the *src* gene. This codes for enzymes (tyrosine-specific protein kinases) involved in the phosphorylation of tyrosine residues in target proteins. Several growth-regulating factors act through specific membrane receptors that have tyrosine-specific protein kinase activity (i.e. they phosphorylate tyrosine residues in target proteins); therefore one result of upregulation of this activity is that normal host cell growth regulation is lost.

More than 20 retroviral oncogenes are now known *(Fig. 3.12)*. Only one retrovirus – human T cell leukemia virus (HTLV 1 and 2) – is of major importance as a cancer-causing virus in man. Paradoxically this neither possesses a viral oncogene nor directly activates a cellular oncogene (see below). In contrast, several retroviruses are known to cause cancers in animals.

Viral oncogenes have probably arisen from incorporation of host oncogenes into the viral genome during viral replication

Oncogenes are designated by short acronyms, preceded by 'v' if a viral oncogene is described (e.g. *v-myc*) or by 'c' for a cellular (host) oncogene (e.g. *c-myc*). DNA probes made from copies of the Rous sarcoma virus *src* oncogene have revealed complementary DNA in both infected and normal chicken cells, as well as in cancerous and normal human cells. This striking finding has since been repeated with many other retroviral oncogene sequences and it is now known that these can make up as much as 0.03–0.3% of the mammalian genome. Oncogene sequences have been identified in a wide variety of animals, from man to fruit flies, implying that they are conserved because of some valuable function. Which came first, host or viral oncogenes? The fact that host oncogenes contain introns, whereas viral oncogenes do not, and that their chromosomal positions are fixed, imply that they, and not the viral forms, are the original genes.

From what we now know about the gene products of viral oncogenes we can guess that cellular oncogenes (or 'proto-oncogenes') probably play an important role in host cell growth regulation. They may code for growth factors themselves, for

EXAMPLES OF RETROVIRAL ONCOGENES			
class of gene product	oncogene	virus	disease
tyrosine kinases	fms ros src yes	FeLV ALV ALV ALV	sarcoma
serine/threonine kinases	mos	MuLV	sarcoma
growth factors	sis	FeLV	sarcoma (platelet-derived growth factor)
growth factor receptor	erbB	ALV	erythroid leukemia (epidermal growth factor)
hormone receptor	erbA	ALV	erythroid leukemia (thyroid hormone)
GTP-binding proteins	Ha-ras Ki-ras	MuLV MuLV	sarcoma erythroid leukemia
DNA-binding proteins	myb myc fos	ALV ALV/FeLV MuLV	myeloblast leukemia carcinoma osteosarcoma

Fig. 3.12 Oncogenes, gene products, viruses known to carry them, and associated animal diseases. (ALV/FeLV/MuLV, avian, feline and murine leukemia viruses; GTP, guanosine triphosphate.)

cell surface receptor molecules that bind specific growth factors, for components of intracellular signalling systems, or for DNA-binding proteins that act as transcription factors.

The Rous sarcoma virus *src* oncogene is incorporated within the viral genome adjacent to the gene coding for viral envelope proteins *(Fig. 3.13)*. Unlike other strongly transforming viruses, the Rous virus has all three genes (*gag, pol and env*) necessary for replication; in the others (termed 'defective' transforming viruses), incorporation of an oncogene results in deletion of genetic material in the regions coding for the *pol* and/or *env* genes, so preventing replication. This becomes possible only with help from genetically complete helper viruses.

Oncogenes can be carried from one cell to another within the same host or from one host to another. This can occur through 'vertical' transmission (from mother to offspring) through passage of viruses in gametes, across the placenta or in milk. It can also occur by 'horizontal' transmission, the virus passing in, for example, saliva and urine (see Chapter 8).

Transformation of a cell occurs:
• When viral oncogenes are incorporated into the host genome (as in Rous sarcoma virus).
• When viral DNA is inserted near to a cellular oncogene.

The former may be due to mutations in the oncogene sequence while in the viral genome, single base changes in cellular oncogenes are known to confer the ability to transform normal cells. The latter may reflect altered expression of the host oncogene through disturbance of normal regulatory influences. Altered expression can occur whether the insertion is of a retroviral oncogene or of non-oncogenic viral DNA; it can also occur as a result of exposure to a variety of carcinogens. The products of cellular oncogenes are normally used in series to regulate cellular proliferation in a carefully controlled manner. Viral oncogene products or overexpressed cellular oncogene products shortcircuit and overload this complex control system, resulting in unregulated cell division.

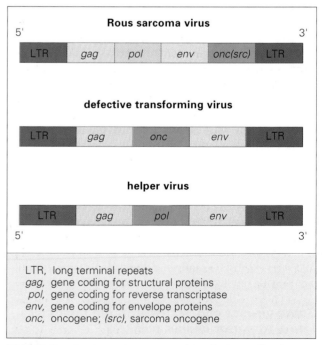

Fig. 3.13 Rous sarcoma virus can transform the host cell and replicate because it has both the oncogene *src* and a complete genome. Some transforming viruses are defective – they carry the oncogene, but lack genes for full replication. Helper viruses can supply these genes.

Major groups of viruses

The classification of viruses into major groups (families) is based upon a few simple criteria (*Fig. 3.14* and the Appendix). These include:

- The type of nucleic acid in the genome.
- The number of nucleic acid strands and their polarity.
- The mode of replication.
- The size, structure and symmetry of the virus particle.

The Bacteria

Compared with the huge numbers of free-living bacteria, relatively few species cause disease. The majority are now well-known and well studied but, nevertheless, new pathogens continue to emerge and the significance of previously unrecognized infections becomes apparent. A good example is infection with *Legionella*, the cause of Legionnaires' disease.

Classification of bacteria uses both phenotypic and genotypic data. For clinical purposes the phenotypic data are of most practical value, and rest on an understanding of bacterial structure and biology.

Structure

Bacteria are 'prokaryotes' and have a characteristic cellular organization

The genetic information of bacteria is carried in a long ds, circular molecule of DNA (*Fig. 3.15*). By analogy with eukaryotes (see Chapter 2) this can be termed a 'chromosome', but there are no introns, the DNA comprising a continuous coding sequence of genes. The chromosome is not localized within a distinct nucleus; no nuclear membrane is present and the DNA is tightly coiled into a region known as the 'nucleoid'. Extrachromosomal DNA may also be present and carried in small circular plasmids. The cytoplasm contains many ribosomes, but no other organelles; many of the metabolic functions performed in eukaryote cells by membrane-bound organelles such as mitochondria are carried out by the cell membrane. In all bacteria except mycoplasmas the cell is surrounded by a complex cell wall. External to this wall may be capsules, flagellae and pili. Knowledge of the cell wall and these external structures is important in diagnosis and pathogenicity and for understanding bacterial biology.

Bacteria are classified according to their cell wall as Gram positive or Gram negative

Gram staining is a basic microbiologic procedure for detection and identification of bacteria (see Chapter 14). The main structural component of the cell wall is a 'peptidoglycan' (mucopeptide or murein), a mixed polymer of hexose sugars (*N*-acetylglucosamine and *N*-acetylmuramic acid) and amino acids:

- In Gram-positive bacteria the peptidoglycan forms a thick (20–80 nm) layer external to the cell membrane, and may contain other macromolecules.
- In Gram-negative species the peptidoglycan layer is thin (5–10 nm) and is overlaid by an outer membrane, anchored to lipoprotein molecules in the peptidoglycan

layer. The principal molecules of the outer membrane are lipopolysaccharides and lipoprotein (*Fig. 3.16*).

The polysaccharides and charged amino acids in the peptidoglycan layer make it highly polar, providing the bacterium with a thick hydrophilic surface. This property allows Gram-positive organisms to resist the activity of bile in the intestine. Conversely, the layer is digested by lysozyme, an enzyme present in body secretions, which therefore has bactericidal properties. Synthesis of peptidoglycan is disrupted by penicillin and cephalosporin antibiotics (see Chapter 30).

In Gram-negative bacteria the outer membrane is also hydrophilic, but the lipid components of the constituent molecules give hydrophobic properties as well. Entry of hydrophilic molecules such as sugars and amino acids is necessary for nutrition and is achieved through special channels or pores formed by proteins called 'porins'. The lipopolysaccharide (LPS) in the membrane confers both antigenic properties (the 'O antigens' from the carbohydrate chains) and toxic properties (the 'endotoxin' from the lipid A component; see Chapter 12).

In the Gram-positive mycobacteria the peptidoglycan layer has a different chemical basis for cross-linking to the lipoprotein layer, and the outer envelope contains a variety of complex lipids (mycolic acids). These create a waxy layer, which alters both the staining properties of these organisms (the so-called acid-fast bacteria) and gives considerable resistance to drying and other environmental factors. Mycobacterial cell wall components also have a pronounced adjuvant activity (i.e. they promote immunologic responsiveness).

External to the cell wall may be an additional capsule of high molecular weight polysaccharides (amino acids in anthrax bacilli) that give a slimy surface. This provides protection against phagocytosis by host cells and is important in determining virulence. With *Streptococcus pneumoniae* infection only a few capsulated organisms can cause a fatal infection, but unencapsulated mutants cause no disease.

Many bacteria possess flagella

Flagella are long helical filaments extending from the cell surface, which enable bacteria to move in their environment. These may be restricted to the poles of the cell, singly (polar) or in tufts (lophotrichous), or distributed over the general surface of the cell (peritrichous). Bacterial flagella are quite different from eukaryote flagella and the forces that result in movement are generated quite differently (being ATP-independent). Motility allows positive and negative responses to chemical stimuli (chemotaxis). Flagella are built of protein components (flagellins), which are strongly antigenic. These antigens, the H antigens, are important targets of protective antibody responses.

Pili are another form of bacterial surface projection

Pili are more rigid than flagella and function in attachment, either to other bacteria (the 'sex' pili) or to host cells (the 'common' pili). Adherence to host cells involves specific interactions between component molecules of the pili (adhesins) and molecules in host cell membranes. For example, the adhesins of *E. coli* interact with fucose/mannose molecules on the surface of intestinal epithelial cells

MAJOR GROUPS OF VIRUSES						
DNA viruses						
virus family	**envelope present**	**capsid symmetry**	**particle size (nm)**	**DNA molecular weight (×10⁻⁶)**	**DNA structure***	**medically important viruses**
Parvoviridae	no	icosahedral	22	2	ss linear	B19 virus
Papovaviridae	no	icosahedral	55	3–5	ds circular, supercoiled	papilloma virus , polyomavirus (JC, BK)
Adenoviridae	no	icosahedral	75	23	ds linear	adenovirus
Hepadnaviridae	yes	icosahedral	42	1.5	ds incomplete circular	hepatitis B virus
Herpesviridae	yes	icosahedral	100**	100–150	ds linear	herpes simplex virus, varicella-zoster virus, cytomegalovirus, Epstein–Barr virus
Poxviridae	yes	complex	250 × 400	125–185	ds linear	smallpox virus, vaccinia virus
RNA viruses						
virus family	**envelope present**	**capsid symmetry**	**particle size (nm)**	**DNA mol. wt (×10⁻⁶)**	**RNA structure***	**medically important viruses**
Picornaviridae	no	icosahedral	28	2–3	ss linear, non-segmented, +ve sense	poliovirus, rhinovirus, hepatitis A virus, enteroviruses
Reoviridae	no	icosahedral	75	15	ds linear, 10 segments	reovirus, rotavirus, Colorado tick fever
Togaviridae	yes	icosahedral	40–70	4	ss linear, non-segmented, +ve sense	rubella virus, yellow fever virus
Retroviridae	yes	icosahedral	100	7†	ss linear, 2 segments, +ve sense	HIV, human T cell leukemia virus
Coronaviridae	yes	helical	100	5	ss linear, non-segmented, +ve sense	coronavirus
Caliciviridae	no	icosahedral	35–40	2.6	ssRNA, +ve sense	Norwalk agent
Orthomyxoviridae	yes	helical	80–120	4	ss linear, 8 segments, –ve sense	influenza virus
Paramyxoviridae	yes	helical	150	6	ss linear, non-segmented, –ve sense	measles, mumps, parainfluenza, respiratory syncytial viruses
Rhabdoviridae	yes	helical	75 × 180	3–4	ss linear, non-segmented, –ve sense	rabies virus
Arenaviridae	yes	helical	80–130	5	ss circular, 2 segments with cohesive ends, –ve sense	lymphocytic choriomeningitis virus
Bunyaviridae	yes	helical	100	5	ss circular, 3 segments with cohesive ends, –ve sense	California encephalitis, sandfly fever viruses
Filoviridae	yes	complex	80 × (800 – 900)	4.2	ssRNA, –ve sense	Marburg, Ebola virus

* ss, single stranded; ds, double stranded
** the herpesvirus nucleocapsid is 100 nm, but the envelope varies in size; the entire virus can be as large as 200 nm in diameter
† retrovirus RNA contains 2 identical molecules of molecular weight 3.5×10^6

Fig. 3.14 Summary of major families of viruses. Prions (agents responsible for kuru, Creutzfeldt–Jakob disease) are not included because they are not viruses and their status remains unclear (see Appendix).

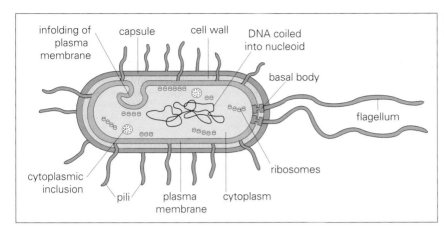

Fig. 3.15 Diagrammatic structure of a generalized bacterium.

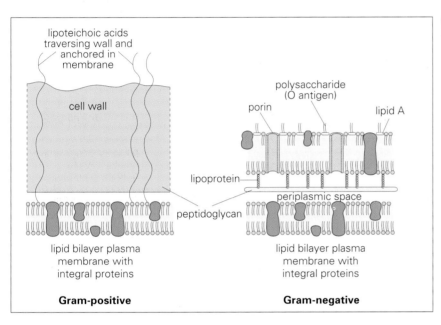

Fig. 3.16 Construction of the cell walls of Gram-positive and Gram-negative bacteria.

(see Chapter 20). The presence of many pili may help to prevent phagocytosis, reducing host resistance to bacterial infection. Although immunogenic, their antigens can be changed, allowing the bacteria to avoid immune recognition. The mechanism of 'antigenic variation' has been elucidated in the gonococci and is known to involve recombination of genes coding for 'constant' and 'variable' regions of pili molecules.

Nutrition
All pathogenic bacteria are heterotrophic
All bacteria obtain energy by oxidizing preformed organic molecules (carbohydrates, lipids and proteins) from their environment. Metabolism of these molecules yields adenosine triphosphate (ATP) as an energy source. Metabolism may be aerobic, where the final electron acceptor is oxygen, or anaerobic, where the final acceptor is an organic molecule:
- In aerobic metabolism, complete utilization of an energy source such as glucose produces 38 molecules of ATP.
- In anaerobic metabolism, respiration is incomplete and only two molecules of ATP are produced.

Anaerobic respiration (fermentation) is therefore less efficient, but can be used where substrates are readily available, as they usually are in the host's body. The requirement for oxygen in respiration may be 'obligate' or it may be 'facultative', some organisms being able to switch between aerobic and anaerobic respiration. Those that use fermentation pathways often use the major product pyruvate in secondary fermentations by which additional energy can be generated.

Bacteria obtain nutrients mainly by taking up small molecules across the cell wall
Bacteria take up small molecules such as amino acids, oligosaccharides and small peptides across the cell wall. Gram-negative species can also take up and use larger molecules after preliminary digestion in the periplasmic space. Uptake and transport of nutrients into the cytoplasm is achieved by the cell membrane, using a variety of transport mechanisms, including facilitated diffusion and active transport. Oxidative metabolism also takes place at the membrane–cytoplasm interface.

Some species require only minimal nutrients in their environment, having considerable synthetic powers, whereas others have complex nutritional requirements. *E. coli*, for example, can be grown in media providing only glucose and inorganic salts; streptococci, on the other hand, will grow only in complex media providing them with many organic compounds.

Growth and division

The growth and division of a bacterium into two identical 'daughter cells' takes *E. coli* only 20–30 minutes, while other bacteria such as *Mycobacterium tuberculosis* grow much more slowly, dividing every 24 hours.

A bacterial cell must duplicate its genomic DNA before it can divide

All bacterial genomes are circular and their replication begins at a single site known as the origin of replication. A multienzyme replication complex binds to the origin and initiates unwinding and separation of the two DNA strands, each of which serves as a template for DNA polymerase. The polymerization reaction involves incorporation of deoxyribonucleotides, which correctly base pair with the template DNA. Two characteristic replication forks are formed, which proceed in opposite directions around the chromosome. The two copies of the genome produced during replication are each comprised of one parental strand and one newly synthesized strand of DNA.

Replication of the genome takes approximately 40 minutes in *E. coli*, so when these bacteria grow and divide every 20–30 minutes they need to initiate new rounds of DNA replication before an existing round of replication has finished. In such instances daughter cells inherit DNA that has already initiated its own replication.

Replication must be accurate

Accurate replication is essential because DNA carries the information that defines the properties and processes of a cell. It is achieved because DNA polymerase is capable of proofreading newly incorporated deoxyribonucleotides and excising those that are incorrect. This reduces the frequency of errors to approximately one mistake (an incorrect base pair) per 10^{10} nucleotides copied.

Cell division is preceded by genome segregation and septum formation

The process of cell division (or septation) involves:
- Segregation of the replicated genomes.
- The formation of a septum in the middle of the cell.
- Division of the cell to give separate daughter cells.

The septum is formed by an invagination of the cytoplasmic membrane and ingrowth of the peptidoglycan cell wall (and outer membrane in Gram-negative bacteria). Septation and DNA replication and genome segregation are not tightly coupled, but are sufficiently well coordinated to ensure that very few daughter cells do not have the correct complement of genomic DNA.

Bacterial growth and division are important targets for antimicrobial agents

Antimicrobials that target the processes involved in bacterial growth and division include:

- Quinolones (nalidixic acid and norfloxacin), which inhibit the unwinding of DNA by DNA gyrase during DNA replication.
- The many inhibitors of peptidoglycan cell wall synthesis (e.g. beta-lactams such as the penicillins, cephalosporins and carbapenems, and glycopeptides such as vancomycin).

Gene expression

Gene expression describes the processes involved in decoding the 'genetic information' contained within a gene to produce a functional protein or RNA molecule.

Most genes are transcribed into mRNA

The overwhelming majority of genes (e.g. up to 98% in *E. coli*) are transcribed into mRNA, which is then translated into proteins. Certain genes, however, are transcribed to produce ribosomal RNA species (5S, 16S, 23S), which provide a scaffold for assembling ribosomal subunits; others are transcribed into transfer RNA (tRNA) molecules, which together with the ribosome participate in decoding mRNA into functional proteins.

Transcription

The DNA is copied by a DNA-dependent RNA polymerase to yield an RNA transcript. The polymerization reaction involves incorporation of ribonucleotides, which correctly base pair with the template DNA.

Transcription is initiated at promoters

Promoters are nucleotide sequences in DNA that can bind the RNA polymerase. The frequency of transcription initiation can be influenced by many factors, for example:
- The exact DNA sequence of the promoter site.
- The overall topology (supercoiling) of the DNA.
- The presence or absence of regulatory proteins that bind adjacent to and may overlap the promoter site.

Consequently, different promoters have widely different rates of transcriptional initiation (of up to 3000-fold). Their activities can be altered by regulatory proteins. σ-factor (a component RNA polymerase) plays an important role in promoter recognition. The presence of several different σ-factors in bacteria enables sets of genes to be switched on simply by altering the level of expression of a particular σ-factor. This is particularly important in controlling the expression of genes involved in spore formation in Gram-positive bacteria.

Transcription usually terminates at specific termination sites

These termination sites are characterized by a series of uracil residues in the mRNA following an inverted repeat sequence, which can adopt a stem-loop structure (which forms as a result of the base-pairing of ribonucleotides) and interfere with RNA polymerase activity. In addition, certain transcripts terminate following interaction of RNA polymerase with the transcription termination protein, rho.

mRNA transcripts often encode more than one protein in bacteria

The DNA encoding such multigene mRNA transcripts (or polycistronic mRNAs) are known as operons (*Fig. 3.17*).

Operons provide a way of ensuring that protein subunits that make up particular enzyme complexes or are required for a specific biological process are synthesized simultaneously and in the correct stoichiometry. For example:

- Most of the subunits of the small and large ribosomal complexes of *E. coli* are encoded by two large operons.
- The proteins required for the uptake and metabolism of lactose are encoded by the *lac* operon.

Many of the proteins responsible for the pathogenic properties of medically important microorganisms are likewise encoded by operons, for example:

- Cholera toxin from *V. cholerae*.
- Fimbriae of uropathogenic *E. coli*, which mediate colonization.

Translation

The exact sequence of amino acids in a protein (polypeptide) is specified by the sequence of nucleotides found in the mRNA transcripts. Decoding this information to produce a protein is achieved by ribosomes and tRNA molecules in a process known as translation. Each three bases (triplet) in the mRNA sequence corresponds to a codon for a specific amino acid.

Translation begins with formation of an initiation complex and terminates at a STOP codon

The initiation complex is comprised of mRNA, ribosome and an initiator tRNA molecule (carrying formylmethionine). Ribosomes bind to specific sequences in mRNA (Shine–Dalgarno sequences) and begin translation at an initiation (START) codon, AUG, which hybridizes with the anti-codon loop of the initiator tRNA molecule. The polypeptide chain elongates as a result of movement of the ribosome along the mRNA molecule and the recruitment of further tRNA molecules (carrying different amino acids), which recognize the subsequent codon triplets.

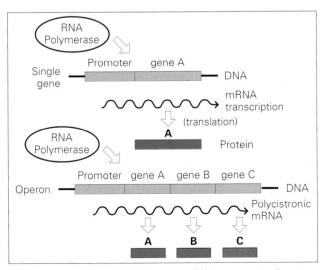

Fig. 3.17 Bacterial genes are present on DNA as separate discrete units (single genes) or as operons (multigenes), which are transcribed from promoters to give monocistronic or polycistronic messneger RNA (mRNA) molecules, respectively. mRNA is translated into protein.

Ribosomes carry out a condensation reaction, which couples the incoming amino acid (carried on the tRNA) to the growing polypeptide chain.

Translation is terminated when the ribosome encounters one of three termination (STOP) codons – UGA, UAA or UAG.

Transcription and translation are important targets for antimicrobial agents

Such antimicrobial agents include:

- Inhibitors of RNA polymerase such as rifampicin.
- An array of bacterial protein synthesis inhibitors including macrolides (erythromycin), aminoglycosides (kanamycin), tetracycline, streptomycin, spectinomycin and chloramphenicol.

Regulation of gene expression
Bacteria adapt to their environment by controlling gene expression

Bacteria show a remarkable ability to adapt to changes in their environment. This is predominantly achieved by controlling gene expression, thereby ensuring that proteins are only produced when and if they are required. For example:

- Bacteria may encounter a new source of carbon or nitrogen and as a consequence switch on new metabolic pathways that enable them to transport and use such compounds.
- When compounds such as amino acids are depleted from a bacterium's environment the bacterium may be able to switch on the production of enzymes that enable it to synthesize the particular molecule it requires *de novo*.

Expression of many virulence determinants by pathogenic bacteria is highly regulated

This makes sense since it conserves metabolic energy and ensures that virulence determinants are only produced when their particular property is needed. For example enterobacterial pathogens are often transmitted in contaminated water supplies. The temperature of such water will probably be lower than 25°C and low in nutrients. However, upon entering the human gut there will be a striking change in the bacterium's environment – the temperature will rise to 37°C, there will be an abundant supply of carbon and nitrogen and a low availability of both oxygen and free iron (an essential nutrient). Bacteria adapt to such changes by switching on or off a range of metabolic and virulence-associated genes.

The analysis of virulence gene expression is one of the fastest growing aspects of the study of microbial pathogenesis. It provides an important insight into how bacteria adapt to the many changes they encounter as they initiate infection and spread into different host tissues.

The most common way of altering gene expression is to change the amount of mRNA transcription

The level of mRNA transcription can be altered by altering the efficiency of binding of RNA polymerase to promoter sites. Environmental changes such as shifts in growth temperature (from 25°C to 37°C) or the availability of oxygen can change the extent of supercoiling in DNA, thereby altering the overall topology of promoters and the efficiency of transcription initiation. However, most instances of transcriptional regulation are mediated by regulatory proteins, which bind specifically to the DNA adjacent to or overlapping the promoter site and alter RNA polymerase binding and transcription. The regions of DNA to which regulatory proteins bind are known as operators or operator sites. Regulatory proteins fall into two distinct classes:

- Those that increase the rate of transcription initiation (activators).
- Those that inhibit transcription (repressors) *(Fig. 3.18)*.

Genes subject to negative regulation bind repressor proteins. Genes subject to positive regulation need to bind activated regulatory protein(s) to promote transcription initiation.

The principles of gene regulation in bacteria can be illustrated by the regulation of genes involved in sugar metabolism

Bacteria use sugars as a carbon source for growth and prefer to use glucose rather than other less well metabolized sugars. When growing in an environment containing both glucose and lactose, bacteria such as *E. coli* preferentially metabolize glucose and at the same time prevent the expression of the *lac* operon, the products of which transport and metabolize lactose *(Fig. 3.19)*. This is known as catabolite repression. It occurs because the transcriptional initiation of the *lac* operon is dependent upon a positive regulator, the cAMP-dependent catabolite activation protein (CAP), which is only activated when cAMP is bound. When bacteria grow on glucose the cytoplasmic levels of cAMP are low and so CAP is not activated. CAP is therefore unable to bind to its DNA binding site adjacent to the *lac* promoter and facilitate transcription initiation by RNA polymerase. When the glucose is depleted, the cAMP concentration rises, resulting in the formation of activated cAMP–CAP complexes, which bind the appropriate site on the DNA, increasing RNA polymerase binding and transcription.

CAP is an example of a global regulatory protein that controls the expression of multiple genes and controls the expression of over 100 genes in *E. coli*. All genes controlled by the same regulator are considered to constitute a regulon *(Fig. 3.18)*. In addition to the influence of CAP on the *lac* operon, the operon is also subject to negative regulation by the lactose repressor protein (LacI, *Fig. 3.19*). LacI is encoded by the *lacI* gene, which is located immediately upstream of the lactose operon and transcribed by a separate promoter. In the absence of lactose LacI binds specifically to the operator region of the *lac* promoter and blocks transcription. An inducer molecule, allolactose (or its non-metabolizable homologue, isopropyl-thiogalactoside – IPTG) is able to bind to LacI causing an allosteric change in its structure. This releases it from the DNA, thereby alleviating the repression. The *lac* operon therefore illustrates the fine tuning of gene regulation in bacteria – the operon is switched on only if lactose is available as a carbon source for cell growth, but remains unexpressed if glucose, the cell's preferred carbon source, is also present.

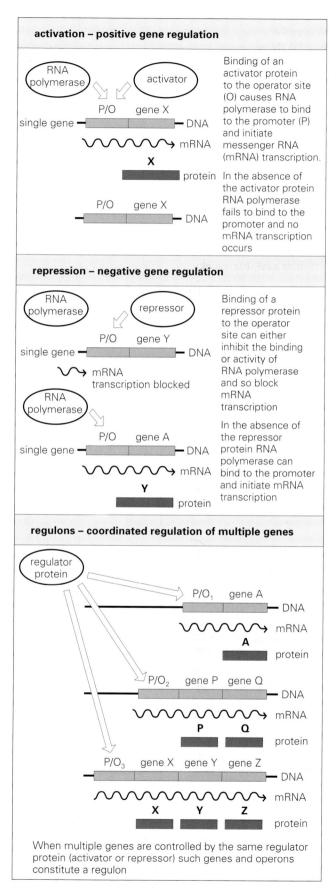

Fig. 3.18 Expression of genes in bacteria is highly regulated, enabling them to switch genes on or off in response to changes in available nutrients or other changes in their environment. Genes and operons controlled by the same regulator constitute a regulon.

Expression of bacterial virulence genes is often controlled by regulatory proteins

An example of such regulation is the production of diphtheria toxin by *Corynebacterium diphtheriae* (see Chapter 15), which is subject to negative regulation if there is free iron in the growth environment. A repressor protein, DtxR, binds iron and undergoes a conformational change that allows it to bind with high affinity to the operator site of the toxin gene and inhibit transcription. When *C. dipththeriae* grow in an environment with a very low concentration of iron (i.e. similar to that of human secretions), DtxR is unable to bind iron and toxin production occurs.

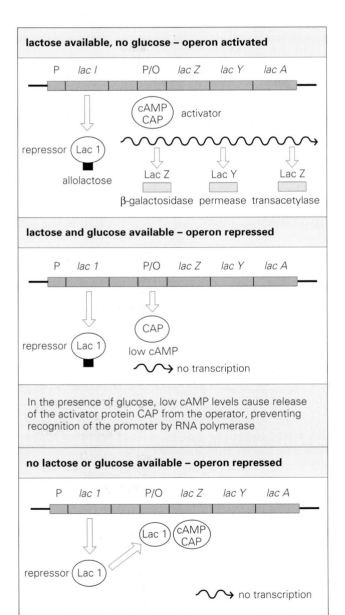

Fig. 3.19 Control of the *lac* operon. Transcription is controlled by the lactose repressor protein (Lac I, negative regulation) and by the catabolite activator protein (CAP, positive regulation). In the presence of lactose as the sole carbon source for growth the *lac* operon is switched on. Bacteria prefer to use glucose rather than lactose, so if glucose is also present the *lac* operon is switched off until the glucose has been used.

Many bacterial virulence genes are subject to positive regulation by 'two-component regulators'

These two-component regulators usually comprise two separate proteins:
- One acting as a sensor to detect environmental changes (such as alterations in temperature).
- The other acting as a DNA-binding protein capable of activating (or repressing in some cases) transcription.

A two-component regulator (encoded by the *bvg* locus) controls expression of a large number virulence genes by *Bordetella pertussis*, the causative agent of whooping cough (see Chapter 17). The sensor protein, BvgS, is a cytoplasmic membrane-located histidine kinase, which senses environmental signals (temperature, Mg^{2+}, nicotinic acid), leading to an alteration in its autophosphorylating activity. In response to positive regulatory signals such as an elevation in temperature, BvgS undergoes autophosphorylation and then phosphorylates, so activating the DNA binding protein BvgA. BvgA then binds to the operators of the pertussis toxin operon and other virulence-associated genes and activates their transcription.

Regulation of virulence genes often involves a cascade of activators

For example:
- BvgA appears to activate the expression of another regulatory protein, which in turn activates the expression of filamentous hemagglutinin, the major adherence factor produced by *B. pertussis*.
- The control of virulence gene expression in *V. cholerae* is under the control of ToxR, a cytoplasmic membrane-located protein, which senses environmental changes. ToxR activates both the transcription of the cholera toxin operon and another regulatory protein, ToxT, which in turn activates the transcription of other virulence genes such as toxin-co-regulated pili, an essential virulence factor required for colonization of the human small intestine.

Mutation and gene transfer

Bacteria are haploid organisms, the chromosomes containing one copy of each gene. Replication of the DNA is a precise process resulting in each daughter cell acquiring an exact copy of the parental genome. Changes in the genome can occur by two processes:
- Mutation.
- Recombination.

These processes result in progeny with phenotypic characteristics that may differ from those of the parent. This is of considerable significance in terms of virulence and drug resistance.

Mutation
Changes in the nucleotide sequence of DNA can occur spontaneously or under the influence of external agents (mutagens)

Point mutations – changes in single nucleotides – alter the triplet code. Such mutations may result in:
- No change in the amino acid sequence of the protein encoded by the gene because the different codons specify the same amino acid and are therefore silent mutations.

- An amino acid substitution in the translated protein, which may or may not alter its stability or functional properties.
- The formation of a STOP codon, causing premature termination and production of a truncated protein.

More comprehensive changes in the DNA involve deletion, replacement, insertion or inversion of several or many bases. The majority of these changes are likely to harm the organism, but a few may be beneficial and confer a selective advantage through the production of different proteins.

Recombination
New genotypes arise when genetic material is transferred from one bacterium to another
In such instances, the transferred DNA either:
- Recombines with the genome of the recipient cell.
- Is on a plasmid capable of replication in the recipient.

Recombination can bring about large changes in the genetic material, and since these events usually involve functional genes, they are likely to be expressed phenotypically. DNA can be transferred from a donor cell to a recipient cell by:
- Transformation.
- Transduction.
- Conjugation.
- Transposition *(Fig. 3.20)*.

Transformation
Some bacteria can be transformed by DNA present in their environment
Certain bacteria such as *Streptococcus pneumoniae, Bacillus subtilis, Haemophilus influenzae* and *Neiserria gonorrhoeae* are naturally 'competent' to take up DNA fragments from related species across their cell walls. Such DNA fragments may be present in the environment of the competent cell as a result of lysis of other organisms, the release of their DNA and its cleavage into smaller fragments. Once taken into the cell, the DNA has to recombine with an homologous segment of the recipient's chromosome to be stably maintained and inherited. If organisms take up completely unrelated DNA the absence of any homology prevents recombination and the DNA is degraded.

Most bacteria are not naturally competent to be transformed by DNA, but competence can be induced artificially by either treating cells with certain bivalent cations and then subjecting them to a heat shock at 42°C or by electric shock treatment (electroporation).

Transformation is a powerful tool for molecular genetic analysis of bacteria.

Transduction
Transduction involves the transfer of genetic material by infection with a bacteriophage
A bacteriophage is a bacteria-infecting virus particle. During bacteriophage replication DNA is packaged into phage capsids (heads), and normally involves incorporation of phage DNA. However, occasionally, host genomic DNA is erroneously packaged, resulting in a 'transducing particle', which can attach to and transduce genomic DNA into a recipient cell. The DNA usually has to be incorporated by homologous

recombination if it is to be stably inherited. This type of gene transfer is known as generalized transduction *(Fig. 3.20)*.

Another form of transduction is exhibited by 'temperate' bacteriophages, which integrate at specialized attachment sites into the bacterial genome, where the phage becomes lysogenic, and is replicated as part of the genome during normal DNA replication. Examples of lysogenic phages include bacteriophage λ and the phage in *C. diphtheriae*, which carries the diphtheria toxin gene. When lysogenic phages enter a lytic cycle to produce numerous phage particles, they are occasionally incorrectly excised from the site of attachment. This can result in phages containing a piece of bacterial genomic DNA adjacent to the attachment site. Infection of a recipient cell then results in a high frequency of recombinants in which donor DNA has recombined with the recipient genome in the vicinity of the attachment site.

Conjugation
Many bacteria possess extrachromosomal DNA in the form of plasmids
In addition to the DNA contained within the chromosome, many bacteria possess plasmids. These are independent, self-replicating, circular units of DNA, some of which are relatively large (60–120 kilobases) while others are quite small (1.5–15 kilobases). Plasmids can carry a wide variety of genes (up to 100 on larger plasmids) and these can confer phenotypic advantages to the host bacterial cell, including for example:
- Virulence genes, which encode toxins and other proteins that increase the virulence of microorganisms.
- Metabolic genes, which encode enzymes for catabolism and degradation of new nutrients.
- Resistance genes, which inhibit the activity of antibiotics.
- Tumorigenic genes, such as those found on the Ti plasmid of *Agrobacterium tumefaciens*, involved in tumor formation in plants.

Plasmids also contain genes for plasmid replication, and in some cases for mediating plasmid transfer between bacteria (*tra* genes). Plasmid replication is similar to the replication of genomic DNA, though there may be some differences. Not all plasmids are replicated bidirectionally – some have a single replication fork, others are replicated like a 'rolling circle'. The number of plasmids per bacterial cell (copy number) varies for different plasmids, ranging from 1–1000 copies/cell. The rate of initiation of plasmid replication determines the plasmid copy number. Some plasmids (broad-host range plasmids) are able to replicate in many different bacterial species, others have a more restricted host range.

Conjugation is a type of bacterial 'mating' in which DNA is transferred from one bacterium to another
Conjugation is dependent upon the *tra* genes encoded by 'conjugative' plasmids and involves the formation of sex pili, allowing bacteria to make cell–cell contact and to transfer a copy of the plasmid DNA into the recipient cell *(Fig. 3.20)*. Occasionally, conjugative plasmids such as the fertility plasmid

(F plasmid or F factor) of *E. coli* integrate into the bacterial genome and such integrated plasmids are called episomes. When an integrated F episome undergoes conjugative transfer, genomic DNA is transferred from the donor cell into the recipient. Such strains, in contrast to cells containing the unintegrated F plasmid mediate high frequency transfer and recombination of genomic DNA (Hfr strains). The circular nature of the bacterial genome and the relative 'map' positions of different genes were established using interrupted mating of Hfr strains. Conjugative plasmids are transferred between cells at high frequency and rapidly spread throughout bacterial populations.

Conjugative transfer of plasmids with resistance genes has been an important cause of the spread of resistance to commonly used antibiotics. When a conjugative plasmid is present in the same cell as a non-conjugative plasmid, the non-conjugative plasmid can sometimes be transferred into the recipient cell as well by a process known as mobilization.

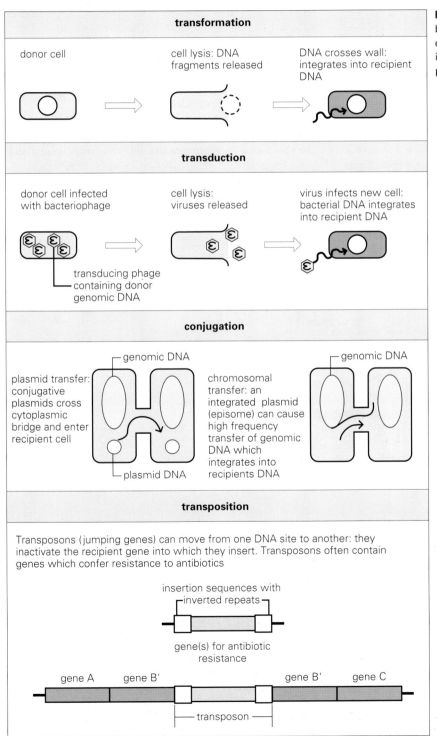

Fig. 3.20 Different ways in which genes can be transferred between bacteria. With the exception of plasmid transfer, donor DNA integrates into the recipient's genome by a process of recombination.

Widespread use of antibiotics has applied a strong selection pressure in favor of bacteria able to resist them

In the majority of cases antibiotic resistance is due to the presence of resistance genes on conjugative plasmids (R plasmids; see Chapter 30). These are known to have existed before the era of mass antibiotic treatments, but they have become widespread in many species as a result of selection. R plasmids may carry genes for resistance to several antibiotics. For example, the common R plasmid – R1 – confers resistance to ampicillin, chloramphenicol, fusidic acid, kanamycin, streptomycin and sulphonamides, and there are many others conferring resistance to a wide spectrum of antibiotics. R plasmids can recombine so that individual plasmids can be responsible for new combinations of multiple drug resistance.

Plasmids can carry virulence genes

Such plasmids may encode toxins and other proteins that increase the virulence of microorganisms. For example:

- The virulent enterotoxinogenic strains of *E. coli* that cause diarrhea produce one of two different types of plasmid-encoded enterotoxin. The enterotoxin alters the secretion of fluid and electrolytes by the intestinal epithelium (see Chapter 20).

- In *Staphylococcus aureus* both an enterotoxin and a number of enzymes involved in bacterial virulence (hemolysin, fibrinolysin) are encoded by plasmid genes.

The production of toxins by bacteria and their pathologic effects are discussed in detail in Chapter 12.

Plasmids are valuable tools for cloning and manipulating genes

Molecular biologists have generated a wealth of recombinant plasmids to use as vectors for genetic engineering *(Fig. 3.21)*. Plasmids can be used to transfer genes across species barriers so that defined gene products can be studied or synthesized in large quantities in different recipient organisms.

Transposition

Transposable elements are DNA sequences that can jump (transpose) from one site to another in the genome of a cell

The most extensively studied transposable elements are those found in *E. coli* and other Gram-negative bacteria; examples are also found in Gram-positive bacteria, yeast, plants and other organisms.

The simplest transposable elements are called 'insertion sequences' (ISs). They are less than 2 kilobases in length and they encode an enzyme (transposase), which is required for

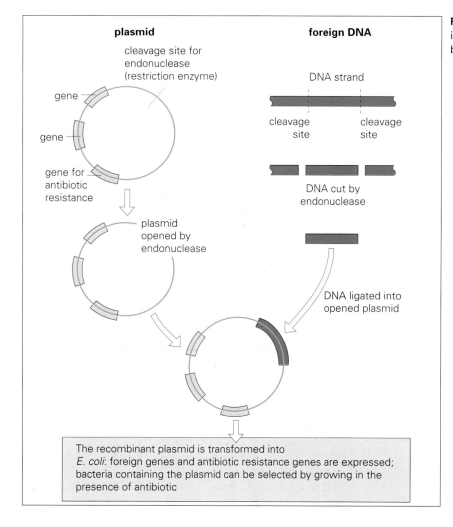

Fig. 3.21 The use of plasmid vectors to introduce foreign DNA in *Escherichia coli* – a basic step in gene cloning.

plasmid foreign DNA

cleavage site for endonuclease (restriction enzyme)

gene

gene

gene for antibiotic resistance

DNA strand

cleavage site   cleavage site

DNA cut by endonuclease

plasmid opened by endonuclease

DNA ligated into opened plasmid

The recombinant plasmid is transformed into *E. coli*: foreign genes and antibiotic resistance genes are expressed; bacteria containing the plasmid can be selected by growing in the presence of antibiotic

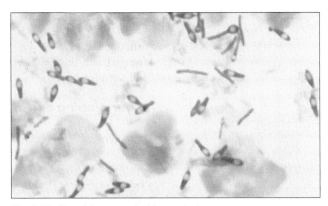

Fig. 3.22 *Clostridium tetani* with terminal spores.

transposition from one DNA site to another. At the ends of ISs there are usually short inverted repeat sequences (23 nucleotides long in IS1), which also play an important role in transposition. In addition, IS elements are flanked by short direct repeat sequences (of genomic DNA). The duplication is generated during the transposition process.

Larger transposable elements (transposons) (over 2 kilobases in length) often contain genes encoding resistance to one or more antibiotics *(Fig. 3.20)*, in addition to the transposase. Furthermore, virulence genes, such as those encoding heat-stable enterotoxin from *E. coli* have been found on transposons.

Transposons can be divided into two classes:
- Those having IS elements at both ends (composite transposons), such as Tn5.
- Simple transposons, such as Tn3.

In Tn5 the DNA segment between the two ISs contains a gene encoding resistance to kanamycin; Tn3 codes for resistance to beta-lactams.

The ease with which transposons move into or out of DNA sequences means that transposition can occur:
- From host genomic DNA harboring a transposon to a plasmid.
- From one plasmid to another plasmid.
- From a plasmid to genomic DNA.

Transposition onto a broad-host range conjugative plasmid can lead to the rapid dissemination of antibiotic resistance among different bacteria.

Survival under adverse conditions
Some bacteria form endospores

Certain bacteria can form highly resistant spores – endospores – within their cells, and these enable them to survive adverse conditions. They are formed when the cells are unable to grow (e.g. when environmental conditions change or when nutrients are exhausted), but never by actively growing cells. The spore has a complex multilayered coat surrounding a new bacterial cell. There are many differences in composition between endospores and normal cells, notably the presence of dipicolinic acid and a high calcium content, both of which are thought to confer the endospore's extreme resistance to heat and chemicals.

Because of their resistance, spores can remain viable in a dormant state for many years, reconverting rapidly to normal existence when conditions improve. When this occurs a new bacterial cell grows out from the spore and resumes vegetative life. Endospores are abundant in soils and those of the *Clostridium* and *Bacillus* are a particular hazard *(Fig. 3.22)*. Tetanus and anthrax caused by these bacteria are both associated with endospore infection of wounds, the bacteria developing from the spores once in appropriate conditions.

Major groups of bacteria
Detailed summaries of members of these major groups are given in *Fig. 14.19* and in the Appendix.

The Fungi

Fungi are eukaryotes, but distinct from plants and animals. Characteristically they are multinucleate or multicellular organisms with a thick cell wall growing as thread-like filaments (hyphae), but many other growth forms occur. Of these the mushroom and the single-celled yeasts are most familiar. Fungi are ubiquitous in the environment and are of enormous importance commercially in baking, brewing and in pharmaceuticals. They also cause significant human infections. Pathogenic species digest material externally by releasing enzymes and also take up nutrients directly from host tissues.

Major groups of disease-causing fungi
Fungal pathogens can be divided on the basis of their growth forms or the type of infection they cause

Fungal pathogens may exist as branched filamentous forms or as yeasts *(Fig. 3.23)*; some show both growth forms in their cycle and are known as 'dimorphic' fungi. In filamentous forms (e.g. *Trichophyton*), the mass of hyphae forms a 'mycelium'. Asexual reproduction results in the formation of sporangia, which liberate the spores by which the fungus is dispersed; spores are a common cause of infection after inhalation. In yeast-like forms (e.g. *Cryptococcus*) the characteristic form is the single cell, which reproduces by division. Budding may also occur, with the 'bud' remaining attached, forming pseudohyphae. Dimorphic forms (e.g. *Histoplasma*) form hyphae at environmental temperatures, but occur as yeast cells in the body, the switch being temperature-induced. *Candida* is an important exception in the dimorphic group, showing the reverse and forming hyphae within the body.

Two types of infection (mycoses) are recognized:
- Superficial mycoses, where the fungus grows at the body surface in skin, hair and nails.
- Deep mycoses, with involvement of internal organs.

The first are usually mild, but the second can be life-threatening. The superficial pathogens are spread by direct contact, whereas the deep mycoses often result from the opportunistic growth of fungi in individuals with impaired immune competence (see Chapter 28). Free-living fungi can also cause disease indirectly when their toxins are present in items used as food (e.g. the aflatoxins).

Many of the fungi that cause disease are free-living organisms and are acquired by inhalation or by entry through wounds. Some are part of the normal flora (e.g.

by growth form

filamentous	yeasts
growing as multinucleate, branching hyphae, forming a mycelium	growing as ovoid or spherical single cells multiply by budding and division

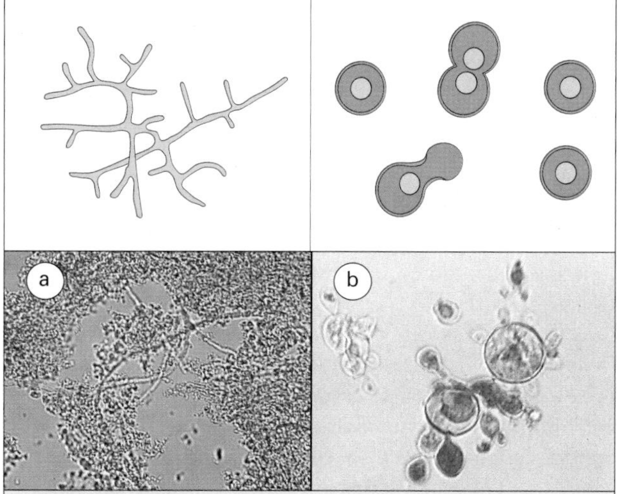

by type of infection

superficial mycoses	deep mycoses
Epidermophyton	Aspergillus
Microsporum	Blastomyces
Trichophyton	Candida
Sporothrix	Coccidioides
	Cryptococcus
	Histoplasma
	Paracoccidioides

Fig. 3.23 Two ways to classify fungi that cause disease – by growth form and by type of infection. (a) Hypahae in skin scraping fromringworm lesion. (Courtesy of DK Banerjee.) (b) Spherical yeasts of *Histoplama*. (Courtesy of Y Clayton and G Midgley.)

Candida) and are innocuous unless the body's defenses are compromised. The filamentous forms grow extracellularly, but yeasts can survive and multiply within macrophages and neutrophils. Neutrophils can play a major role in controlling the establishment of invading fungi. Species that are too large for phagocytosis can be killed by extracellular factors released from phagocytes as well as by other components of the immune response. Some species, notably *Cryptococcus neoformans*, prevent phagocytic uptake because they are surrounded by a polysaccharide capsule (see Chapter 22).

The major groups of fungi causing human disease are shown in *Figure 3.24*. *Pneumocystis*, an organism previously thought to be a protozoan is now believed to be a fungus, but is considered below under protozoa for convenience.

The Protozoa

Protozoa can infect all the major tissues and organs of the body

Protozoa are single-celled animals. Many species are important parasites of humans, the infections being most prevalent in tropical and subtropical regions, but also occurring in temperate regions.

IMPORTANT FUNGAL DISEASES				
type	**anatomic location**	**representative disease**	**genus of causative organism(s)**	**growth form**
superficial cutaneous	hair shaft, dead layer of skin	tinea versicolor	*Malassezia*	Y
	epidermis, hair, nails	dermatophytosis (ringworm)	*Microsporum, Trichophyton epidermophyton*	F
subcutaneous	subcutis	sporotrichosis mycetoma	*Sporothrix* several genera	Y* F
deep systemic	internal organs	coccidioidomycosis histoplasmosis blastomycosis paracoccidioidomycosis	*Coccidioides* *Histoplasma* *Blastomyces* *Paracoccidioides*	** Y Y Y
opportunistic	internal organs	cryptococcosis candidiasis aspergillosis	*Cryptococcus* *Candida* *Aspergillus*	Y Y† F*

Y, yeast; F, filamentous; * growth form in the body; † also forms pseudohyphae

** *Coccidioides* has an unusual growth form with yeast-like endospores within a spherule

Fig. 3.24 Summary of fungi that cause important human diseases.

Transmission of protozoan parasites occurs in many ways, the two commonest being injection by the bites of blood-sucking insects and accidental ingestion of infective stages. The geographic restriction of some species reflects both the distribution of vector insect species and the climatic conditions (primarily temperature) necessary for the parasites to complete their development in the insect. Orally acquired infections are favored by low standards of social and personal hygiene, and by increased survival of infective stages in warm damp conditions.

Protozoa infect body tissues and organs as:
• Intracellular parasites in a wide variety of cells.
• Extracellular parasites in the blood, intestine or urinogenital system *(Fig. 3.25)*.

Intracellular species obtain nutrients from the host cell by direct uptake or by ingestion of cytoplasm. Extracellular species feed by direct nutrient uptake or by ingestion of host cells. Reproduction in humans is usually asexual, by binary or multiple division of growing stages (trophozoites). Sexual reproduction is normally absent or restricted to the insect vector phase; *Cryptosporidium* is exceptional in undergoing sexual reproduction in humans. Asexual reproduction gives the potential for a rapid increase in number, particularly where host defense mechanisms are impaired. For this reason some protozoans are most pathogenic in the very young (e.g. *Toxoplasma* in neonates) and in immunocompromised individuals (e.g. *Cryptosporidium* and *Pneumocystis* in AIDS patients).

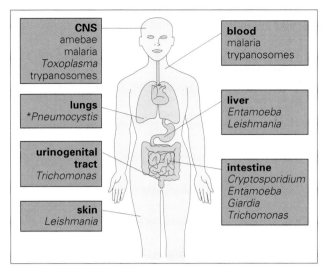

Fig. 3.25 The occurrence of protozoan parasites in the body. (*Included for convenience – now considered a fungus.) (CNS, central nervous system)

Protozoa have evolved many sophisticated strategies to avoid immune recognition of their plasma membrane

The interface between host and extracellular protozoa is the parasite's plasma membrane and examples of strategies

location	species	mode of transmission	disease
	**FEATURES OF MEDICALLY IMPORTANT PROTOZOA**		
intestinal tract	*Entamoeba histolytica* *Giardia lamblia* *Cryptosporidium* spp.	ingestion of cysts in food	amebiasis giardiasis cryptosporidiosis
urinogenital tract	*Trichomonas vaginalis*	sexual	trichomoniasis
blood and tissue	*Trypanosoma* spp. *T. cruzi*	reduviid bug	trypanosomiasis Chagas' disease
	T. gambiense *T. rhodesiense*	tsetse fly	sleeping sickness
	Leishmania spp. *L. donovani*	sand fly	visceral leishmaniasis (kala-azar)
	L. tropica, L. mexicana *L. braziliensis*	sand fly	cutaneous leishmaniasis mucocutaneous leishmaniasis

	Plasmodium spp.
	  P. vivax, P. ovale
	  P. malariae
		Anopheles mosquito	malaria

	P. falciparum	*Anopheles* mosquito	malaria
	Toxoplasma gondii	ingestion of cysts in raw meat; contact with soil contaminated by cat feces	toxoplasmosis
	Pneumocystis carinii	inhalation	pneumonia

Fig. 3.26 Summary of the location, transmission and diseases caused by protozoan parasites.

to avoid immune recognition of this surface include the following:
- Trypanosomes undergo repeated antigenic variation of surface antigens.
- Malaria parasites show polymorphisms in dominant surface antigens.
- Amebae can consume complement at the cell surface.

Although intracellular stages are removed from direct contact with antibody, complement and phagocytes, their antigens may be expressed at the surface of the host cell, which can then be a target for cytotoxic effectors. Survival within cells, particularly within macrophages (*Leishmania*, *Toxoplasma*) involves a variety of devices to evade or inactivate the harmful effects of intracellular enzymes or reactive oxygen and nitrogen metabolites. Protozoa of medical importance are summarized in *Figure 3.26*.

The Helminths

The term 'helminth' is used for all groups of parasitic worms. Three main groups are important in humans:
- The tapeworms (Cestoda).
- The flukes (Trematoda or Digenea).
- The roundworms (Nematoda).

The first two belong to the Platyhelminthes or flatworms, the third are included in a separate phylum.

Helminths are generally large organisms with a complex body organization

Although invading larval stages may measure only 100–200 μm adult worms may be centimeters or even meters long. Infections are commonest in warmer countries, but intestinal species also occur in temperate regions.

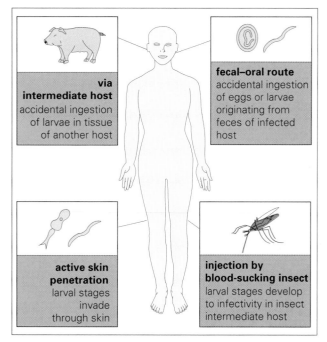

Fig. 3.27 How helminth parasites enter the body.

Transmission occurs in four distinct ways (*Fig. 3.27*):
- By swallowing infective eggs or larvae via the fecal–oral route.
- By swallowing infective larvae in the tissues of another host.
- By active penetration of the skin by larval stages.
- In the bite of a blood-sucking insect.

The greater frequency of helminths in tropical and subtropical regions reflects the climatic conditions that favor survival of infective stages, the socioeconomic conditions that facilitate fecal–oral contact, the practises involved in food preparation and consumption, and the availability of suitable vectors. Elsewhere, infections are commonest in children, in individuals closely associated with domestic animals and in individuals with particular food preferences.

Many helminths live in the intestine, while others live in the deeper tissues. Almost all organs of the body can be parasitized. Flukes and nematodes actively feed on host tissues or on the intestinal contents; tapeworms have no digestive system and absorb pre-digested nutrients.

The majority of helminths do not replicate within the host. In its simplest form, as in intestinal worms, sexual reproduction results in the production of eggs, which are released from the host in fecal material. In others, eggs and larvae may accumulate within the host, but do not mature. Certain tapeworm larval stages can reproduce asexually in man. The nematode *Strongyloides* is exceptional in that eggs produced in the intestine can hatch there, releasing infective larvae, which reinvade the body – the process of 'autoinfection'. A similar phenomenon occurs with the tapeworm *Taenia solium*.

The outer surfaces of helminths provide the primary host–parasite interface

In tapeworms and flukes the surface is a complex plasma membrane, and in both there are protective mechanisms to prevent the host damaging the outer surface. The nematode outer surface is a tough collagenous cuticle, which, although antigenic, is largely resistant to immune attack. However, smaller larval stages may be damaged by host granulocytes and macrophages. Worms release large amounts of soluble antigenic material in their excretions and secretions, and this plays an important role both in immunity and pathology.

The larvae of flukes and tapeworms must pass through one or more intermediate hosts, but those of nematodes can develop within a single host

Platyhelminths (flatworms) have flattened bodies with muscular suckers and/or hooks for attachment to the host. Most flukes are hermaphrodites, except the schistosomes, which have separate sexes. The reproductive organs of tapeworms are replicated along the body (the strobila) in a series of identical segments or 'proglottids'. The terminal 'gravid' proglottids become filled with mature eggs, detach and pass out in the feces. The eggs of both flukes and tapeworms develop into larvae that must pass through one or more intermediate hosts and develop into other larval stages before the parasite is again infective to humans. The tapeworm *Hymenolepis nana* is exceptional and can go through a complete cycle from egg to adult in the same host.

Nematodes (roundworms) have long cylindrical bodies and generally lack specialized attachment organs. The sexes are separate – most liberate fertilized eggs, but some release early-stage larvae directly into the host's body. Development from egg or larva to adult can be direct and occur in a single host, or may be indirect, requiring development in the body of an intermediate host. Classification of nematodes is complex and for practical purposes only two categories need be considered:

- Those that mature within the gastrointestinal tract (some of which may migrate through the body during development).
- Those that mature in deeper tissues.

Helminths and disease
Adult tapeworms are acquired by eating undercooked or raw meat containing larval stages
Tapeworms frequently infect humans, but are relatively harmless despite their potential for reaching a large size. Humans can also act as the intermediate hosts for certain species, and the development of larval stages in the body can cause severe disease (*Fig. 3.28*).

The most important flukes are those causing schistosomiasis
Several species of fluke can mature in humans, developing in the intestine, lungs, liver and blood vessels. The most important, both in terms of prevalence and pathology, are the blood flukes or schistosomes, the cause of schistosomiasis or bilharzia. Three main species – *Schistosoma haematobium*, *Schistosoma japonicum* and *Schistosoma mansoni* – are responsible for human disease (*Fig. 3.29*).

Certain nematodes that infect man are highly specific, others are zoonoses
Several of the many species of nematode that infect man are highly specific and can mature in no other host. Others have a much lower host specificity, being acquired accidentally as zoonoses, with humans acting either as the intermediate or the final host after picking up infection from domestic animals or in food (*Fig. 3.30*).

HUMAN TAPEWORM INFECTIONS			
species	acquired from	other hosts	site in humans
adult worms			
Taenia saginata	larvae in beef	none	intestine
Taenia solium	larvae in pork	none	intestine
Diphyllobothrium latum	larvae in fish	fish-eating mammals	intestine
Hymenolepis nana	eggs, or larvae in beetles	rodents	intestine
Hymenolepis diminuta*	larvae in insects	rats, mice	intestine
Dipylidium caninum*	larvae in fleas	dogs, cats	intestine
larval worms			
Taenia solium (cysticercosis)	eggs in food or water contaminated with human feces	pigs	brain, eyes
Echinococcus granulosus (hydatid disease)	eggs passed by dogs	sheep	liver, lung, brain
Echinococcus multilocularis*	eggs passed by carnivores	rodents	liver
Pseudophyllid tapeworms* (sparganosis)	larvae in other hosts	many vertebrates	subcutaneous tissues, eye
Taenia multiceps*	eggs passed by dogs	sheep	brain, eye, subcutaneous tissue
* rare infections			

Fig. 3.28 Summary of the location, transmission and other hosts used by tapeworms that infect humans.

HUMAN FLUKE INFECTIONS		
species	acquired from	site in humans
Schistosoma haematobium		blood vessels of bladder
Schistosoma japonicum	penetration of skin by larval stages released from snails	blood vessels of intestine
Schistosoma mansoni		blood vessels of intestine
Clonorchis sinensis	ingesting fish infected with larval stages	liver
Fasciola hepatica	ingesting vegetation (cress) with larval stages	liver
Paragonimus westermani	ingesting crabs infected with larval stages	lungs

Fig. 3.29 Summary of the location and transmission of flukes that infect humans.

HUMAN NEMATODE INFECTIONS		
species	acquired by	site in humans
transmitted person-to-person		
Ascaris lumbricoides	ingestion of eggs	small intestine
Enterobius vermicularis	ingestion of eggs	large intestine
Hookworms Ancylostoma duodenale	skin penetration	small intestine
Necator americanus	by infective larvae	small intestine
Strongyloides stercoralis	skin penetration by infective larvae; autoinfection	small intestine (adults) general tissues (larvae)
Trichuris trichiura	ingestion of eggs	large intestine
transmitted person-to-person via arthropod vector		
Brugia malayi	bite of mosquito carrying infective larvae	lymphatics (adults) blood (larvae)
Onchocerca volvulus	bite of Simulium fly carrying infective larvae	skin (larvae, adults) eye (larvae)
Wuchereria bancrofti	bite of mosquito carrying infective larvae	lymphatics (adults) blood (larvae)
Loa loa	bite of deer fly carrying infective larvae	tissues
zoonoses transmitted from animals		
Angiostrongylus cantonensis	ingestion of larvae in snails, crustacea	CNS (larvae)
Anisakis simplex	ingestion of larvae in fish	stomach, small intestine (larvae)
Capillaria phillipinensis	ingestion of larvae in fish	small intestine (adults, larvae)
Toxocara canis*	ingestion of eggs passed by dogs	tissues, CNS (larvae)
Trichinella spiralis*	ingestion of larvae in pork, wild mammals	small intestine (adults) muscles (larvae)

* these species are the commonest in this group

Fig. 3.30 Summary of the location and transmission of nematodes that infect humans. (CNS, central nervous system.)

The Arthropods

Many insects feed on human blood,

Such insects include mosquitoes, midges, biting flies, bugs, fleas and ticks. Some mites also feed in this way – chiggers, the larvae of trombiculid mites, are a familiar example. The head and body forms of the louse *Pediculus humanus* and the crab louse *Phthirus pubis* have more permanent contact with the human, reproducing on the body or in clothing as well as feeding on blood. Only the scabies mite *Sarcoptes scabiei* lives permanently on man, burrowing into the superficial layers of skin to feed and lay eggs. Heavy infections can build up, particularly on individuals with reduced immune responsiveness, causing a severe inflammatory condition (see Chapter 23).

Arthropod infestation carries the additional hazard of disease transmission

Arthropods transmit pathogens of all major groups, from viruses to worms: some (e.g. mosquitoes and ticks) transmit a wide variety of organisms *(Fig. 3.31)*. The ability to transmit infections acquired from animals poses a constant threat of zoonoses to humans. Some, such as yellow fever, have been known for a century, whereas others, such as the viral encephalitides and Lyme disease, have been recognized only comparatively recently (1920s and 1975 respectively).

The Normal Flora

The preceding sections have focused on organisms that are quite clearly parasites or pathogens. Their presence is often associated with pathologic changes and they are rarely found in healthy individuals. Other organisms covered in this chapter may cause disease under certain circumstances (e.g. in the newborn or in stressed, traumatized or immunocompromised individuals), but usually coexist quite peacefully with their host. Many of these form what is termed the 'indigenous' or 'normal' flora of the body – a collection of species routinely found in the normal healthy individual.

The normal flora is acquired rapidly during and shortly after birth and changes continuously throughout life

The organisms present at any given time reflect the age, nutrition and environment of the individual. It is therefore difficult to define the normal flora very precisely because it is to a large extent environmentally determined. This is well illustrated by data from NASA astronauts who were rendered relatively bacteriologically sterile by antibiotic treatment before their space flights. It took only six weeks after the flight for their flora to repopulate, and the repopulating species were precisely those of their immediate neighbors.

INFECTIOUS DISEASES TRANSMITTED BY ARTHROPODS		
	disease	**arthropod vector**
viruses arboviruses	dengue fever yellow fever encephalitides hemorrhagic fevers	mosquitoes mosquitoes mosquitoes, ticks ticks, mosquitoes
bacteria *Yersinia pestis* *Borrelia recurrentis* *Borrelia burgdorferi*	plague relapsing fever Lyme disease	fleas soft ticks hard ticks
rickettsias *R. prowazeki* *R. mooseri* *R. rickettsia* *R. akari*	epidemic typhus endemic (murine) typhus spotted fever rickettsial pox	lice, ticks fleas ticks mites
protozoa *Trypanosome cruzi* *T.b. rhodesiense* *T.b. gambiense* *Plasmodium* spp. *Leishmania* spp.	American trypanosomiasis (Chagas' disease) African trypanosomiasis (sleeping sickness) malaria leishmaniasis	reduviid bugs tsetse flies mosquitoes sandflies
worms *Wuchereria* and *Brugia* *Onchocerca*	lymphatic filariasis onchocerciasis	mosquitoes *Simulium* flies

Fig. 3.31 Summary of infectious diseases transmitted by arthropods.

The bowel flora of children in developing countries is quite different from that of children in developed countries. In addition, breastfed infants have lactic acid streptococci and lactobacilli in their gastrointestinal tract, whereas bottlefed children show a much greater variety of organisms.

The term 'flora' is used because the majority of the organisms, that occur where the body communicates with the external environment, are bacteria

It has been estimated that humans have approximately 10^{13} cells in the body and something like 10^{14} bacteria associated with them, the majority in the large bowel. Members of groups such as viruses, fungi and protozoa are also regularly found in healthy individuals, but form only a minor component of the total population of resident organisms.

The organisms occur in those parts of the body that are exposed to, or communicate with, the external environment, namely the skin, nose and mouth, and intestinal and urinogenital tracts. Internal organs and tissues are normally sterile. The main organisms found in these sites are shown in *Figure 3.32*.

Different regions of the skin support different flora

Exposed dry areas have relatively few resident organisms on the surface, whereas moister areas (axillae, perineum, between the toes, scalp) support much larger populations. *Staphylococcus epi-*

dermidis is one of the commonest species, making up some 90% of the aerobes and occurring in densities of 10^3–$10^4/cm^2$; *Staph. aureus* may be present in the moister regions.

Anaerobic diphtheroids occur below the skin surface in hair follicles, sweat and sebaceous glands, *Propionibacterium acnes* being a familiar example. Changes in the skin occurring during puberty often lead to increased numbers of this species, which can be associated with acne. A number of fungi, including *Candida*, occur on the scalp and around the nails. They are infrequent on dry skin, but can cause infection in moist skin folds (intertrigo).

Both the nose and mouth can be heavily colonized by bacteria

Common bacteria colonizing these areas are streptococci, staphylococci, diphtheroids and Gram-negative cocci. Some of the species found in healthy individuals are potentially pathogenic (e.g. *Staph. aureus*, *Strep. pneumoniae*, *Streptococcus pyogenes*, *Neisseria meningitidis*, *Lactobacillus*, *Candida*).

The mucous membranes of the mouth can have the same microbial density as the large intestine, numbers approaching $10^{11}/g$ wet weight of tissue.

Dental caries is one of the commonest infectious diseases in developed countries

The surfaces of the teeth and the gingival crevices carry large numbers of anaerobic bacteria. Plaque is a film of bacterial

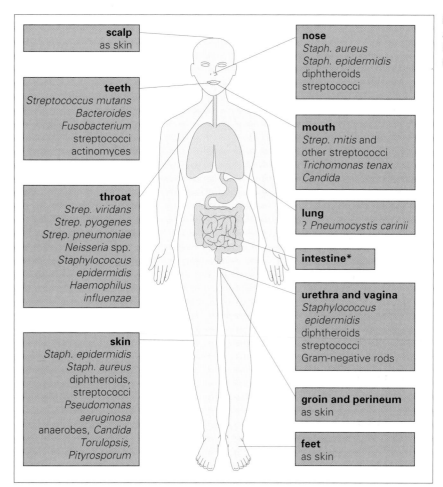

scalp
as skin

teeth
Streptococcus mutans
Bacteroides
Fusobacterium
streptococci
actinomyces

throat
Strep. viridans
Strep. pyogenes
Strep. pneumoniae
Neisseria spp.
Staphylococcus
epidermidis
Haemophilus
influenzae

skin
Staph. epidermidis
Staph. aureus
diphtheroids,
streptococci
Pseudomonas
aeruginosa
anaerobes, Candida
Torulopsis,
Pityrosporum

nose
Staph. aureus
Staph. epidermidis
diphtheroids
streptococci

mouth
Strep. mitis and
other streptococci
Trichomonas tenax
Candida

lung
? Pneumocystis carinii

intestine*

urethra and vagina
Staphylococcus
epidermidis
diphtheroids
streptococci
Gram-negative rods

groin and perineum
as skin

feet
as skin

Fig. 3.32 Examples of organisms that occur as members of the normal flora and their location on the body. (*Those found in the intestine are detailed in *Fig. 3.34.*)

cells anchored in a polysaccharide matrix, which the organisms secrete. When teeth are not cleaned regularly, plaque can accumulate rapidly and the activities of certain bacteria, notably *Streptococcus mutans*, can lead to dental decay (caries), as acid fermented from carbohydrates can attack dental enamel. The prevalence of dental decay is linked with diet.

The pharynx and trachea carry their own normal flora

The flora of the pharynx and trachea may include both α- and β-hemolytic streptococci as well as a number of anaerobes, staphylococci (including *Staph. aureus*), *Neisseria* and diphtheroids. The respiratory tract is normally quite sterile, despite the regular intake of organisms by breathing. However substantial numbers of clinically normal people may carry the fungus *Pneumocystis carinii* in their lungs.

In the gut the density of microorganisms increases from the stomach to the large intestine

Stomach contents harbor only transient organisms, the acidic pH providing an effective barrier. However, the gastric mucosa may be colonized by acid-tolerant lactobacilli and streptococci. The upper intestine is only lightly colonized (10^4 organisms/g), but populations increase markedly in the ileum, where streptococci, lactobacilli, enterobacteriaceae and *Bacteroides* may all be present. Bacterial numbers are very high (estimated at 10^{11}/g) in the large bowel and many species can be found *(Fig. 3.33)*. The vast majority (95–99%) are anaerobes, *Bacteriodes* being especially common and a major component of fecal material. Harmless protozoans can also occur in the intestine (e.g. *Entamoeba coli*) and these can be considered as part of the normal flora, despite being animals.

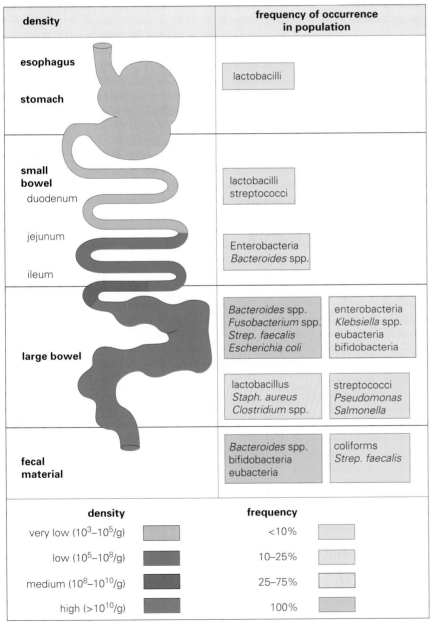

Fig. 3.33 The longitudinal distribution, frequency of occurrence and densities of the bacteria making up the normal flora of the human gastrointestinal tract.

The urethra is lightly colonized in both sexes, but the vagina supports an extensive flora of bacteria and fungi

The urethra in both sexes is relatively lightly colonized, although *Staph. epidermidis*, *Strep faecalis* and diphtheroids may be present. In the vagina the composition of the bacterial and fungal flora undergoes age-related changes:

- Before puberty the predominant organisms are staphylococci, streptococci, diphtheroids and *E. coli*.
- Subsequently *Lactobacillus aerophilus* predominates, its fermentation of glycogen being responsible for the maintenance of an acid pH, which prevents overgrowth by other vaginal organisms.

A number of fungi occur, including *Candida*, which can overgrow to cause the pathogenic condition 'thrush' if the vaginal pH rises and competing bacteria diminish. The protozoan *Trichomonas vaginalis* may also be present in healthy individuals.

Advantages and disadvantages of the normal flora
Some of the species of the normal flora are positively beneficial to the host

The importance of these species for health is sometimes revealed quite dramatically under stringent antibiotic therapy. This can drastically reduce their numbers to a minimum and the host may then be overrun by introduced pathogens or by overgrowth of organisms normally present in small numbers. After treatment with clindamycin, overgrowth by *Clostridium difficile*, which survives treatment, can give rise to pseudomembranous colitis.

Ways in which the normal flora prevent colonization by potential pathogens include the following:

- Skin bacteria produce fatty acids, which discourage other species from invading.
- Gut bacteria release a number of factors with antibacterial activity (bacteriocins, colicins) as well as metabolic waste products that help prevent the establishment of other species.
- Vaginal lactobacilli maintain an acid environment, which suppresses growth of other organisms.
- The sheer number of bacteria present in the normal flora of the intestine means that almost all of the available ecologic niches become occupied; these species therefore outcompete others for living space.

Gut bacteria also release organic acids, which may have some metabolic value to the host; they also produce B vitamins and vitamin K in amounts that are large enough to be valuable if the diet is deficient. The antigenic stimulation provided by the intestinal flora helps to ensure the normal development of the immune system.

What happens when the normal flora is absent? Germ-free animals tend to live longer, presumably because of the complete absence of pathogens, and develop no caries (see Chapter 15). However, their immune system is less well developed and they are vulnerable to introduced microbial pathogens. At the time of birth humans are germ free, but acquire the normal flora during and immediately after birth, with the accompaniment of intense immunologic activity.

The disadvantages of the normal flora lie in the potential for spread into previously sterile parts of the body

This may happen when:

- The intestine is perforated or the skin is broken.
- During extraction of teeth (when viridans streptococci may enter the bloodstream).
- Organisms such as *E. coli* from the perianal skin ascend the urethra and cause urinary tract infection.

Overgrowth by potentially pathogenic members of the normal flora can occur when the composition of the flora changes (e.g. after antibiotics) or when:

- The local environment changes (e.g. increases in stomach or vaginal pH).
- The immune system becomes ineffective (e.g. AIDS, clinical immunosuppression).

Under these conditions, the potential pathogens take the opportunity to increase their population size or invade tissues, so becoming harmful to the host. An account of diseases associated with such opportunistic infections is given in Chapter 28.

- Organisms that cause infectious diseases can be grouped into six main categories – viruses, bacteria, fungi, protozoa, helminths and arthropods.
- Each group has distinctive characteristics (structural and molecular make-up, biochemical and metabolic strategies, reproductive processes), which determine how the organisms interact with their hosts, and how they cause disease.
- Some organisms (the normal flora) can be positively beneficial to the host. These live on or within the body without causing disease, and play an important role in protecting the host from pathogenic microbes.

Further Reading

Cann AJ. *Principles of Molecular Virology,* 2nd edition. Academic Press, 1997.

Collier, LH ed. *Topley and Wilson's Microbiology and Microbiol Infections*, 9th edition. London: Edward Arnold, 1998.

Dale JW. *Molecular Genetics of Bacteria,* 2nd edition. Chichester: John Wiley & Sons, 1994.

Introduction

In the preceding chapters, we have outlined some of the fundamental characteristics of the myriad types of micro- and macroparasites that may infect the body. We now turn to consider the ways in which the body seeks to defend itself against infection from these organisms.

The body has both 'innate' and 'adaptive' immune defenses

When an organism infects the body, the defense systems already in place may well be sufficient to prevent replication and spread of the infectious agent, thereby preventing development of disease. These established mechanisms are referred to as constituting the 'innate' immune system. However, should innate immunity be insufficient to parry the invasion by the infectious agent, the so-called 'adaptive' immune system then comes into action, although it takes time to reach its maximum efficiency (*Fig. 4.1*). When it does take effect, it generally eliminates the infective organism, allowing recovery from disease.

The main feature distinguishing the adaptive response from the innate mechanism is that specific memory of infection is imprinted on the adaptive immune system, so that should there be a subsequent infection by the same agent, a particularly effective response comes into play with remarkable speed. It is worth emphasizing, however, that there is close synergy between the two systems, with the adaptive mechanism greatly improving the efficiency of the innate response.

The contrasts between these two systems are set out in *Figure 4.2*. On the one hand, the soluble factors such as lysozyme and complement, together with the phagocytic cells, contribute to the innate system, while on the other the lymphocyte-based mechanisms that produce antibody and T lymphocytes are the main elements of the adaptive immune system. Not only do these lymphocytes provide improved resistance by repeated contact with a given infectious agent, but the memory with which they become endowed shows very considerable specificity to that infection. For instance, infection with measles virus will induce a memory to that microorganism alone and not to another virus such as rubella.

Defense Against Entry into the Body

A variety of biochemical and physical barriers operate at the body surfaces

Before an infectious agent can penetrate the body, it must overcome biochemical and physical barriers that operate at the body surfaces. One of the most important of these is the skin, which is normally impermeable to the majority of infectious agents. Many bacteria fail to survive for long on the skin because of the direct inhibitory effects of lactic acid and fatty acids present in sweat and sebaceous secretions and the lower pH to which they give rise (*Fig. 4.3*). However, should

there be skin loss, as can occur in burns for example, infection becomes a major problem.

The membranes lining the inner surfaces of the body secrete mucus, which acts as a protective barrier, inhibiting the adherence of bacteria to the epithelial cells, thereby preventing them from gaining access to the body. Microbial and other foreign particles trapped within this adhesive mucus may be removed by mechanical means such as ciliary action, coughing and sneezing. The flushing action of tears, saliva and urine, are other mechanical strategies that help to protect the epithelial surfaces. In addition, many of the secreted body fluids contain microbicidal factors, for example the acid in gastric juice, spermine and zinc in semen, lactoperoxidase in milk and lysozyme in tears, nasal secretions and saliva.

The phenomenon of microbial antagonism associated with the normal bacterial flora of the body is explained in Chapter 3. These commensal organisms suppress the growth of many potentially pathogenic bacteria and fungi at superficial sites first by virtue of their physical advantage of previous occupancy, especially on epithelial surfaces, second by competing for essential nutrients, or third by producing inhibitory substances such as acid or colicins. The latter are a class of bactericidins that bind to the negatively charged surface of susceptible

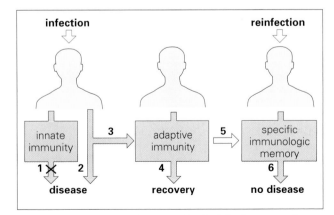

Fig. 4.1 Innate and adaptive immunity. An infectious agent first encounters elements of the innate immune system. These may be sufficient to prevent disease (1), but if not, disease may result (2). The adaptive immune system is then activated (3) to produce recovery (4) and a specific immunologic memory (5). Following reinfection with the same agent, no disease results (6) and the individual has acquired immunity to the infectious agent.

COMPARISON OF INNATE AND ADAPTIVE IMMUNE SYSTEMS		
	innate immune system	**adaptive immune system**
major elements		
soluble factors	lysozyme, complement, acute phase proteins e.g. C-reactive protein, interferon	antibody
cells	phagocytes natural killer cells	T lymphocytes
response to microbial infection		
first contact	+	+
second contact	+	++++
	non-specific no memory	specific memory
	resistance not improved by repeated contact	resistance improved by repeated contact

Fig. 4.2 Comparison of innate and adaptive immune systems. Innate immunity is sometimes referred to as 'natural' and adaptive as 'acquired'. There is considerable interaction between the two systems. 'Humoral' immunity due to soluble factors contrasts with immunity mediated by cells. Primary contact with antigen produces weak adaptive and non-adaptive responses, but if the same antigen persists or is encountered a second time the specific response to that antigen is much enhanced.

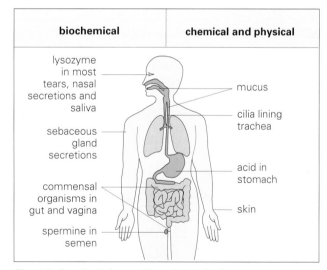

biochemical	chemical and physical

lysozyme in most tears, nasal secretions and saliva

sebaceous gland secretions

commensal organisms in gut and vagina

spermine in semen

mucus

cilia lining trachea

acid in stomach

skin

Fig. 4.3 Exterior defenses. Most of the infectious agents encountered by an individual are prevented from entering the body by a variety of biochemical and physical barriers. The body tolerates a variety of commensal organisms, which compete effectively with many potential pathogens.

bacteria and form a voltage-dependent channel in the membrane, which kills by destroying the cell's energy potential.

Defenses Once the Microorganism Penetrates the Body

Despite the general effectiveness of the various barriers, microorganisms successfully penetrate the body on many occasions. When this occurs two main defensive strategies come into play based on:

- The destructive effect of soluble chemical factors, such as bactericidal enzymes.
- The mechanism of phagocytosis, involving engulfment and killing of microorganisms by specialized cells.

Professional phagocytes

Perhaps because of the belief that professionals do a better job than amateurs, the cells that shoulder the main burden of our phagocytic defenses have been labelled 'professional phagocytes'. These consist of two major cell families, as originally defined by Elie Metchnikoff, the Russian zoologist (see panel):

- The large macrophages.
- The smaller polymorphonuclear granulocytes, which are generally referred to as polymorphs or neutrophils because their cytoplasmic granules do not stain with hematoxylin and eosin.

Elie Metchnikoff (1845–1916)

This perceptive Russian zoologist can legitimately be regarded as the father of the concept of cellular immunity in which it is recognized that certain specialized cells mediate the defense against microbial infections. He was intrigued by the motile cells of transparent starfish larvae and made the critical observation that a few hours after introducing a rose thorn into the larvae the rose thorn became surrounded by the motile cells. He extended his investigations to mammalian leukocytes, showing their ability to engulf microorganisms, a process that he termed 'phagocytosis' (literally, eating by cells).

Because he found this process to be even more effective in animals recovering from an infection, he came to the conclusion that phagocytosis provided the main defense against infection. He defined the existence of two types of circulating phagocytes: the polymorphonuclear leukocyte, which he termed a 'microphage', and the larger 'macrophage'.

Although Metchnikoff held the somewhat polarized view that cellular immunity based upon phagocytosis

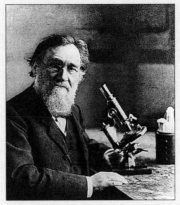

Fig. 4.4 Elie Metchnikoff (1845–1916). (Courtesy of the Wellcome Institute Library, London.)

provided the main, if not the only, defense mechanism against infectious microorganisms, we now know that the efficiency of the phagocytic system is enormously enhanced through cooperation with humoral factors, in particular antibody and complement.

As a very crude generalization, it may be said that the polymorphs provide the major defense against pyogenic (pus-forming) bacteria, while the macrophages are thought to be at their best in combatting organisms capable of living within the cells of the host.

Macrophages are widespread throughout the tissues

Macrophages originate as bone marrow promonocytes, which develop into circulating blood monocytes *(Fig. 4.5)* and finally become the mature macrophages, which are widespread throughout the tissues and collectively termed the 'mononuclear phagocyte system' *(Fig. 4.6)*.

These macrophages are present throughout the connective tissue and are associated with the basement membrane of small

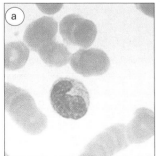
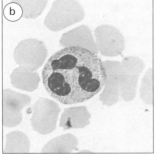

Fig. 4.5 Phagocytic cells. (a) Blood monocytes and (b) polymorphonuclear neutrophils, both derived from bone marrow stem cells. (Courtesy of PM Lydyard.)

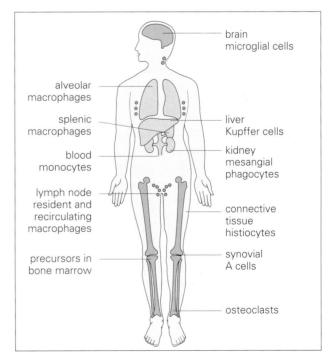

Fig. 4.6 The mononuclear phagocyte system. Tissue macrophages are derived from blood monocytes, which are manufactured in the bone marrow.

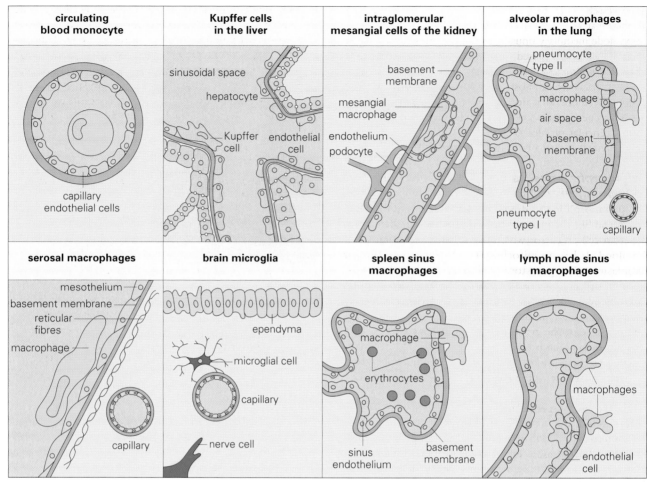

Fig. 4.7 Cellular disposition of mononuclear phagocytes.

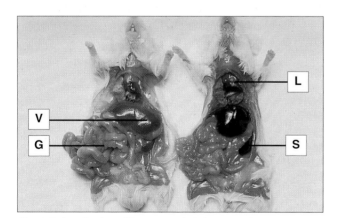

Fig. 4.8 Localization of intravenously injected particles in the mononuclear phagocyte system. (Right) A mouse was injected with fine carbon particles and killed five minutes later. Carbon accumulates in organs rich in mononuclear phagocytes – lungs (L), liver (V), spleen (S) and areas of the gut wall (G). (Left) Normal organ color shown in a control mouse. (Courtesy of PM Lydyard.)

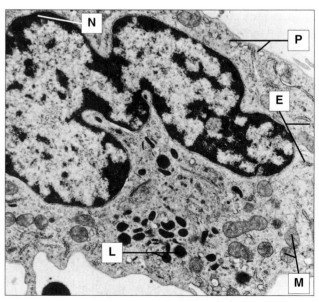

Fig. 4.9 Monocyte (×8000), with 'horseshoe' nucleus (N). Phagocytic and pinocytic vesicles (P), lysosomal granules (L), mitochondria (M) and isolated profiles of rough-surfaced endoplasmic reticulum (E) are evident. (Courtesy of B Nichols. Copyright Rockefeller University Press.)

blood vessels. They are particularly concentrated in the lung (alveolar macrophages), liver (Kupffer cells), and the lining of lymph node medullary sinuses and splenic sinusoids *(Fig. 4.7)* where they are well placed to filter off foreign material *(Fig. 4.8)*. Other examples are the brain microglia, kidney mesangial cells, synovial A cells and osteoclasts in bone. In general, these are long-lived cells that depend upon mitochondria for their metabolic energy and show elements of rough-surfaced endoplasmic reticular profiles *(Fig. 4.9)* related to the formidable array of different secretory proteins that these cells generate.

Polymorphs possess a variety of enzyme-containing granules

The polymorph is the dominant white cell in the bloodstream and like the macrophage shares a common hemopoietic stem cell precursor with the other formed elements of the blood. It has no mitochondria, but uses its abundant cytoplasmic glycogen stores for its energy requirements; therefore, glycolysis enables these cells to function under anaerobic conditions, such as those in an inflammatory focus. The polymorph is a non-dividing, short-lived cell with a segmented nucleus; the cytoplasm is characterized by an array of granules, including:

- The primary azurophilic granule, which contains myeloperoxidase, some lysozyme and families of cationic proteins.
- The secondary 'specific' granules associated with lactoferrin and lysozyme.
- The tertiary granules typical of the conventional lysosome with acid hydrolases *(Fig. 4.10)*.

Phagocytosis

The first event in the uptake and digestion of a microorganism by the professional phagocyte involves the attachment of

the microbe to the surface of the cell *(Fig. 4.11)*. The attachment itself usually represents a somewhat primitive recognition mechanism, probably involving carbohydrate elements on the infectious agent. The attached particle may then initiate the ingestion phase by activating anactin–myosin contractile system, which sends arms of cytoplasm around the particle until it is completely enclosed within a vacuole (phagosome; *Figs 4.11, 4.12)*. Shortly afterwards, the

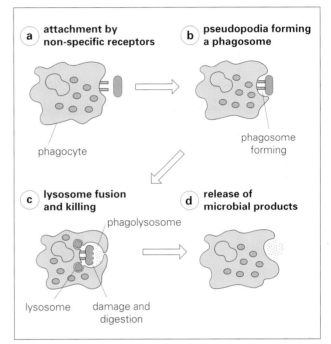

Fig. 4.11 Phagocytosis. Phagocytes attach to microorganisms (blue icon) via their non-specific cell surface receptors (a). If the membrane now becomes activated by the attached infectious agent, the pathogen is taken into a phagosome by pseudopodia, which extend around it (b). Once inside the cell, lysosomes fuse with the phagosome to form a phagolysosome (c). The infectious agent is then killed by a battery of microbicidal degradation mechanisms and the microbial products are released (d).

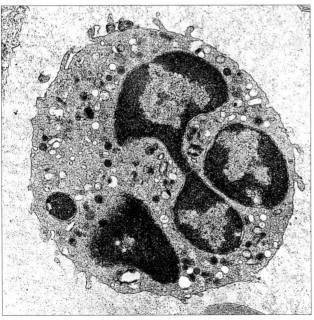

Fig. 4.10 Neutrophil. The multi-lobed nucleus and cytoplasmic granules are well displayed. (Courtesy of D McLaren.)

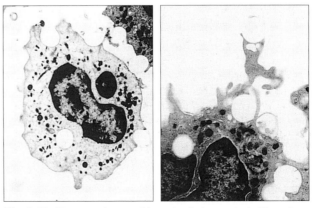

Fig. 4.12 Electron micrographic study of phagocytosis. These two micrographs show human phagocytes engulfing latex particles. ×3000 (a); ×4500 (b). (Courtesy of CHW Horne.)

cytoplasmic granules fuse with a phagosome and discharge their contents around the incarcerated microorganism, which is then the target of a dastardly array of killing mechanisms.

The killing process

As phagocytosis is initiated, there is a vigorous burst of oxygen consumption resulting from a dramatic increase in activity of the hexose monophosphate shunt. This generates NADPH and reduces molecular oxygen through a unique plasma membrane reduced nicotinamide adenine dinu-cleotide phosphate (NADPH) oxidase to a series of powerful microbicidal agents, namely superoxide anion, hydrogen peroxide, singlet oxygen and hydroxyl radicals (*Fig. 4.13*; see also Chapter 9). Subsequently, the peroxide, in association with myeloperoxidase, generates a potent halogenating system from halide ions, which is capable of killing both bacteria and viruses.

As superoxide anion is formed, the enzyme superoxide dismutase acts to convert it to molecular oxygen and hydrogen peroxide, but in the process consumes hydrogen

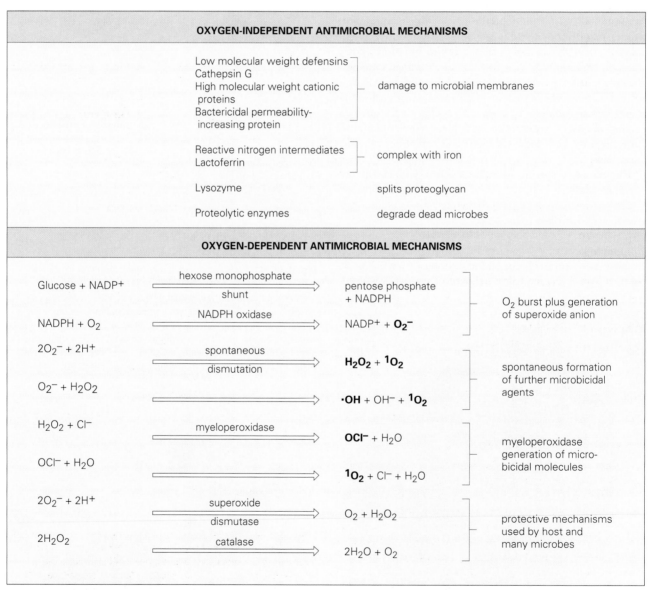

Fig. 4.13 Antimicrobial mechanisms in phagocytic vacuoles. Microbicidal species in bold letters. O_2^-, superoxide anion; $^1O_2$, singlet (activated) oxygen; $\cdot OH$, hydroxyl free radical. Reactive nitrogen intermediates such as nitric oxide (NO) are derived from asparagine.

NADPH, reduced nicotinamide adenine dinucleotide phosphate; NAPD$^+$, oxidized NADPH; H_2O_2, hydrogen peroxide.

ions. Therefore initially there is a small increase in pH, which facilitates the antibacterial function of the families of cationic proteins derived from the phagocytic granules. These molecules damage microbial membranes by the action of cathepsin G and by direct adherence to the microbial surface. Other granule-derived factors are:

- Lactoferrin and reactive nitrogen intermediates like nitric oxide, which through their ability to complex iron, deprive bacteria of an essential growth element.
- Lysozyme, which splits the proteoglycan cell wall of bacteria.

The pH now falls and the dead or dying microorganism are extensively degraded by acid hydrolytic enzymes, and the degradation products released to the exterior.

Recruitment of defensive phagocytes
Phagocytes are mobilized and targeted onto the microorganism by chemotaxis

Phagocytosis cannot occur unless the bacterium first attaches to the surface of the phagocyte, and clearly this cannot happen unless both have become physically close to each other. There is therefore a need for a mechanism that mobilizes phagocytes from afar and targets them onto the bacterium. Many bacteria produce chemical substances, such as formyl methionyl peptides, which directionally attract leukocytes, a process known as 'chemotaxis'. However, this is a relatively weak signalling system and evolution has provided the body with a far more effective magnet that uses a complex series of proteins collectively termed 'complement'.

Activation of the complement system

Complement resembles blood clotting, fibrinolysis and kinin formation in being a major triggered enzyme cascade system. Such systems are characterized by their ability to produce a rapid, highly amplified response to a trigger stimulus mediated by a cascade phenomenon in which the product of one reaction is the enzymic catalyst of the next. The most abundant and most central component is C3 (complement components are designated by the letter 'C' followed by a number) and the cleavage of this molecule is at the heart of all complement-mediated phenomena.

In normal plasma, C3 undergoes spontaneous activation at a very slow rate to generate the split product C3b. This is able to complex with another complement component, factor B, which is then acted upon by a normal plasma enzyme, factor D, to produce the C3 splitting enzyme C3bBb. This C3 convertase can then split new molecules of C3 to give C3a (a small fragment), and further C3b. This represents a positive feedback circuit with potential for runaway amplification; however, the overall process is restricted to a tick-over level by powerful regulatory mechanisms, which break the unstable soluble-phase C3 convertase into inactive cleavage products *(Fig. 4.14)*.

In the presence of certain molecules, such as the carbohydrates on the surface of many bacteria, the C3 convertase can become attached and stabilized against breakdown. Under these circumstances, there is active generation of

new C3 convertase molecules, and what is known as the 'alternative' complement pathway can swing into full tempo (see Chapter 5).

Complement synergizes with phagocytic cells to produce an acute inflammatory response

Activation of the alternative complement pathway with a consequent splitting of very large numbers of C3 molecules has important consequences for the orchestration of an integrated antimicrobial defense strategy *(Fig. 4.15, see overleaf)*. Large numbers of C3b produced in the immediate vicinity of the microbial membrane, bind covalently to that surface and act as opsonins (molecules that make the particle they coat more susceptible to engulfment by phagocytic cells; see

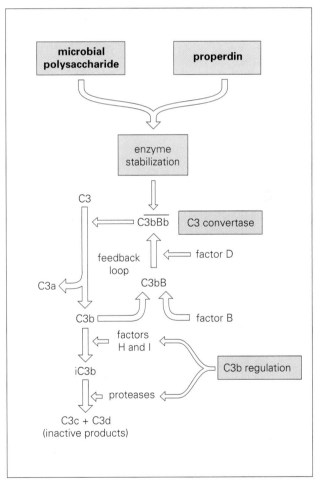

Fig. 4.14 Activation of complement by microorganisms. C3b is formed by the spontaneous breakdown of C3 complexes with factor B to form C3bB which is split by factor D to produce a C3 convertase capable of further cleaving C3. The convertase is heavily regulated by factor H and I but can be stabilized on the surface of microbes and properdin. The horizontal bar indicates an enzymically active complex.

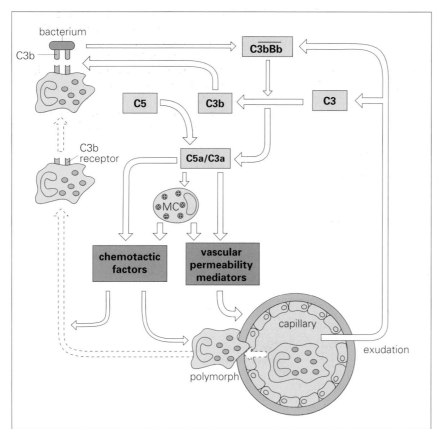

Fig. 4.15 The defensive strategy of the acute inflammatory reaction initiated by bacterial activation of the alternative complement pathway. Activation of the C3bBb C3 convertase by the bacterium leads to the generation of C3b (which binds to the bacterium), C3a and C5a, and recruitment of mast cell (MC) mediators. These in turn cause capillary dilatation and exudation of plasma proteins, and chemotactic attraction and adherence of polymorphs to the C3b-coated bacterium. The polymorphs are then activated for the final kill.

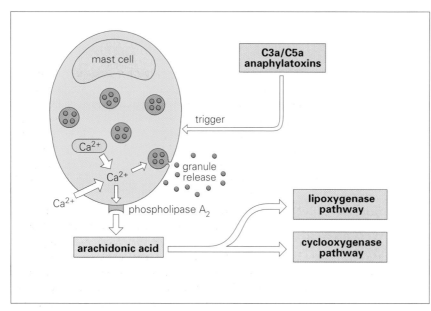

Fig. 4.16 Triggering of a mast cell leading to release of mediators by two major pathways: (a) release of pre-formed mediators present in the granules, and (b) the metabolism of arachidonic acid produced through activation of phospholipase A_2. Intracellular calcium (Ca^{2+}) and cyclic adenosine monophosphate (cAMP) are central to the initiation of these events but details are still unclear.

below). This C3b, together with the C3 convertase, acts on the next component in the sequence, C5, to produce a small fragment, C5a, which together with C3a, has a direct effect on mast cells to cause their degranulation. Consequently, mediators of vascular permeability body factors chemotactic for polymorphs are released. The nature of this degranulation process and of the products to which it gives rise are shown in *Figures 4.16–4.17*, while the circulating equivalent of the tissue mast cell (*Figures 4.18* and *4.19*) the basophil, is shown in *Figure 4.20*.

The vascular permeability mediators increase the permeability of capillaries by modifying the intercellular forces

MAST CELL MEDIATORS

	pre-formed	effect
granule release	histamine	vasodilation, increased capillary permeability, chemokinesis, bronchoconstriction
	heparin	anticoagulant
	tryptase	activates C3
	β-Glucosaminidase	splits off glucosamine
	ECF	eosinophil chemotaxis
	NCF	neutrophil chemotaxis
	platelet activating factor	mediator release
	newly synthesized	**effect**
lipoxygenase pathway	leukotrienes C4 and D4 (SRS-A) leukotriene B4	vasoactive, bronchoconstriction, chemotaxis and/or chemokinesis
cyclooxygenase pathway	prostaglandins thromboxanes	affect bronchial muscle, platelet aggregation and vasodilation

Fig. 4.17 Mediators released by mast cell triggering. Chemotaxis refers to directed migration of granulocytes up the concentration gradient of the mediator, whereas chemokinesis describes randomly increased motility of these cells. (ECF, eosinophil chemotactic factor; NCF, neutrophil chemotactic factor, SRS-A, slow reacting substance of anaphylaxis.)

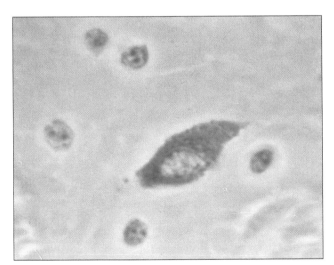

Fig. 4.18 Histologic appearance of a human (gut) connective tissue mast cell showing the dark blue cytoplasm with brownish granules. Alcian blue and Safranin, ×600. (Courtesy of TSC Orr.)

between the endothelial cells of the vessel wall. This allows the exudation of fluid and plasma components, including more complement, to the site of the infection. These mediators *(Fig. 4.17)* also upregulate molecules such as intercelllar adhesion molecule-1 (ICAM-1) and endothelial cell leukcyte adhesion molecule-1 (ELAM-1), which bind to specific complementary molecules on the polymorphs and encouage them to stick to the walls of the capillaries, a process termed 'margination'.

The chemotactic factors, on the other hand, provide a chemical gradient which attracts marginated polymorphonuclear leukocytes from their intravascular location, through the walls of the blood vessels, and eventually leads them to the site of the C3b-coated bacteria that initiated the whole activation process. Polymorphs have a well-defined receptor for C3b on their surface and as a result the opsonized bacteria adhere very firmly to the surface of these newly arrived cells.

The processes of capillary dilatation (erythema), exudation of plasma proteins and of fluid (edema) due to hydrostatic and osmotic pressure changes, and the accumulation of neutrophils, are collectively termed the 'acute inflammatory response', and result in a highly effective way of focusing phagocytic cells onto complement-coated microbial targets.

It also seems clear that the macrophage can be stimulated by certain bacterial toxins such as the lipopolysaccha-

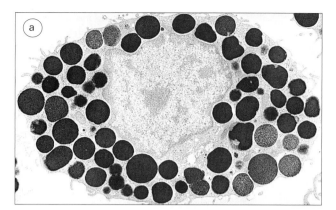

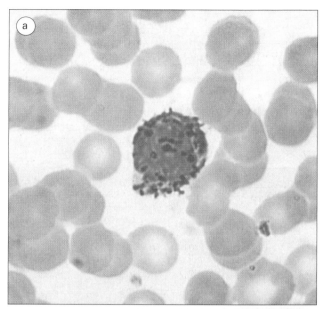

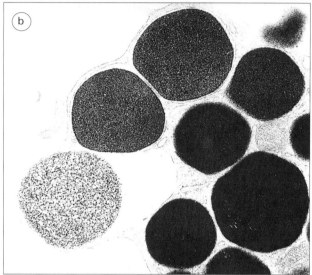

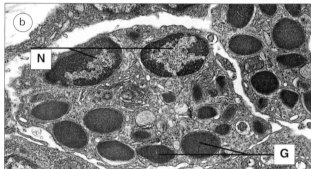

Fig. 4.19 Electron micrographs of rat peritoneal mast cells. These show (a) the undegranulated cell with its electron-dense granules ×6000 and (b) a granule in the process of exocytosis ×30 000 (Courtesy of TSC Orr.)

Fig. 4.20 Morphology of the basophil. (a) This blood smear shows a typical basophil with its deep violet–blue granules. Wright's stain, ×1500. (b) Electron micrograph showing the ultrastructure of the basophil. Basophils in guinea pig skin showing the nuclei (N) and characteristic randomly distributed granules (G). ×6000. (Courtesy of D McLaren.)

rides (LPS), by the action of C5a, and by the phagocytosis of C3b-coated bacteria, to secrete other potent mediators of acute inflammation, which reinforce the mast-cell directed pathway *(Fig. 4.21)*.

C9 molecules form the 'membrane attack complex', which is involved in cell lysis

We have already introduced the idea that following the activation of C3, the next component to be cleaved is C5; the larger C5b fragment that results becomes membrane bound. This subsequently binds components C6, C7 and C8, which form a complex capable of inducing a critical conformational change in the terminal component C9. The unfolded C9 molecules become inserted into the lipid bilayer and polymerize to form an annular 'membrane attack complex' (MAC) *(Figs 4.22, 4.23)*. This behaves as a transmembrane channel that is fully permeable to electrolytes and water; because of the high internal colloid osmotic pressure of cells, there is a net influx of sodium (Na^+), and this frequently leads to lysis.

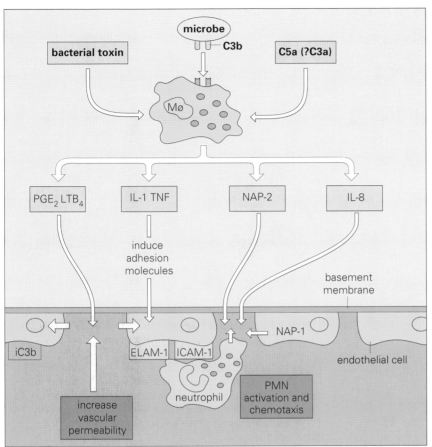

Fig. 4.21 A role for the macrophage (Mø) in the initiation of acute inflammation. Stimulation induces macrophage secretion of mediators. Blood neutrophils stick to the adhesion molecules on the endothelial cell and use them to provide traction as they force their way between the cells, through the basement membrane (with the help of secreted elastase) and up the chemotactic gradient. During this process they become progressively activated by neutrophil activating peptide-1 (NAP-1). (PGE₂, prostaglandin E$_2$; LTB$_4$, leukotriene B$_4$; IL-1, interleukin-1; TNF, tumor necrosis factor; ELAM-1, endothelial cell leukocyte adhesion molecule-1; ICAM-1, intercellular adhesion molecule-1; IC3b, opsonic fragment of third complement component)

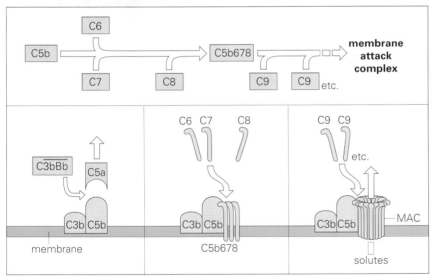

Fig. 4.22 Assembly of the C5b-9 membrane attack complex (MAC). Recruitment of a further C3b into the C3bBb enzymic complex generates a C5 convertase which cleaves C5a from C5 and leaves the remaining C5b attached to the membrane. Once C5b is membrane bound, C6 and C7 attach themselves to form the stable complex, C5b67, which interacts with C8 to yield C5b678. This unit has some effect in disrupting the membrane, but primarily causes the polymerization of C9 to form tubules traversing the membrane. The resulting tubule is referred to as a MAC. Disruption of the membrane by this structure permits the free exchange of solutes, which is primarily responsible for cell lysis.

Acute phase proteins

Certain proteins in the plasma, collectively termed 'acute phase proteins', increase in concentration in response to early 'alarm' mediators such as interleukin-1 (IL-1), IL-6 and tumour necrosis factor (TNF), released as a result of infection or tissue injury *(Fig. 4.21)* Many acute phase reactants such as C-reactive protein (CRP) increase dramatically *(Fig. 4.24)*, while others show more moderate rises, usually less than five-fold *(Fig. 4.25)*. In general, these proteins are thought to have defensive roles.

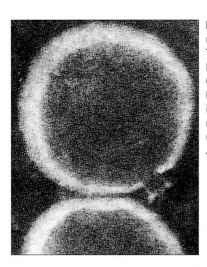

Fig. 4.23 Electron micrograph of the MAC. The funnel-shaped lesion is due to a human C5b-9 complex that has been reincorporated into lecithin liposomal membranes. ×234 000. (Courtesy of J Tranum-Jensen and S Bhakdi.)

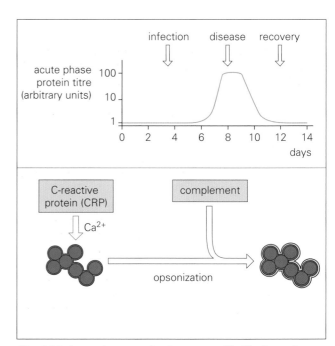

Fig. 4.24 Acute phase proteins, here exemplified by C-reactive protein (CRP), are serum proteins that increase rapidly in concentration (sometimes up to 100-fold) following infection (graph). They are important in innate immunity to infection. CRP recognizes and binds in a calcium (Ca^{2+}) dependent fashion to molecular groups found on a wide variety of bacteria and fungi. In particular, it binds the phosphocholine moiety of pneumococci. The CRP acts as an opsonin and activates complement with all the associated sequelae.

ACUTE PHASE PROTEINS PRODUCED IN RESPONSE TO INFECTION IN THE HUMAN	
acute phase reactant	**role**
dramatic increases in concentration:	
C-reactive protein	fixes complement, opsonizes
mannose binding protein	fixes complement, opsonizes
α_1 acid glycoprotein	transport protein
serum amyloid A protein	?
moderate increases in concentration:	
α_1 proteinase inhibitors	inhibits bacterial proteases
α_1 anti-chymotrypsin	inhibits bacterial proteases
C3, C9, factor B	increase complement function
caeruloplasmin	O_2 scavenger
fibrinogen	coagulation
angiotensin	blood pressure
haptoglobin	binds hemoglobin
fibronectin	cell attachment

Fig. 4.25 Acute phase proteins produced in response to infection in the human. (Adapted from Stadnyk and Gauldie, 1991.)

Other extracellular antimicrobial factors

There are many microbicidal agents that operate at short range within phagocytic cells, but also appear in various body fluids in sufficient concentration to have direct inhibitory effects on infectious agents. For example, lysozyme is present in fluids such as tears and saliva in amounts capable of acting against the proteoglycan wall of susceptible bacteria. Similarly, lactoferrin may appear in the blood in sufficient concentration to complex iron and deprive bacteria of this important growth factor. Whether agents that normally act over a short-range, such as reactive oxygen metabolites or TNF (a cytotoxic molecule produced by macrophages and other cell types), can reach concentrations in the body fluids

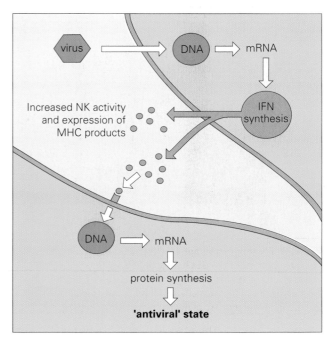

Fig. 4.26 The action of interferon (IFN). Virus infecting a cell induces the production of IFN. This is released and binds to IFN receptors on other cells. The IFN induces the production of antiviral proteins, which are activated if virus enters the second cell. (NK, natural killer; MHC, major histocompatibility complex.)

that are adequate to allow them to act at a distance from the cell producing them, will be discussed in chapter 9, particularly when considering the mechanisms by which the blood-borne forms of parasites such as malaria are attacked.

Interferons are a family of broad-spectrum antiviral molecules

Interferons (IFNs) are widespread throughout the animal kingdom and are discussed further in Chapter 9. They were first recognized by the phenomenon of viral interference, in which a cell infected with one virus is found to be resistant to superinfection by a second unrelated virus. Leukocytes produce many different αIFNs (IFNα), while fibroblasts and probably all cell types synthesize IFNβ. A third type (IFNγ) is not a component of the innate immune system and will be discussed in Chapter 5 as a member of the important cytokine family.

When cells are infected by a virus, they synthesize and secrete IFN, which binds to specific receptors on nearby uninfected cells. The bound IFN exerts its antiviral effect by facilitating the synthesis of two new enzymes, which interfere with the machinery used by the virus for its own replication. The mechanism of action of IFN is discussed more fully in Chapter 9; the net result is to set up a cordon of infection-resistant cells around the site of virus infection, so restraining its spread *(Fig. 4.26)*. IFN is highly effective *in vivo* as supported by experiments in which mice injected with an antiserum to murine IFN were found to be killed by several hundred times less virus than was needed to kill the controls. It should be emphasized, however, that IFN seems to play a significant role in recovery from, rather than prevention of, viral infections.

Extracellular killing
Natural killer cells attach to virally infected cells, allowing them to be differentiated from normal cells

There is a widely held view that viruses represent fragments of the genome of multicellular organisms that have achieved

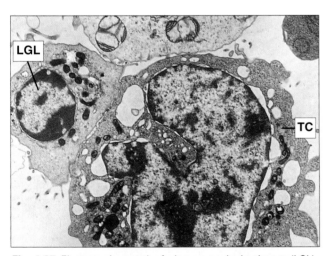

Fig. 4.27 Electron micrograph of a large granular lmphocyte (LGL) killing a tumor cell (TC). LGLs bind to and kill IgG antibody-coated (see *Fig. 5.14*), and even non-coated, tumor cells. It is essential for the membranes of the two cells to be closely apposed in order for the LGL to deliver the 'kiss of death'. ×4500. (Courtesy of P Lydyard.)

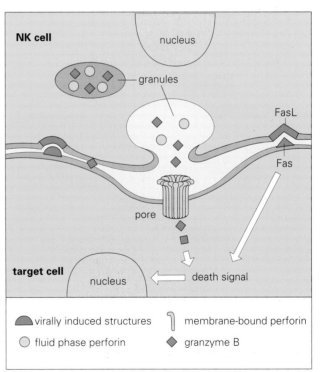

Fig. 4.28 Schematic model of lysis of virally infected target cell by a natural killer (NK) cell. As the NK cell receptors bind to the surface of the virally infected cell, there is exocytosis of granules and release of cytolytic mediators into the intercellular cleft. A calcium (Ca^{2+})-dependent conformational change in the perforin enables it to insert and polymerize within the membrane of the target cell to form a transmembrane pore, which leads to cell lysis. This allows entry of granzyme B into the target cell where it causes programmed cell death (apoptosis). A back-up cytolytic system uses engagement of the Fas receptor with its ligand (FasL), which can also trigger apoptosis involving a calcium-independent fragmentation of nuclear DNA.

the ability to exist in an extracellular state. The small number of genes present in the viral genome, however, do not include those required for viral replication. Accordingly, it is essential for viruses to penetrate the cells of an infected host in order to subvert the cells' replicative machinery towards viral replication. Clearly, it is in the interests of the host to try to kill such infected cells before the virus has had a chance to reproduce. Natural killer (NK) cells are cytotoxic cells that appear to have evolved to carry out just such a task. These are large granular lymphocytes (LGLs) *(Fig. 4.27)* that attach themselves to structures, presumably glycoproteins, on the surface of virally infected cells and allow them to be differentiated from normal cells; activation of the NK cell results in the extracellular release of its granule contents into the space between the target and effector cells. These contents include perforin molecules, which resemble C9 in many respects, especially in their ability to insert into the membrane of the target cell and polymerize to form annular transmembrane pores, like the MAC. This permits the entry of another granule protein, granzyme B, which leads to death of the target cell by apoptosis (programmed cell death) *(Fig. 4.28)*.

Subsidiary cytotoxic mechanisms may involve molecules resembling TNF. TNF was first recognized as a product of activated macrophages. These cells are known to be capable of killing certain other cells, particularly some tumor cells, presumably by the production of a cell poison.

Yet a further mode of cytotoxicity can be turned on by the activated macrophage, involving the direct 'burning' of the surface of another cell by means of a stream of reactive oxygen intermediates, produced at the macrophage membrane by the respiratory oxygen burst, as discussed previously (see p. 52).

Eosinophils act against large parasites

It takes little imagination to realize that professional phagocytes are far too small to be capable of physically engulfing large parasites such as helminths. An alternative strategy, such as killing by an extracellular broadside of the type discussed above, would seem to be a more appropriate form of defense. Eosinophils appear to have evolved to fulfil this role. These polymorphonuclear relatives of the neutrophil have distinctive cytoplasmic granules, which stain strongly with acidic dyes *(Fig. 4.29)* and have a characteristic ultrastructural appearance. A major basic protein (MBP) has been identified in the core of the granule, while the matrix has been shown to contain an eosinophilic cationic protein, a peroxidase and a perforin-like molecule. The cells have surface receptors for C3b and when activated generate copious amounts of active oxygen metabolites.

Many helminths can activate the alternative complement pathway but, although resistant to C9 attack, their coating with C3b allows adherence to the eosinophils through their C3b surface receptors. Once activated, the eosinophil launches its extracellular ammunition, which includes the release of major basic proteins and the cationic protein to damage the parasite membrane, with a possibility of a further 'chemical burn' from the oxygen metabolites and 'leaky porous plug' formation by the perforins.

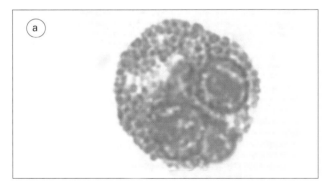

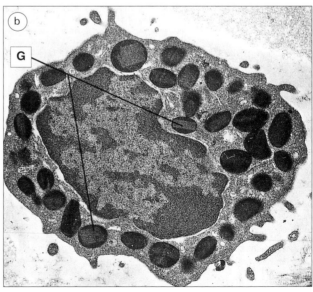

Fig. 4.29 The eosinophil granulocyte is capable of extracellular killing of parasites (e.g. worms) by releasing its granule contents. (a) Morphology of the eosinophil. This blood smear enriched for granulocytes shows an eosinophil with its multilobed nucleus and heavily-stained cytoplasmic granules. Leishman's stain. ×1800. (Courtesy of P Lydyard.) (b) Electron micrograph showing the ultrastructure of a guinea pig eosinophil. The mature eosinophil contains granules (G) with central crystalloids. ×8000. (Courtesy of D McLaren.)

- The innate system of immune defense consists of a formidable barrier to entry and second-line phagocytes and circulating soluble factors. Colonization of the body by normally non-pathogenic ('opportunistic') microorganisms occurs whenever there is a hereditary or acquired deficiency in any of these functions.
- The main phagocytic cells are **polymorphonuclear neutrophils** and **macrophages**. Organisms adhere to their surface, activate the engulfment process and are taken inside the cell where they fuse with cytoplasmic granules. A formidable array of oxygen-dependent and oxygen-independent microbicidal mechanisms then come into play.
- The complement system, a multicomponent triggered enzyme cascade, is used to attract phagocytic cells to the microbes and engulf them.
- The most abundant complement component, C3, is split by a convertase enzyme formed from its own cleavage product C3b and factor B and stabilized against breakdown caused by factors H and I through association with the microbial surface. As it is formed, C3b becomes covalently linked to the microorganism.
- The next most abundant component, C5, is activated to yield a small peptide, C5a, while residual C5b binds to the surface of the microorganism and assembles the terminal components C6–9 into a MAC, which is freely permeable to solutes and can lead to osmotic lysis. In addition, C5a is a potent chemotactic agent for polymorphs and greatly increases capillary permeability.
- C3a and C5a act on mast cells causing the release of further mediators such as histamine, LTB_4 and TNF, with effects on capillary permeability and adhesiveness and neutrophil chemotaxis. They also activate neutrophils, which bind to the C3b-coated microbes by their surface C3b receptors and then ingest them.
- The influx of polymorphs and increase in vascular permeability constitute the potent antimicrobial acute inflammatory response.
- Inflammation can also be initiated by tissue macrophages, which subserve a similar role to that of the mast cell since signalling by bacterial toxins, C5a or by C3b-coated bacteria adhering to surface complement receptors on tissue macrophages causes the release of TNF, LTB_4, PGE_2, NCF and a neutrophil activating peptide.
- Other humoral defenses include the acute phase proteins such as CRP and the IFNs, which can block viral replication.
- Virally infected cells can be killed by LGLs with NK activity.
- Extracellular killing can also be effected by C3b-bound eosinophils, which may be responsible for the failure of many large parasites to establish a foothold in potential hosts.
- It is probably true to say that engulfment and killing by phagocytic cells is the mechanism used to dispose of the majority of microbes, and the mobilization and activation of these cells by orchestrated responses such as the acute inflammatory response (*Fig. 4.30*) is a key feature of innate immunity. However, not every organism is readily susceptible to phagocytosis or even to killing by complement or lysozyme and this brings us to the role of the adaptive immune response, which is explored in Chapter 5.

1. What is the essential difference between innate and adaptive immunity?
2. What mechanisms are used by phagocytic cells to kill microorganisms they have engulfed?
3. How does complement contribute to defense against infection?
4. What are the innate defenses against viral infection?

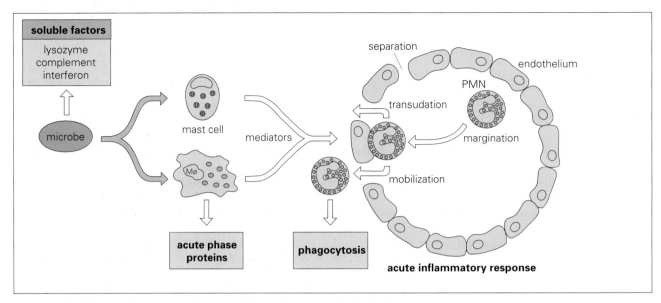

Fig. 4.30 Mobilization of defensive components of innate immunity. Microbes, either through complement activation or through direct effects on manophages, release mediators which increase capillary permeability to allow transudation of plasma bactericidal molecules, and chemotactically attract plasma polymorphs to the infection site.

Further Reading

Nichols B, Bainton DF, Farquhar MG. Differentiation of monocytes: origin, nature and fate of their azurophil granules. *J Cell Biol* 1971;**50**:498–515.

Roitt IM, Brostoff J, Male D. *Immunology*, 5th edition. London: Mosby International, 1998.

Stadnyk AW, Gauldie J. The acute phase protein response during parasitic infection. *Immunol Today* 1991;**7**: A7–A12.

Wilson GS, Miles AA, Parker MT, eds. *Topley and Wilson's Principles Of Bacteriology, Virology And Immunity*, 7th edition. Baltimore: Williams and Wilkins, 1983.

Adaptive Responses Provide a Quantum Leap in Effective Defense

Introduction

Infectious agents frequently find ways around the innate defenses

In Chapter 4, we discussed the many ways in which the primary or innate defenses of the body may counteract microbial infection. However, infectious agents frequently find ways around these defenses as there is a huge number of different microorganisms surrounding us and they have a powerful ability to mutate. For example:

- The surface of some microbes fails to activate the alternative complement pathway.
- Other microbes can activate the alternative complement pathway, but do so at the end of flagellae, so that the membrane attack complex is planted at a site distant from the body of the organism and therefore causes no damage.
- In other cases, microorganisms taken into the body of the macrophage develop subterfuges that prevent the development of the awesome battery of microbicidal mechanisms that the macrophage normally expresses (see Chapter 9).
- Cells infected with certain viruses may prove to be resistant to the cytotoxic action of natural killer cells or the viruses may be only weak stimulators of interferon, so that cell-to-cell transmission of the virus proceeds unchecked.
- Yet another microbial subterfuge is the production of bacterial toxins that can kill the phagocyte if not neutralized.

Adaptive responses act against microorganisms that overcome the innate defenses

It is clear that the body needs to provide immune defenses that can be 'tailor-made' to each individual variant of the different species of microorganisms. Ideally, these should link the organism directly into the various killing mechanisms of the innate system. In this chapter, we shall see how evolution has achieved this by inserting specific recognition sites on antibody molecules and on certain lymphocytes. When an infectious agent enters the body, the lymphocytes respond to it and produce a reaction that is specific for that particular microorganism. Furthermore, the magnitude of this response increases with time, often to quite high levels, so that we speak of it as an 'adaptive' or 'acquired' response. We know that the body produces millions of different antibodies, which as a population are capable of recognizing virtually any pathogen that has arisen or might arise.

The Role of Antibodies

The acute inflammatory response
Antibodies act as adaptors to focus acute inflammatory reactions

Antibodies *(Figs 5.1* and *5.2)* are synthesized by host B lymphocytes (so-called because they mature in the bone marrow) when they make contact with an infectious microbe, which acts as a foreign antigen (i.e. it generates antibodies). Each antibody has a recognition site that is complementary in shape to the surface of the foreign antigen and enables it to bind with varying degrees of strength to that antigen. Other sites on the antibody molecule are specialized for functions such as activating the complement

system and inducing phagocytosis by macrophages and polymorphs *(Fig. 5.3)*. Therefore, when a microbial antigen is coated with several of these adaptor antibody molecules, they induce complement fixation and phagocytosis, processes that the microbe may well have evolved to try and avoid. In this way, the reluctant microorganism becomes drawn into the innate defense mechanism of the acute inflammatory response. We will now examine the ways in which antibody can mediate these different phenomena.

Antibody complexed with antigen activates complement through the 'classical' pathway

When antibody molecules bind an antigen, the resulting complex activates the first component of complement, C1, converting it into an esterase. This initiates a second route of complement activation *(Fig. 5.4)* termed the 'classical' pathway, mainly because scientists discovered it before the 'alternative' pathway (see Chapter 4), although the evidence indicates that the alternative pathway is of greater antiquity in evolutionary terms. The activated first component splits off a small peptide from each of the succeeding components C4 and C2, the residual fragments forming a composite, the C4b2b complex. The C4b2b complex has the enzymatic ability or property of a C3 convertase. It has a similar function to the alternative pathway C3 convertase, C3bBb, and the sequence of events following the splitting of C3 is indistinguishable from that occurring in the alternative pathway. C3a and C5a anaphylatoxins are formed and C3b binds to the surface of the microbe–antibody complex *(Fig. 5.5)*. Subsequently, the later components are assembled into a membrane attack complex (MAC) (see *Fig. 4.22)*, which may help to kill the microorganism if it has been focused onto a vulnerable site.

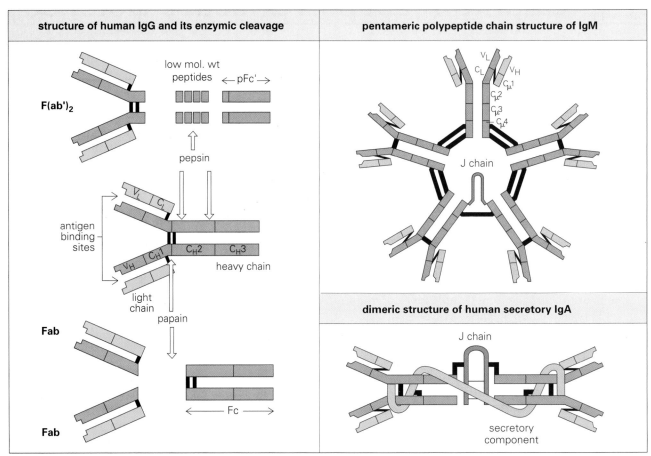

Fig. 5.1 The structure of immunoglobulins. The basic structure of immunoglobulins is a unit consisting of two identical light polypeptide chains and two identical heavy polypeptide chains linked together by disulfide bonds (black bars). Each chain is made up of individual globular domains. Different antibodies have different V_L and V_H domains, which are therefore highly variable, whereas the remaining domains (C_L and C_H1 etc.) are relatively constant in amino acid structure. Cleavage of human immunoglobulin G (IgG) by pepsin induces a divalent antigen-binding fragment, $F(ab')_2$ and a pFc' fragment composed of two terminal C_H3 domains. Papain produces two univalent antigen binding fragments, Fab, and an Fc portion containing the C_H2 and C_H3 heavy chain domains. Polymerisation of the basic immunoglobulin units to form IgM and IgA is catalyzed by the J (joining) chain. The portion of the transporter (which transfers IgA across the mucosal cell to the lumen) which remains attached to the IgA is termed 'secretory piece'.

BIOLOGICAL PROPERTIES OF MAJOR IMMUNOGLOBULIN CLASSES IN THE HUMAN					
designation	IgG	*IgA	IgM	IgD	IgE
major characteristics	most abundant internal Ig	protects external surfaces	very efficient against bacteremia	mainly lymphocyte receptor	initiates inflammation, raised in parasitic infections causes allergy symptoms
antigen binding	++	++	++	++	++
complement fixation (classical)	++	−	+++	+	−
cross placenta	++	−	−	−	−
fix to homologous mast cells and basophils	−	−	−	−	++
binding to macrophages and polymorphs	+++	+	−	−	+

Fig. 5.2 Biologic properties of major immunoglobulin (Ig) classes in the human.
(* Dimer in external secretion carries secretory component; IgA dimer and IgM contain J chains.)

The acute inflammatory reaction can also be initiated by antibody bound to mast cells

A specialized antibody, immunoglobulin E (IgE), has a backbone site with a high affinity for specific receptors on the surface of mast cells. When microbial antigen attaches to these cell-bound antibodies the surface receptors are cross-linked and transduce a signal to the interior of the cell. This signal

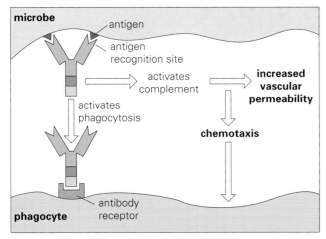

Fig. 5.3 The antigen adaptor molecule. Antibodies (anti-foreign bodies) are produced by host lymphocytes on contact with invading microbes, which act as antigens (i.e. generate antibodies). Each antibody *(Fig. 5.1)* has a recognition site (Fab) enabling it to bind antigen, and a backbone structure (Fc) capable of some secondary biologic action such as activating complement and phagocytosis.

leads to the release of mediators capable of increasing vascular permeability and inducing polymorph chemotaxis *(Fig. 5.6)*.

Activation of phagocytic cells
Antigen–antibody complexes activate phagocytic cells

Other sites on the backbone of certain types of antibody molecule bind to specialized receptors on the surface of phagocytic cells. If there is more than one antibody in the antigen–antibody complex, these receptors are cross-linked so inducing the cell to put out arms of cytoplasm, which enclose the complex in a phagocytic vacuole *(Fig. 5.7)*. Note also that there is a 'bonus effect' of multivalent binding of reversible ligand–receptor links; for example, the association constant for a complex binding through two antibody molecules to the phagocyte is the product rather than the sum of the individual association constants.

Blocking microbial reactions
Antibodies block microbial interactions by combining with one of the reacting molecules

For example, an antibody directed against the influenza hemagglutinin will prevent the virus from attaching to its specific receptor on a cell, making it unable to infect that cell *(Fig. 5.8)*. Likewise, antibodies to an essential transport molecule on a bacterial surface can prevent the uptake of that nutrient and cause a metabolic block. As a final example, an antibody to a bacterial toxin will prevent damage to the cells with which the toxin would otherwise interact.

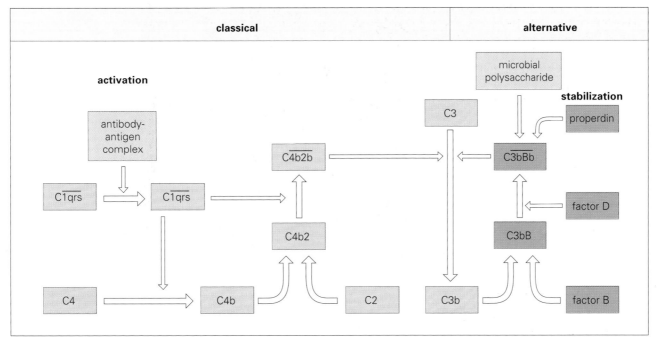

Fig. 5.4 The complex of antibody with microbial antigen activates the first component of the 'classical' pathway leading to cleavage of C3 through the C4b2b C3 convertase. This contrasts with the activation of the 'alternative' pathway, which depends upon stabilization of the C3 convertase (C3bBb) on the microbial surface. The classical pathway is in general antibody dependent, the alternative pathway is not. A bar (‾) indicates an active complex.

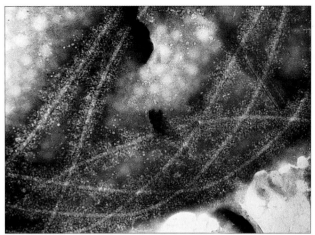

Fig. 5.5 Electron microscopy of C3-coated salmonella flagellae. The flagellae have been incubated with anti-flagella antibody and complement. The electron-dense material extending 30 nm on either side of each flagellum is believed to be C3b. The interpretation of this is that complement fixation by antibody results in a heavy macromolecular coating of C3b on biologic membranes to which complement has been fixed. ×700 000. (Courtesy of A Feinstein and E Munn.)

The Role of T Lymphocytes

Defense against intracellular organisms

Viruses and many different species of microorganisms can live within cells where they are shielded from attack by antibody. The body has therefore evolved a defense system against such organisms based upon the T lymphocyte, so-called because it matures in the thymus gland.

T lymphocytes bind to peptide derived from intracellular organisms complexed with major histocompatability complex

As microorganisms go through their various life cycles they sometimes die within the cells they infect. The proteins derived from these dead organisms are fragmented by intracellular enzymes ('processing') and the peptides are incorporated into cytoplasmic vacuoles where they associate with a molecule of the major histocompatibility complex (MHC) *(Fig. 5.9)*. (MHC molecules were originally discovered

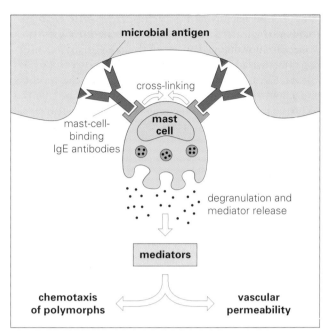

Fig. 5.6 Degranulation of mast cells by interaction of microbial antigen with specific antibodies of the IgE class, which bind to special receptors on the mast cell surface. The cross-linking of receptors caused by this interaction leads to the release of mediators, which induce an increase in vascular permeability and attract polymorphs – that is, they provoke an acute inflammatory reaction at the site of the microbial antigen.

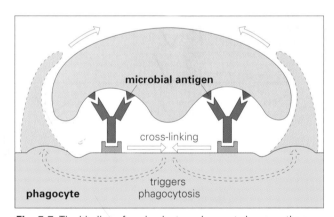

Fig. 5.7 The binding of a microbe to a phagocyte by more than one antibody cross-links the antibody receptors on the phagocyte surface and triggers phagocytosis of the microorganism.

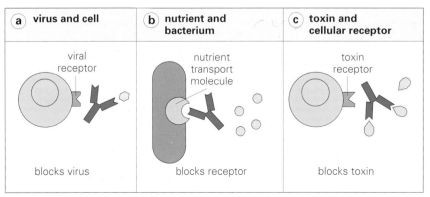

Fig. 5.8 Because of its size, antibody can block interactions between (a) a virus and a cell, (b) a nutrient and a bacterium and (c) a toxin and a cellular receptor.

because of their ability to bring about the most violent rejection of grafts interchanged between members of the same species. We now know that one of their important functions is to act as surface markers. Class I MHC molecules are present on virtually every cell in the body and can therefore be used as a marker for a 'cell'. Class II MHC molecules appear mainly on macrophages and B cells.)

A specialized T cell receptor (TCR) on the T lymphocyte *(Fig. 5.10)*, which is analogous to an antibody molecule in its ability to recognize foreign antigen, is specialized for binding to the complex of MHC molecule and peptide derived from the intracellular organism *(Fig. 5.11)*. Therefore, when it recognizes these two moieties together the T lymphocyte binds to an infected cell of a type indicated by the class of the MHC. The T lymphocyte then becomes activated and, depending upon its particular characteristics, sets off an effector mechanism to deal with the intracellular microorganisms, as explained below.

T lymphocytes help macrophages kill intracellular parasites

The task of recognizing macrophages that have unwelcome guests, such as *Listeria* or tubercle bacilli living within them,

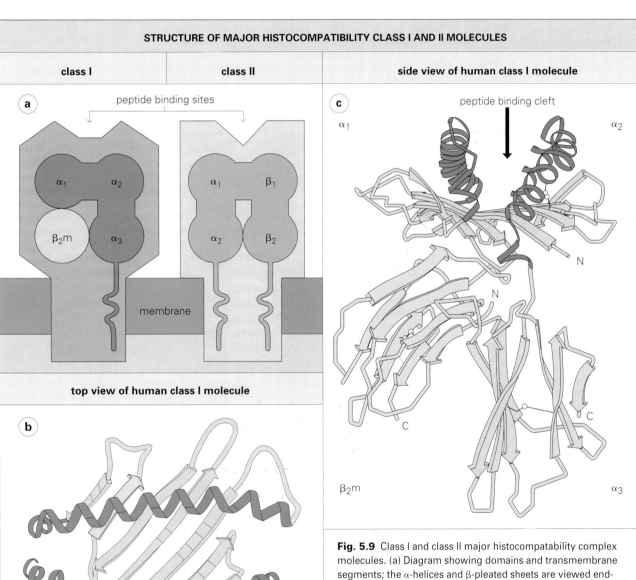

STRUCTURE OF MAJOR HISTOCOMPATIBILITY CLASS I AND II MOLECULES

Fig. 5.9 Class I and class II major histocompatability complex molecules. (a) Diagram showing domains and transmembrane segments; the α-helices and β-pleated sheets are viewed end-on. (b) Top surface of human class I molecule (HLA-A2) based on X-ray crystallographic structure. The strands making the β-pleated sheet are shown as thick grey arrows in the amino to carboxyl direction, α-helices are represented as helical ribbons. The inside facing surfaces of the two helices and the upper surface of the β-pleated sheet form a cleft. The two black spheres represent an intrachain disulfide bond. (c) Side view showing the cleft and the typical immunoglobulin folding of the α3 and β2-microglobulin (β2m) domains (four antiparallel β-strands on one face and three on the other). (Adapted from PI Bjorkman *et al*, 1987, with permission.)

falls to a subset of lymphocytes called the T helper (TH1) cells. When a specific TH1 cell combines with a complex of class II MHC molecule and microbial peptide on the surface of an infected macrophage, the T cell is triggered to release macrophage activating factors, notably interferon (IFNγ) (see Chapter 9). This unleashes previously suppressed microbicidal mechanisms within the macrophage, so leading to the death of the intracellular parasites *(Fig. 5.12)*.

T lymphocytes inhibit intracellular replication of viruses

Cells infected with virus express complexes consisting of class I MHC and a virally-derived peptide on their surface. These are recognized by the specific receptors on cytotoxic T (Tc) cells, all which are therefore led into close proximity to their virally infected target. The target cell is then killed by similar extracellular mechanisms to those described in Chapter 4.

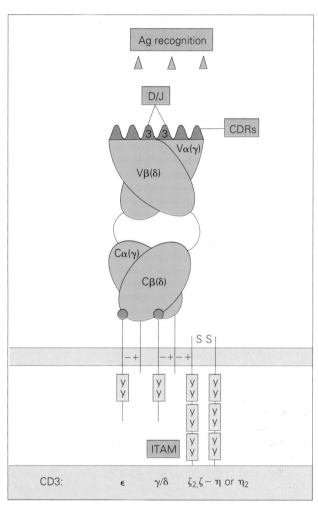

Fig. 5.10 The T cell receptor (TCR)/CD3 complex. The TCR resembles the immunoglobulin Fab antigen-binding fragment in structure. The variable and constant segments of the TCR2 α and β chains (VαCα/VβCβ) and the corresponding TCR1 γ and δ chains belong structurally to the immunoglobulin family. The complementarity determining regions (CDR) make contact with the antigen (MHC/peptide, *Fig. 5.11*). The TCRα and β CDR3 loops encoded by *D/J* genes are both short: the TCRγ CDR3 is also short with a narrow length distribution, but the δ loop is long with a broad length distribution, resembling the immunoglobulin light and heavy chain CDR3s, respectively. Negative charges on transmembrane segments of the five invariant chains of the CD3 complex contact the opposite charges on the TCR Cα and Cβ chains, conceivably as depicted in the inset figure. The cytoplasmic domains of the CD3 peptide chains contain immunoreceptor tyrosine-based activation motifs (ITAM), which contact the src oncogene family protein tyrosine kinases. Try not to confuse the TCRγδ and the CD3γδ chains.

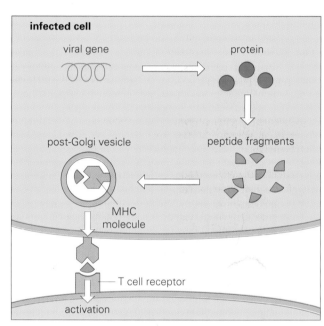

Fig. 5.11 T lymphocytes are activated when their specific cell surface receptors recognize an infected cell by binding to a surface major histocompatibility complex (MHC) molecule that is associated with a peptide fragment of a degraded intracellular microorganism. T helper cells recognize peptide plus class II MHC molecule and cytotoxic T cells recognize peptides plus class I MHC molecule.

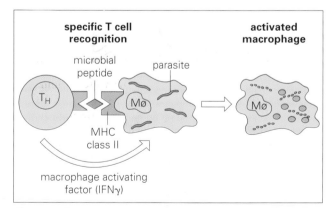

Fig. 5.12 T helper (TH) cells trigger the killing of parasites within macrophages (Mø). Recognition of the infected macrophage by the TH cell TCR results in lymphocyte activation with release of IFNγ. This then activates the macrophage, which turns on its microbicidal mechanisms to kill the intracellular parasite. Whereas the TH1 subset of helper cells produces interleukin-2 (IL-2) and cytokines such as IFNγ (see *Fig. 6.8*), which mediate chronic inflammatory reactions, another subset, TH2, secretes IL-4, IL-5 and IL-6 and helps B cells make antibody.

Since the virally derived peptides appear on the cell surface at a very early stage of infection, the Tc cells kill the cell before the virus has had an opportunity to replicate significantly and the host has won an important battle. The NK cell fulfils a similar function as the Tc cell, but because it lacks the specialized receptors for recognizing the particular viral peptide in association with class I MHC, its chances of binding strongly to the surface of the infected target cell are much less than those of the Tc cell. However, it is of interest that both the Tc cell and the TH cell are capable of releasing IFNs, which markedly improve the performance of the NK cell, so making a useful integrated system. An important additional responsibility of these IFNs is to render adjacent cells resistant to replication of viral particles, which gain entrance through intercellular transport mechanisms *(Fig. 5.13)*.

Extracellular Attack on Large Infectious Agents

Defensive cells attack the antibody-coated surfaces of parasites

Where a parasite is demonstrably larger than a phagocytic cell, it is physically impossible for phagocytosis to occur. However, it is still possible for the defensive cells to deliver an extracellular attack on the surface of the parasite. This can occur through the phenomenon of 'antibody-dependent cell-mediated cytotoxicity' (ADCC) in which effector cells bind through their surface receptors to antibody molecules coating the target cell *(Fig. 5.14)*. The result of this interaction is to induce activation of the effector cell and the release of materials to damage the parasite target. Major cell types that indulge in this type of activity are:

- The macrophage.
- The eosinophil.
- The NK cell, which in this context of ADCC, is often referred to as a K cell.

Local Defenses at Mucosal Surfaces

The immune mechanisms involving the acute inflammatory response and T cell-mediated systems operate well within the milieu of the body. It is worth examining, however, the special nature of the defenses required to protect the body at the mucosal surfaces, which face the exterior for example in the lung and the gastrointestinal tract *(Fig. 5.15)*.

The first line of defense aims to prevent the microbe from adhering to the mucosal surface

Adhesion to the mucosal surface is a prerequisite for penetrating the body. To prevent this there is the innate mechanism of mucus production. In addition, a special antibody, IgA, is synthesized by the lymphoid aggregates, some of which are organized (adenoids, tonsil, Peyer's patches), while others are less organized (lamina propria, lung, urinogenital tract). Together these lymphoid aggregates constitute the

mucosal-associated lymphoid tissue (MALT). The IgA is then actively transported by a carrier molecule into the lumen and is associated with the mucosal surface in a high concentration where it continues to bear a portion of the carrier called 'secretory piece' (see *Fig. 5.1*). When coated with such IgA antibodies, the adhesion of infectious agents to the mucosa is greatly diminished, but they can still be captured by local macrophages with surface receptors for IgA. Mast cells tend to cluster in the submucosal region and, should a microorganism break through the mucosal barrier, it could encounter a mast cell that has bound the specialized IgE antibody to its surface; on reaction with this surface antibody, the mast cell is triggered to release mediators of the acute inflammatory reaction. By increasing vascular permeability,

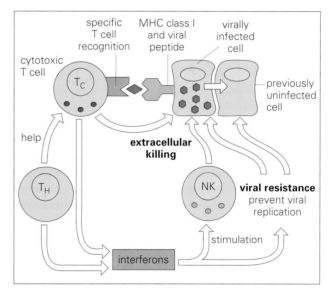

Fig. 5.13 Cytotoxic T (Tc) cells specifically recognize and kill virally infected cells before the virus replicates. Natural killer (NK) cells can do the same, though far less effectively; however their activity is enhanced by interferons (IFNs) produced by Tc and TH cells. Local production of IFNs also prevents adjacent cells from becoming infected by intercellular viral transport.

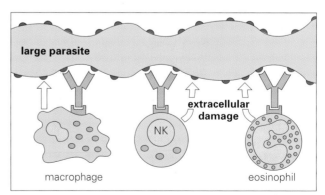

Fig. 5.14 Antibody-dependent cell-mediated cytotoxicity. Different effector cells bind to the parasite surface through their receptor for antibody and damage the parasite target. The antibodies mostly belong to the IgG class (see *Figs 5.1* and *5.2*).

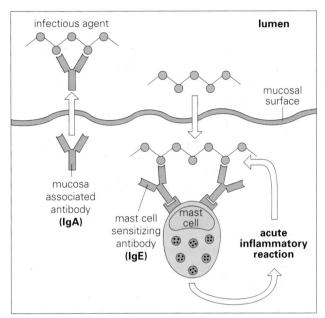

Fig. 5.15 Defense of body mucosal surfaces. A specialized antibody associated with the mucosal surface – secretory immunoglobulin A (IgA) – blocks adherence of the microbe to the mucosa and hence entry into the body. An infectious agent gaining entrance to the body will fire IgE-sensitized mast cells, which cluster beneath the surface and generate a protective local acute inflammatory response by attracting complement-fixing antibodies, complement and polymorphs from the blood.

these mediators will bring about the flooding of the site with plasma proteins, including other classes of antibody and complement, while chemotactic agents will attract polymorphonuclear leukocytes.

Defenses against larger parasites in the gut lumen

The presence of larger parasites, such as nematodes, within the lumen of the gut poses special problems. It is thought that antigens derived from the nematode may penetrate the submucosal space and activate T and B cells and degranulate sensitized mast cells. The latter will produce an acute inflammation at the mucosal surface and almost certainly lead to an outflow of antibody, complement and probably effectors of ADCC into the lumen. In the lumen, the antibody, complement and effectors of ADCC can then interact with the parasite and inflict metabolic damage. In the meantime, the interaction with sensitized T_H cells will lead to the release of soluble factors termed lymphokines, which include a mediator capable of stimulating the goblet cells lining the intestinal villi. The goblet cells then release their mucins into the lumen where they coat the damaged parasite and facilitate expulsion from the body (*Fig. 5.16*).

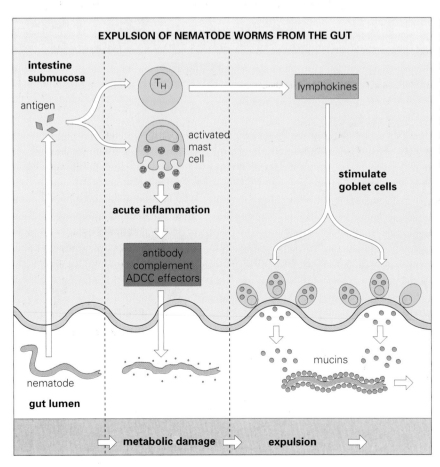

Fig. 5.16 Expulsion of nematode worms from the gut. Worm antigen is thought to trigger an acute inflammatory reaction in the submucosa. This facilitates the recruitment of complement and possibly antibody-dependent cell-mediated cytotoxicity effectors, which damage the parasite. Soluble factors (lymphokines), released by antigen-specific triggering of T helper cells, stimulate the secretion of mucins by goblet cells, which coat the worm and aid its expulsion.

- The evolution of the adaptive response has provided the body with a powerful series of mechanisms that extend and exploit the innate mechanisms of defense. Thus, this lymphocyte-mediated response greatly augments the innate defense against each particular infecting organism.
- In most cases, the effector mechanisms lead the organism back into the innate systems of defense such as phagocytosis, complement activation and macrophage intracellular killing.
- Taking an overall view of the adaptive responses, humoral immunity mediated by antibody produced by B lymphocytes is effective in neutralizing bacterial toxins, and by interacting with complement, mast cells and polymorphs, which produces the acute inflammatory reaction (Fig. 5.17). This response is especially effective against extracellular microbes, and the quantum leap provided by antibody in the clearance of extracellular bacteria from the blood is clearly shown in the example in Figure 5.18.
- In contrast, the T cell-mediated response is directed to intracellular organisms. The TH cells interact with macrophages by producing lymphokines, firstly chemotactic factors and secondly IFNγ, which activate phagocytic cells to switch on their intracellular antimicrobial mechanisms. Tc cells are effective against viruses, killing virally infected targets and preventing the spread of virus through the local production of IFNs.
- Figure 5.19 emphasizes the close interactions between innate and acquired mechanisms leading to defense against extracellular microorganisms on the one hand, and intracellular infections on the other. In keeping with these concepts, deficiencies in humoral immunity from whatever cause, predispose the individual to infection by extracellular organisms, whereas defects in T cell-mediated responses are primarily associated with intracellular infections.
- The first contact with antigen evokes a response that leaves behind a memory of the encounter so that the subsequent response to a second contact with antigen is more powerful and evolves more rapidly than on the first occasion. The cellular bases for these phenomena are explained in Chapter 6. The production of memory by a primary interaction with antigen provides the basis for vaccination, where the first contact is with an avirulent form of the microorganism or its component antigens.
- The other point to stress at this stage is the specificity of memory – infection with measles, for example, produces a subsequent immunity to that virus, but does not afford protection against an unrelated virus such as mumps.

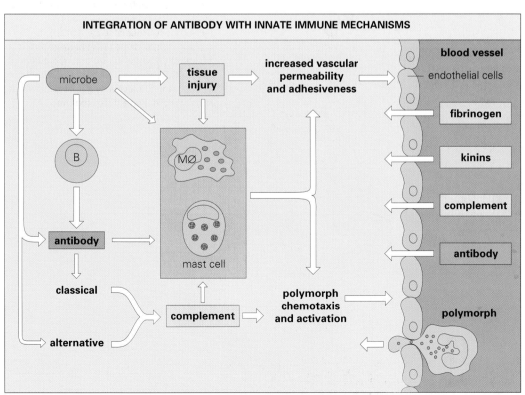

Fig. 5.17 Integration of antibody with the innate immune mechanisms leading to the production of a protective acute inflammatory reaction. The activated endothelial cells allow exudation of soluble proteins from the circulation and express accessory molecules, which aid the binding of the polymorphs to the capillary wall and their subsequent escape into the infected site. (MØ, macrophage.)

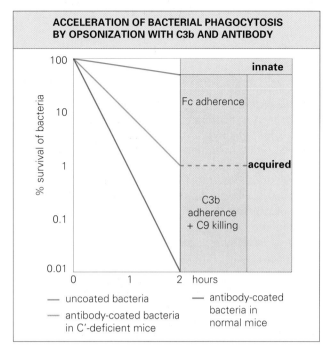

Fig 5.18 The slow rate of phagocytosis of uncoated bacteria (innate immunity) is increased many times by acquired immunity through coating with antibody and then C3b (opsonization). Killing may also take place through the C5-9 terminal complement components. This is a hypothetical, but realistic situation; the natural proliferation of the bacteria has been ignored.

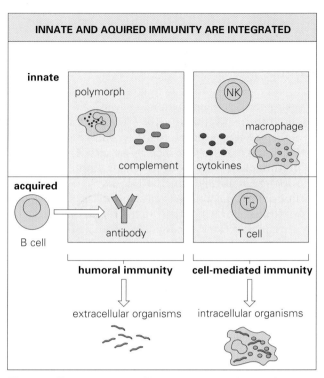

Fig. 5.19 The mechanisms of innate and acquired immunity are integrated to provide the basis for humoral and cell-mediated immunity respectively. Thus, deficiencies of humoral immunity predispose to infection with extracellular organisms and deficiencies of T cell-mediated responses are associated primarily with intracellular infections.

1. What are the features of the antibody molecule that make it so effective in defense against infection?
2. What are the advantages of having different immunoglobulin classes?
3. How do T cells recognize intracellular infections?
4. What are the effector functions of T cells?
5. How is the triad of antibody, complement and polymorphonuclear leukocytes integrated to produce an acute inflammatory response?

Further Reading

Goldschmeider I, Gotschilich EC, Artenstein MS. Human immunity to the meningococcus. I. The role of humoral antibodies. *J Exp Med* 1969;**129**:1307.
Griffiths GM. The cell biology of CTL killing. *Curr Opin Immunol* 1995;**7**:343.

Law SKA, Reid KBM. *Complement*. In: *Focus Series*. Male DK, ed. Oxford: IRL Press, 1988.
Roitt IM, Brostoff J, Male DK, eds. *Immunology*, 5th edition. London: Mosby International Ltd, 1997.

Introduction

As we saw in the last chapter, adaptive immune responses are generated by lymphocytes which are derived from stem cells differentiating within the primary lymphoid organs (bone marrow and thymus). From there they colonize the secondary lymphoid tissues where they mediate the immune responses to antigens *(Fig. 6.1)*. The lymph nodes are concerned with responses to antigens which drain into them from the tissues, while the spleen is concerned primarily with antigens which reach it from the bloodstream. In addition, unencapsulated aggregates of lymphoid tissue termed 'mucosa-associated lymphoid tissue' or MALT, lie in the mucosal surface where they have the job of responding to antigens from the environment by producing antibodies for mucosal secretions.

B and T Cell Receptors

B and T cells can be distinguished by their surface markers

As they differentiate into populations with differing functions, B and T cells acquire molecules on their surface that reflect these specializations. It is possible to produce homogeneous antibodies of a single specificity – termed 'monoclonal antibodies' – that can recognize such surface markers. When laboratories from all over the world compared the monoclonal antibodies they had raised, it was found that groups or clusters of monoclonal antibodies were each recognizing a common molecule on the surface of the lymphocyte. Each surface component so defined, was referred to as a 'CD' molecule *(Fig. 6.2)*, where CD refers to a 'cluster determinant'.

Each lymphocyte expresses a receptor of unique specificity on its surface

Among the surface markers on the B and T cells referred to above are the antigen receptors on the plasma membrane. B cells possess surface immunoglobulin whereas the T cell receptor (TCR) on the surface of the T lymphocyte acts as an antigen recognition unit (see *Chapter 5, Fig. 5.10*). We now know that despite the very large number of different components that could be combined together in multiple ways to give a diversity of surface receptors, each B lymphocyte rearranges its germline genes coding for these receptors so that it selects one and only one of the specificities for each receptor polypeptide chain. It then expresses that receptor molecule on its surface *(Fig. 6.3)*. Once this occurs, the other genes coding for these antigen receptors in the lymphocyte are no longer used. In other words, following this genetic rearrangement process, the lymphocyte becomes committed to the synthesis and expression of a single receptor type. An analogous process occurs in the rearrangement of the αβ and γδ genes coding for the TCR. Just as for B cells, each T cell expresses one and only one specific combination of receptor peptides, and therefore shows a single specificity to which it is committed for the whole of its lifespan.

Clonal Expansion of Lymphocytes

Antigen selects and clonally expands lymphocytes bearing complementary receptors

As there is such a large number of different possible specificities that lymphocytes can express, perhaps of the order of millions, there must of necessity be only a relatively small number that have a particular specificity. Thus, when a microbe invades the body, the total number of lymphocytes initially committed to recognizing the antigens that go to make up the microbial constitution are relatively small, and must be expanded if there is to be a sufficient number to protect the host. Evolution has provided a masterful solution to this problem. When a microbe enters the body, its component antigens combine with only those lymphocytes whose surface receptors are complementary to the shape of these antigens. The cells that bind the antigen become activated and proliferate clonally under the influence of soluble growth factors termed cytokines (see section on cytokines below) to form a large population of cells derived from the original *(Fig. 6.4)*.

In the case of B cells, a large proportion of the clonally expanded lymphocytes become plasma cells, dedicated to the synthesis and secretion of antibodies. Since these plasma cells are derived from a parent cell that is already committed to the production of only one specific antibody, the final product is identical to the molecule that was posted on the surface of the original antigen-recognizing cell. We therefore have the production of large amounts of antibody which, like that on the surface of the parent cell, must combine with the invading antigen *(Fig. 6.4)*.

A similar process of clonal selection and expansion occurs with T cells, producing a large number of effectors with the same specificity as the original parent cell; some of these cells release cytokines, whereas others have cytotoxic functions so that they act as effectors of T cell-mediated immunity. In the case of both B and T cells, a fraction of the clonally expanded population become resting memory cells *(Fig. 6.4)*. Thus, more cells are capable of recognizing the microbial antigen in

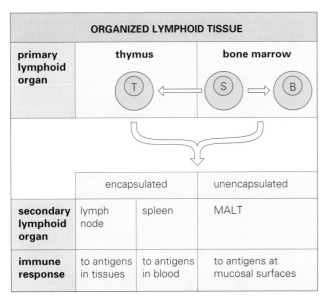

ORGANIZED LYMPHOID TISSUE			
primary lymphoid organ	thymus	bone marrow	
	encapsulated		unencapsulated
secondary lymphoid organ	lymph node	spleen	MALT
immune response	to antigens in tissues	to antigens in blood	to antigens at mucosal surfaces

Fig. 6.1 Organized lymphoid tissue. Stem cells (S) arising in the bone marrow differentiate into immuno-competent B and T cells in the primary lymphoid organs. These cells then colonize the secondary lymphoid tissues where immune responses are organized. (MALT, mucosa-associated lymphoid tissue.)

any subsequent infection than in the initial virgin population that existed before the primary infection occurred.

Role of Memory Cells

Secondary immune responses are bigger and brisker than primary responses

The increased number of lymphocytes specific for a given antigen present in the memory pool produced by the primary response give rise to a much stronger antibody response on second contact with antigen. This provides the principal for vaccination *(Fig. 6.5)*. The microbe or antigen to be used for vaccination is modified in such a way that it no longer produces disease or damage, but still retains the majority of its antigenic shapes. The primary response produced by the vaccination gives rise to a pool of memory cells, which can generate an abundant secondary response on subsequent contact with the antigen during a natural infection.

T-independent and T-dependent Antigens

Some antigens stimulate B cells without the need for intervention by T lymphocytes

These so-called T-independent antigens are of two main types:
- The first type contain molecular features that enable them to stimulate a wide variety of B cells independently of their specific antigen receptors; they are therefore referred to as 'polyclonal activators'. Those B cells carrying surface receptors that recognize epitopes on the polyclonal

SURFACE MARKERS ON B AND T CELLS			
function/identity	**CD designation**	**B cells**	**T cells**
antigen receptors			
Surface immunoglobulin	—	+ +	–
T cell $\alpha\beta$, $\gamma\delta$	—	–	+ +
TCR signal transducer	CD3	–	+ +
receptors for			
Sheep red cells (rosettes: antigen non-specific)	CD2	–	+ +
MHC class II (mainly T helpers)	CD4	–	+ +
MHC class I (cytotoxic/suppressors)	CD8	–	+ +
Complement (CR2)	CD21	+ +	–
Complement (CR1)	CD35	+ +	+
FcγII	CDw32	+ +	–
Fcϵ	CD23	+	–
IL–2 (α-chain)	CD25	act*	act*
MHC			
Class I	—	+ +	+ +
Class II	—	+ +	act*
other markers			
Differentiation marker	CD5	subset	+ +
Restricted leukocyte common antigen	CD45R	+	memory
* activated cells only			

Fig. 6.2 Surface markers on T and B cells. (IL, interleukin; MHC, major histocompatability complex; TCR, T cell receptor; Fc, dimer of immunoglobulin heavy chain excluding the Fab V_H and C_H1 domains in *Fig. 5.1*.)

activator attract the molecule to their surfaces and are preferentially stimulated relative to the remainder of the B cell population *(Fig. 6.6)*.
- The second type of T-independent antigen involves repeating determinants, which can cross-link immunoglobulin receptors on the B cell and apparently stimulate the lymphocyte directly *(Fig. 6.6)*.

One feature of both these types of T-independent antigen is that they give rise mainly to low affinity IgM rather than IgG antibody responses and rarely induce a memory response.

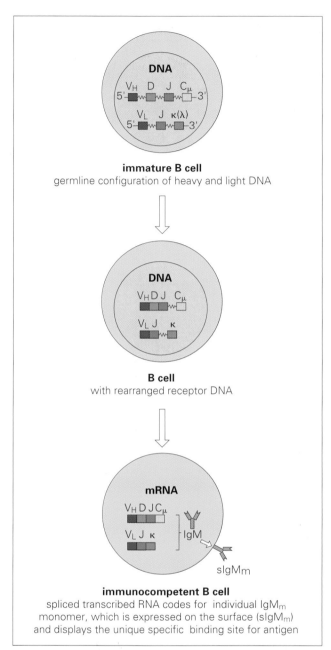

Fig. 6.3 Differentiation events leading to the expression of unique IgM on the surface of an immunocompetent B lymphocyte. Leader sequences have been omitted for simplicity.

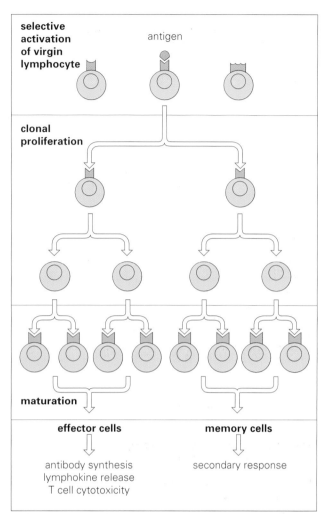

Fig. 6.4 Generation of a large population of effector and memory cells after primary contact of B or T cell with antigen. A fraction of the progeny of the original antigen-reactive lymphocytes become non-dividing memory cells, whereas the others become the effector cells of humoral or cell-mediated immunity. Memory cells require fewer cycles before they develop into effectors, thus shortening the reaction time for the secondary response.

Antibody production frequently requires T cell help

The majority of antigens will stimulate B cells only if they have the assistance of T lymphocyte helper (TH) cells. The sequence of events is as follows:

- In stage 1, the antigen is processed by an antigen-presenting cell (APC), which degrades it and places a peptide derived from it on its surface in association with major histocompatibility complex (MHC) class II molecules (*Fig. 6.7*), as discussed in Chapter 5. This complex is recognized by, and primes, a TH cell with a complementary receptor on its surface.

- In stage 2, a B cell with surface receptors complementary to an epitope on the original antigen, captures the antigen on its receptor, internalizes it and after processing also presents a derived peptide on its surface in association with endogenous MHC class II molecules. This is the complex against which the TH cell was originally primed and recognition of the processed antigen by the primed TH causes stimulation of the B cell with subsequent activation, proliferation and maturation.

It should be noted that although the TH cell recognizes a processed determinant of the antigen, the B cell is programmed to make only antibody with the same specificity as its surface receptor, and therefore the antibodies that finally

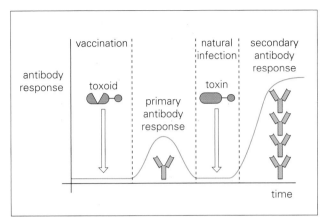

Fig. 6.5 Primary and secondary responses. The antibody response on the second contact with antigen is more rapid and more intense. Therefore, following vaccination with a benign form of the antigen (a chemically modified form of tetanus toxin in the example shown) to produce a primary response, subsequent contact with antigen in the form of a natural infection evokes the more efficient secondary response.

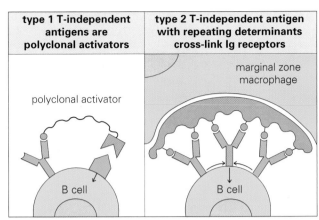

Fig. 6.6 B cell activation by T-independent antigens. The requirements for an antigen-presenting cell (APC) for type 2 antigens is still uncertain. (Ig, immunoglobulin.)

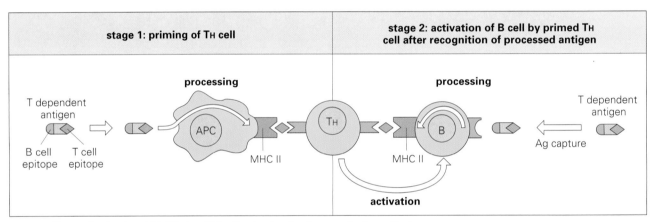

Fig. 6.7 The mechanism by which T helper (TH) cells stimulate B cells to synthesize antibody to T-dependent antigens. See text for a detailed description of the sequence of events. (Ag, antigen; APC, antigen-presenting cell; MHC, major histocompatability complex.)

result will be directed against the epitope on the antigen recognized by the B cell surface receptor.

Cytokines

Cytokines are soluble intercellular communication factors in the immune response

Interactions between the APC, the TH cell and the B cell are effected by the recognition of processed antigen in association with MHC class II molecules by the TCR, as indicated in *Figure 6.7*. Following this recognition process, the cells act on each other by releasing soluble factors termed cytokines *(Fig. 6.8)*, which react with appropriate complimentary surface receptors on the target cell . As can be seen from *Figure 6.9*, the APC provides an important triggering factor for the TH cell [i.e inter-

lukin-1 (IL-1)]. In the activated T cell, the gene encoding the IL-2 receptor (IL-2R) is derepressed and the IL-2R molecule is expressed on the surface of the lymphocytes. A subpopulation of TH cells is also induced to synthesize IL-2, which acts as a growth factor for T cells by combining with the IL-2R causing proliferation. Other cytokines are produced *(Fig. 6.8)* and among other things play a role:

• In the activation, proliferation and maturation of B cells.
• In the switch of B cells from IgM production.
• Perhaps in the generation of mutations in the variable region of the immunoglobulin gene, leading to the possibility of the selection of high-affinity antibody molecules during the immune response.

The formation of memory B cells is also almost certainly under the influence of T lymphocyte control. *Figure 6.9* clearly shows the broad sweep of the cytokine network and the involvement of many different cell types.

CYTOKINES: HORMONES OF THE IMMUNE SYSTEM		
factor	source	actions
IL-1 α/β	macrophages	inflammatory
IL-2	T cells	T and B cell proliferation
IL-3	T cells	pluripotent growth
IL-4	T cells	T and B proliferation, activation of macrophages
IL-5	T cells	eosinophil differentiation, B cell growth
IL-6	T cells	B cell differentiation
IL-7	T cells	B and T cell proliferation
IL-8	T cells	PMN activation
IL-9	T cells	mast cell growth
IL-10	T cell/B cell, macrophages	inhibition of TH1 cytokine production
IL-11	BM stromal cells	induction acute phase proteins
IL-12	Monocytes, Mφ	induction of TH1 cells
IL-13	T	inhibits mononuclear phagocyte inflammation: proliferation and differentiation B-cells
IL-16	CD8 T, CD4 (not preformed)	Chemotaxis CD4 T cells and esoinophils
IFNα	multiple	antiviral
IFNβ	multiple	antiviral
IFNγ	T cells,	antiviral, activation of macrophages, inhibition of TH2 cells
	NK cells	MHC induction
TNFα	monocytes	cytotoxicity, cachexia, fever
TNFβ	T cells	cytotoxicity, cachexia, fever
TGFβ	T cell/macrophages	inhibits activation of NK cells, and T cells, macrophages; inhibits proliferation of B and T cells
GM-CSF	T cells	growth of granulocytes and monocytes
G-CSF	macrophages	growth of granulocytes
M-CSF	macrophages	growth of monocytes
steel factor	BM stromal cells	stem cell division (c-kit ligand)

Fig. 6.8 Known cytokines and their actions. (G-CSF, granulocyte colony stimulating factor; GM-CSF, granulocyte macrophage colony stimulating factor; IFN, interferon; IL, interleukin; M-CSF, macrophage colony stimulating factor; NK, natural killer cell; PMN, polymorphonuclear lymphocyte; TGF, transforming growth factor; TNF, tumor necrosis factor.)

Regulatory Mechanisms

Unlimited expansion of clones must be checked by regulatory mechanisms

Once lymphocyte clones are activated by antigen, they clearly cannot be allowed to go on dividing indefinitely, otherwise they would completely fill the body of the host. There are therefore several mechanisms regulating the expansion of these dividing lymphocytes.

One of the most important factors controlling the immune response is the concentration of antigen. There is of course a distinct evolutionary advantage in a system where the immune response is switched on by antigen and switched off when the antigen is no longer present. It is perhaps not surprising then that selective processes have guided the production of such a system in which the immune response is antigen-driven through the direct effect of antigen on the lymphocyte receptors. As the antigen is eliminated by metabolic catabolism and by clearance through the immune response, the drive to the immune system disappears.

Antibody itself has feedback potential

IgM produced early in the response has a positive feedback, stimulating the response in its fledgling stages. In contrast, IgG in sufficient concentrations produces negative feedback and acts to downregulate the immune response. There is also considered to be a population of T suppressor (Ts) cells, which act to downregulate both TH cells and B cells, whether through antigen-specific or idiotype-specific mechanisms. The epitopes on one lymphocyte receptor (idiotype) recognized by the receptor on another lymphocyte (the anti-idiotype) can form a network of interactions through which suppression may be mediated (Fig. 6.10).

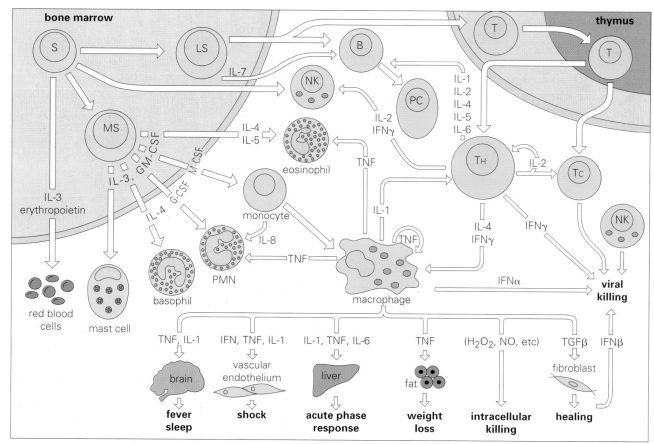

Fig. 6.9 Cellular interactions mediated by cytokines. T helper (TH) cells tend to skew into two major subsets: TH1, producing interleukin-2 (IL-2) and interferon-γ (IFN$_\gamma$), which activate macrophage-mediated chronic inflammatory reactions, and TH2, producing IL-4, IL-5 and IL-6, which act to support B cell antibody responses. (H$_2$O$_2$, hydrogen peroxide; LS, lymphoid stem cell; MS, myeloid stem cell; NK, natural killer cell; NO, nitric oxide; PC, plasma cell; PNM, polymormpho-nuclear lyphocyte; S, stem cell; TNF, tumor necrosis factor) (Adapted from JHL Playfair , 1996.)

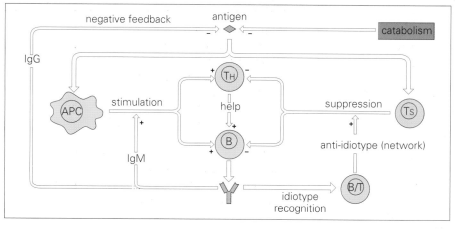

Fig. 6.10 Regulation of the immune response. T help for cell-mediated immunity is subject to similar regulation. The recruitment of B cells by anti-idiotype T helper (TH) cells and direct activation of anti-idiotype T suppressor (Ts) cells by idiotype-positive TH cells have been omitted for the sake of clarity. (APC, antigen-presenting cell.)

Tolerance Mechanisms

Tolerance mechanisms prevent immunologic self-reactivity

To avoid reaction against the body's own components, it is essential for the immune system to develop non-reactivity or 'tolerance' to self molecules. In essence, it is thought that cells that are autoreactive are either:

- Eliminated by some form of clonal deletion.
- Made anergic early in the life of the cell.
- Sometimes silenced through Ts systems later in life *(Fig. 6.11)*.

T cells are more readily tolerized than B cells at a given antigen concentration

There is extremely good evidence that self molecules in the thymus can lead to the deletion or 'anergy' of the specific T

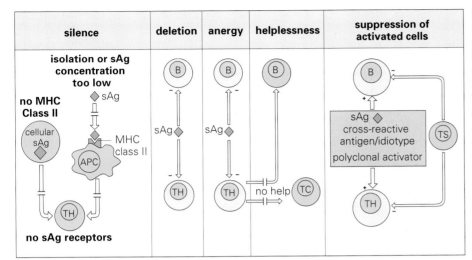

silence	deletion	anergy	helplessness	suppression of activated cells

Fig. 6.11 Mechanisms of self-tolerance. Self antigens (sAg) will not provoke a response if there is insufficient processed peptide–complex major histocompatability/(MHC) class II molecules or if there are no autoreactive T cells. Both B and T cells can be silenced by clonal deletion or made anergic (still living, but unresponsive) by contact with self antigen. B cells and cytoxic T (Tc) cells cannot function without T cell help. Inadvertent stimulation of available autoreactive cells may be checked by T suppressor (Ts) cells. Cells that are dead, unreactive or suppressed are shown in gray. (APC, antigen-presenting cell.) (Modified from IM Roitt , 1997.)

cell clone. B cells in contact with a relatively high concentration of self proteins are also subject to clonal deletion or anergy, but there is less need to tolerize other B cells in the sense that autoreactive B cells directed to thymus-dependent antigens will be unable to respond (helpless) if the corresponding TH cells to that molecule have been tolerized, be it through clonal deletion or T suppression (Fig. 6.11).

Unresponsiveness will also result if self components cannot be seen or recognized by the immune system. This may occur because over a long period of time the repertoire has lost the genes giving rise to autoreactive receptors. However, even if autoreactive T cells are present, they will not be activated if the self antigen is not presented in processed form in combination with MHC class II molecules in adequate concentrations. Therefore, they will also be unable to react with the whole molecules that constitute the surface array on cells that do not express class II. Since most cells express class I molecules, it seems reasonable to assume that the cytotoxic T (Tc) cells capable of reacting against cells expressing processed intracellular components have been deleted, are helpless or are suppressed.

- Each lymphocyte expresses either antibody or a TCR with a single specificity for antigen.
- A lymphocyte bearing a complementary antibody or TCR on its surface will bind antigen, be activated, proliferate to form a clone, and differentiate into antibody-forming cells or effectors of cell-mediated immunity, and also form a large pool of memory cells.
- Second contact with antigen stimulates the pool of memory cells to produce a larger and faster response than the primary reaction. Therefore, vaccination with a benign form of the antigen prepares the individual for an effective response on second contact with the antigen during a natural infection.
- Many antigens require T cell help before they can activate B cells, and the interactions are mediated by a variety of soluble cytokines.
- Unlimited expansion of clones is restricted by antigen concentration, antibody feedback T cell suppression and apoptosis.
- Reactivity to self is prevented by a variety of tolerance mechanisms.

1. What are the advantages of each B lymphocyte expressing a single antibody specificity on its surface?
2. How do TH cells function in antibody production?
3. Define the term cytokine and describe the main effects that this class of molecule mediates.
4. What are the main factors regulating adaptive immune responses?
5. How does the body normally avoid making autoreactive responses?

Further Reading

Playfair JHL. *Immunology At A Glance,* 6th edition. Oxford: Blackwell Science, 1996.

Roitt IM. *Essential Immunology* 9th edition,. Oxford: Blackwell Science, 1997.

Roitt IM, Brostoff J, Male DK, eds. *Immunology,* 5th edition. London: Mosby International, 1997.

2

the conflicts

Conflicts: Background to the Infectious Diseases

Introduction

Vertebrates have been continuously exposed to microbial infections throughout their hundreds of millions of years of evolution. Disease or death was the penalty for inadequate defenses. Therefore they have developed:
- Highly efficient methods for recognizing foreign invaders.
- Effective inflammatory and immune responses to restrain the growth and spread of foreign invaders and to eliminate them from the body.

The fundamental bases of these defenses has been described in Chapters 4 and 5. If these defenses were completely effective, microbial infections would be scarce and terminated rapidly as microorganisms would not be allowed to persist in the body for long periods.

Microbes rapidly evolve characteristics that enable them to overcome the host's defenses

Microorganisms faced with the antimicrobial defenses of the host species have evolved and developed a variety of characteristics that enable them to bypass or overcome these defenses and carry out their obligatory steps *(Fig. 7.1)*. Unfortunately microorganisms evolve with extraordinary speed in comparison with their hosts. This is partly because they multiply much more rapidly, the generation time of an average bacterium being one hour or less compared with about 20 years for the human host. Rapid evolutionary change is also favored in bacteria that can hand over genes (carried on plasmids) directly to other bacteria, including unrelated bacteria. Antibiotic resistance genes, for instance, can then be transferred rapidly between species. This rapid rate of evolution ensures that microbes are always many steps ahead of the host's antimicrobial defenses. Indeed if there are possible ways around the established defenses, microorganisms are likely to have discovered and taken advantage of them. Infectious microorganisms therefore owe their success to this ability to adapt and evolve, exploiting weak points in the host's defenses, as outlined in *Figures 7.2–7.4*. The host in turn has had to respond to such strategies.

Host–Parasite Relationships

The speed with which host adaptive responses can be mobilized is crucial

Every infection is a race between the capacity of the microorganism to multiply, spread and cause disease and the ability of the host to control and finally terminate the infection

OBLIGATORY STEPS FOR INFECTIOUS MICROORGANISMS		
step	**requirement**	**phenomenon**
attachment ± entry into body	evade natural protective and cleansing mechanisms	entry (infection)
local or general spread in the body	evade immediate local defenses	spread
multiplication	increase numbers (many will die in the host, or en route to new hosts)	multiplication
evasion of host defenses	evade immune and other defenses long enough for the full cycle in the host to be completed	microbial answer to host defenses
shedding from body (exit)	leave body at a site and on a scale that ensures spread to fresh hosts	transmission
cause damage in host	not strictly necessary but often occurs*	pathology, disease

Fig. 7.1 Successful infectious microorganisms must take certain obligatory steps. (*The last step, causing damage in the host, is not strictly necessary, but a certain amount of damage may be essential for shedding. The outpouring of infectious fluids in the common cold or diarrhea for instance, or the trickle from vesicular or pustular lesions, is required for transmission to fresh hosts.)

HOST DEFENSES AND THE MICROBES ANSWER

	defense	microbial answer	mechanism	example
mechanical and other barriers	microbe rinsed away from epithelial surface by host secretions (plus ciliary activity in respiratory tract)	bind firmly to epithelial surface	surface molecule on microbe attaches to 'receptor' molecule on host epithelial cell	influenza, Rhinovirus chlamydia, Gonococcus
		interfere with ciliary activity	produce ciliotoxic/ciliostatic molecule	*Bordetella pertussis* pneumococcus, Pseudomonas
	host cell membrane as barrier to intracellular microbe	traverse host cell membrane	fusion protein in viral envelope	influenza, HIV
		suffer uptake by phagocyte and resist killing	see above	see above
		enter cell by active penetration	microbial enzymes mediate cell penetration	trypanosomes, *Toxoplasma gondii*
phagocytic and immediate host defenses	microbe ingested and killed by phagocyte	interfere with function (e.g. chemotaxis) of phagocyte or kill it (before or after phagocytosis)	release leucocidins, antiphagocytic haemolysins etc.	staphylococci, Streptococci shigella, *E. coli*, Pseudomonas
		inhibit phagocytosis	microbial outer wall or capsule impedes phagocytosis	pneumococci, *Treponema pallidum, H. influenzae*
		inhibit lysosomal fusion	microbe liberates molecule form phagosome	*M tuberculosis, Toxoplasma gondii*
		resist killing and multiply in phagocyte	unknown; may involve exit from phagosome (listeria)	*Brucella* sp., *Listeria monocytogenes* measles, dengue viruses
	host molecules (lactoferrin, transferrin etc.) restrict availability of free iron needed by microbe	microbe competes with host for iron	microbe possesses avidly iron-binding molecules (siderophores)	pathogenic neisseria *E. coli*, Pseudomonas
	complement activated with anti-microbial effects	interfere with alternate pathway complement activation	fully sialylated bacterial surface	K antigen of *E. coli*, Group B meningococcus
		inactivate complement components	production of an elastase	*Pseudomonas aeruginosa*
		interfere with complement-mediated phagocytosis	C3b receptor on microbe competes with that on phagocyte complement access blocked	*Candida albicans, Toxoplasma gondii* M protein of *Strep. pyogenes*
	infected host produces interferons to inhibit virus replication	induce a poor interferon response	HBc of hepatitis B suppresses IFN-β production	hepatitis B, rotaviruses
		enjoy insensitivity to interferons	prevent activation of interferon-induced enzymes	adenovirus

immune defenses			
infected host produces antimicrobial antibody	destroy antibody	bacterium liberates IgA protease	gonococcus, *H. influenzae* streptoccocci
	fail to induce protective antibody	Infection lymphoid cells?	scrapie agents
	display Fc receptor on microbial surface	antibody bound to microbe in upside down position	staphylcocci (Protein A), Trypanosomes certain streptococci; herpes simplex virus cytomegalovirus
	microbial antigen (polysaccharide) project beyond microbial surface	C activation occurs away from microbial surface and C-mediated damage thus avoided	Gram-negative bacteria
	avoid immune recognition	acquire coating of host molecules	hydatid disease, Schistosomiasis
infected host produces antimicrobial cell-mediated immune response	invade T cells, and interfere with their function or kill them	virus envelope molecule binds to CD4 on helper T cell surface	HIV
	switch on T cells or B cells non-specifically, non-productively	Polyclonal activation of B cells Polyclonal activation of T cells by release of T cell mitogens	EB virus, *Mycoplasma pneumoniae* staphylococcal toxins
antimicrobial immune response recognizes infected cells and destroys them, or liberates cytokines with antimicrobial effects	microbe in cell fails to display microbial antigens on cell surface	antiviral antibody modulates and removes viral antigens	measles
		viral antigens not synthesized	herpes simplex virus in sensory neurones
		virus inhibits transport of MHC class 1 molecules to cell surface thus avoiding recognition by T cell	cytomegalovirus, adenovirus
antimicrobial immune responses	infect glands or epithelial surfaces relatively inaccessible to circulating antibody or immune cells	virus has tropism for cells in glands or on surfaces	cytomegalovirus, Rabies virus (salivary glands)
	suppress immune responses	invade immune tissues	HIV, measles
	vary microbial antigens either in individually infected host, or during spread in host community	switch on different surface antigens	*Trypanosoma* sp., *Borrelia recurrentis*
		mutation genetic recombination	influenza virus, streptococci, gonococci

Fig. 7.2 Host defenses and microbial evasion strategies: mechanical and other barriers. Microbes evolve fast and are generally one step ahead in this ancient conflict, but it must be remembered that the antimicrobial defenses themselves represent the host's answer to invading microbes.

(Fig. 7.3). For instance, a 24-hour delay before an important host response comes into operation can give a decisive advantage to a rapidly growing microorganism. From the host's point of view, it may allow enough damage to cause disease. More importantly from the microbe's point of view, it may give the microbe the opportunity to be shed from the body in larger amounts or for an extra day or two. A microbe that achieves this will be rapidly selected for in evolution.

Adaptation by both host and parasite leads to a more stable balanced relationship

The picture of conflict between host and parasite, usually and appropriately described in military terms, is central to an understanding of the biology of infectious disease. As with military conflicts, adaptation on both sides (see panel) tends to lessen the damage and incidence death in the host population, leading to a more stable and balanced relationship. The successful parasite gets what it can from the host without causing too much damage, and in general the more ancient the relationship the less the damage. Many microbial parasites, not only the normal flora (see Chapter 3), but also polioviruses, meningococci and pneumococci and others, live for the most part in peaceful coexistence with their human host.

Some microorganisms remain at body surfaces, perhaps spreading locally, but failing to invade deeper tissues. These include the common cold viruses, wart viruses, mycoplasmas and skin fungi. Often the disease is mild, but severe illness can occur when powerful toxins are produced and act either locally (cholera) or at distant sites (diphtheria).

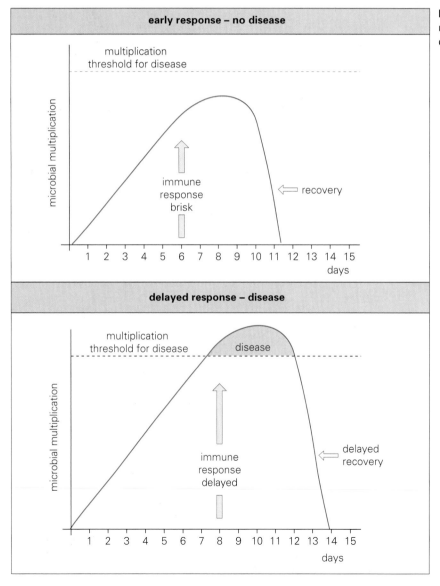

Fig. 7.3 Every infection is a race. Delays in mobilizing host adaptive defenses can lead to disease or death.

Myxomatosis

Myxomatosis provides a well-studied classic example of the evolution of an infectious disease in a highly susceptible population. Myxomavirus, which is spread mechanically by mosquitoes, normally infects South American rabbits (*Sylvilagus brasiliensis*), but they remain perfectly well, developing only a virus-rich skin swelling at the site of the mosquito bite. The same virus in the European rabbit (*Oryctolagus cuniculus*) causes a rapidly fatal disease.

Myxomavirus was successfully introduced into Australia in 1950 as an attempt to control the rapidly increasing rabbit population. Initially, more than 99% of infected rabbits died (*Fig. 7.4*), but then two fundamental changes occurred:

- First, new, less lethal strains of virus appeared and replaced the original strain. This occurred because rabbits infected with these strains survived for longer and their virus was therefore more likely to be transmitted.

- Second, the rabbit population changed its character, as those that were genetically more susceptible to the infection were eliminated. In other words, the virus selected out the more resistant host, and the less lethal virus strain proved to be a more successful parasite. If the rabbit population had been eliminated the virus would also have died out, but the host–parasite relationship

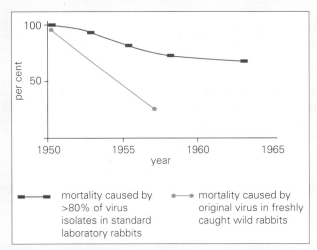

Fig. 7.4 Myxomatosis is the best-studied example of the appearance of a highly lethal microbe in a host population that gradually settles down to a state of more balanced pathogenicity. *Vibrio cholerae* has progressed in this direction, and perhaps HIV is destined to tread the same path.

quite rapidly settled down to reach a state of better balanced pathogenicity. And, of course, Australia's rabbit problem remained unsolved.

Four types of infection can be distinguished

The four types of infecting microorganisms (*Fig. 7.3*) are:

- Microorganisms with specific mechanisms for attaching to, or penetrating, the body surfaces of normal healthy hosts (most viruses and certain bacteria).

- Microorganisms introduced into normal healthy hosts by biting arthropods (malaria, plague, typhus, yellow fever).

- Microorganisms introduced into otherwise normal healthy hosts via skin wounds or animal bites (*Clostridia*, rabies, *Pasteurella multocida*).

- Microorganisms able to infect a normal healthy host only when surface or systemic defenses are impaired (see Chapter 28) – as occurs with burns, insertion of foreign bodies (cannulas and catheters), urinary tract infections in men (stones, enlarged prostate, see Chapter 18), bacterial pneumonia following initial viral damage (post-influenza) or depressed immune responses (immunosuppressive drugs or diseases such as AIDS).

Causes of Infectious Diseases

More than 100 microbes quite commonly cause infection

Humans are host to many different microorganisms. In addition to the scores of microbes that form the normal flora there are more than 100 that quite commonly cause

infection, some of them remaining in the body for many years afterwards, and several hundred others that are responsible for less common infections. Against this rich background of parasitic activity, how do we prove that a

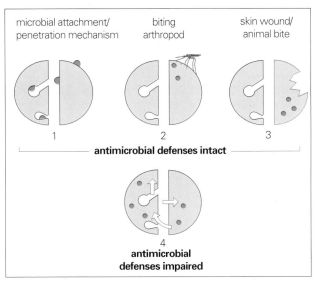

Fig. 7.5 Four types of microbial infection can be distinguished. Surface or systemic defenses of the host can be impaired in a variety of ways.

certain microorganism is the culprit in a given disease? In some instances (anthrax, cholera, tetanus) the causative microorganism is identified and incriminated at an early stage, but in the case of glandular fever and viral hepatitis it is not so easy.

Koch's postulates to identify the microbial causes of specific diseases

In 1890, Robert Koch (see panel) set out as 'postulates' the following criteria he felt to be necessary for a microorganism to be accepted as the cause of a given disease:

- The microbe must be present in every case of the disease.
- The microbe must be isolated from the diseased host and grown in pure culture.
- The disease must be reproduced when a pure culture is introduced into a non-diseased susceptible host.
- The microbe must be recoverable from an experimentally-infected host.

However, modifications were needed in order to include certain bacterial diseases and the new world of viral diseases. The microbe could not always be grown in the laboratory (*Treponema pallidum*, wart viruses), and for certain microbes – hepatitis B, Epstein–Barr virus (EBV) – there were (initially) no susceptible animal species. The criteria were modified therefore on several occasions to accommodate these problems and finally reformulated and brought up to date by A S Evans in 1976.

In the early days of microbiology, Koch's postulates brought a welcome clarity. The germ theory of disease causation had only recently been set out following Koch's classic studies on anthrax (1876) and tuberculosis (1882), and methods for isolating microbes in pure culture and identifying them were only just being developed.

Nowadays conclusions about causation are reached using enlightened common sense

Nowadays, with our vastly increased technology and understanding of infection, those attempts to make lists and apply rigid criteria may seem old fashioned. Perhaps we can now reach conclusions about causation using common sense . For instance, we recognize that diseases sometimes do not appear until many years after a specific-infection (subacute sclerosing panencephalitis, Creutzfeldt–Jakob disease; see Chapter 22). Nevertheless, gray areas remain, especially in diseases of possible or probable microbial etiology where the microbe does not act alone. Cofactors or genetic and immunologic factors in the host may play a vital part. Examples include:

- The cancers associated with viruses (hepatitis B, genital wart viruses, EBV).

Robert Koch (1843–1910)

In 1876, while in general practise in Berlin, Robert Koch *(Fig. 7.6)* isolated the anthrax bacillus, and became the first to show a specific organism as the cause of a disease. In 1882 he discovered *Mycobacterium tuberculosis* as the cause of tuberculosis. He then went on to lead the 1883 expedition to Egypt and India, and discovered the cause of cholera – *Vibrio cholerae*.

Koch was the founder of the 'germ theory' of disease, which maintained that certain diseases were caused by a single species of microbe. In 1890, he set out his 'postulates' as ground rules (see text). New techniques were necessary to meet the exacting requirements of the postulates, and Koch became the first to grow bacteria in 'colonies', initially on potato slices and later, with his pupil Petri, on solid gelatin media.

Koch himself could not reproduce cholera in animals, however, and not all microbes could be cultivated. His neat rules therefore had to be modified. Nevertheless, he brought order and clarity to medicine – until then diseases were attributed to miasmas or mists, to punishments from the Gods or devils, or to unfortunate conjunctions of the stars and planets. However, there was resistance to his ideas. A distinguished Munich physician, Max Von Petternkofer, believed that he had put paid to the new theory when he drank a pure culture of *V. cholerae* and suffered no more than mild diarrhea!

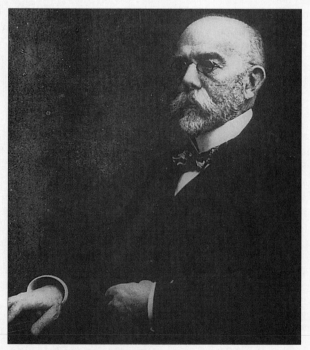

Fig. 7.6 Robert Koch (1843–1910).

The Biologic Response Gradient   89

- Diseases of possible microbial origin where a number of different microbes may be involved (postviral fatigue syndrome, exacerbations of multiple sclerosis).
- Diseases that might be infectious, but occur in only a very small proportion of genetically predisposed individuals (rheumatoid arthritis, juvenile diabetes mellitus).

Possible problems in assigning disease etiology

Finally, there are two interesting possibilities that could give problems in assigning disease etiology, although neither have yet been shown to apply to human disease:

- First, in some infections the DNA of the causative virus is integrated into the genome of the host, and is transmitted vertically. It therefore behaves as a genetic attribute. This is known to occur, for instance, with mammary tumor virus in mice.
- Second, the causative microbe triggers off the disease process and then disappears completely from the body and is no longer detectable. This is known to be the case in the cerebellar hypoplasia occurring in hamsters and cats after intrauterine infection with parvovirus. There are no known examples in humans.

The Biologic Response Gradient

It is uncommon for a microbe to cause exactly the same disease in all infected individuals

Hence a physician must be able to make a diagnosis when only some of the possible signs and symptoms are present. The exact clinical picture depends upon many variables such as infecting dose and route, age, sex, presence of other microbes, nutritional status and genetic background. Infections such as measles or cholera give a fairly consistent disease picture, but others such as syphilis cause such a wide spectrum of pathology that Sir William Osler (1849–1919) stated that 'He who knows syphilis, knows medicine'.

There is great variation not only in the nature, but also in the severity of clinical disease. Many infections are asymptomatic in more than 90% of individuals, the clinically characterized illness applying to only an occasional unfortunate host (Fig. 7.7). This illness can be mild or severe. Asymptomatically, infected individuals are important because although they develop immunity and resistance to reinfection, they are not identified, move normally in the community and can infect others. Clearly there is little point in isolating a clinically-infected patient when there is a high frequency of asymptomatically-infected individuals in the community. This phenomenon can be represented as an iceberg (Fig. 7.8).

FREQUENCY OF CLINICALLY-APPARENT DISEASE	
infection	approximate % with clinically-apparent disease*
Pneumocystis carinii	0
poliomyelitis (child)	0.1–1.0
Epstein–Barr virus (1–5 year old child)	1.0**
rubella	50
influenza (young adult)	60
whooping cough typhoid malaria anthrax	>90
gonorrhoea (adult male) measles	99
rabies HIV (?)	100

* on primary infection
** 30–75% in young adults

Fig. 7.7 The likelihood of developing clinical disease often depends upon age and sex, as shown. When there is a lengthy incubation period the proportion with clinical disease may increase with time, from a few per cent to (probably) 100% in the case of HIV.

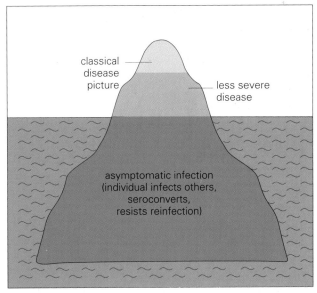

Fig. 7.8 The 'iceberg' concept of infectious disease.

- Faced with host defenses (see Chapters 4–6), the microbes (see Chapters 1–3) have developed mechanisms to bypass them, and in turn the host defenses have had to be modified, although slowly, in response.
- There is a conflict between the microbe and host, and every infectious disease is the result of this ancient conflict. Details of the host–microbe conflict will now be given (see Chapters 8–12), followed by an outline of diagnostic methods (see Chapters 13, 14), and then a central account of infectious diseases according to the body systems involved (see Chapters15–28).
- Speed matters. Every infection is a race between microbial replication and spread and the mobilization of host responses.
- There are four types of infection depending upon whether host defenses are intact or impaired.
- It is sometimes difficult to incriminate a specific microbe as the cause of a disease.
- Microbes do not necessarily produce the same disease in all infected individuals. A biologic response gradient causes a spectrum that can range from an asymptomatic to a lethal infection.

1. How could you prove that a virus was the cause of diabetes mellitus?
2. Everyone dies after developing rabies, so how is this infection maintained in nature?
3. List the steps that a successful microbe must accomplish in the host. Which are the most important?
4. If a virus, for example myxomavirus, has gene products that interfere with immune responses or with the action of a cytokine how could you show that this really mattered in the infected host?
5. Since every infection is a race, what is it that prevents all microbes from completing their infection within a few days?
6. Phagocytes have impressive antimicrobial powers yet many microbes seem to multiply in them. Why is this?

Further Reading

Burnet FM, White DO. *The Natural History of Infectious Disease,* 4th edition. Cambridge: Cambridge University Press, 1972

Falkow W. Koch's postulates applied to microbial pathogenicity. *Rev Inf Dis* **10**:S274, 1988.

Mims CA, Dimmock NJ, Nash A, Stephen J. *Mims' Pathogenesis of Infectious Disease,* 4th edition. London: Academic Press, 1995.

Smith GA. Virus strategies for evasion of the host response to infection. *Trends Microbiol* 1994; **2**:81–88.

Introduction

Microorganisms must attach to, or penetrate, the host's body surfaces

The mammalian host can be considered as a series of body surfaces *(Fig. 8.1)*. To establish themselves on or in the host, microorganisms must either attach to, or penetrate, one of these body surfaces. The outer surface, covered by skin or fur, protects and isolates the body from the outside world, forming a dry, horny, relatively impermeable outer layer. Elsewhere, however, there has to be more intimate contact and exchange with the outside world. Therefore in the alimentary, respiratory and urinogenital tracts, where food is absorbed, gases exchanged and urine and sexual products released, the lining consists of one or more layers of living cells. In the eye, the skin is replaced by a transparent layer of living cells, the conjunctiva. Well-developed cleansing and defense mechanisms are present at all these body surfaces and entry of microorganisms always has to occur in the face of these natural mechanisms. Successful microorganisms therefore possess efficient mechanisms for attaching to, and often traversing, these body surfaces.

Receptor molecules

There are often specific molecules on microbes that bind to receptor molecules on host cells, either at the body surface (viruses, bacteria) or in tissues (viruses). These receptor molecules, of which there may be more than one, are not, of course, present for the benefit of the virus or other infectious agent; they have specific functions in the life of the cell. Very occasionally the receptor molecule is present only in certain cells, which are then uniquely susceptible to infection. Examples include the CD4 molecule for HIV and the C3d receptor (CR_2) for Epstein–Barr virus. In these cases the presence of the receptor molecule determines virus tropism and accounts for the distinctive pattern of infection. Receptors are therefore critical determinants of cell susceptibility, not only at the body surface, but in all tissues. After binding to the susceptible cell, the microorganism can multiply at the surface (mycoplasma, *Bordetella pertussis*) or enter the cell and infect it (viruses, chlamydia; see Chapter 10).

Exit from the body

Microorganisms must also exit from the body if they are to be transmitted to a fresh host. They are either shed in large numbers in secretions and excretions or are available in the blood for uptake, for example by blood-sucking arthropods and needles.

Sites of Entry

Skin

Microorganisms gaining entry via the skin may cause a skin infection or infection elsewhere

Microorganisms infecting or entering the body via the skin are listed in *Figure 8.2*. On the skin, microorganisms other than residents of the normal flora (see Chapter 3) are soon inactivated, especially by fatty acids (skin pH is about 5.5), and probably by substances secreted by sebaceous and other

glands, and materials produced by the normal flora of the skin. Skin bacteria may enter hair follicles or sebaceous glands to cause styes and boils, or teat canals to cause staphylococcal mastitis.

Several types of fungi (the dermatophytes) infect the non-living keratinous structures (stratum corneum, hair, nails) produced by the skin. Infection is established as long as the parasites rate of downward growth into the keratin exceeds the rate of shedding of the keratinous product. When the latter is very slow, as in the case of nails, the infection is more likely to become chronic.

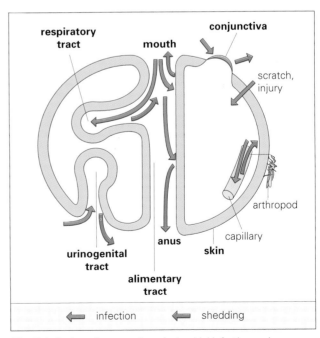

Fig. 8.1 Body surfaces as sites of microbial infection and shedding.

MICROORGANISMS THAT INFECT VIA THE SKIN		
microorganism	**disease**	**comments**
arthropod-borne viruses	various fevers	150 distinct viruses, transmitted by bite of infected arthropod bites
rabies virus	rabies	bite from infected animals
wart viruses	warts	infection restricted to epidermis
staphylococci	boils, etc	commonest skin invaders
Rickettsia	typhus, spotted fevers	infestation with infected arthropod
Leptospira	leptospirosis	contact with water containing infected animals' urine
streptococci	impetigo, erysipelas	concurrent pharyngeal infection in one-third of cases
Bacillus anthracis	cutaneous anthrax	systemic disease following local lesion at inoculation site
Treponema pallidum and *T. pertenue*	syphilis, yaws	warm, moist skin more susceptible
Yersinia pestis, Plasmodia	plague, malaria	bite from infected rodent flea or mosquito
Trichophyton spp. and other fungi	ringworm, athletes foot	infection restricted to skin, nails, hair
Ankylostoma duodenale (or *Necator americanus*)	hookworm	silent entry of larvae through skin of e.g. foot
filarial nematodes	filariasis	bite from infected mosquito, midge, blood-sucking fly
Schistosoma spp.	schistosomiasis	larvae (cercariae) from infected snail penetrate skin during wading or bathing

Fig. 8.2 Microorganisms that infect via the skin. Some remain restricted to the skin (wart viruses, ringworm), while others enter the body after growth in the skin (syphilis) or after mechanical transfer across the skin (arthropod-borne infections, schistosomiasis).

Wounds, abrasions or burns are more common sites of infection. Even a small break in the skin can be a portal of entry if virulent microorganisms such as streptococci, leptospira or hepatitis B virus are present at the site. A few microbes, such as leptospira or the larvae of *Ankylostoma* and *Schistosoma*, are able to traverse the unbroken skin by their own activity.

Biting arthropods

Biting arthropods such as mosquitoes, ticks, fleas and sandflies (see Chapter 26) penetrate the skin during feeding and can thus introduce infectious agents or parasites into the body. The arthropod transmits the infection and is an essential part of the life cycle of the microorganism. Sometimes the transmission is mechanical, the microorganism contaminating the mouth parts without multiplying in the arthropod. In most cases, however, the infectious agent multiplies in the arthropod and as a result of millions of years of adaptation causes little or no damage to that host. After an incubation period it appears in the saliva or feces and is transmitted during a blood feed. The mosquito for instance, injects saliva directly into host tissues as an anticoagulant, whereas the human body louse defecates as it feeds and *Rickettsia rickettsii*, which is present in the feces, is introduced into the bite wound when the host scratches the affected area.

The conjunctiva

The conjunctiva can be regarded as a specialized area of skin. It is kept clean by the continuous flushing action of tears, aided every few seconds by the windscreen wiper action of the eyelids. Therefore the microorganisms that infect the normal conjunctiva (chlamydia, gonococci) must have efficient attachment mechanisms (see Chapter 16). Interference with local defenses due to decreased lacrimal gland secretion or conjunctival or eyelid damage allows even non-specialist microorganisms to establish themselves.

Respiratory tract

Some microorganisms can overcome the respiratory tract's cleansing mechanisms

Air normally contains suspended particles, including smoke, dust and microorganisms. Efficient cleansing mechanisms (see Chapters 15 and 17) deal with these constantly inhaled particles. With about 500–1000 microorganisms per m^3 inside buildings, and a ventilation rate of 6 l/min at rest, as many as 10 000 microorganisms per day are introduced into the lungs. In the upper or lower respiratory tract inhaled microorganisms, like other particles, will be entrapped in mucus, carried to the back of the throat by ciliary action, and swallowed. Those that invade the normal healthy respiratory tract have developed specific mechanisms to avoid this fate.

Interfering with cleansing mechanisms

The ideal strategy is to attach firmly to the surfaces of cells forming the mucociliary sheet. Specific molecules on the organism (often called adhesins) bind to receptor molecules on the susceptible cell *(Fig. 8.3)*. Examples of such respiratory infections are given in *Figure 8.4*.

Inhibiting ciliary activity is another way of interfering with cleansing mechanisms. This helps invading microorganisms establish themselves in the respiratory tract. *B. pertussis* for instance not only attaches to respiratory epithelial cells, but also interferes with ciliary activity, while other bacteria *(Fig. 8.5)* produce various ciliostatic substances of generally unknown nature.

Avoiding destruction by alveolar macrophages

Inhaled microorganisms reaching the alveoli encounter alveolar macrophages, which remove foreign particles and keep the air spaces clean. Most microorganisms are destroyed by these macrophages, but one or two pathogens have learnt either to avoid phagocytosis or to avoid destruction after phagocytosis. Tubercle bacilli, for instance, survive in the macrophages and respiratory tuberculosis is thought to be initiated in this way. The vital role of macrophages in antimicrobial defenses is dealt with more thoroughly in Chapter 9.

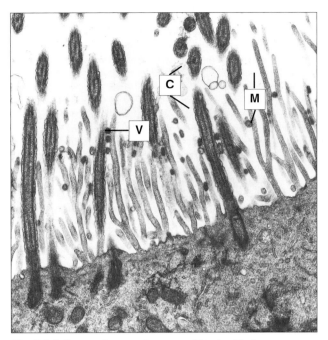

Fig. 8.3 Influenza virus attachment to ciliated epithelium. Influenza virus particles (V) attached to cilia (C) and microvilli (M). Electron micrograph of thin section from organ culture of guinea pig trachea one hour after addition of the virus. (Courtesy of RE Dourmashkin.)

Alveolar macrophages are damaged following inhalation of toxic asbestos particles and certain dusts, and this leads to increased susceptibility to respiratory tuberculosis.

MICROBIAL ATTACHMENT IN THE RESPIRATORY TRACT			
microorganism	disease	microbial adhesin	receptor on host cell
influenza virus	influenza	hemagglutinin	neuraminic acid-containing glycoprotein
rhinovirus, coxsackie A viruses	common cold	capsid protein	ICAM-1-type molecule
parainfluenza virus type 1 respiratory syncytial virus	respiratory illness	envelope protein	glycoside
Mycoplasma pneumoniae	atypical pneumonia	mycoplasmal molecule on 'foot'	neuraminic acid
Haemophilus influenzae Strep pneumoniae Klebsiella pneumoniae	respiratory disease	surface molecule	carbohydrate sequence in glycolipid
measles virus	measles	hemagglutinin	CD46

Fig. 8.4 Microbial attachment in the respiratory tract. (ICAM-1 intercellular adhesion molecule-1, CD46 = membrane cofactor protein involved in complement regulation.)

INTERFERENCE WITH CILIARY ACTIVITY IN RESPIRATORY INFECTIONS		
cause	**mechanisms**	**importance**
infecting bacteria interfere with ciliary activity (B. pertussis, H influenzae, P. aeruginosa, M. pneumoniae)	production of ciliostatic substance (tracheal cytotoxin from B. pertussis, at least 2 substances from H influenzae, at least 7 from P. aeruginosa	++
viral infection	ciliated cell dysfunction or destruction by influenza, measles	+++
atmospheric pollution (automobiles, cigarette smoking, etc.)	acutely impaired mucociliary function	?+
inhalation of unhumidified air (indwelling tracheal tubes, general anesthesia)	acutely impaired mucociliary function	+
chronic bronchitis cystic fibrosis	chronically impaired mucociliary function	+++

Fig. 8.5 Interference with ciliary activity in respiratory infections. Although microbes can actively interfere with ciliary activity (first item), a more general impairment of mucociliary function also acts as a predisposing cause of respiratory infection.

Gastrointestinal tract

Some microorganisms can survive the intestine's defenses of acid, mucus and enzymes

Apart from the general flow of intestinal contents, there are no particular cleansing mechanisms in the intestinal tract, except in so far as diarrhea and vomiting can be included in this category. Under normal circumstances, multiplication of resident bacteria is counterbalanced by their continuous passage to the exterior with the rest of the intestinal contents. Ingestion of a small number of non-pathogenic bacteria followed by growth in the lumen of the alimentary canal produces only relatively small numbers within 12–18 hours, the normal intestinal transit time.

Infecting bacteria must attach themselves to the intestinal epithelium *(Fig. 8.6)* if they are to establish themselves and multiply in large numbers. They will then avoid being carried straight down the alimentary canal to be excreted with the rest of the intestinal contents. The concentration of microorganisms in feces depends on the balance between the production and removal of bacteria in the intestine. Therefore *Vibrio cholerae (Figs 8.7, 8.8)* and the rotaviruses both establish specific binding to receptors on the surface of intestinal epithelial cells. For *V. cholerae*, establishment in sur-

face mucus may be sufficient for infection and pathogenicity. The fact that certain microbes infect mainly the large bowel *(Shigella* spp.) or small intestine (most salmonellae, rotaviruses) indicates the presence of specific receptor molecules on epithelial cells in these sections of the alimentary canal.

Crude mechanical devices for attachment

Crude mechanical devices are used for the attachment and entry of certain parasitic protozoans and worms. *Giardia lamblia*, for example, has specific molecules for adhesion to the microvilli of epithelial cells, but also has its own microvillar sucking disc. Hookworms attach to the intestinal mucosa by means of a large mouth capsule containing hooked teeth or cutting plates. Other worms (e.g. *Ascaris*) maintain their position by 'bracing' themselves against peristalsis, while tapeworms adhere closely to the mucus covering the intestinal wall, the anterior hooks and sucker playing a relatively minor role for the largest worms. A number of worms actively penetrate into the mucosa as adults (*Trichinella, Trichuris*) or traverse the gut wall to enter deeper tissues (e.g. the embryos of *Trichinella* released from the female worm and the larvae of *Echinococcus* hatched from ingested eggs).

MICROBIAL ATTACHMENT IN THE INTESTINAL TRACT			
microorganism	**disease**	**attachment site**	**mechanism**
poliovirus	poliomyelitis	intestinal epithelium	viral capsid protein reacts with specific receptor on cell (perhaps ICAM*)
rotavirus	diarrhea	intestinal epithelium	viral outer capsid protein binds to glypolipid receptor on cell
Vibrio cholerae	cholera	intestinal epithelium	specific bacterial molecule (adhesin)** binds to fucose/ mannose receptor on cell
Escherichia coli (certain strains)	diarrhea		
Salmonella typhi	enteric fever		
Shigella spp.	dysentery	colonic epithelium	unknown***
Giardia lamblia	diarrhea	duodenal, jejunal epithelium	protozoa bind to mannose-D phosphate on host cell; also have mechanical sucker
Entamoeba histolytica	dysentery	colonic epithelium	lectin on surface of amoebae binds to asialofetuin on host cell
Ankylostoma duodenale	hookworm	intestinal epithelium	four hooks

* intracellular adhesion molecule; has important functions in inflammatory and 'social' life of cells; acts as receptor molecule for poliovirus on cells *in vitro*
** often on pili or fimbriae (e.g. up to 200 pili, each bearing adhesins, on *E. coli*)
*** after attachment *Shigella* (and other pathogenic bacteria) induces epithelial cell to engulf it

Fig. 8.6 Microbial attachment in the intestinal tract.

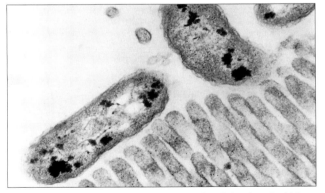

Fig. 8.7 Attachment of *Vibrio cholerae* to brush border of rabbit villus. Thin section electron micrograph, ×10 000. (Courtesy of ET Nelson.)

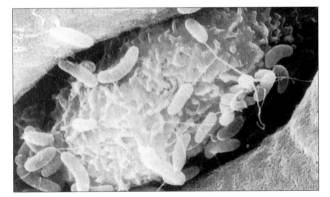

Fig. 8.8 Adherence of *Vibrio cholerae* to M cells in human ileal mucosa. (Courtesy of T Yamamoto.)

Mechanisms to counteract mucus, acids, enzymes and bile

Successful intestinal microbes must counteract or resist mucus, acids, enzymes and bile.

Mucus protects epithelial cells, perhaps acting as a mechanical barrier to infection. It may contain molecules that bind to microbial adhesins, therefore blocking attachment to host cells. It also contains secretory IgA antibodies, which protect the immune individual against infection. Motile microorganisms (*V. cholerae*, salmonellae and certain strains of *Escherichia coli*) can propel themselves through the mucus layer and are therefore more likely to reach epithelial cells to make specific attachments; *V. cholerae* also produces a mucinase, which probably helps its passage through the mucus. Non-motile microorganisms, in contrast, rely on random and passive transport in the mucus layer.

As might be expected, microorganisms that infect by the intestinal route are often capable of surviving in the presence of acid, proteolytic enzymes and bile. This also applies to microorganisms shed from the body by this route *(Fig. 8.9)*.

All organisms infecting by the intestinal route must run the gauntlet of acid in the stomach. The fact that tubercle bacilli resist acid conditions favors the establishment of intestinal tuberculosis, but most bacteria are acid sensitive and prefer slightly alkaline conditions. For instance, volunteers who drank different doses of *V. cholerae* contained in 60 ml saline showed a 10 000-fold increase in susceptibility to cholera when 2 g of sodium bicarbonate was given with the bacteria. The minimum disease-producing dose was 10^8 bacteria without bicarbonate and 10^4 bacteria with bicarbonate. Similar experiments have been carried out in volunteers with *Salmonella typhi* and the minimum infectious dose of 1000–10 000 bacteria was again significantly reduced by the ingestion of sodium bicarbonate.

When the infecting microorganism penetrates the intestinal epithelium (*Shigella*, *S. typhi*, hepatitis A and other enteroviruses) the final pathogenicity depends upon:

* Subsequent multiplication and spread.
* Toxin production.
* Cell damage.
* Inflammatory and immune responses.

Microbial exotoxin, endotoxin and protein absorption

Microbial exotoxins, endotoxins and proteins can be absorbed from the intestine on a small scale. Diarrhea generally promotes the uptake of protein, and absorption of protein also takes place more readily in the infant, which in some species needs to absorb antibodies from milk. As well as large molecules, particles the size of viruses can also be taken up from the intestinal lumen. This occurs in certain sites in particular, such as those where Peyer's patches occur. Peyer's patches are isolated collections of lymphoid tissue lying immediately below the intestinal epithelium, which in this region is highly specialized, consisting of so-called M cells. M cells take up particles and foreign proteins and deliver them to underlying immune cells with which they are intimately associated by cytoplasmic processes.

Urinogenital tract

Microorganisms gaining entry via the urinogenital tract can spread easily from one part of the tract to another

The urinogenital tract is a continuum, so microorganisms can spread easily from one part to another and the distinction between vaginitis and urethritis, or between urethritis and cystitis is not always easy or necessary (see Chapters 18 and 19).

Vaginal defenses

The vagina has no particular cleansing mechanisms and repeated introductions of a contaminated, sometimes

MICROBIAL SUCCESS IN THE GASTROINTESTINAL TRACT		
property	**examples**	**consequence**
specific attachment to intestinal epithelium	poliovirus, rotavirus, *Vibrio cholerae*	microorganism avoids expulsion with other gut contents and can establish infection
motility	*V. cholerae*, certain *Escherichia coli* strains	bacteria travel through mucus and are more likely to reach susceptible cell
production of mucinase (neuraminidase)	*V. cholerae*	may assist transit through mucus
acid resistance	*Mycobacterium tuberculosis*	encourages intestinal tuberculosis (acid labile microorganisms depend on protection in food bolus or in diluting fluid) increased susceptibility in individuals with achlorhydria
	enteroviruses (hepatitis A, poliovirus, coxsackieviruses, echoviruses)	infection and shedding from gastrointestinal tract
bile resistance	*Salmonella*, *Shigella*, enteroviruses	intestinal pathogens
	Enterococcus faecalis, *E. coli*, *Proteus*, *Pseudomonas*	establish residence
resistance to proteolytic enzymes	reoviruses in mice	permits oral infection
anaerobic growth	*Bacteroides fragilis*	most common resident bacteria in anaerobic environment of colon

Fig. 8.9 Microbial properties that aid success in the gastrointestinal tract.

pathogen-bearing foreign object (the penis), makes the vagina particularly vulnerable to infection, forming the basis for sexually transmitted diseases (see Chapter 19). Nature has responded by providing additional defenses. During reproductive life, the vaginal epithelium contains glycogen due to the action of circulating estrogens, and certain lactobacilli colonize the vagina, metabolizing the glycogen to produce lactic acid. As a result the normal vaginal pH is about 5.0, which inhibits colonization by all except the lactobacilli and certain other streptococci and diphtheroids. Normal vaginal secretions contain up to 10^8/ml of these commensal bacteria. If other microorganisms are to colonize and invade they must either have specific mechanisms for attaching to vaginal or cervical mucosa or take advantage of minute local injuries during coitus (genital warts, syphilis) or impaired defenses (presence of tampons, estrogen imbalance). These are the microorganisms responsible for sexually transmitted diseases.

Urethral and bladder defenses

The regular flushing action of urine is a major urethral defense and urine in the bladder is normally sterile.

The bladder is more than an inert receptacle and in its wall there are intrinsic, but poorly understood, defense mechanisms. These include a protective layer of mucus and the ability to generate inflammatory responses and produce secretory antibodies and immune cells.

Mechanism of urinary tract invasion

The urinary tract is nearly always invaded from the exterior via the urethra and an invading microorganism must first and foremost avoid being washed out during urination. Specialized attachment mechanisms have therefore been developed by successful invaders (e.g. gonococci, *Fig. 8.10*). A defined peptide on the bacterial pili binds to a carbohydrate polymer on the urethral cell, and the cell is then induced to engulf the bacterium. This is referred to as parasite-directed endocytosis and also occurs with chlamydia.

Sexual anatomy is a major determinant of urinogenital infection *(Fig. 8.11)*. Spread to the bladder is no easy task in the male, where the flaccid urethra is 20 cm long. Therefore urinary infections are rare in males unless organisms are introduced by catheters or when the flushing activity of urine is impaired (see Chapter 18). Things are different in females. Not only is the urethra much shorter (5 cm), but it is also very close to the anus *(Fig. 8.11)*, which is a constant source of intestinal bacteria. Urinary infections are about 14 times more common in women and at least 20% of women have a symptomatic urinary tract infection at some time during their life. The invading bacteria often begin their invasion by colonizing the mucosa around the urethra and probably have special attachment mechanisms to cells in this area. Bacterial invasion is favored by the mechanical deformation of the urethra and surrounding region that occurs during sexual intercourse, which can lead to urethritis and cystitis. Bacteriuria is about 10 times more common in sexually active women than in nuns.

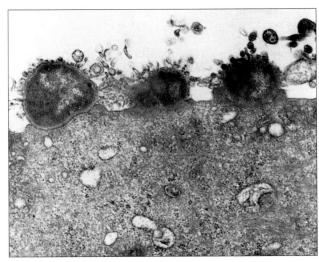

Fig. 8.10 Adherence of gonococci to the surface of a human urethral epithelial cell. (Courtesy of PJ Watt.)

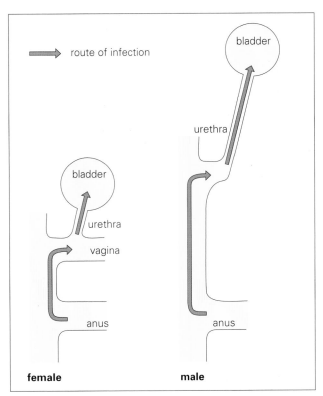

Fig. 8.11 The female urinogenital tract is particularly vulnerable to infection, due mainly to topographic considerations as the urethra is shorter and nearer to the anus.

Oropharynx

Microorganisms can invade the oropharynx when mucosal resistance is reduced

Commensal microorganisms in the oropharynx are described in Chapter 15.

Oropharyngeal defenses

The flushing action of saliva provides a natural cleansing mechanism (about 1 l/day is produced, needing 400 swallows), aided by masticatory and other movements of the tongue, cheek and lips. On the other hand, material borne backwards from the nasopharynx is firmly wiped against the pharynx by the tongue during swallowing and microbes therefore have an opportunity to enter the body at this site. Additional defenses include secretory IgA antibodies, antimicrobial substances such as lysozyme, the normal flora, and the antimicrobial activities of leukocytes present on mucosal surfaces and in saliva.

Mechanisms of oropharyngeal invasion

Attaching to mucosal or tooth surfaces is obligatory for invading microorganisms (and also for residents). For instance, different types of streptococci make specific attachments via lipoteichoic acid molecules on their pili to the buccal epithelium and tongue (resident *Streptococcus salivarius*), to teeth (resident *S. mutans*), or to pharyngeal epithelium (invading *S. pyogenes*).

\multicolumn{5}{c}{TYPES OF INFECTION AND THEIR ROLE IN TRANSMISSION}
type of infection	host defenses	microbial evasion mechanism	examples	value of infection in transmission
respiratory tract	mucociliary clearance	adhere to epithelial cells interfere with ciliary action	influenza virus pertussis	essential
	alveolar macrophage	replicate in alveolar macrophage	*Legionella*, tuberculosis	essential
intestinal tract	mucus, peristalsis	adhere to epithelial cells	rotavirus, *Salmonella*	essential
	acid, bile	resist acid, bile	poliovirus	essential
liver	Kupffer cells and endothelial cells	localize in sinusoid bypass Kupffer cells and endothelial cells	hepatitis viruses	essential: • microbe from liver → bile → gut (hepatitis A); • microbe from liver → blood (hepatitis B, yellow fever)
reproductive tract	flushing action of urine and sexual secretions, mucosal defenses	adhere to urethral/vaginal epithelial cells	gonococcus, *Chlamydia*	essential
urinary tract	flushing action of urine	adhere to urethral/epithelial cells	*Escherichia coli*	no value
		reach urine from tubular epithelium	polyomavirus	valuable
central nervous system	enclosed in bony 'box' of skull and vertebral column	reach CNS via nerves or blood vessels that enter skull or vertebral column	bacterial meningitis, viral encephalitis (e.g. rabies)	no value (except rabies)
skin, mucosa	layers of constantly shed cells (mucosa) dead keratinized cell layers (skin)	invade skin/mucosa from below	varicella, measles	essential
		infect basal epidermal layer	papillomaviruses	essential
		infect via minor abrasions	staphylococci, streptococci	valuable
		penetrate intact skin	schistosomiasis, ankylostomiasis, anthrax	essential
vascular system	skin	injection of microbe by biting vector replication blood cells or in vascular endothelial cells	malaria, yellow fever	essential

Fig. 8.12 Types of infection. For each type of host defense the successful microbe has an answer, which may or may not be important for transmission.

Factors that reduce mucosal resistance allow commensal and other bacteria to invade, as in the case of gum infections due to vitamin C deficiency or *Candida* invasion (thrush) due to changed resident flora after broad-spectrum antibiotics. When salivary flow is decreased for 3–4 hours, as between meals, there is a fourfold increase in the number of bacteria in saliva (see Chapter 15). In dehydrated patients salivary flow is greatly reduced and the mouth soon becomes overgrown with bacteria. As at all body surfaces, there is a shifting boundary between good behavior by residents and tissue invasion according to changes in host defenses.

Exit and Transmission

Microorganisms have a variety of mechanisms to ensure exit from the host and transmission

Successful microbes must leave the body and then be transmitted to fresh hosts. Highly pathogenic microbes (e.g. Ebola virus, *Legionella pneumophila*) will have little impact on host populations if their transmission is uncommon or ineffective. Nearly all microbes are shed from body surfaces, this being the route of exit to the outside world. Some,

MICROBIAL RESISTANCE TO DRYING AS A FACTOR IN TRANSMISSION		
stability on drying	**examples**	**consequence**
stable	tubercle bacilli staphylococci	spread more readily in air (dust, dried droplets)
	clostridial spores anthrax spores histoplasmal spores	spread readily from soil
unstable	*Neisseria meningitidis* streptococci *Bordetella pertussis* common cold viruses influenza virus measles	require close (respiratory) contact
	gonococci HIV *Treponema pallidum*	require close (sexual) contact
	polioviruses hepatitis A *Vibrio cholerae* leptospira	spread via water, food
	yellow fever virus malaria trypanosomes	spread via vectors (i.e. remain in a host)
	larvae/eggs of worms	need moist soil (except pinworms)

Fig. 8.13 Microbial resistance to drying as a factor in transmission. Microbes that are already dehydrated such as spores and artificially freeze-dried viruses are also more resistant to thermal inactivation. Spores can survive for years in soil.

however, are extracted from inside the body by vectors, for example the blood-sucking arthropods that transmit yellow fever, malaria and filarial worms. *Figure 8.12* lists the types of infection and their value in the transmission of the microbe and provides a summary of the host defenses and the ways in which they are evaded. Transfer from one host to another forms the basis for the epidemiology of infectious disease (see Chapter 33).

Transmission depends upon three factors:
- The number of microorganisms shed.
- The microorganism's stability in the environment.
- The number of microorganisms required to infect a fresh host (the efficiency of the infection).

Number of microorganisms shed

Obviously the more virus particles, bacteria, protozoa and eggs that are shed, the greater the chance of reaching a fresh host. There are, however, many hazards. Most of the shed microorganisms die, and only an occasional one survives to perpetuate the species.

Stability in the environment

Microorganisms that resist drying spread more rapidly in the environment than those that are sensitive to drying *(Fig. 8.13)*. Microorganisms also remain infectious for longer periods in the external environment when they are resistant to thermal inactivation. Certain microorganisms have developed special forms (e.g. clostridial spores, amebic cysts) that enable them to resist drying, heat inactivation and chemical insults, and this testifies to the importance of stability in the environment. If still alive, microorganisms are more thermostable when they have dried. Drying directly from the frozen state (freeze-drying) can make them very resistant to environmental temperatures. The fact that spores and cysts are dehydrated accounts for much of their stability. Microorganisms that are sensitive to drying depend upon close contact, vectors, or contamination of food and water for spread.

Number of microorganisms required to infect a fresh host

The efficiency of the infection varies greatly between microorganisms, and helps explain many aspects of transmission. For instance, volunteers ingesting 10 *Shigella dysenteriae* bacteria (from other humans) will become infected, whereas as many as 10^6 *Salmonella* spp. (from animals) are needed to cause food poisoning. The route of infection also matters. A single tissue culture infectious dose of a human rhinovirus instilled into the nasal cavity causes a common cold, and although this dose contains many virus particles, about 200 such doses are needed when applied to the pharynx. As few as 10 gonococci can establish an infection in the urethra, but many thousand times this number are needed to infect the mucosa of the oropharynx or rectum.

Other factors affecting transmission

Genetic factors in microorganisms also influence transmission. Some strains of a given microorganism are therefore more readily transmitted than others, although the exact mechanism is often unclear. Transmission can vary independently of the ability to do damage and cause disease (pathogenicity or virulence).

Activities of the infected host may increase the efficiency of shedding and transmission. Coughing and sneezing are reflex activities that benefit the host by clearing foreign material from the upper and lower respiratory tract, but they also benefit the microorganism. Strains of microorganism that are more able to increase fluid secretions or irritate respiratory epithelium will induce more coughing and sneezing than those less able and will be transmitted more effectively. They will therefore be positively selected for. Similar arguments can be applied to the equivalent intestinal activity – diarrhea. Although diarrhea eliminates the infection more rapidly (prevention of diarrhea often prolongs intestinal infection), from the microbe's point of view it is a highly effective way of contaminating the environment and spreading to fresh hosts.

Microorganisms can be transmitted to humans by humans, vertebrates and biting arthropods

Types of Transmission

Transmission is most effective when it takes place directly from human to human. The commonest, worldwide infections are spread by the respiratory, fecal–oral or venereal routes. A separate set of infections are acquired from animals, either directly from vertebrates (the zoonoses) or from biting arthropods. Infections acquired from other species are either not transmitted or transmit very poorly from human to human. Types of transmission are illustrated in Figure 8.14.

Transmission from the respiratory tract
Respiratory infections spread rapidly when people are crowded together indoors
An increase in nasal secretions with sneezing and coughing promotes effective shedding from the nasal cavity. In a sneeze *(Fig. 8.15)* up to 20 000 droplets are produced, and during a common cold, for instance, many of them will contain virus particles.

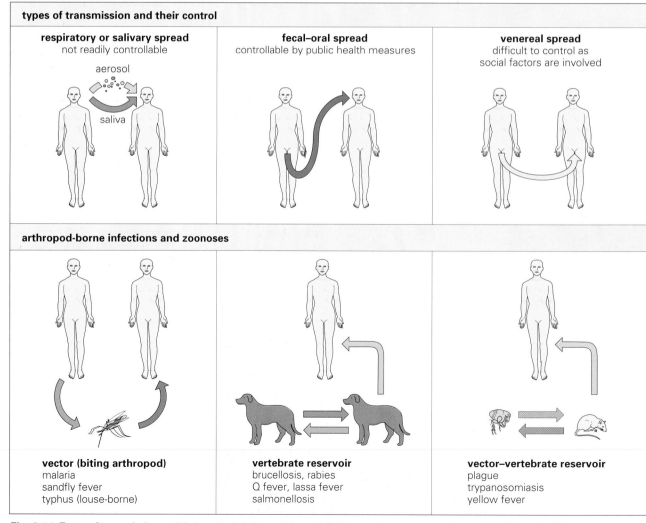

Fig. 8.14 Types of transmission and their control. Arthropod-borne infections and zoonoses can be controlled by controlling vectors or by controlling animal infection. There is virtually no person to person transmission of these infections.

A smaller number of microorganisms (hundreds) are expelled from the mouth, throat, larynx and lungs during coughing (whooping cough, tuberculosis). Talking is a less important source of airborne particles, but does produce them, especially when the consonants f, p, t and s are used. It is surely no accident that many of the most abusive words in the English language begin with these letters, so that a spray of droplets (possibly infectious) is delivered with the abuse!

The size of inhaled droplets determines their initial localization. The largest droplets fall to the ground after traveling approximately 4 m and the rest settle according to size. Those up to 10 mm in diameter can be trapped on the nasal mucosa. The smallest (1–4 mm diameter) are kept suspended for an indefinite period by normal air movements, and it is particles of this size that are likely to pass the turbinate baffles in the nose and reach the lower respiratory tract.

When people are crowded together indoors respiratory infections spread rapidly, for example the common cold in schools and offices and meningococcal infections in military recruits. This is perhaps why respiratory infections are common in winter. The air in ill-ventilated rooms is also more humid, favoring survival of suspended microorganisms such as streptococci and enveloped viruses. Air conditioning is another factor, as the dry air leads to impaired mucociliary activity. Respiratory spread is, in one sense, unique. Material from one person's respiratory tract can be taken up almost immediately into the respiratory tract of other individuals. This is in striking contrast to the material expelled from the gastrointestinal tract, and helps explain why respiratory infections spread so rapidly when people are indoors.

Handkerchiefs, hands and other objects can carry respiratory infection such as common cold viruses from one individual to another, although coughs and sneezes provide a more dramatic route. Transmission from the infected conjunctiva is referred to in Chapter 16.

The presence of receptors *(Fig 8.4)* and local temperature as well as initial localization can determine which part of the respiratory tract is infected. For instance, it can be assumed that rhinoviruses arrive in the lower respiratory tract on a large scale, but fail to grow there because, like leprosy bacilli, they prefer the cooler temperature of the nasal mucosa.

Transmission from the gastrointestinal tract
Intestinal infection spreads easily if public health and hygiene are poor

The spread of an intestinal infection is assured if public health and hygiene are poor, the microbe appears in the feces in sufficient numbers and there are susceptible individuals in the vicinity. Diarrhea gives it an additional advantage, and the key role of diarrhea in transmission has been referred to above. During most of human history there has been a large scale recycling of fecal material back into the mouth and this continues in developing countries. The attractiveness of the fecal–oral route for microorganisms and parasites is reflected in the great variety that are transmitted in this way.

Intestinal infections have been to some extent controlled in developed countries. The great public health reforms of the nineteenth century led to the introduction of adequate sewage disposal and a supply of purified water. For instance, in England 200 years ago there were no flushing toilets and no sewage disposal and much of the drinking water was contaminated. Cholera and typhoid spread easily, and in London the Thames became an open sewer. Nowadays, as in other cities, a complex underground disposal system separates sewage from drinking water. Intestinal infections are still transmitted in developed countries, but via food and fingers rather than by water and flies. Therefore, although each year in the UK there are dozens of cases of typhoid

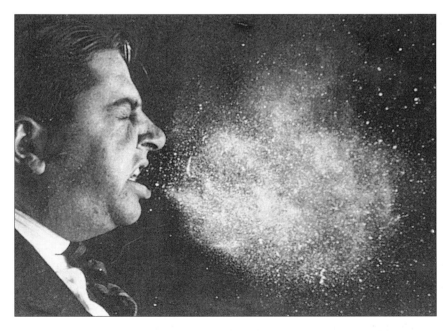

Fig. 8.15 Droplet dispersal following a violent sneeze. Most of the 20 000 particles seen are coming from the mouth. (Courtesy of the American Association for the Advancement of Science.)

acquired on visits to developing countries, the infection is not transmitted to others.

The microorganisms that appear in feces usually multiply in the lumen or wall of the intestinal tract, but there are a few that are shed into bile. For instance, hepatitis A (enterovirus 72) enters bile after replicating in liver cells.

Transmission from the urinogenital tract
Urinogenital tract infections are often sexually transmitted

Urinary tract infections are common, but most are not spread via urine. Urine can contaminate food, drink and living space. Those infections that are spread by urine are listed in *Figure 8.16*.

Sexually transmitted diseases (STDs)

Microorganisms shed from the urinogenital tract are often transmitted as a result of mucosal contact with susceptible individuals. They are therefore transmitted as a result of sexual activity. If there is a discharge, organisms are carried over the epithelial surfaces and transmission is more likely. Some of the most successful sexually transmitted microorganisms (gonococci, chlamydia) therefore induce a discharge. Other microorganisms are transmitted effectively from mucosal sores (ulcers), for example *Treponema pallidum* and herpes simplex virus. The human papillomaviruses are transmitted from genital warts or from foci of infection in the cervix where the epithelium, although apparently normal, is dysplastic and contains infected cells (see Chapter 19).

The transmission of STDs is determined by social and sexual activity. Recent changes in the size of the human population and way of life have had a dramatic effect on the epidemiology of STDs. People now have an increased number of sexual partners due to increasing population density, increased movement of people, the decline of the idea that sexual activity is sinful and the knowledge that (except AIDS) STDs are treatable and pregnancy is avoidable. In addition, the contraceptive pill has favored the spread of STDs by discouraging the use of mechanical barriers to conception. Condoms have been shown to reliably retain herpes simplex virus, HIV, chlamydia and gonococci in simulated coital tests of the syringe and plunger type (see Chapter 19).

STDs are, however, transmitted with far less speed and efficiency than respiratory or intestinal infections. Influenza can be transmitted to a multitude of others during one hour in a crowded room or a rotavirus to a score of children during a morning at kindergarten, but STDs can only spread to each person by a separate sexual act. Promiscuity is therefore essential. Frequent sexual activity is not enough without promiscuity because stable partners can do no more than infect each other. The increased general level of promiscuity in society together with the huge numbers of sexual partners of certain individuals such as prostitutes has led to a dramatic rise in the incidence of STDs.

As almost all mucosal surfaces of the body can be involved in sexual activity, microorganisms have had increasing opportunity to infect new body sites. The meningococcus, a nasopharyngeal resident, has therefore sometimes been recovered from the cervix, the male urethra, and the anal canal, while occasionally gonococcus and chlamydia infect the throat and anal canal. The possibilities are illustrated in all their complexity in *Figure 8.17*, apparently limited only by anatomic considerations. It is no surprise that genito-oro-anal contacts have sometimes allowed intestinal infections such as salmonella, giardia, hepatitis A, shigella, and pathogenic amoebae to spread directly between individuals despite good sanitation and sewage disposal.

HUMAN INFECTIONS TRANSMITTED VIA URINE		
infection	details	value in transmission
schistosomiasis	parasite eggs excreted in bladder	+++
typhoid	bacterial persistence in bladder scarred by schistosomiasis	+
polyomavirus infection	commonly excreted in urine in normal pregnancy	?
cytomegalovirus infection	commonly excreted in infected children	?
leptospirosis	infected rats and dogs excrete bacteria in urine	++
lassa fever (and South American hemorrhagic fevers)	persistently infected rodent excretes virus in urine	+++

Fig. 8.16 Human infections transmitted via urine. Schistosomiasis is the major infection transmitted in this way, the eggs undergoing development in snails before reinfecting humans. Viruses are shed in the urine after infecting tubular epithelial cells in the kidney.

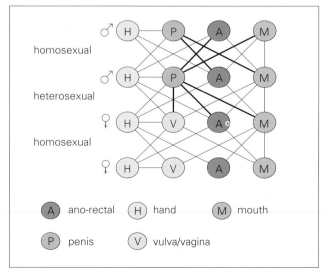

Fig. 8.17 The mechanisms of sexual transmission of infection. (Redrawn from Wilcox, 1981.)

Semen as a source of infection
It might be expected that semen is involved in the transmission of infection, and this is the case in viral infections of animals such as blue tongue and foot and mouth disease. In humans, cytomegalovirus is often present in large quantities in semen, and the fact that it is also recoverable from the cervix suggests that it is sexually transmitted. Hepatitis B and HIV are also present in semen, and although the quantities are probably small, this presence plays a role in both homosexual and heterosexual transmission.

Perinatal transmission
The female genital tract can also be a source of infection for the newborn child (see Chapter 21). During passage down an infected birth canal microorganisms can be wiped onto the conjunctiva of the infant or inhaled, leading to a variety of conditions such as conjunctivitis, pneumonia and bacterial meningitis.

Transmission from the oropharynx
Oropharyngeal infections are often spread in saliva
Saliva is often the vehicle of transmission. Microorganisms such as streptococci and tubercle bacilli reach saliva during upper and lower respiratory tract infections, while certain viruses infect the salivary glands and are transmitted in this way. Paramyxovirus, herpes simplex virus, cytomegalovirus and human herpesvirus type 6 are shed into saliva. In young children, fingers and other objects are regularly contaminated by saliva and each of these infections is acquired by this route. Epstein–Barr virus is also shed into saliva, but is to be transmitted less effectively, perhaps because it is present only in cells or in small amounts. In developed countries people often escape infection during childhood, and become infected as adolescents or adults during the extensive salivary exchanges (mean 4.2 ml/h) that accompany deep kissing (see Chapter 24). Saliva from animals is the source of a few infections and these are included in *Fig. 8.18*.

Transmission from the skin
Skin can spread infection by shedding or direct contact
Dermatophytes (ringworm fungi) are shed from skin and also from hair and nails, the exact source depending on the type of fungus (see Chapter 23). Skin is also an important source of certain other bacteria and viruses, as outlined in *Figure 8.19*.

Shedding to the environment
The normal individual sheds desquamated skin scales into the environment at a rate of about 5×10^8/day, the rate

HUMAN INFECTIONS TRANSMITTED VIA SALIVA	
microorganism	comments
herpes simplex paramyxovirus	infection generally during childhood
cytomegalovirus Epstein–Barr virus	adolescent/adult infection is common
rabies virus	shed in saliva of infected dogs, wolves, jackals, vampire bats, etc
Pasteurella multocida	bacteria in upper respiratory tract of dogs, cats, etc appears in saliva and transmitted via bites, scratches
Streptobacillus moniliformis	present in rat saliva and infects man (rat bite fever)

Fig. 8.18 Human infections transmitted via saliva.

INFECTIONS TRANSMITTED FROM THE SKIN		
microorganism	disease	comments
staphylococci	boils, carbuncles, etc, neonatal skin sepsis	pathogenicity varies, skin lesions or nose picking are common sources of infection
Treponema pallidum	syphilis	mucosal surfaces more infectious than skin
Treponema pertenue	yaws	regular transmission from skin lesions
Streptococcus pyogenes	impetigo	vesicular (epidermal) lesions crusting over, common in children in hot, humid climates
Staphylococcus aureus	impetigo	less common; bullous lesions, especially in newborn
dermatophytes	skin ringworm	different species infect skin, hair, nails
herpes simplex virus	herpes simplex, cold sore	up to 10^6 infectious units per ml of vesicle fluid
varicella-zoster virus	varicella, zoster	vesicular skin lesions occur but transmission is usually respiratory*
coxsackievirus A16	hand, foot and mouth disease	vesicular skin lesions but transmission fecal and respiratory
papilloma-viruses	warts	many types**
Leishmania tropica	cutaneous leishmaniasis	skin sores are infectious
Sarcoptes scabei	scabies	eggs from burrows transmitted by hand (also sexually)

Fig. 8.19 Human infections transmitted from the skin. (*Except in zoster, where a localized skin eruption occurs and the respiratory tract is generally unaffected. **Generally direct contact but plantar warts are commonly spread following contamination of floors.)

depending upon physical activities such as exercise, dressing and undressing. The fine white dust that collects on indoor surfaces, especially in hospital wards, consists largely of skin scales. Staphylococci are present, and different individuals show great variation in staphylococcal shedding, but the reasons are unknown.

Transmission by direct contact or by contaminated fingers is much more common than following release into the environment, and microorganisms transmitted in this way include potentially pathogenic staphylococci and human papillomaviruses.

Transmission in milk

Milk is produced by a skin gland. Microorganisms are rarely shed into human milk and examples include paramyxovirus, cytomegalovirus and human T cell lymphotropic virus 1 (HTLV1), but milk from cows, goats and sheep can be important sources of infection *(Fig. 8.20)*. Other bacteria can be introduced into milk after collection.

Transmission from blood
Blood can spread infection via arthropods or needles

Blood is often the vehicle of transmission. Microorganisms and parasites spread by blood-sucking athropods (see below) are effectively shed into the blood. Infectious agents present in blood (hepatitis viruses, HIV) are also transmissible by needles, either in transfused blood or when contaminated needles are used for injections or intravenous drug misuse. Blood

is also the source of infection in transplacental transmission and this generally involves initial infection of the placenta (see Chapter 21).

Vertical and horizontal transmission
Vertical transmission takes place between parents and their offspring

When transmission is direct from parents to offspring via for example sperm, ovum, placenta *(Fig. 8.21)*, milk or blood, it is referred to as vertical. This is because it can be represented as a vertical flow down a page *(Fig. 8.22)* just like a family pedigree. Other infections, in contrast, are said to be horizontally transmitted, with an individual infecting unrelated individuals by contact, respiratory or fecal–oral spread. Vertically transmitted infections can be subdivided as shown in *Figure 8.23*. Strictly speaking, these infections are able to maintain themselves in the species without spreading horizontally as long as they do not affect the viability of the host. Various retroviruses are known to maintain themselves vertically in animals (e.g. mammary tumor virus in milk, sperm and ovum of mice), but this does not appear to be important in humans, except possibly for HTLV1, where milk transfer seems to be important. There are, however, many retrovirus sequences present in the normal human genome. These DNA sequences are too incomplete to produce infectious virus particles, but can be regarded as amazingly successful parasites. They presumably do no harm and survive within the human species, watched over, conserved and replicated as part of our genetic constitution.

HUMAN INFECTIONS TRANSMITTED VIA MILK		
microorganism	type of milk	importance in transmission
mumps virus	human	–
cytomegalovirus	human	–
HIV	human	–
HTLV1	human	+
Brucella	cow, goat, sheep	++
Mycobacterium bovis	cow	++
Coxiella burnetii (Q fever rickettsia)	cow	+
Campylobacter jejuni	cow	++
Salmonella spp.		
Listeria monocytogenes		
Staphylococcus spp.	cow	+
Streptococcus pyogenes		
Yersinia enterocolitica		

Fig. 8.20 Human infections transmitted via milk. Human milk is rarely a significant source of infection. All microbes listed are destroyed by pasteurization.

TRANSPLACENTAL TRANSMISSION OF INFECTION	
microorganism	effect
rubella virus cytomegalovirus	placental lesion, abortion, stillbirth, malformation
HIV	childhood AIDS
hepatitis B virus	antigen carriage in infant, but most of these infections are perinatal or postnatal
Treponema pallidum	stillbirth, congenital syphilis with malformation
Listeria monocytogenes	meningoencephalitis
Toxoplasma gondii	stillbirth, CNS disease

Fig. 8.21 Human infections transmitted via the placenta.

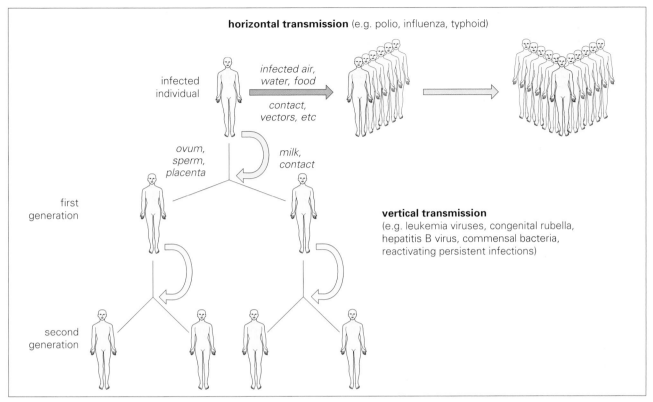

horizontal transmission (e.g. polio, influenza, typhoid)

infected individual

infected air, water, food

contact, vectors, etc

ovum, sperm, placenta

milk, contact

first generation

vertical transmission
(e.g. leukemia viruses, congenital rubella, hepatitis B virus, commensal bacteria, reactivating persistent infections)

second generation

Fig. 8.22 Vertical and horizontal transmission by infection. Most infections are transmitted horizontally, as might be expected in crowded human populations. Vertical transmission becomes more important in small isolated communities (see Chapter 11).

Transmission from Animals

Humans and animals share a common susceptibility to certain pathogens

Humans live in daily contact, directly or indirectly, with a wide variety of other animal species, both vertebrate and invertebrate, not only sharing a common environment, but also a common susceptibility to certain pathogens. The degree to which animal contacts transmit infection depends upon the type of environment (urban/rural, tropical/temperate, hygienic/insanitary) and on the nature of the contact. Close contact is made with vertebrate animals used for food or as pets, and with invertebrate animals adapted to live or feed on the human body. Less intimate contact is made with many other species, which nevertheless may transmit pathogens equally well. For convenience, animal-transmitted infections can be divided into two categories:

• Those involving arthropod and other invertebrate vectors.
• Those transmitted directly from vertebrates (zoonoses).

More detailed accounts of these infections are given in Chapters 25 and 26.

Invertebrate vectors
Insects, ticks and mites – the bloodsuckers – are the most important vectors spreading infection

By far the most important vectors of disease belong to these three groups of arthropods. Many species are capable of transmitting infection and a wide range of organisms is transmitted *(Fig. 8.24)*. In the past, insects have been responsible for some of the most devastating epidemic diseases, for example fleas and plague and lice and typhus. Even today one of the world's most important infectious diseases – malaria – is transmitted by the anopheles mosquito. The distribution and epidemiology of these infections are

TYPES OF VERTICAL TRANSMISSION		
type	**route**	**examples**
prenatal	placenta	rubella cytomegalovirus syphilis toxoplasmosis
perinatal	infected birth canal	gonococcal/ chlamydial conjunctivitis
postnatal	milk or direct contact	cytomegalovirus hepatitis B
germline	viral DNA sequences in human genome	many retroviruses

Fig. 8.23 Types of vertical transmission.

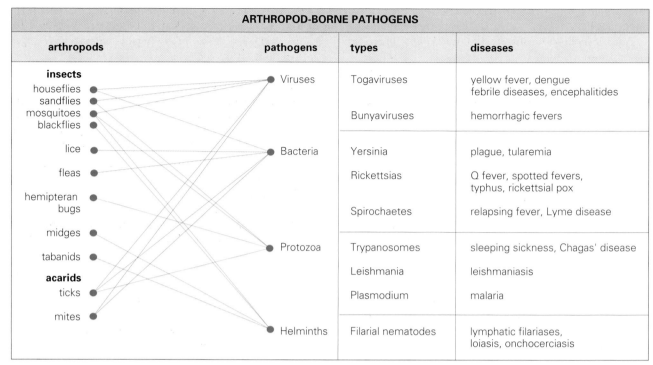

ARTHROPOD-BORNE PATHOGENS			
arthropods	**pathogens**	**types**	**diseases**
insects houseflies sandflies mosquitoes blackflies	Viruses	Togaviruses Bunyaviruses	yellow fever, dengue febrile diseases, encephalitides hemorrhagic fevers
lice fleas hemipteran bugs	Bacteria	Yersinia Rickettsias Spirochaetes	plague, tularemia Q fever, spotted fevers, typhus, rickettsial pox relapsing fever, Lyme disease
midges tabanids **acarids** ticks mites	Protozoa Helminths	Trypanosomes Leishmania Plasmodium Filarial nematodes	sleeping sickness, Chagas' disease leishmaniasis malaria lymphatic filariases, loiasis, onchocerciasis

Fig. 8.24 Arthropod-borne pathogens. Mosquitoes are a major source of infection. Note that, with the exception of pneumonic plague, none are transmitted from human to human.

determined by the climatic conditions that allow the vectors to breed and the organism to complete its development in their bodies. Some diseases are therefore purely tropical and subtropical, for example malaria, sleeping sickness and yellow fever while others are much more widespread, for example plague and typhus.

Passive carriage

Insects may carry pathogens passively on their mouth parts, on their bodies, or within their intestines. Transfer onto food or onto the host occurs directly as a result of the insect feeding, regurgitating or defecating. Many important diseases, such as trachoma, can be transmitted in this way by common species such as houseflies and cockroaches.

Blood-feeding species have mouthparts adapted for penetrating skin in order to reach blood vessels or to create small pools of blood *(Fig. 8.25)*. The ability to feed in this way provides access to organisms in the skin or blood. The mouthparts can act as a contaminated hypodermic needle, carrying infection between individuals.

Biologic transmission

This is much more common, the blood-sucking vector acting as a necessary host for the multiplication and development of the pathogen. Almost all of the important infections (listed in *Fig. 8.25*) are transmitted in this way. The pathogen is reintroduced into the human host, after a period of time, at the next blood meal. Transmission can be by direct injection, usually in the vector's saliva (malaria, yellow fever), or by contamination from feces or regurgitated blood deposited at the time of feeding (typhus, plague).

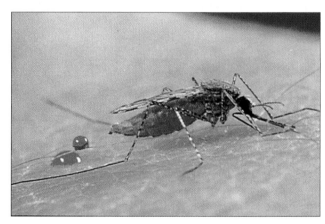

Fig. 8.25 Female *Anopheles* mosquito feeding. (Courtesy of CJ Webb.)

Other invertebrate vectors spread infection either passively or by acting as an intermediate host

Many invertebrates used for food convey pathogens *(Fig. 8.26)*. Perhaps the most familiar are the shellfish (molluscs and crustacea) associated with food poisoning and acute gastroenteritis. These aquatic animals accumulate viruses and bacteria in their bodies, taking them in from contaminated waste, and transferring them passively. In other cases the relationship between the pathogen and the invertebrate is much closer. Many parasites, especially worms, must undergo part of their development in the invertebrate before being able to infect a human. Humans are infected when they eat the invertebrate (intermediate) host. Dietary habits are therefore important in infection.

Aquatic molluscs (snails) are necessary intermediate hosts for schistosomes – the blood flukes. They become infected by larval stages, which hatch from eggs passed into water in the urine or feces of infected people. After a period of development and multiplication large numbers of infective stages (cercariae) escape from the snails. These can rapidly penetrate through human skin, initiating the infection that will result in adult flukes occupying visceral blood vessels (see Chapter 3).

Transmission from vertebrates
Many pathogens are transmitted directly to humans from vertebrate animals

Strictly, the term zoonoses can apply to any infection transmitted to humans from infected animals, whether this is direct (by contact or eating) or indirect (via an invertebrate vector). Here, however, zoonoses are used to describe infections of vertebrate animals that can be transmitted directly. Many pathogens are transmitted in this way (*Fig. 8.27*) by a variety of different routes including contact, inhalation, bites, scratches, contamination of food or water, and ingestion as food.

The epidemiology of zoonoses depends upon the frequency and the nature of contact between the vertebrate and the human hosts. Some are localized geographically, being dependent for example upon local food preferences. Where these involve eating uncooked animal products such as fish or amphibia, a variety of parasites (especially tapeworms and nematodes) can be acquired. Others are associated with occupation, for example if this involves contact with raw animal products (butchers in the case of toxoplasmosis and Q fever) or frequent contact with domestic stock (farm workers

in the case of brucellosis and dermatophyte fungi). In urban areas, zoonoses are most likely to be acquired by eating or drinking infected animal products or by contact with dogs, cats and other domestic pets.

Domestic pets or pests?
Dogs and cats are the commonest domestic pets, and both are reservoirs of infection for their owners (*Fig. 8.28*). The pathogens concerned are spread by contact, bites and scratches, by vectors, and by contamination with fecal material. Major infections transmitted in these ways include:
- Toxocariasis from dogs.
- Toxoplasmosis from cats.
  Both are almost universal in their distribution.
  Humans may acquire hydatid disease from tapeworm eggs passed in dog feces where dogs are used for herding

ZOONOSES-HUMAN INFECTIONS TRANSMITTED FROM VERTEBRATES		
pathogens	**vertebrate vector**	**diseases**
viruses		
arenaviruses	mammals	Lassa fever, lymphocytic choriomeningitis, Bolivian hemorrhagic fever
poxviruses	mammals	cowpox, orf
rhabdoviruses	mammals	rabies
bacteria		
Bacillus anthracis	mammals	anthrax
Brucella	mammals	brucella
Chlamydia	birds	psittacosis
Leptospira	mammals	leptospirosis (Weil's disease)
Listeria	mammals	listeriosis
Salmonella	birds, mammals	salmonellosis
Mycobacterium tuberculosis	mammals	tuberculosis
fungi		
Cryptococcus	birds	meningitis
dermatophytes	mammals	ringworm
protozoa		
Cryptosporidium	mammals	cryptosporidiosis
Giardia	mammals	giardiasis
Toxoplasma	mammals	toxoplasmosis
helminths		
Ankylostoma	mammals	hookworm disease
Echinococcus	mammals	hydatid disease
Taenia	mammals	tapeworms
Toxocara	mammals	toxocariasis (visceral larval migrans)
Trichinella	mammals	trichinellosis

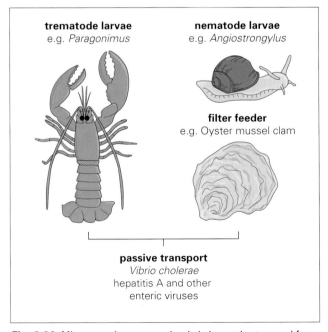

trematode larvae e.g. *Paragonimus*

nematode larvae e.g. *Angiostrongylus*

filter feeder e.g. Oyster mussel clam

passive transport *Vibrio cholerae* hepatitis A and other enteric viruses

Fig. 8.26 Microorganisms transmitted via invertebrates used for food. Filter-feeding molluscs living in estuaries near sewage outlets are a common source of infection.

Fig. 8.27 Human infections transmitted directly from vertebrates (birds and mammals).

domestic animals and have access to infected carcasses. In rural areas of many countries this has been, or remains, an important infection.

Many species of birds are kept as pets and some can pass on serious infections to those in contact with them. Contact is usually through inhalation of infected particulate material. Perhaps the most important of these is psittacosis caused by *Chlamydia psittaci*, which despite the common name 'parrot fever' can be acquired from many avian species.

The recent trend in developed countries towards keeping unusual or exotic pets (especially reptiles, exotic birds and mammals) raises new risks of zoonotic infection. Many reptiles, for example, pass human-infective *Salmonella* spp. in their droppings. Exotic birds and mammals can carry a range of viruses that could be transmitted under the correct conditions. Diagnosis of infections under these circumstances can be difficult if the physician does not know of the existence of such pets.

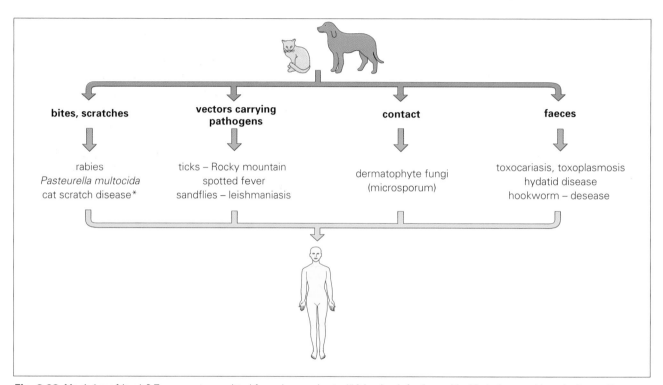

Fig. 8.28 Man's best friends? Zoonoses transmitted from dogs and cats. (*A benign infection, with skin lesions and lymphadenopathy, shown to be due to a newly discovered bacterium, *Afipia catei*.)

- To establish infection in the host, microbes must attach to, or pass across, body surfaces.
- Many microbes have developed chemical or mechanical mechanisms to attach themselves to the surface of the respiratory, urinogenital and alimentary tracts. In the skin they generally depend upon entry via small wounds or arthropod bites.
- Microbes must exit from the body after replication in order to be transmitted to fresh hosts. This also takes place across body surfaces.
- Efficient shedding of microbes from the skin or respiratory, urinogenital or alimentary tracts or delivery into the blood or dermal tissues for uptake during arthropod feeding are vital stages in their life cycles.
- Many human infections come from animals, either directly (zoonoses) or indirectly (via blood-sucking arthropods), and the incidence of these infections depends upon exposure to infected animals or arthropods.

1. Place the following types of transmission in order according to the speed with which the infection generally spreads in the community: sexual, fecal–oral, respiratory, zoonotic.
2. Why are so many arthropod-borne infections and zoonoses not transmitted directly from human to human?
3. Would you expect urine to be an effective vehicle for transmitting an infection? If not, why not?
4. Could you transmit a respiratory infection to others if you did not cough or sneeze?
5. List the routes and the tissues or the cells involved in vertical transmission.
6. Is there anything to stop a microbe, transmitted by the sexual route, that attaches and infects urethral epithelial cells from doing the same to respiratory epithelial cells?

Further Reading

Cohen MS, Sparling PF. Mucosal infection with Neisseria gonorrhoeae. *J Clin Investig* 1992;**89**:1699–1705.

Falkow S. Bacterial entry into eukaryotic cells. *Cell* 1991;**65**:1099–1102.

Haywood AM. Virus receptors: binding, adhesion, strengthening and changes in viral structure. *Virology* 1994;**68**:1–5.

Mims CA. The transmission of infection. *Rev Med Microbiol* 1995;**6**:217–227.

Mims CA, Dimmock NJ, Nash A, Stephen J. Mims' Pathogenesis of Infectious Disease, 4th edition. London: Academic Press, 1995.

Warren KS. The control of helminths; non-replicating infectious agents of man. *Am Rev Publ Health* 1981;**2**:101–116.

Introduction

The barrier effects of the skin and mucous membranes and their adjuncts such as cilia have already been referred to (see Chapter 8). We now turn to the back-up mechanisms called rapidly into play when an organism has penetrated these barriers – namely complement, the phagocytic and cytotoxic cells, and a variety of cytotoxic molecules, the most important of which are listed in *Figure 9.1*. While they lack the dramatic specifity and memory of adaptive (i.e. lymphocyte-based) immune mechanisms, these natural defenses are vital to survival – particularly in invertebrates, where they are the only defense against infection, adaptive responses having evolved only with the earliest vertebrates.

Complement

The alternative pathway of complement activation is part of the early defense system

The basic biology of the complement system and its role in inducing the inflammatory response and promoting chemo-

CYTOTOXIC MOLECULES		
host component		effective against
major cell source	molecule	
liver cells macrophage	complement C1–3 complement C5–9 C-reactive protein	bacteria, fungi *Neisseria* streptococci
macrophage neutrophil	reactive oxygen intermediates (plus peroxidase)	bacteria, fungi malaria
macrophage	lysozyme interferon (α,β) tumour necrosis factor arginase reactive nitrogen intermediates	Gram-positive bacteria viruses viruses, bacteria, malaria schistosome worms leishmania, malaria
neutrophil	defensins cathepsins lactoferrin	bacteria, fungi bacteria, fungi bacteria, yeasts
eosinophil	cationic proteins	schistosome
T lymphocyte	cytokines	viruses some bacteria, fungi, protozoa
natural killer cell	perforins	viruses
liver, fat	high density lipoprotein low density lipoprotein (oxidized)	trypanosomes malaria

Fig. 9.1 Some important cytotoxic molecules that operate against infectious organisms.

taxis, phagocytosis and vascular permeability have been described in Chapter 4. Here we are concerned with its ability to directly damage microorganisms as part of the early response to infection. Contrary to what might be expected from the dramatic lysis of many kinds of bacteria in the test tube, the action of complement *in vivo* is restricted mainly to the *Neisseria*. This is evidenced by the inability of patients deficient in C5, C6, C7, C8 or C9 to eliminate gonococci and meningococci, with the increased risk of developing septicemia or becoming a carrier.

The lack of effect of complement in other infections may be due to escape strategies by the microorganism. For example, the insertion of the C567 complex is prevented by the long side chains of the cell wall polysaccharides of smooth strains of salmonellae and by the capsules of staphylococci, which, unlike the cell wall, do not activate complement *(Fig. 9.2)*.

Mammalian cells such as the neutrophil can avoid lysis by isolating bound complement molecules to a small portion of membrane and budding this off, and some microorganisms can do the same. Certain bacteria, for example streptococci and campylobacter, actively inhibit complement activation, while a covering of non-complement fixing antibody, for example IgA, is yet another way of avoiding lysis. Anti-complement activity is also a feature of several protozoan and helminthic infections, for example infections with *Leishmania* and the hydatid worm *Echinococcus granulosus*.

It should be emphasized that only the alternative pathway of complement activation forms part of this natural 'early defense' system. Activation through the classical pathway occurs only after an antibody response has been made. It is not surprising to learn, therefore, that the alternative pathway appears to have evolved first.

C-reactive Protein

C-reactive protein is an antibacterial agent produced by liver cells in response to cytokines

Among the acute phase proteins produced in the course of most inflammatory reactions, C-reactive protein (CRP) is particularly interesting in being an antibacterial agent, albeit of very restricted range. CRP is a pentameric β-globulin, somewhat resembling a miniature version of IgM (molecular weight

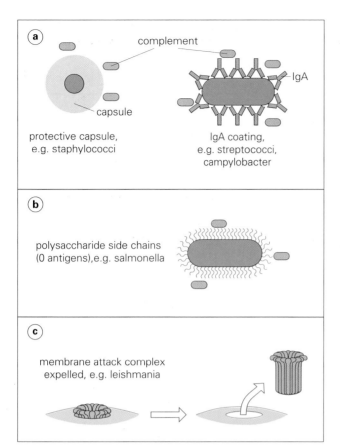

Fig. 9.2 Three ways by which microorganisms can avoid damage by complement. (a) Failure to trigger complement. (b) Protection of the membrane from attack. (c) Expulsion of the membrane attack complex C5–9.

130 000 compared with 900 000 for IgM). It reacts with phosphorylcholine in the wall of some streptococci and subsequently activates both complement and phagocytosis. CRP is produced by liver cells in response to cytokines, particularly interleukin-6 (IL-6, see Chapter 6), and levels can rise as much as 1000-fold in 24 hours – a much more rapid response than that of antibody. Therefore, CRP levels are often used to monitor inflammation, for example in rheumatic diseases. Most of the other acute phase proteins are produced in increased amounts early in infection, but an antimicrobial role for these has not been proved. Indeed it has been suggested that they may be taken up by certain parasites and used to protect the parasite from immune attack or to help the parasite gain access to cells. However, some acute phase proteins may be responsible for reducing pathology by binding toxic bacterial products such as lipopolysaccharide.

Phagocytosis

Phagocytes engulf, kill and digest would-be parasites

Perhaps the greatest danger to the would-be parasite is to be recognized by a phagocytic cell, engulfed, killed and digested. A description of the various stages of phagocytosis is given in Chapter 4. Phagocytes (principally macrophages) are normally found in the tissues where invading microorganisms are more likely to be encountered. In addition, phagocytes present in the blood (principally the polymorphonuclear leukocytes – PMNs) can be rapidly recruited into the tissues when and where required. Only about 1% of the normal adult bone marrow reserve of 3×10^{12} PMNs is present in the blood at any one time, representing a turnover of about 10^{11} PMNs per day. Most macrophages remain within the tissues and well under 1% are present in the blood as monocytes. PMNs are short lived, but macrophages can live for many years (see below).

Successful parasites have evolved numerous ingenious antiphagocytic devices

Antiphagocytic devices *(Fig. 9.3)* range from killing or inhibiting the phagocyte itself, via more subtle ways of eluding contact, to protection against intracellular death allowing the microorganism to survive within the phagocyte – a very serious challenge to the host. The ways in which some of these parasite strategies can be countered by the development of adaptive immune responses (antibody and T cells) are described in Chapter 5.

Intracellular killing by phagocytes
Phagocytes kill organisms using either an oxidative or a non-oxidative mechanism

The mechanisms by which phagocytes kill the organisms they ingest are traditionally divided into oxidative and non-oxidative, depending upon whether the cell consumes oxygen in the process. Respiration in PMNs is non-mitochondrial and anaerobic, and the burst of oxygen consumption, the so-called 'respiratory burst' *(Fig. 9.4)*, that accompanies phagocytosis represents the generation of microbicidal reactive oxygen intermediates (ROIs).

Oxidative killing involves the use of ROIs

The importance of ROIs in bacterial killing was revealed by the discovery that PMNs from patients with chronic granulomatous disease (CGD) did not consume oxygen after phagocytosing staphylococci. Patients with CGD have one of three kinds of genetic defect in a PMN membrane enzyme system involving nicotinamide adenine dinucleotide phosphate (NADPH) oxidase. The normal activity of this system is the progressive reduction of atmospheric oxygen to water with the production of ROIs such as the superoxide ion, hydrogen peroxide and free hydroxyl radicals, all of which can be extremely toxic to microorganisms.

CGD patients are unable to kill staphylococci and certain other bacteria and fungi, which consequently cause deep chronic abscesses. They can, however, deal with catalase-negative bacteria such as pneumococci because these produce, and do not destroy, their own hydrogen peroxide in sufficient amounts to interact with the cell myeloperoxidase, producing the highly toxic hypochlorous acid (HOCl; *Fig. 9.4*). The defective PMNs from CGD patients can be readily

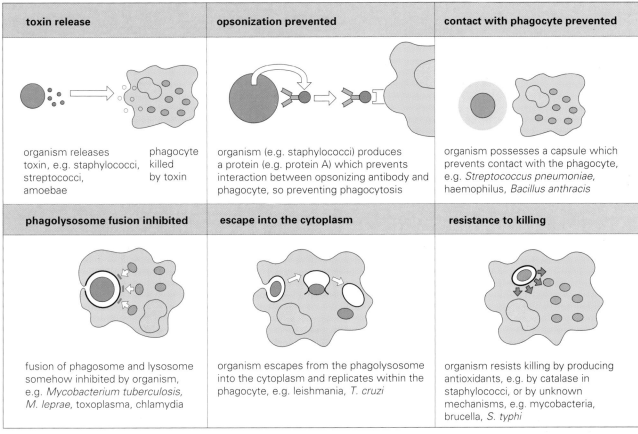

toxin release	opsonization prevented	contact with phagocyte prevented
organism releases toxin, e.g. staphylococci, streptococci, amoebae	phagocyte killed by toxin	organism (e.g. staphylococci) produces a protein (e.g. protein A) which prevents interaction between opsonizing antibody and phagocyte, so preventing phagocytosis	organism possesses a capsule which prevents contact with the phagocyte, e.g. *Streptococcus pneumoniae*, haemophilus, *Bacillus anthracis*

phagolysosome fusion inhibited	escape into the cytoplasm	resistance to killing
fusion of phagosome and lysosome somehow inhibited by organism, e.g. *Mycobacterium tuberculosis*, *M. leprae*, toxoplasma, chlamydia	organism escapes from the phagolysosome into the cytoplasm and replicates within the phagocyte, e.g. leishmania, *T. cruzi*	organism resists killing by producing antioxidants, e.g. by catalase in staphylococci, or by unknown mechanisms, e.g. mycobacteria, brucella, *S. typhi*

Fig. 9.3 Various mechanisms adopted by microorganisms to avoid phagocytosis.

identified *in vitro* by their failure to reduce the yellow dye nitroblue tetrazolium to a blue compound (the 'NBT test', see Chapter 14).

The way in which ROIs actually kill microorganisms is controversial

ROIs can damage cell membranes (lipid peroxidation), DNA and proteins (including vital enzymes), but in some cases it may be the altered pH that accompanies the generation of ROIs that does the damage. Killing of some bacteria and fungi (e.g. *Escherichia coli*, *Candida*) occurs only at an acid pH, while killing of others (e.g. staphylococci) occurs at an alkaline pH.

It is not surprising that bacteria produce molecules that inactivate ROIs, and of these catalase and superoxide dismutase are the best documented *(Fig. 9.5)*.

Non-oxidative killing involves the use of the phagocyte's cytotoxic granules

Oxygen is not always available for killing microorganisms; indeed some bacteria grow best in anaerobic conditions (e.g. the *Clostridia* of gas gangrene), and oxygen would in any case be in short supply in a deep tissue abscess. Phagocytic cells therefore contain a number of other cytotoxic molecules. The best studied are the proteins in the various PMN granules *(Fig. 9.6)*, which act on the contents of the phagosome as the granules fuse with it.

Another phagocytic cell, the eosinophil, is particularly rich in cytotoxic granules *(Fig. 9.6)*. The highly cationic (i.e. basic) contents of these granules give them their characteristic acidophilic staining pattern. Five distinct eosinophil cationic proteins are known and seem to be particularly toxic to parasitic worms, at least *in vitro*. Because of the enormous difference in size between parasitic worms and eosinophils, this type of damage is limited to the outer surfaces of the parasite. The eosinophilia typical of worm infections is presumably an attempt to cope with these large and almost indestructible parasites. It has recently been shown that both the production and level of activity of eosinophils is regulated by T cells and macrophages and mediated by cytokines such as interleukin-5 (IL-5) and tumor necrosis factor (TNF).

Monocytes and macrophages also contain cytotoxic granules, but their contents are less well characterized. Unlike PMNs *(Fig. 9.7)*, macrophages contain little or no myeloperoxidase, but secrete large amounts of lysozyme. Lysozyme is an antibacterial molecule maintained at a concentration of about 30 mg/ml in serum, though this concentration can increase to as high as 800 mg/ml in rare cases of monocytic leukemia. Macrophages also differ from PMNs in being extremely sensitive to activation by bacterial products (e.g. lipopolysaccharide [LPS]) and T cell products e.g. interferon (IFN) γ. Activated macrophages have a greatly enhanced ability to kill both intracellular and extracellular targets.

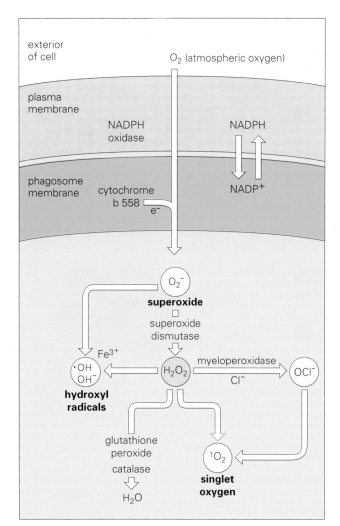

Fig. 9.4 The principal molecules involved in the respiratory burst. Oxygen is progressively reduced by the addition of electrons (e^-).

SOME ORGANISMS KILLED BY REACTIVE OXYGEN AND NITROGEN SPECIES		
Bacteria	**Fungi**	**Protozoa**
Staphylococcus aureus	*Candida albicans*	*plasmodium*
Escherichia coli	*aspergillus*	*leishmania*
Serratia marcescens		(nitric oxide)

Fig. 9.5 Organisms killed by reactive oxygen species.

PMN AND EOSINOPHIL GRANULE CONTENTS		
PMN		**eosinophil**
primary (azurophil)	**specific (heterophil)**	
myeloperoxidase	lysozyme	eosinophil
acid hydrolases	lactoferrin	peroxidase
cathepsins G, B, D	alkaline phosphatase	cationic proteins
defensins	NADPH oxidase	ECP
BPI	collagenase	MBP
cationic proteins	histaminase	neurotoxin
lysozyme		lysophospholipase

Fig. 9.6 Contents of ploymorphonuclear leukocytes (PMN) and eosinophil granules. (BPI, bactericidal permeability increasing protein; ECP, eosinophil cationic protein; NADPH, nicotinamide adenine dinucleotide phosphate; MBP, major basic protein).

A major secreted product of the activated macrophage is cytotoxic nitric oxide

A major secreted product of the activated macrophage is nitric oxide (NO), one of the reactive nitrogen intermediates (RNIs) generated during the conversion of arginine to citrulline by arginase. NO is strongly cytotoxic to a variety of cell types, and RNIs are generated in large amounts during infections (e.g. leishmaniasis, malaria). Arginase can also cause damage by leading to a deprivation of arginine, which is an essential amino acid for some viruses (e.g. herpes simplex) and parasites (e.g. the liver fluke *Schistosoma*).

Cytotoxicity by Lymphoctyes and Natural Killer Cells

Cytotoxic T lymphocytes kill by inducing 'leaks' in the target cell

The well-known cytotoxic or 'killer' Tc lymphocyte (CTL) is unusual in that both antigen-specific recognition and killing of the target are carried out by the same cell. The recognition step, involving an antigenic fragment that becomes associated with a class I major histocompatability complex (MHC) molecule, is discussed in Chapter 5, and displays the high degree of specificity characteristic of adaptive responses. The killing mechanism, however, is relatively non-specific. It appears to involve the induction of 'leaks' in the target cell by the insertion of perforin, a 66 kD molecule that is structurally and functionally similar to the terminal complement component C9 (77 kD; *Fig. 9.8*). Other molecules, including cytokines such as TNF and lymphotoxin may also be involved, and their effects may be either direct or indirect. Target cell death may be due to:

• Leakage.
• Fragmentation of DNA.
• Induction of apoptosis—a 'suicide' program built into all cells.

These mechanisms are thought to operate principally against virus-infected cells, but some cells infected with other intracellular parasites, including mycobacteria (e.g. *Mycobacterium leprae* in Schwann cells) and even protozoa (e.g. *Theileria parva* in lymphocytes) may also be susceptible. Both CD8-positive and CD4-positive T cells have been implicated. Recent experiments with genetically engineered virus–cytokine constructs in T cell-depleted mice indicate that in some cases cytokine release alone may be sufficient for virus killing in the absence of T cells.

PMN AND MACROPHAGES COMPARED		
	PMN	**macrophage**
site of production	bone marrow	bone marrow, tissues
duration in marrow	14 days	54 hours
duration in blood	7–10 hours	20–40 hours (monocyte)
average life span	4 days	months–years
numbers in blood	$(2.5–7.5) \times 10^9/l$	$(0.2–0.8) \times 10^9/l$
marrow reserve	10 x blood	–
numbers in tissues	(transient)	100 x blood
principal killing mechanisms	oxidative non-oxidative	oxidative nitric oxide cytokines
activated by	TNF	TNF, IFN-γ, IL-4 GM-CSF microbial products (e.g. LPS)
important deficiencies	CGD myeloperoxidase chemotactic Chediak–Higashi	lipid storage diseases
major secretory products	lysozyme	over 80, including: lysozyme cytokines (TNF, IL-1) complement factors

Fig. 9.7 The major phagocytic cells, PMNs and macrophages, differ in a number of important respects. (CGD, chronic granulomatous disease; GM-CSF, granulocyte-macrophage colony-stimulating factor; IFN, interferon; IL, interleukin; LPS, lipopolysaccharide; TNF, tumor necrosis factor.)

Natural killer cells are a rapid but non-specific means of controlling viral and other intracellular infections

The mechanism of killing of the large granular lymphocytes (LGLs) – usually referred to as natural killer (NK) cells – appears to resemble that of CTLs fairly closely. The vital difference is the NK cells' lack of an antigen-specific receptor and therefore the absence of specificity, memory and MHC-restriction in their response. Indeed, it seems that NK cells may be best at recognizing cells that do not express MHC antigens (the 'missing self' hypothesis). NK cells are thought of as a more rapid but less specific means of controlling viral and other intracellular infections. Their importance is highlighted by the ability of mice lacking both T and B cells (severe combined immunodeficiency or 'SCID') to control some virus infections, and the same is probably true for SCID in man. Recently, it has been shown that like T cells, NK cells can secrete IFN and other cytokines (see below). This further increases the resemblance between T and NK cells.

Cytotoxic Lipids

As already mentioned, one of the targets of the toxic ROIs is lipid in cell membranes. ROIs are normally extremely short lived (fractions of a second), but their toxicity can be greatly prolonged by interaction with serum lipoproteins to form lipid peroxides. Lipid peroxides are stable for hours and can pass on the oxidative damage to cell membranes, both of the parasite (e.g. malaria-infected red cell) and of the host (e.g. vascular endothelium). The cytotoxic activity of normal serum to some blood trypanosomes has been traced to the high density lipoproteins, and in cotton rats to a macroglobulin.

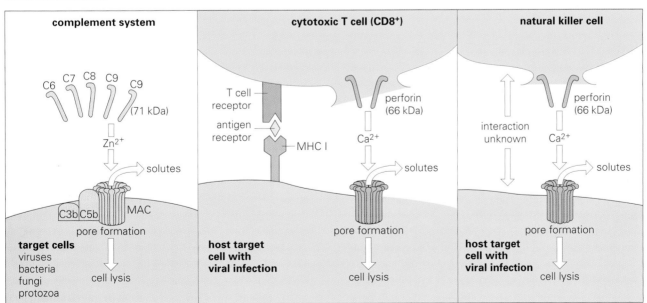

Fig.9.8 Comparison of cytotoxic cells and the lytic mechanisms of the complement system. (Ca^{2+}, calcium; MAC, major attack complex; MHC, major histocompatability complex; Zn^{2+}, zinc.)

HUMAN INTERFERONS			
	IFNα	**IFNβ**	**IFNγ**
alternative name	'leukocyte' IFN	'fibroblast' IFN	'immune' IFN
principal source	all cells	all cells	T lymphocytes
inducing agent	viral infection (or dsRNA)	viral infection (or dsRNA)	antigen (or mitogen)
number of species	22*	1	1
chromosomal location of gene(s)	9	9	12
antiviral activity	+++	+++	+
immunoregulatory activity:			
macrophage action	–	–	++
MHC I upregulation	+	+	+
MHC II upregulation	–	–	+
* each species coded by a different gene			

Fig. 9.9 Human interferons (IFNs). (dsRNA, double stranded ribonucleic acid; MHC, major histocompatability complex.)

Cytokines

Cytokines contribute to both infection control and infection pathology

Early studies with supernatants from cultures of lymphocytes and macrophages revealed a family of non-antigen-specific molecules with diverse activities, including both cell to cell communication and cytotoxicity. These are now collectively known as 'cytokines', and their role in infectious disease is being very actively studied. The way in which these molecules acquired their sometimes rather misleading names and the bewildering overlap of function between molecules of quite different structure are described in detail in Chapter 6.

Cytokines are of importance in infectious disease for two contrasting reasons:
- They can contribute to the control of infection.
- They can contribute to the development of pathology.

The latter harmful aspect – of which TNF in septic shock is a good example – is discussed in Chapter 12. The beneficial effects can be direct or more often indirect via the induction of some other antimicrobial process.

IFNs

The best-established antimicrobial cytokines are the IFNs (*Fig. 9.9*). The name is derived from the demonstration in 1957 that virus-infected cells secreted a molecule that interfered with viral replication in bystander cells. IFN of all three types (α, β and γ) interact with specific receptors on most cells, one for α and β and another for γ, following which they induce an antiviral state via the generation of at least two types of enzyme, a protein kinase and a 2',5'-oligoadenylate synthetase. Both of these enzymes result in the inhibition of viral RNA translation and therefore of protein synthesis (*Fig. 9.10*).

IFNα and IFNβ constitute a major part of the early response to viruses

IFNα and IFNβ are produced rapidly within 24 hours of infection, and constitute a major part of the early response to viruses. IFNγ is mainly a T cell product and is therefore produced later, although in some cases an early IFNγ response may be mounted by NK cells.

IFNs can also inhibit virus assembly at a later stage (e.g. retroviruses), while many of the other effects of IFN also contribute to the antiviral state, for example the enhancement of cellular MHC expression and the activation of NK cells and macrophages (*Fig. 9.11*). Unlike cytotoxic T cells, IFN normally inhibits viruses without damaging the host cell. Some intracellular organisms (e.g. *Leishmania*) can counteract the effect of IFNγ on MHC expression, thereby facilitating their own survival.

Although best known for their antiviral activity, IFNs have recently been shown to be induced by, and active against, a wide range of organisms, including rickettsia, mycobacteria and several protozoa. The lack of any clearcut IFN deficiency syndromes makes it hard to assess their importance in isolation, but this may in fact be an indication that IFN deficiency is incompatible with survival. In animal experiments, treatment with antibodies to IFN greatly increases susceptibility to viral infection and, conversely, treatment with IFN has proved useful for some human virus infections, notably chronic hepatitis B (see Chapter 30).

Other cytokines
TNF can directly or indirectly kill virally-infected cells

TNF has been shown to kill cells infected with a number of viruses, though in some cases this may be secondary to the

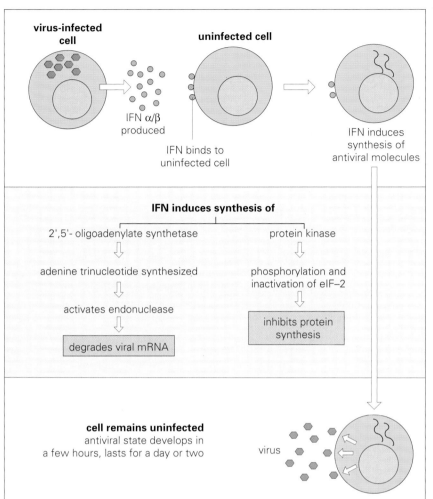

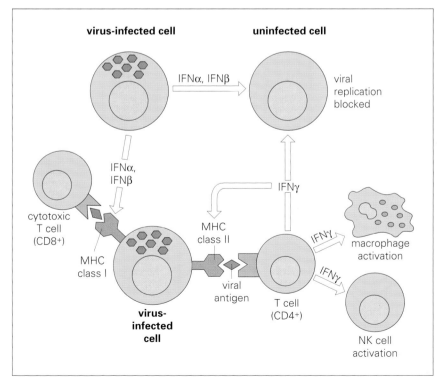

Fig. 9.10 The molecular basis of interferon (IFN) action.

Fig. 9.11 The multiple activities of interferons (IFNs) in viral immunity. (MHC, major histocompatability complex; NK, natural killer.)

induction of IFN. A striking example of a potentially useful role for TNF in infection is the inhibition of the proliferation of B lymphocytes by Epstein–Barr virus (EBV). EBV infection in people with malaria can lead to Burkitt's lymphoma, a monoclonal tumor of B cells, and TNF levels have been shown to be raised in malaria: conceivably, this is part of an attempt to prevent the development of the lymphoma. However, TNF is also thought to contribute to the pathology of malaria as well as that due to bacterial endotoxins (see Chapter 12). This illustrates the often confusing role that cytokines play in infectious diseases of all kinds – 'enough is enough' and 'too much is dangerous' seem to be the rules for these powerful molecules. Paradoxically TNF concentration is raised in HIV infection and has been found to enhance the replication of HIV in T cells – a 'positive feedback' with worrying potential.

Most interleukins contribute to protection in one or more infectious diseases

In all cases this protection against infectious disease is derived from the activation of macrophages, B cells, eosinophils, and other effector cells. Needless to say, parasites have found ways to avoid such activation. For example the South American trypanosome *Trypanosoma cruzi* can downregulate receptors for IL-2, while in malaria, circulating soluble IL-2 receptors can block the normal T cell activation by IL-2. *Pseudomonas* bacteria secrete proteolytic enzymes that cleave IL-2 and IFNγ, and it seems likely that many similar evasive mechanisms will become evident as systems for the detection of cytokines, their receptors, and their natural inhibitors become more sophisticated. There is currently great interest in the potential of IL-12 as an activator of NK cells.

Fever

A raised temperature almost invariably accompanies infection (see Chapter 27). In many cases the cause can be traced to the release of cytokines such as IL-1 or TNF, which play important roles in both immunity and pathology (see Chapter 11). However, the interesting question as to whether the raised temperature itself is of benefit to the host remains.

It is probably unwise to generalize about the benefit or otherwise of fever

Several microorganisms have been shown to be susceptible to high temperature. This was the basis for the 'fever therapy' of syphilis by deliberate infection with blood-stage malaria, and the malaria parasite itself may also be damaged by high temperatures, though it is obviously not totally eliminated. In general, however, one would predict that successful parasites were those that were adapted to survive episodes of fever; indeed the 'stress' or 'heat-shock' proteins produced by both mammalian and microbial cells in response to stress of many kinds, including heat, are thought to be part of their protective strategy. On the other hand, several host immune mechanisms might also be expected to be more active at higher temperatures: examples are complement activation, lymphocyte proliferation and the synthesis of proteins such as antibody and cytokines.

- Protection against infectious organisms that penetrate the outer barriers of the skin and mucous membranes is mediated by a variety of early defence mechanisms.
- These early defence mechanisms occur more rapidly though are less specific than the adaptive mechanisms based on lymphocyte responses.
- Important early defence mechanisms include the acute phase response, the complement system, IFNs, phagocytic cells and NK cells. Together these act as a first line of defence during the initial hours or days of infection.

1. What distinguishes killing by T cells and NK cells?
2. How do IFNs lead to the elimination of viruses?
3. What are acute phase proteins and what is their significance?
4. How may a microorganism escape being phagocytosed and killed?

Further Reading

Baron S, Tyring SK, Fleischmann WR *et al.* The interferons. Mechanisms of action and clinical applications. *J Am Med Assoc* 1991;**266(10)**:1375–1383.

Clas F, Loos M. Complement and bacteria. In: Whaley K (ed.). *Complement in Health and Disease.* Lancaster: MTP Press, 1987.

Cooper NR. Complement evasion mechanisms of microorganisms. *Immunol Today* 1991;**12**:327–331.

Liew FY, Cox FEG. Non-specific defence mechanism: the role of nitric oxide. *Immunol Today* 1991;**12(3)**:A17–A21.

Morgan BP. Complement membrane attack on nucleated cells: resistance, recovery and non-lethal effects. *Biochem J* 1989;**264**:1–14.

Pepys MB. Aspects of the acute phase response: the C-reactive protein system. In: *Clinical Aspects of Immunology,* 4th edition. Oxford: Blackwell Science Publications, 1982.

Introduction

An infection may be a surface infection or a systemic infection

Many successful microorganisms multiply in epithelial cells at the site of entry on the body surface, but fail to spread to deeper structures or through the body. Local spread takes place readily on a fluid-covered mucosal surface, often aided by ciliary action, and large-scale movements of fluid spread the infection to more distant areas on the surface. This is obvious in the gastrointestinal tract. In the upper respiratory tract, high 'winds' (coughing, sneezing) can splatter infectious agents onto new areas of mucosa, or into the openings of sinuses or the middle ear, while the gentler downward trickle of mucus during sleep may seed an infectious agent into the lower respiratory tract. As a result, large areas of the body surface can be involved within a few days, with shedding to the exterior. There is not enough time for a primary immune response to be generated, and therefore non-adaptive responses – interferon, natural killer cells – are more important in controlling the infection. These surface infections therefore show a 'hit-and-run' pattern.

In contrast, other microorganisms spread systemically through the body via lymph or blood. They often undergo a complex or stepwise invasion of various tissues before reaching the final site of replication and shedding to the exterior (e.g. measles, typhoid). Surface and systemic infections and their consequences are compared in *Figure 10.1*.

Features of Surface and Systemic Infections

A variety of factors determine whether an infection is a surface or a systemic infection

What prevents surface infections from spreading more deeply? Why do the microbes that cause systemic infections leave the relatively safe haven of the body surface to spread through the body, where they will bear the full onslaught of host defenses? These are important questions. For instance, what are the factors that persuade meningococci residing harmlessly on the nasal mucosa to invade deeper tissues, reach the blood and meninges, and cause meningitis (see Chapter 22)? The answer is not known.

Temperature is one factor that can restrict microbes to body surfaces. Rhinovirus infections, for instance, are restricted to the upper respiratory tract because they are temperature sensitive, replicating efficiently at 33°C, but not at the temperatures encountered in the lower respiratory tract (37°C). *Mycobacterium leprae* is also temperature sensitive, which accounts for its replication being more or less limited to nasal mucosa, skin and superficial nerves.

The site of budding is a factor that can restrict viruses to body surfaces. Influenza and parainfluenza viruses invade surface epithelial cells of the lung, but are liberated by budding from the free (external) surface of the epithelial cell, not from the basal layer from where they could spread to deeper tissues (*Fig. 10.2*).

Many microorganisms are obliged to spread systemically because they fail to spread and multiply at the site of initial infection, the body surface. In the case of measles or typhoid, there is, for unknown reasons, next to no replication at the site of initial respiratory or intestinal infection. Only after spreading through the body systemically are large numbers of micro-

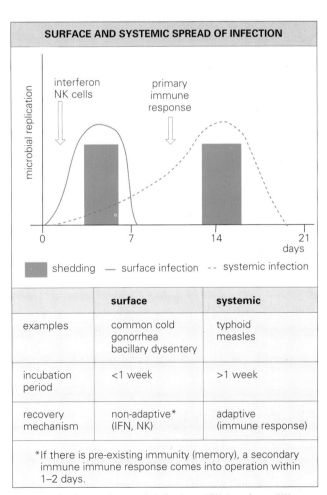

SURFACE AND SYSTEMIC SPREAD OF INFECTION

		surface	systemic
examples		common cold gonorrhea bacillary dysentery	typhoid measles
incubation period		<1 week	>1 week
recovery mechanism		non-adaptive* (IFN, NK)	adaptive (immune response)

*If there is pre-existing immunity (memory), a secondary immune immune response comes into operation within 1–2 days.

Fig. 10.1 Surface and systemic infections. (IFN, interferon; NK, natural killer.)

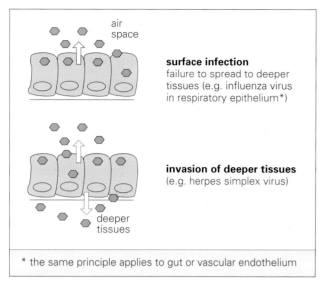

Fig. 10.2 Topography of virus release from epithelial surfaces can determine the pattern of infection.

organisms delivered back to the same surfaces, where they multiply and are shed to the exterior. Other microorganisms need to spread systemically because they have committed themselves to infection by one route while major replication and shedding occurs at a different site. The microbe must reach the replication site, and there is then no need for extensive replication at the site of initial infection. For instance, mumps and hepatitis A viruses infect via the respiratory and alimentary routes, respectively, but must spread through the body to invade and multiply in salivary glands (mumps) and liver (hepatitis A).

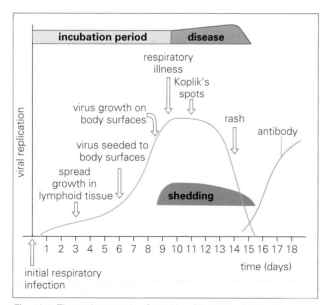

Fig. 10.4 The pathogenesis of measles. Virus invades body surfaces via blood vessels, and reaches surface epithelium first in the respiratory tract where there are only 1–2 layers of epithelial cells and then in mucosae (Koplik's spots) and finally in the skin (rash).

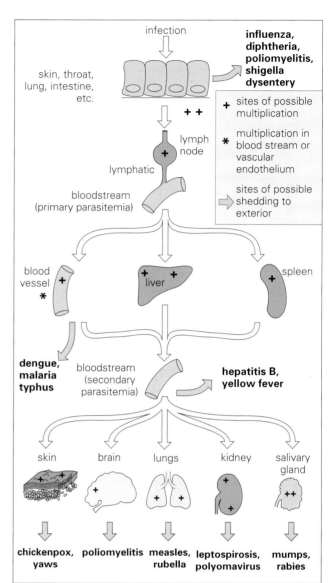

Fig. 10.3 The spread of infection throughout the body. Bone marrow and muscle are possible sources for secondary parasitemia in addition to blood vessels, liver and spleen.

In systemic infections there is a stepwise invasion of different tissues of the body

This stepwise invasion is illustrated in *Figure 10.3* and such infections include measles (*Fig. 10.4*) and typhoid (*Fig. 10.5*). Although the final sites of multiplication may be essential for microbial shedding and transmission (e.g. measles), they are sometimes completely unnecessary from this point of view (e.g. meningococcal meningitis, paralytic poliomyelitis). These microbes are not shed to the exterior after multiplying in the meninges or spinal cord.

For the microbe, systemic spread is fraught with obstacles and a major encounter with immune and other defenses is inevitable. Microorganisms have therefore been forced to develop strategies for bypassing or countering these defenses (see Chapter 11).

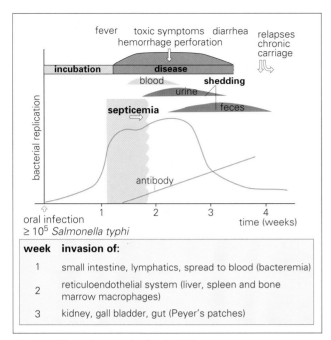

week   invasion of:

week	invasion of:
1	small intestine, lymphatics, spread to blood (bacteremia)
2	reticuloendothelial system (liver, spleen and bone marrow macrophages)
3	kidney, gall bladder, gut (Peyer's patches)

Fig. 10.5 The pathogenesis of typhoid fever.

REPLICATION RATES OF MICROORGANISMS

microorganism	situation	mean doubling time
most viruses	in cell*	< 1 h
many bacteria e.g. *Escherichia coli* staphylococci	*in vitro*	20–30 min
Salmonella typhimurium	*in vitro* *in vivo*	30 min 5–12 h
Mycobacterium tuberculosis	*in vitro* *in vivo*	24 h many days
Mycobacterium leprae[†]	*in vivo*	2 weeks
Treponema pallidum[†]	*in vivo*	30 h
Plasmodium falciparum	*in vitro/in vivo* (erythrocyte or hepatic cell)	8 h

* but some viruses show greatly delayed replication or delayed spread from cell to cell

[†] cannot be cultivated *in vitro*

Fig. 10.6 Replication rates of different microorganisms.

Rapid replication is essential for surface infections

The rate of replication of the infecting microorganism is of central importance, and doubling times vary from 20 minutes to several days *(Fig. 10.6)*. Hit-and-run (surface) infections need to replicate rapidly, whereas a microorganism that divides every few days (e.g. *Mycobacterium tuberculosis*) is likely to cause a slowly evolving disease with a long incubation period. Microorganisms nearly always multiply faster *in vitro* than they do in the intact host, as might be expected if host defenses are performing a useful function. In the host, microorganisms are phagocytosed and killed and the supply of nutrients may be limited. The net increase in numbers is slower than in laboratory cultures where microbes are not only free from attack by host defenses, but also every effort has been made to supply them with optimal nutrients, susceptible cells, and so on.

Mechanisms of Spread through the Body

Spread to lymph and blood
Invading microbes encounter a variety of defences on entering the body

After traversing the epithelium and its basement membrane at the body surface, invading microbes face the following defences:

- Tissue fluids containing antimicrobial substances (antibody, complement).
- Local macrophages (histiocytes) – subcutaneous and submucosal macrophages are a threat to microbial survival.
- The physical barrier of local tissue structure – local tissues consist of various cells in a hydrated gel matrix and although viruses can spread by stepwise invasion of cells, invasion is more difficult for bacteria and those that spread

effectively sometimes possess special spreading factors (e.g. streptococcal hyaluronidase).

- The lymphatic system – the rich network of the lymphatic system soon conveys microorganisms to the battery of phagocytic and immunologic defenses awaiting them in the local lymph node *(Fig. 10.7)*. Macrophages, strategically placed in the marginal and other lymph sinuses, constitute an efficient filtering system for lymph.

The infection may be halted at any stage, but by multiplying locally or in lymph nodes and by evading phagocytosis the microorganism can ultimately reach the bloodstream. Therefore, a minor injury to the skin, followed by a red streak (inflamed lymphatic) and a tender, swollen local lymph node are classic signs of streptococcal invasion. Most bacteria cause a great deal of inflammation when they invade in this way. In the early stages lymph flow increases, but eventually if there is enough inflammation and tissue damage in the node itself, the flow of the lymph may cease. In contrast, viruses and other intracellular microorganisms often invade lymph and blood silently and asymptomatically during the incubation period; this is facilitated when they infect monocytes or lymphocytes without initially damaging them.

Spread from blood
The fate of microorganisms in the blood depends upon whether they are free or associated with circulating cells

Viruses or small numbers of bacteria can enter the blood without causing a general body disturbance. For instance transient bacteremias are fairly common in normal individuals (e.g. they may occur after defecation or brushing teeth), but

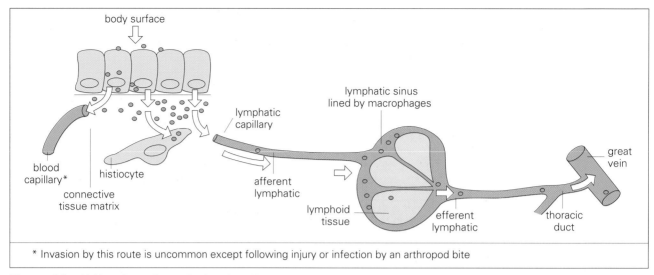

* Invasion by this route is uncommon except following injury or infection by an arthropod bite

Fig. 10.7 Microbial invasion and spread to lymph and blood.

the bacteria are usually filtered out and destroyed in macrophages lining the liver and spleen sinusoids. Under certain circumstances the same bacteria have a chance to localize in less well defended sites, such as congenitally abnormal heart valves in the case of viridans streptococci causing infective endocarditis, or in the ends of growing bones in the case of *Staphylococus aureus* osteomyelitis.

If microorganisms are free in the blood they are exposed to body defences such as antibodies and phagocytes. However, if they are associated with circulating cells, the associated cell can protect them from host defenses and carry them around the body. For example, many viruses such as Epstein–Barr virus (EBV) and rubella and intracellular bacteria *(Listeria, Brucella)* are present in lymphocytes or monocytes and, if not damaged or destroyed, these 'carrying cells' protect and transport them. Malaria infects erythrocytes and a few viruses infect platelets.

On entering the blood, microorganisms are exposed to macrophages of the reticuloendothelial system (see Chapter 4). Here in the sinusoids, where blood flows slowly, they are often phagocytosed and destroyed. But certain microorganisms survive and multiply in these cells (*Salmonella typhi*, *Leishmania donovani*, yellow fever virus). The microorganism may then:
- Spread to adjacent hepatic cells in the liver (hepatitis viruses), or splenic lymphoid tissues (measles virus).
- Re-invade the blood (*S. typhi*, hepatitis viruses).

Fig. 10.8 Circulating micoorganisms that invade organs via small blood vessels.

CIRCULATING MICROBES THAT INVADE ORGANS VIA SMALL BLOOD VESSELS		
microbe	**disease**	**principal organs invaded***
viruses hepatitis B rubella varicella–zoster virus polio mumps	hepatitis B congenital rubella chickenpox poliomyelitis mumps	liver placenta (fetus) skin, respiratory tract brain, spinal cord parotid, mammary glands
bacteria *Rickettsia rickettsi* *Treponema pallidum* *Neisseria meningitidis*	Rocky Mountain spotted fever secondary syphilis meningitis	skin skin, mucosae meninges
protozoa *Trypanosoma cruzi* *Plasmodium* spp.	Chagas' disease malaria	heart, skeletal muscle liver
helminths *Schistosoma* spp. (larvae) *Ascaris lumbricoides* (larvae) *Ancylostoma duodenale* (larvae)	schistosomiasis ascariasis hookworm	veins of bladder, bowel lung lung
* in liver, sinusoids; elsewhere, capillaries, venules		

Each circulating microorganism invades characteristic target organs and tissues

If uptake by reticuloendothelial macrophages is not complete within a short time or if large numbers of microorganisms are present in the blood, there is an opportunity for localization elsewhere in the vascular system. Why each circulating microorganism invades characteristic target organs and tissues *(Fig. 10.8)* is not completely understood, but may be due to:

- Specific receptors for the microorganism, leading to localization on the vascular endothelium of certain target organs.
- Random localization in organs throughout the body, only some of them being suitable for subsequent colonization and replication.

Circulating microbes also localize in sites where there is local inflammation because of the slower flow and sticky endothelium in inflamed vessels

After localization and organ invasion, the replicating microbe is shed from the body if the organ has a surface with access to the outside world *(Fig. 10.3)*. It may also be shed back into the bloodstream, either directly or via the lymphatic system.

Spread via nerves
Certain viruses spread via peripheral nerves from peripheral parts of the body to the central nervous system and vice versa

Tetanus toxin reaches the central nervous system (CNS) by this route. Rabies, herpes simplex virus (HSV) and varicella–zoster virus (V-ZV) travel in axons (see Chapters 8 and 22) and although the rate is slow, being accounted for by axonal flow (up to 10 mm/hour), this movement is important in the pathogenesis of these infections. Rabies not only reaches the CNS largely by peripheral nerves, but takes the same route from the CNS when it invades the salivary glands. Few, if any, host defenses are in a position to control this type of viral spread once nerves are invaded. Routes of invasion of the CNS are illustrated in *Figure 10.9*.

An uncommon route of spread to the CNS is via olfactory nerves with axons terminating on olfactory mucosa. For instance, certain free living ameba (e.g. *Naegleria* spp.) found in sludge at the bottom of freshwater pools may take this route

and cause meningoencephalitis in swimmers (see Chapter 22). Viruses and bacteria in the nasopharynx (e.g. meningococci, poliovirus) generally spread to the CNS via the blood.

Spread via cerebrospinal fluid
Once microorganisms have crossed the blood–cerebrospinal barrier they spread rapidly in the cerebrospinal fluid spaces

Such microorganisms can then invade neural tissues (echoviruses, mumps virus) as well as multiply locally (*Neisseria meningitidis, Haemophilus influenzae, Streptococcus pneumoniae*) and possibly infect ependymal and meningeal cells.

Spread via other routes
Rapid spread from one visceral organ to another can take place via the pleural or peritoneal cavity

Both the pleural and peritoneal cavities are lined by macrophages, as if in expectation of such invasion, and the peritoneal cavity contains an antimicrobial armory, consisting of the omentum (the 'abdominal policeman'), and many lymphocytes, macrophages and mast cells. Injury or disease in an abdominal organ provides a source of infection for peritonitis, as do chest wounds or lung infections for pleurisy.

Genetic Determinants of Spread and Replication

The pathogenicity of a microorganism is determined by the interplay of a variety of factors

These factors are referred to in Chapters 7 and 12. A distinction is sometimes made between pathogenicity and virulence: virulence implies a quantitative measure of pathogenicity. For instance, it can be expressed as the number of organisms necessary to cause death in 50% of individuals or lethal dose 50 (LD50). Nearly all pathogenicity factors are controlled by host and microbial genes. It has long been known that there are host genetic influences on susceptibility to infectious disease, and that mutations in microorganisms affect their pathogenicity. Within the past 15 years some of these genetic factors have been revealed by the application of molecular genetics techniques and as a result it is increasingly possible to identify the specific gene products involved. Progress has also been made, though with greater difficulty, in understanding the mode of action of these gene products.

Genetic determinants in the host
The ability of a microorganism to infect and cause disease in a given host is influenced by the genetic constitution of the host

At a relatively gross level, some human pathogens either do not infect other species or infect only closely related primates (e.g. measles, trachoma, typhoid, hepatitis B, warts), whereas others infect a very wide range of hosts (rabies, anthrax). Also, within a given host species, there are genetic determinants of susceptibility. The best examples are found in animals, but there are examples for human disease (see below). One example at the

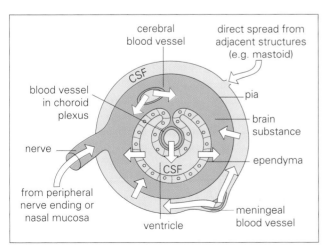

Fig. 10.9 Routes of microbial invasion of the central nervous system. (CSF, cerebrospinal fluid.)

molecular level is the sickle cell gene and susceptibility to malaria. Malaria merozoites (see Chapter 24) parasitize red blood cells and metabolize hemoglobin, freeing heme and using globin as a source of amino acids. The sickle cell gene causes a substitution of the amino acid valine for glutamic acid at one point in the β-polypeptide chain of the hemoglobin molecule. The new hemoglobin (hemoglobin S) becomes insoluble when reduced, and precipitates inside the red cell envelope, distorting the cell into the shape of a sickle. In homozygous individuals there are two of these genes and the individual has the disease sickle cell anemia, but in the heterozygote (sickle cell trait) the gene is less harmful, and provides resistance to severe forms of falciparum malaria, which ensures its selection in endemic malarial regions. The gene would be eliminated from populations after 10–20 generations unless it conferred some advantage. Restriction endonuclease analyses of the gene in Indian and West African populations have revealed that it arose independently in these malarious countries. Homozygotes, however, show increasing susceptibility to other infections, particularly *Strep. pneumoniae*, as a result of splenic dysfunction following repeated splenic infarcts.

Susceptibility often operates at the level of the immune response

A poor immune response to a given infection can lead to increased susceptibility to disease, whereas an immune response that is too vigorous may lead to immunopathologic disease (see Chapter 12). Of particular importance are the major histocompatibilty complex (MHC) genes on chromosome 6, coding for MHC class II (HLA A–D) antigens and controlling specific immune responses (see Chapters 5 and 6). For example, susceptibility to leprosy (see Chapter 23) is strongly influenced by MHC class II genes. People with HLA DR3 are more susceptible to tuberculoid leprosy, whereas those with HLA DQ1 are more susceptible to lepromatous leprosy.

Studies of identical twins (see panel) provide evidence that genetic determinants affect susceptibility to tuberculosis. The present day European population shows considerable resistance to this disease. During the great epidemics of pulmonary tuberculosis in Europe in the seventeenth, eighteenth and nineteenth centuries, genetically susceptible individuals were weeded out. In 1850 mortality rates in Boston, New York, London, Paris and Berlin were over 500/100 000, but with improvements in living conditions these fell to 180/100 000 by 1900, and they have fallen even more since then. However, previously unexposed populations, especially in Africa and the Pacific Islands, show much greater susceptibility to respiratory tuberculosis. In the Plains Indians living in the Qu'Appelle Valley reservation in Saskatchewan, Canada, in 1886, tuberculosis spread through the body to infect glands, bones, joints and meninges, giving a death rate of 9000/100 000.

Genetic determinants in the microbe
Virulence is likely to be coded for by more than one microbial gene

Virulence is determined by numerous factors such as adhesion, penetration into cells, antiphagocytic activity, production of toxins and interaction with the immune system. Consequently different genes and gene products are probably involved at different stages in pathogenesis.

Under natural circumstances microorganisms are constantly undergoing genetic change, especially mutations. The single-stranded RNA viruses in particular show very high mutation rates. Some of these mutations affect surface antigens, which undergo rapid selection in the host under immune pressure (antibody, cell-mediated immunity), as in the case of the rapidly evolving M proteins of streptococci, and the capsid proteins of picornaviruses. In addition, genetic changes in bacteria are often due to acquisition or loss of extrachromosomal genetic elements called 'plasmids' (see Chapter 3).

Changes in the virulence of a microorganism take place during artificial culture in the laboratory. For instance, in the classical procedure for obtaining a live vaccine (see Chapter 29), a microorganism is repeatedly grown (passaged) *in vitro*

Genetically determined susceptibility to infection

There are several classic examples of susceptibility to infectious disease determined by unidentified but presumably genetic factors in the human host:

The Lubeck disaster due to vaccination with virulent tubercle bacilli

In Lubeck, Germany, in 1926, living virulent tubercle bacilli instead of attenuated (vaccine) bacilli were inadvertently given to 249 babies. There were 76 deaths, but the rest, who developed only minor lesions, survived and were alive and well 12 years later. Each received the same inoculum, and it seems likely that the differences in outcome were largely due to genetic factors in the host.

A military misfortune due to contamination of yellow fever vaccine with hepatitis B virus

In 1942, more than 45 000 US military personnel were vaccinated against yellow fever, but were inadvertently injected at the same time with hepatitis B virus present as a contaminant in the human serum used to stabilize the vaccine. There were 914 clinical cases of hepatitis, of which 580 were mild, 301 moderate and 33 severe. Even with a given batch of vaccine the incubation period varied from 10–20 weeks. Serologic tests were not then available so the number of subclinical infections is unknown. In this case both physiologic and genetic influences on susceptibility may have played a part.

Identical twins are affected similarly by respiratory tuberculosis

A study of tuberculosis in twins when at least one twin had the disease, showed that for identical twins, the other twin was affected in 87% of cases. With non-identical twins the equivalent figure was only 26%. In addition, the identical twins had a similar type of clinical disease.

and this generally leads to reduced pathogenicity in the host. The new strain is then referred to as 'attenuated' *(Fig. 10.10)*.

Our understanding of the genetic basis for microbial pathogenicity had advanced rapidly in recent years due to DNA cloning and genetic manipulation techniques. For instance, by introducing or deleting/inactivating genome segments, the virulence genes can be identified. Examples are shown in *Figure 10.11*. For many viruses the nucleic acid sequence of the entire genome has been established and functions are slowly being assigned to specific sequences.

Other Factors Affecting Spread and Replication

Various other factors have an influence on susceptibility to infectious disease *(Fig. 10.12)*. In most cases it is not known whether this involves differences in microbial spread and replication or differences in host immune and inflammatory reponses. Infections in hosts with immunologic and other defects are described in Chapter 26.

The brain can influence immune responses

When stress (a loosely used word) is associated with malnutrition or crowding it may be difficult to disentangle the separate influences of these various factors on susceptibility to infection, as in the case of tuberculosis. The brain can, however, influence immune responses, acting via the hypothalamus, pituitary and adrenal cortex. It has long been known that glucocorticoids, which have powerful actions on immune cells, are needed for resistance to infection and trauma. A shortage of glucocorticoids, as in Addison's disease, or an excess, as with steroid therapy, results in increased susceptibility to infection *(Fig. 10.12)*. In addition, the brain, the endocrine and the immune systems often use the same molecular messengers – cytokines, peptide hormones, neurotransmitters. Neural cells, for instance, have receptors for interferons and for interleukins (IL) – IL-1, IL-2, IL-3, IL-6 – and thymic lymphocytes can produce prolactin and growth hormone. Immune–neuroendocrine cross-talk now has molecular respectability and provides an acceptable basis for the influence of the brain on immunity and infectious disease.

ATTENUATION OF PATHOGENS *IN VITRO*		
pathogen	**passage**	**attenuated (live) product**
Mycobacterium bovis	10 years of repeated passage in glycerin–bile–potato medium	bacille Calmette–Guérin (BCG) vaccine
rubella virus	27 passages in human diploid cells	rubella vaccine (Wistar RA 27/3)

Fig. 10.10 Examples of attenuation of pathogens following repeated passage *in vitro*.

THE MOLECULAR BASIS OF MICROBIAL PATHOGENICITY		
microorganism	**gene or gene product**	**effect on virulence**
Streptococcus pyogenes	M protein; 60 mm long coiled coil extending from bacterial cell wall with N terminal hypervariable domain amino acid sequence overlap with host components (myosin, tropomyosin, keratin, etc.)	antiphagocytic role; inhibit opsonization; exact mechanism unknown autoimmune complication
Yersinia enterocolitica	invasion (inv) gene codes for 92 kD protein on bacterial surface	required for uptake of bacteria into epithelial cells and macrophages of Peyer's patches
Shigella spp.	ipa B (**i**nvasion **p**lasmid **a**ntigen B) gene	mediates lysis of vacuolar membrane and escape of bacteria into cytoplasm of colonic epithelial cells*
Leishmania donovani	Arg–Gly–Asp sequence of gp63 surface protein	binds to C3b receptor on macrophage and thereby infects this cell
Neisseria gonorrhoeae	genes for proteins of pili (fimbriae) and for certain outer membrane proteins	proteins mediate attachment to mucosal cells, independent control of each gene makes *N. gonorrhoeae* the 'master chameleon', altering its surface antigens to evade host immune responses
herpes simplex virus type I	gene for envelope glycoprotein C (gC)	gC acts as receptor for C3b, blocking the classical pathway and enabling virus or virus-infected cell to resist lysis by complement plus antibody
* Shigellae enter gut wall via M cells in Peyer's patches, then invade colonic epithelial cells from basolateral surfaces. In this, as in other bacterial infections, invasiveness depends upon coordinated expression of many different genes.		

Fig. 10.11 Examples of the molecular basis of microbial pathogenicity.

HOST FACTORS INFLUENCING SUSCEPTIBILITY TO INFECTIOUS DISEASE			
factor	**example**	**alteration in susceptibility**	**mechanism**
pregnancy	hepatitis viruses	more lethal outcome	?increased metabolic burden for liver in pregnancy
	urinary infections	pyelonephritis more common	reduced peristalsis in ureter
malnutrition	measles	more severe; more lethal	vitamin A deficiency; depressed (CMI)
age	respiratory syncytial virus	more severe; more lethal in infant	small diameter of airways
	mumps, chicken-pox, Epstein–Barr virus infection	more severe in adult	?increased immunopathology
atmospheric pollution	raised sulfur dioxide levels	excess acute respiratory disease	?interference with mucociliary defenses
	silicosis	increased susceptibility to tuberculosis	?damage to lung macrophages
foreign bodies	necrotic bone fragments	chronic osteomyelitis more common	antimicrobial defenses less effective in necrotic tissue
	necrotic tissue	increased susceptibility to *Clostridium perfringens*	anaerobic necrotic tissues favour bacterial growth
stress, hormones	glucocorticoid production:- *decreased* (Addison's disease)	increased susceptibility to infection	hypersensitivity to inflammatory/immune responses?
	increased (steroid therapy)	increased susceptibility to infection	reduction in protective immune/inflammatory responses

Fig. 10.12 Host factors influencing susceptibility to infectious disease. (CMI, cell-mediated immunity.)

- Infections restricted to the body surfaces (common cold, shigella dysentery) have shorter incubation periods than systemic infections (measles, typhoid), and adaptive (immune) host responses tend to be less important.
- Microbes with a slow growth rate (e.g. *M. tuberculosis*) tend to cause more slowly evolving diseases.
- Spread through the body takes place primarily via lymph and blood. The fate of circulating microbes depends upon whether they are free or present in circulating blood cells.
- Uptake by reticuloendothelial cells in liver and spleen focuses infection into these organs, but specific localization in the vascular bed of other organs (e.g. mumps virus in salivary glands, meningococci in meninges) is not understood.
- Viruses can spread in either direction along nerve axons, and this is important in the pathogenesis of recurrent HSV infection, zoster and rabies.
- Pathogenicity and virulence are strongly influenced by genetic factors in the host (e.g. tuberculosis in identical twins) and by genetic factors in the microbe (e.g sickle cell trait in falciparum malaria).

1. What are the routes by which microbes can reach a) the salivary glands and b) the liver?
2. Is invasion of the CNS ever of any value from the microbe's point of view?
3. Give examples of microbes that a) travel free in the plasma and b) travel in association with blood cells. What are the consequences in each case?
4. Why can tuberculosis and leprosy bacilli not cause rapid 'hit and run' infections?
5. Give an example of a change in a single human gene that causes an important change in susceptibility to an infectious disease.

Further Reading

Alonzo de Velasco E, Verheul AF, Verhoef J, Snippe H. *Streptococcus pneumoniae*: virulence factors, pathogenesis and vaccines. *Microbiol Rev* 1995;**59**:591–603.

Griffin JW, Watson DF. Axonal transport in neurologic disease. *Ann Neurol* 1988;**23**:3–13.

Mims CA, Dimmock NJ, Nash A, Stephen J. *Mims' Pathogenesis of Infectious Disease*, 4th edition. London: Academic Press, 1995.

Savino W, Dardenne M. Immune–neuroendocrine interactions. *Immunol Today* 1995;**16**:318–322.

Townsend GC, Scheld WM. *In vitro* models of the blood–brain barrier to study bacterial meningitis. *Trends Microbiol* 1995;**3**:441–445.

Parasite Survival Strategies and Persistent Infections

Introduction

Most common infectious organisms have developed 'answers' to host defenses
So far we have concentrated on the battery of mechanisms available to the host, both natural and adaptive, to keep out and destroy the parasite. Powerful as these are, they are obviously not 100% effective, otherwise healthy people would never have infections. In fact, most of the common infectious organisms described in this book have developed 'answers' to host defenses because their ability to survive as human parasites has depended upon this. They successfully infect humans and are of concern to the physician precisely because they have developed strategies for evading or actively interfering with host defenses.

The evasive strategies adopted by microbes to avoid natural non-adaptive innate defenses such as phagocytes and complement have been outlined in Chapter 9. These include:

- Killing phagocytes.
- Avoiding being killed by phagocytes.
- Producing iron-binding molecules.
- Interfering with ciliary action.

Strategies to evade adaptive defenses are more sophisticated than those for evading innate defenses

The success of microbes in evading or interfering with adaptive (immune) defenses is discussed in this chapter. The strategies involved are more sophisticated than those evading innate defenses because lymphocytes are programmed so that their cell receptors can recognize virtually any shape (B cells) or amino acid sequence (T cells), provided it is not identical to self, for example:

- The polysaccharide capsules of bacteria prevent non-immune contact between phagocytes and the bacterial cell wall, but are quickly recognized as foreign by B cell surface receptors (immunoglobulin), leading to the formation of antibody with consequent opsonization and phagocytosis of the bacteria.
- Many microorganisms such as bacteria and fungi can resist intracellular destruction by macrophages, but their peptides are presented in association with major histocompatability complex (MHC) molecules on the macrophage surface, and their presence is detected by T cells. A new set of cytotoxic and other immune mechanisms are then brought into action.

In both these examples the lymphocytes are behaving like a highly specialized and sharply observant secret police force in contrast to the everyday activities of the more pedestrian macrophage.

Parasite Survival Strategies

Parasite survival strategies can take as many forms as there are parasites, but they can be usefully classified according to the immune component that is evaded and the means

selected to do this (see Chapter 7). As a result, the microbe is able to undergo what are often quite lengthy periods of growth and spread during the incubation period before being shed and transmitted to the next host, as occurs in hepatitis B and tuberculosis. Shedding of the microbe for just a few extra days after clinical recovery gives more extensive transmission in the community and this is a worthwhile result.

Some microbes are able to persist in the host

Certain microbes are able to remain (persist) in the host for many years, often for life. From the microbe's point of view, persistence is worthwhile only if shedding occurs during the persistence. Persistent microbes fall into two categories:

- Those that are shed more or less continuously, such as the Epstein–Barr virus (EBV) into saliva, hepatitis B virus into blood and eggs into feces in various helminth infections.
- Those that are shed intermittently, such as herpes simplex virus (HSV), polyomaviruses, typhoid bacilli, tubercle bacilli and malaria parasites.

Viruses are particularly good at thwarting immune defenses

Viruses are able to thwart immune defenses for a number of reasons:

- Their invasion of tissues and cells is often 'silent'. Unlike most bacteria they do not form toxins, and as long as they do not cause extensive cell destruction there is no sign of illness until the onset of immune and inflammatory responses, sometimes several weeks after infection as occurs in hepatitis B virus and EBV infections.
- Viruses such as rubella virus, wart viruses, hepatitis B virus and EBV can infect cells for long periods without adverse effects on cell viability.
- In addition viruses establish intimate molecular relationships with the infected cell. Their replication depends on this intimacy and it means that many viruses can engineer subtle changes in cell function such as interfering with the production or action of interferons (rotaviruses, adenoviruses).

Virus latency is based on the intimate molecular relationship with the infected cell. The viral genome continues to be present in the host without producing antigens or infectious material, and only does so very occasionally, when the virus reactivates (becomes patent).

Strategies for evading host defenses

One strategy for evading microorganisms is to cause a rapid 'hit and run' infection. The microbe invades, multiplies and is shed within a few days, before immune defenses have had time to come into action. Infections of the body surfaces (rhinoviruses, rotaviruses) come into this category. Otherwise, the principal strategies employed by parasites to elude the lymphocyte (as discussed in the following pages) are:

- Concealment of antigens.
- Antigenic variation.
- Immunosuppression.

Concealment of Antigens

A spy in a foreign country can conceal his presence from the police by hiding, by never venturing out of doors, or by adopting the disguise of a native. Parasites have the same choice. Places to hide include the interior of host cells (though the MHC molecules act as 'informers' for this compartment, picking up and transporting microbial peptides to the cell surface where they will be recognized), and particular sites in the body where lymphocytes do not normally circulate ('privileged sites', the equivalent of 'no-go' areas).

Remaining inside cells without their antigens being displayed on the surface prevents recognition

If a microbe can remain inside cells without allowing its antigens to be displayed on the cell surface, it will remain unrecognized ('incognito') as far as immune defenses are concerned. Specific antibody and T cell responses may be induced, but the microbe inside the cell is unaffected. Persistent latent viruses such as HSV in sensory neurones behave in this way. During reactivation, of course, re-exposure and boosting of immune defenses is inevitable.

Other strategies are possible. Several viruses (HIV in macrophages, coronaviruses) display their proteins 'secretly' on the walls of intracellular vacuoles instead of at the cell surface, and bud into these vacuoles. Adenoviruses have taken more active steps to avoid antigen display. One of the adenoviral proteins (E19) combines with class I MHC molecules and prevents their passage to the cell surface so that infected cells are not recognized by cytotoxic T cells.

Colonizing privileged sites keeps the microbe out of reach of circulating lymphocytes

The vast numbers of microbes that colonize the skin and the intestinal lumen, together with those that are shed directly into external secretions, are effectively out of reach of circulating lymphocytes. They are exposed to secretory antibodies, which although able to bind to the microbe (e.g. influenza virus) and render it less infectious, are generally unable to kill the microbe or control its replication in or on the epithelial

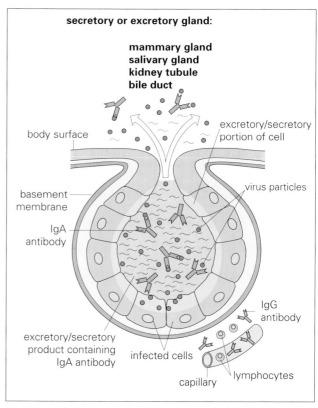

Fig. 11.1 Viral infection of cell surfaces facing the external world. Infection of the surface epithelium of, for instance, a secretory or excretory gland allows direct shedding of the virus to the exterior, as well as avoidance of host immune defenses.

surface *(Figs 11.1, 11.2)*. A local inflammatory response, however, can enhance host defenses.

Within the body it is more difficult to avoid lymphocytes and antibodies, but certain sites are safer than others. These include the central nervous system, joints, testes and placenta. Here lymphocyte circulation is less intense and there is more restricted access of antibodies and complement. However, as soon as inflammatory responses are induced then lymphocytes, monocytes and antibodies are rapidly delivered and the site loses its privilege.

Additional privileged sites can be created by the infectious organism itself. A good example is the hydatid cyst that develops in liver, lung or brain around growing colonies of the tapeworm *Echinococcus granulosus (Fig. 11.3)* inside which the worms can survive even though the blood of the host contains protective levels of antibody.

Perhaps the most highly privileged site of all is host DNA and this is occupied by the retroviruses. Retroviral RNA is transcribed by the reverse transcriptase into DNA as a necessary part of the replicative cycle and this then becomes integrated into the DNA of the host cell (see Chapter 19). As long as there is no cell damage and viral products are not expressed on the cell surface where they can be recognized by immune defenses, the virus enjoys total anonymity. This is what makes complete cure and complete removal of virus from a patient infected with HIV such a daunting task. The

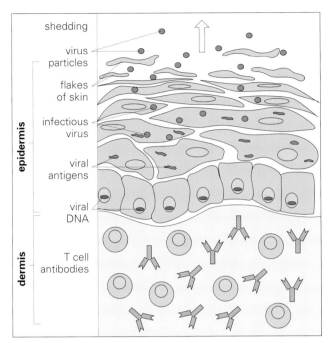

Fig. 11.2 Wart virus replication in epidermis – a privileged site? Cell differentiation such as keratinization controls virus replication, and as a result virus matures when it is physically removed from immune defenses.

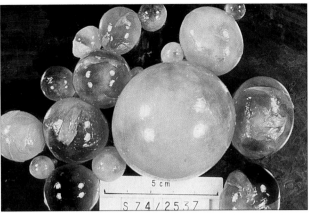

Fig. 11.3 Hydatid cysts. Multiple, thin-walled, fluid-filled cysts in a surgical specimen. The lung is a common site. (Courtesy of JA Innes.)

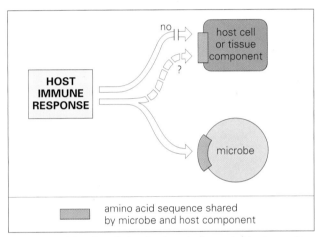

Fig. 11.4 Molecular mimicry by the microbe probably does not restrain the immune response, but host cells and tissue can then be subject to immune damage, for example rheumatic heart disease following streptococcal infection is caused by antibodies reacting with meromyosin, the cross-reacting determinant.

intragenomic site becomes even more privileged if the egg or sperm is infected. The viral genome will then be present in all embryonic cells and transferred from one generation to another as if it were the host's own DNA. Luckily this does not happen with HIV or with human T cell lymphotropic virus (HTLV) 1 and 2. However, the 'endogenous' retroviruses of humans present in profusion as DNA sequences in our genome, but not expressed as antigens, come into this category. They are part of our inheritance. This surely represents the ultimate, the final logical step in parasitism, at the borderline between infection and heredity.

Mimicry sounds like a useful strategy, but does not prevent the host from making an antimicrobial response

If the microbe can in some way avoid inducing an immune response, this can be regarded as a 'concealment' of its antigens. One method is by mimicking host antigens (*Fig. 11.4*). Numerous examples are known of parasite-derived molecules that resemble those of the host (*Fig. 11.5*). In the case of viral proteins, mimicry based on amino acid sequence homology (sharing of 8–10 consecutive amino acids) is seen to be common when computer comparisons are made between viral and host proteins. Perhaps the most celebrated example, however, is the cross-reaction between group A beta-hemolytic streptococci and human myocardium. This cross-reaction underlies the development of rheumatic heart disease following repeated streptococcal infection due to antibody made against the cross-reacting determinant meromyosin (*see Fig. 11.4*). The

fact that the host makes such autoantibodies shows that in this case mimicry does not protect the bacteria. The conclusion is that although mimicry sounds like a useful strategy for microbes and occurs quite frequently, it does not prevent the host from making an antimicrobial autoimmune response.

Microbes can conceal themselves by taking up host molecules to cover their surface

This is illustrated in *Figure 11.5*. A superb example of this is the blood-fluke *Schistosoma*, which acquires a complete surface coat of host blood group glycolipids, MHC antigens and immunoglobulin molecules from the plasma. Such a worm must indeed be virtually invisible even to a lymphocyte. For unknown reasons, however, this strategy is essentially restricted to worms.

The uptake of immunoglobulin molecules by the microbe seems to be a more widespread phenomenon. A number of viruses and bacteria code for Fc receptors, which are displayed

MIMICRY AND UPTAKE OF HOST ANTIGENS		
antigen	parasite	corresponding host antigen
mimicry	Epstein–Barr virus	human fetal thymus*
	streptococci	cardiac muscle (meromyosin)
	klebsiella	HLA-B27**
	Mycobacterium tuberculosis	65 kDa heat shock protein
	Neisseria meningitidis	embryonic brain
	treponema	cardiolipin†
	Mycoplasma pneumoniae	erythrocytes††
	plasmodia	thymosin-α_1
	Trypanosoma cruzi	heart, nerve
	schistosoma	glutathione transferase
antigen uptake	cytomegalovirus	β_2-microglobulin
	schistosoma	glycolipids, HLA, Ig etc.
	filarial nematodes	albumin

*   also cross-reacts with erythrocytes of certain species and is the basis for the Paul Bunnell (heterophil antibody) test
** possible basis for ankylosing spondylitis
†   basis for Wassermann-type antibody test for syphilis
†† basis for cold agglutinin test

Fig. 11.5 Some examples of mimicry or uptake of host antigens by parasites. (HLA, human lymphocyte antigen; Ig, immunoglobulin.)

on their surface and bind immunoglobulin molecules of all specificities in an immunologically useless upside-down position (*Fig. 11.6*, and see below). This prevents the access of specific antibodies or T cells to the microbe or the infected cell.

Tolerizing the host prevents the induction of an immune response

An alternative strategy for the microbe is to avoid inducing an immune response or to induce a poor response. There are four possible methods:

- Infection during early embryonic life.
- The production of large quantities of the microbial antigen or of antigen–antibody complexes.
- Exploiting 'gaps' in the host's immune repertoire.
- Upsetting the balance between antibody and cell-mediated immune responses – between T helper cells (TH) 1 and 2 responses.

Infection during early embryonic life

Before development of the immune system, a time when antigens present are regarded as 'self', infection could possibly result in immune tolerance. However, in the case of intrauterine infection with cytomegalovirus (CMV), rubella virus and syphilis, the fetus does eventually produce IgM antibody, which is detectable in umbilical cord blood. But cell-mediated responses are more seriously impaired. Children with congenital CMV or rubella fail to develop lymphoproliferative

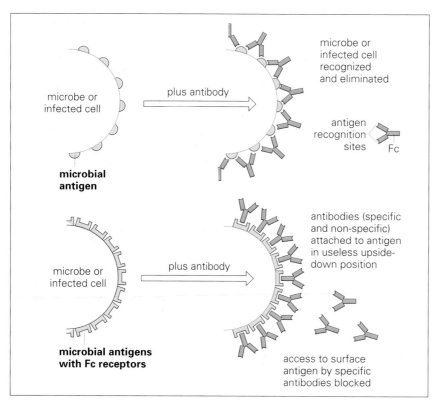

Fig. 11.6 The production of Fc receptors is of some benefit to microbes, for example staphylococci, streptococci, herpes simplex virus, varicella–zoster virus and cytomegalovirus.

responses to CMV or rubella antigens and consequently take years to clear the virus from the body (see Chapter 21). In some cases infection in the neonatal period is more likely to result in tolerance than infection in later life. Therefore, neonatal infection with hepatitis B virus frequently results in permanent carriage of the virus, though the mechanism is unknown.

Production of large quantities of microbial antigen or antigen–antibody complexes

Large quantities of microbial antigen or antigen–antibody complexes circulating in the body can cause immune tolerance to that antigen. Anergy, as evidenced by normal antibody but depressed cell-mediated immune responses, is seen in disseminated coccidiomycosis and cryptococcosis, and in visceral and diffuse cutaneous leishmaniasis, in each case associated with large amounts of microbial antigen in the circulation.

Exploiting 'gaps' in the host's immune repertoire

There are likely to be certain peptides to which the host makes a poor immune response, based on the nature of the host's MHC class II molecules. These represent genetically determined 'gaps' in the host's immune repertoire, and microbes, as they evolve, might be be expected to match these peptides. In other words, microbes may be constantly 'probing' the immune repertoire of the host, seeking out weaknesses. There is no proof that this occurs, but it is conceivable, for instance, that the great susceptibility of African people to tuberculosis is due to a genetically determined, poor cell-mediated immune response to key tubercular antigens. Europeans show greater resistance due to the 'weeding out' of genetically susceptible individuals over hundreds of years. It has been estimated that 30% of all adult deaths in Europe in the nineteenth century were due to tuberculosis.

Upsetting the balance between antibody and Tн1 and Tн2 responses

Resistance to infection often depends upon a suitable balance between antibody and Tн1 and Tн2 responses (see Chapter 5). Good defense against tuberculosis and herpesviruses needs cell-mediated immunity whereas antibody is required for good defense against polioviruses or *Streptococcus pneumoniae*. By inducing an ineffective type of response a microbe can promote its own survival.

Antigenic Variation

Reverting to the image of a spy in foreign territory, there is another way to confuse the enemy – by repeated changes in appearance. The African trypanosome, the causative organism of sleeping sickness, does this, and so do a wide range of viruses, bacteria and protozoa. Antigenic variation can occur:

- During the course of infection in a given individual.
- During spread of the microbe through the host community *(Fig. 11.7)*.

As a strategy for evading host immune responses, antigenic variation depends upon variation occurring in antigens whose recognition is involved in protection. Antigenic variation is common as the microbe passes through the host community and it tends to be more important in longer-lived hosts, such as humans in whom microbial survival is favored by multiple reinfections during the lifetime of a given individual. Also it is more common in infections limited to respiratory or intestinal epithelium where the incubation period is less than one week and the microbe can commonly infect, multiply and be shed from the body before a significant secondary immune response is generated. During systemic infections (measles, mumps, typhoid) the incubation period is longer and secondary responses have more opportunity to come into action and control an infection by an antigenic variant. Accordingly, antigenic variation is not an important feature of these systemic infections.

At the molecular level there are three main mechanisms for antigenic variation:

- Mutation.
- Recombination.
- Gene switching.

The best known example of mutation is the influenza virus

As the influenza virus spreads through the community there are repeated mutations in the genes coding for hemagglutinin and neuraminidase (see Chapter 17), causing small antigenic changes that are sufficient to reduce the effectiveness of B and T cell memory built up in response to earlier infections. This is called 'antigenic drift'. Human rhinoviruses and enteroviruses are evolving rapidly and show a similar drift. Antigenic drift could account for the

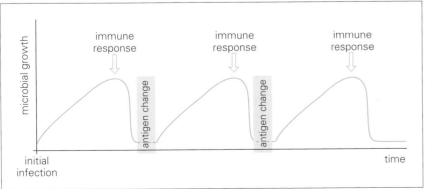

Fig. 11.7 Antigenic variation as a microbial strategy. The change in antigens may take place in the originally infected individual enabling the microbe to undergo renewed growth (e.g. trypanosomiasis), or it may take place as the microbe passes through the host population, enabling it to reinfect a given individual (e.g. influenza).

wealth of antigenic types of staphylococci, streptococci and pneumococci. During poliovirus epidemics, mutations occur at the rate of about two base substitutions per week, some of them involving the main antigenic sites on the virus. HIV (see Chapter 19) undergoes antigenic drift, but in this case it occurs during infection of a given individual, which helps to explain the difficulties experienced by the immune system in controlling this infection. Mutations affecting the epitopes recognized by cytotoxic T (Tc) cells are the source of 'escape mutants'.

The classic example of recombination involves influenza A virus

More extensive and sudden alterations in antigens can take place by the exchange of genetic material between two different microbes. The classic example is genetic 'shift' in influenza A virus, in which human and avian virus strains recombine (see Chapter 17). As a result, a completely new strain of influenza A virus suddenly emerges, brandishing a hemagglutinin or neuraminidase of avian origin. This new virus, not previously experienced by the present population, gives rise to an influenza pandemic.

Gene switching was first demonstrated in African trypanosomes

Gene switching represents the most dramatic form of antigenic variation and was first demonstrated in the African trypanosomes, *Trypanosoma gambiense* and *T. rhodesiense* (see Chapter 00). These organisms carry genes for about 1000 quite distinct surface molecules known as variant-specific glycoproteins, which cover almost the entire surface and are immunodominant. The trypanosome can switch from the use of one gene to another, much as a B cell does with the immunoglobulin heavy chain constant genes. The effect on the host is a sequence of unrelated infections at approximately weekly intervals. This enables the trypanosome to persist while the immune system is constantly trying to catch up with it. The main stimulus for each gene switch is possibly the antibody response itself, but the exact mechanism is not clear. About 10% of the trypanosome genome consists of surface coat genes, but this is a worthwhile investment for the parasite.

Gene switching is thought to result in the relapsing persistent course of certain infections

Gene switching is also thought to be responsible for the relapsing persistent course of certain other infections, including *Borrelia recurrentis* (relapsing fever) and brucellosis. It is also important in gonorrhea, not because of antigenic variation, but because changes in bacterial properties are desirable at different stages of the infection. For instance, attachment to urethral epithelium is vital early in infection by *Neisseria gonorrhoeae*, but attachment to phagocytes is less desirable. Hence there is a switching of genes coding for the pilin and outer membrane proteins that mediate attachment. However, gonococci also show great antigenic variation as they circulate through the host community and this is achieved by genetic rearrangements and recombinations in the repertoire of pilin genes.

Immunosuppression

Many virus infections cause a general temporary immunosuppression

A large variety of microorganisms cause immunosuppression in the infected host. As a subversive strategy this makes sense, but the extent to which the microbe benefits is often debatable. The host shows a depressed immune response to antigens of the infecting microbe (antigen-specific suppression) or, more commonly, both to antigens of the infecting microbe and unrelated antigens. HIV is one of the most spectacular, but by no means the only microbe that interferes with the immune system in this way *(Fig. 11.8)*. The mechanism is generally not understood, but it often involves invasion of the immune system by the microbe – in other words 'to evade, invade'.

Clearly it would benefit the microbe if most responses to its own but not to other antigens were suppressed, but this is uncommon. However, a general immunosuppression, as long as it is temporary, might give the microbe enough time to grow, spread and be shed before being eliminated. This is what happens in many virus infections. A lasting general immunosuppression would be detrimental to the microbe because susceptibility to other infections would cause unnecessary damage to the host species. From this point of view HIV has certainly overstepped the mark.

Different microbes have different immunosuppressive effects

Immunosuppression by microbes often involves actual infection of immune cells, either :
- T cells (HIV, measles).
- B cells (EBV) .
- Macrophages (HIV, leishmania).
- Dendritic cells (HIV).

This may result in impaired cell function, such as blocking of cell division, blocking of release of interleukin-2 (IL-2) or other cytokines, or in cell death.

Additional immunosuppressive actions taken by microbes include the release of immunosuppressive molecules. For instance, the gp41 polypeptide formed by HIV acts as an 'immunologic anesthetic', temporarily blocking T cell function. Other microbes (poxviruses, herpesviruses, *T. cruzi*) release molecules that interfere with the action of complement or with immunologically important cytokines such as IL-2, IFNs or tumor necrosis factor (TNF). There is no doubt that other examples will be discovered in the future.

Certain microbe toxins are immunosuppressants

A particularly dramatic form of immune interference is practised by the staphylococci. Many strains liberate exotoxins (staphylococcal enterotoxin, epidermolytic toxin and toxic shock syndrome toxin) that are responsible for disease. At first sight, producing these toxins seems to be of no advantage to the staphylococci, but it is now recognized that they have extremely powerful immunomodulatory actions – they are the most potent T cell mitogens known, and act at picomolar concentrations. They function as 'superantigens' and

DEPRESSED IMMUNE RESPONSES CAUSED BY MICROBIAL INFECTIONS			
parasite		feature of immunosuppression	mechanism
viruses	HIV	↓Ab ↓CMI long lasting	↓CD4$^+$ T cells immunosuppressive molecule (gp41) ↓ antigen presentation by infected APC polyclonal activation of B cells
	Epstein–Barr virus	↓CMI temporary	includes polyclonal activation of infected B cells
	measles	↓CMI temporary	differentiation blocked in infected T and B cells
	cytomegalovirus	↓CMI temporary	unknown; infection of very occasional mononuclear cells
	varicella–zoster virus mumps	↓CMI temporary	infection of T cells
bacteria	*M. leprae* (lepromatous leprosy)	↓CMI	polyclonal activation of B cells induction of suppressor T cells
protozoa	*Trypanosoma* *Plasmodia* *Toxoplasma* *Leishmania*	↓Ab ↓CMI	?
Ab, antibody; CMI, cell-mediated immunity; APC, antigen-presenting cell			

Fig. 11.8 Depressed immune responses in microbial infections. In most cases the mechanisms are unclear, but possible important factors are listed. For HIV, the depressed responses are seen later, after initial neutralizing antibody and cytotoxic cell responses. There are at least nine possible mechanisms involved in HIV immunosuppression, but decreased numbers of CD4$^+$ T cells is probably the most important.

after binding to class II MHC molecules on antigen-presenting cells, act as polyclonal activators of T cells (*see Fig. 11.9*). A large proportion (2–20%) of all T cells respond by dividing and releasing cytokines; only 0.001–0.01% are capable of doing this in response to a regular antigen.

It would be logical to presume that these toxins, which are coded for by plasmids, were acquired by the parasite to upset immune responses and therefore help in the eternal battle with host defenses. As if to confirm this, it has been found that similar molecules are produced by certain streptococci and mycoplasmas.

Possible mechanisms by which the staphylococcal toxins may interfere with immune defenses include:

- Excessive local liberation of cytokines by activated cells, upsetting the delicate balance of immune regulation.
- Killing of T cells or other immune cells.
- Polyclonal activation, diverting T cells of all specificities into immunologically unproductive activity (see *Fig. 11.9*).

Less dramatic polyclonal activation is seen in many other infections. Microbes may cause polyclonal activation of B cells as well as T cells, for example in EBV and HIV infections, and this can be interpreted as an 'immunodiversion' by the infecting microbe. One consequence is that a range of 'irrelevant', sometimes autoimmune, antibodies are formed (e.g. heterophil antibodies in EBV infection).

Some microbes interfere with the local expression of the immune response in tissues

Some microbes do not interfere with the development of an immune response, but actively interfere with its expression in tissues. For instance *N. gonorrhoeae*, *S. pneumoniae* and many strains of *Haemophilus influenzae* liberate a protease that cleaves human IgA antibody. These bacteria are residents or invaders of mucosae where IgA antibodies operate, and the ability to produce such an enzyme seems unlikely to be an accident.

An equally worthwhile local interference practised by so many different infectious agents that it is likely to be significant, is the production by the microbe of Fc receptor molecules (see *Fig. 11.6*). The best known example is protein A, a cell wall protein excreted from virulent staphylococci that inhibits the phagocytosis of antibody-coated bacteria, as shown in *Figure 11.6*. Certain herpesviruses (HSV, varicella–zoster virus (VZV), CMV) code for molecules that act as Fc receptors for IgG, and streptococci produce an Fc receptor for IgA.

Other examples include:

- The production by *Pseudomonas* of an elastase that inactivates the C3b and C5a components of complement and hence tends to inhibit opsonic and other host defense functions of complement.

- HSV production of a molecule, gC (glycoprotein C), that functions as a receptor for C3b. It is present on the virus particle and on the infected cell and interferes with complement activation, protecting both the virus and the infected cell from destruction by antibody and complement.

Unfortunately, although the above phenomena look convincingly like microbial adaptations for upsetting host defenses, it is not always easy to prove that this is the case.

Immune system function depends on the local liberation of cytokines, which bind to receptor molecules on other immune cells. The larger viruses (poxviruses, herpesviruses) often encode their own versions of these cytokines (e.g. an IL-10 homolog by EBV) or receptor molecules, and therefore interfere with the immune system communication network.

Various viruses evade IFNs by either failing to induce adequate amounts (hepatitis B) or developing resistance to their antiviral action (rotaviruses, adenoviruses).

Persistent Infections

Persistent infections represent a failure of host defenses

One way of looking at persistent infections (Fig. 11.10) is to regard them as failures of host defenses. Host defenses are designed to control microbial growth and spread and to eliminate the microbe from the body. The microbe may persist:

- In a flagrantly defiant infectious form, as with hepatitis B

in the blood or the schistosome in the blood vessels of the alimentary tract or bladder.
- In a form with low or partial infectivity, for instance adenoviruses in the tonsils and adenoids.
- In a completely non-infectious form, often without producing any microbial antigens. Latent virus infections are classic examples of this type of persistence. In the case of HSV, viral DNA persists for many years, probably for life, in sensory neurones in the dorsal root ganglia.

The molecular basis for viral latency has still not been elucidated. It involves special adaptations by the virus to the state of latency – in the case of HSV and VZV there are 'latency-associated transcripts' produced in infected neurones that are needed to maintain this delicate type of intracellular parasitism.

Latent infections can become patent

Latent infections are so-called because they can become patent. This is where they become of immense medical interest. The legacy of latent herpesvirus infections in man is described in Chapter 24. Different patterns of acute and persistent infections are illustrated in *Figure 11.11*. During their persistence, such infections are not important causes of acute illness and by their nature cannot be acutely lethal. Persistent infections are important for four main reasons:

- They can be reactivated (*Fig. 11.12*, see below).
- They are sometimes associated with chronic disease, as in the case of chronic hepatitis B infections, subacute sclerosing panencephalitis following measles, and AIDS.

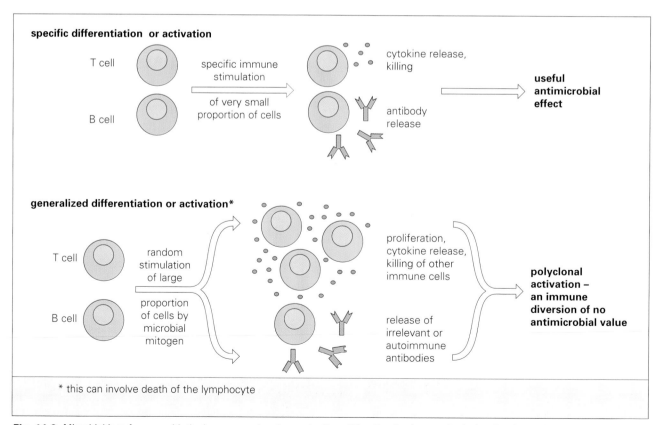

Fig. 11.9 Microbial interference with the immune system by production of T or B cell mitogens (polyclonal activators).

- They are sometimes associated with cancers such as hepatocellular carcinoma with hepatitis B virus and Burkitt's lymphoma and nasopharyngeal carcinoma with EBV.
- From the microbial viewpoint, they enable the infectious agent to persist in the host community (see panel).

Reactivation
Reactivation is clinically important in immunosuppressed individuals

Reactivation occurs in immunocompromised patients, and is of major clinical importance in those immunosuppressed as a result of chronic disease or infection (AIDS), tumors (leukemias, lymphomas), or in those immunosupressed by the physician following transplantation (Fig. 11.13). Reactivation also occurs during naturally occurring periods of immunocompromise, the most important of these being pregnancy and old age. From the microbe's point of view, latency is an adaptation that allows reactivation with renewed growth and shedding of the infectious agent during these naturally-occurring periods.

Features of reactivation in herpesvirus infections are described in Chapters 19, 23 and 24. We still know very

PERSISTENT INFECTIONS					
	microorganism	site of persistence	infectiousness of persistent microorganism	consequence	shedding of microorganism to exterior
viruses	herpes simplex	dorsal root ganglia	–	activation, cold sore	+
		salivary glands	+	none known	+
	varicella zoster	dorsal root ganglia	–	activation, zoster	+
	cytomegalovirus	lymphoid tissue	–	activation ± disease	+
	Ebstein–Barr virus	lymphoid tissue	–	lymphoid tumor	–
		epithelium	–	nasopharyngeal carcinoma	–
		salivary glands	+	none known	+
	hepatitis B	liver (virus shed into blood)	+	chronic hepatitis: liver cancer	+
	adenoviruses	lymphoid tissue	–	none known	+
	polyomaviruses BK and JC (man)	kidney	–	activation (pregnancy, immunosuppression)	+
	T cell leukemia viruses	lymphoid and other tissues	±	late leukemia, neurologic disease	–
	paramyxovirus	brain	±	subacute sclerosing panencephalitis	–
	HIV	lymphocytes macrophages	+	chronic disease	+
chlamydia	trachoma	conjunctiva	+	chronic disease and blindness	?
rickettsia	Rickettsia prowazeki	lymph node	?	activation	+
bacteria	Salmonella typhi	gall bladder urinary tract	+	intermittent shedding in urine, feces	+
	Mycobacterium tuberculosis	lung or lymph node (macrophages?)	?	activation, tuberculosis in middle aged	+
	Treponema pallidum	disseminated	±	chronic disease	–
protozoa	Plasmodium vivax	liver	?	activation, clinical malaria	+
	Toxoplasma gondii	lymphoid tissue muscle brain	±	activation, neurologic disease	–
	Trypanosoma cruzi	blood macrophages	±	chronic disease	–

Fig. 11.10 Examples of persistent infections in humans. Shedding to the exterior takes place either directly, for example via skin lesions, saliva or urine, or indirectly via the blood (hepatitis B, malaria).

little about reactivation mechanisms at the molecular level, as might be expected in view of our ignorance about the latent state itself.

It is useful to distinguish two stages in reactivation

The first event (stage A) in reactivation *(Fig. 11.14)*, the resumption of viral activity in the latently infected cell, is the most mysterious stage. In the case of HSV, this can be triggered by sensory stimuli arriving in the neurone (from skin areas responding to sunlight) and also by certain fevers (i.e. during other infections) or by hormonal influences. Little more than this is known!

The second event (stage B) involves the spread and replication of the reactivated virus. HSV must travel down the sensory axon to the skin or mucosal surface, infect and spread in subep-

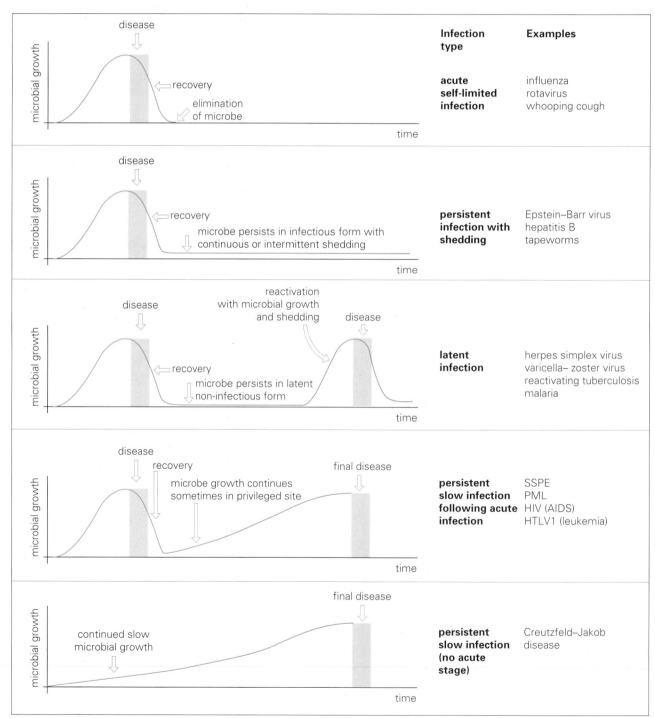

Fig. 11.11 Patterns of acute and persistent infections. For some microbes (e.g. CMV, tuberculosis) the distinction between persistence in infectious form and true latency is not clear. (HTLV1, human T cell leukemia virus1; PML, progressive multifocal leukencephalopathy; SSPE, subacute sclerosing panencephalitis.)

ithelial tissues and then in the epithelium, finally forming a virus-rich vesicle (more than one million infectious units/ml of vesicle fluid). All this takes at least 3–4 days. Stage B is less mysterious than stage A and can be controlled by the immune system. Therefore, cold sores may be associated with poor lymphocyte responses to HSV antigens, and zoster with declining cell-mediated responses (specifically to VZV antigens) in old people.

Stage A probably occurs more frequently than stage B, because immune defenses often arrest the process during stage B before final production of the lesion. Hence as many as 10–20% of HSV reactivation episodes are thought to be 'non-lesional' with burning, tingling, and itching at the site, but no signs of a cold sore. Also, zoster may involve no more than the sensory prodrome associated with virus reactivation and replication in sensory neurones; skin lesions are prevented by host defenses.

Reactivation of EBV and CMV with appearance of the virus in saliva (EBV) or blood (CMV) is generally asymptomatic. In immunologically-deficient individuals, however, reactivation may progress to cause clinical disease; either hepatitis and pneumonitis in the case of CMV or the rarer hairy tongue leukoplakia due to EBV (see Chapter 24).

Persistence is of survival value for the microbe

Persistence without any further shedding as occurs in subacute sclerosing panencephalitis and progressive multifocal leukencephalopathy (see Chapter 22) is of no survival value, but there are obvious advantages if the microbe is also shed, either continuously or intermittently. This is especially true when the host species consists of small isolated groups of individuals (Fig. 11.12). Measles, for instance, is not normally a persistent infection. It only infects humans, does not survive for long outside the body and has nowhere else to go (i.e. there is no animal reservoir). Without a continued supply of fresh susceptible humans the virus could not maintain itself and would become extinct. There has to be, at all times, someone acutely infected with measles. From studies of island communities it is clear that you need a minimum of about 500 000 humans to maintain measles without reintroduction from outside. In paleolithic times, when humans lived in small isolated groups, measles could not have existed in its present form.

In contrast, persistent and latent infections are admirably adapted for survival under these circumstances. VZV can maintain itself in a community of less than 1000 individuals. Children get chickenpox, the virus persists in latent form in sensory neurones and, later in life, the virus reactivates to cause shingles. By this time a new generation of susceptible individuals has appeared and the shingles vesicles provide a fresh source of virus.

Serologic studies show that the viral infections prevalent in small, completely isolated Indian communities in the Amazon basin are persistent or latent (e.g. due to adenoviruses, polyomaviruses, papillomaviruses, herpesviruses) rather than non-persistent (e.g. due to influenza, measles, poliovirus). The same principles apply to non-viral infections. Those present in small communities are either persistant/latent (typhoid respiratory tuberculosis) or have an animal reservoir for maintenence of the microbe.

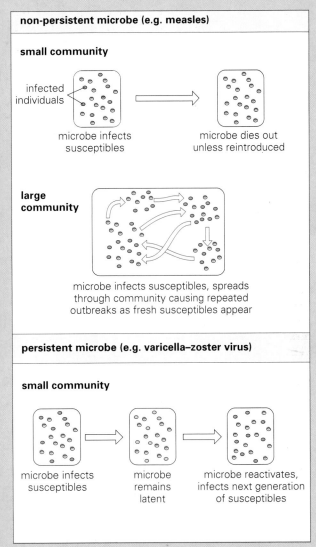

Fig. 11.12 Persistence is a microbial survival strategy.

REACTIVATION OF PERSISTENT INFECTIONS		
circumstance	**infectious agent**	**site of shedding**
old age	varicella–zoster virus	skin vesicles
	tuberculosis	saliva
pregnancy	polyomaviruses (BK, JC)	urine
	cytomeglovirus	cervix
	herpes simplex virus 2	cervix
	Epstein–Barr virus	saliva
leukemias, lymphomas (e.g. Hodgkins' disease)	varicella–zoster virus	skin vesicles
	polyomavirus (JC)	CNS (PML)*
post-transplant immunosuppression	herpes simplex virus	skin/mucosal lesions
	varicella–zoster virus	skin vesicles
	wart viruses	skin
	cytomeglovirus	viremia, pneumonitis*
	Epstein–Barr virus	saliva
	hepatitis B	blood
HIV infection	*Pneumocystis carinii*	lung*
	Toxoplasma gondii	CNS*
	varicella–zoster virus	skin vesicles
	herpes simplex virus	skin/mucosal lesions
	Mycobacterium tuberculosis polyomavirus (JC)	lung CNS (PML)*

* no shedding from these sites

Fig. 11.13 Reactivation of persistant infections. (PML, progressive multifocal leukencephalopathy.)

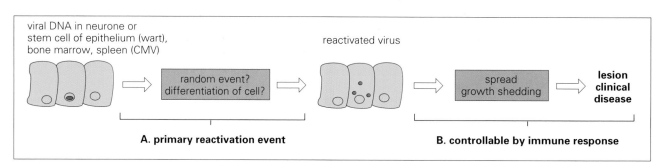

Fig. 11.14 Two stages in reactivation of latent viruses. (CMV, cytomegalovirus.)

- Many successful parasites have adopted strategies for evading immune responses. These enable them to stay in the body long enough to complete their business of infection and shedding to fresh hosts. Some parasites persist indefinitely in the body.
- Mechanisms of immune evasion include:
  a. Concealing parasite antigens from the host (staying inside host cells, infecting 'privileged sites').
  b. Changing parasite antigen, either in the infected individual (trypanosomiasis) or during spread through the host population (influenza).
  c. Direct action on immune cells (e.g. HIV on CD4$^+$ T cells) or on immune signaling systems (e.g. production of fake cytokine or cytokine receptor molecules).
  d. Local interference with immune defenses (production of IgA proteases, Fc receptors).
- During persistent infections the microbe may continue to multiply and be able to infect others (HIV, hepatitis B).
- Alternatively, during persistent infections the microbe enters into a latent state and later in life reactivates with renewed multiplication and the ability to infect others (herpes viruses).

1. Could molecular mimicry be a mere biologic accident? If it were, would you expect it to be more common with short (4–5) than with long (7–8) amino acid sequences?
2. Why should antigenic variation involve especially the outer (surface) molecules of a parasite?
3. Based on your understanding of herpesvirus latency:
   a. Could you catch shingles after contact with a case of chickenpox?
   b. Could you develop a cold sore after contact with a patient with a cold sore?
4. Under what circumstances might a wart virus in the epidermis be exposed to immune defenses?

Further Reading

Fitzpatrick DR, Bielefeldt–Ohmann H. Mechanisms of herpes virus immuno-evasion. *Microb Pathogen* 1991;**10**:253–259.
Garcia–Blanco MA, Cullen BR. Molecular basis of latency in pathogenic human viruses. *Science* 1991;**254**:815–820.
Lower R, Lower J, Kurth R. The viruses in all of us: characteristics and biologic significance of human retrovirus sequences. *Proc Nat Acad Sci* 1996;**93**:5177–5184.

Maizels RM, Bundy DAP, Selkirk ME *et al*. Immunologic modulation and evasion by helminth parasites in human populations. *Nature* 1993;**365**:797–805.
Smith GL. Virus strategies for evasion of the host response to infection. *Trends Microbiol* 1994;**2**:81–88.

Introduction

Symptoms of infections are produced by the microorganisms or the host's immune responses

Symptoms that appear rapidly after the acquisition of an infection are usually due to the direct action of the invading microbe or its secretions. Thus a virus in a cell may cause metabolic 'shut-down' or lyse the cell. Bacteria, however, provoke most of their acute effects by releasing toxins, but may also cause distress by inducing inflammation. The inflammatory response is, of course, an important component of host protection, vascular permeability being vital for the rapid mobilization of cells such as neutrophils, and serum components such as complement and antibody. Inflammation is therefore intrinsically a healthy sign and it is interesting that some virulent bacteria (e.g. staphylococci) can to some extent inhibit the inflammatory response.

Often, however, pathologic changes are secondary to the activation of immunologic mechanisms that are normally thought of as protective. These may involve the natural or the adaptive immune system or, more usually, both *(Fig. 12.1)*. Tissue damage resulting from adaptive immune responses is usually referred to as 'immunopathology' and is quite common in infectious diseases, particularly those that are chronic and persistent. The immunologic basis of these mechanisms of tissue damage is described in Chapter 6.

Pathology Due to Direct Effects of the Microorganism

Direct effects may result from cell rupture, organ blockage or pressure effects

Organisms that multiply in cells and subsequently spread usually do so by rupturing the cell. Many viruses and some intracellular bacteria and protozoa behave in this way

(Fig. 12.2). It is important to realize that many others do not. For example, viruses or bacteria may remain latent (e.g. herpes simplex virus and varicella-zoster virus in nerve ganglia and *Mycobacterium tuberculosis* in macrophages), and many viruses can bud from a cell without disrupting it. The type of cell infected may also have an influence on survival of the organism, thus HIV lyses T cells, but persists in macrophages. Other direct effects include:

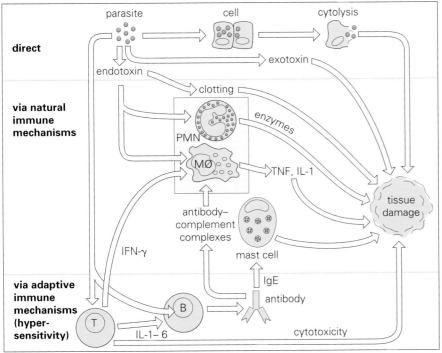

Fig. 12.1 Pathologic effects of infection: a general scheme. Infectious parasitic organisms can cause disease directly (top) or indirectly via overactivation of various immune mechanisms, either natural (center) or adaptive (bottom). (IFN, interferon; IL, interleukin; MØ, macrophage; PMN, polymorphonuclear leukocyte.)

ORGANISMS THAT DIRECTLY DAMAGE TISSUE		
organism	**cell or tissue damaged**	**mechanism**
viruses poliovirus rhinovirus HIV coxsackievirus rotavirus	neurones URT mucosa CD4, T cells, macrophages, pancreatic β cells, heart enterocytes	cytopathic
bacteria *Streptococcus mutans* mycobacteria	teeth macrophages	acid production damaged macrophage releases cytokines
fungi *Histoplasma*	macrophages	damaged macrophage releases cytokines
protozoa *Plasmodium*	erythrocytes	damaged erythrocyte removed
helminths *Ascaris* *Echinococcus*	intestinal occlusion biliary occlusion hydatid cyst	mechanical mechanical, inflammation pressure effects

Fig. 12.2 Many organisms directly damage or destroy the tissues they infect. This is especially common with cytopathic viruses. (URT, upper respiratory tract.)

- Blockage of major hollow viscera by worms.
- Blockage of lung alveoli by dense growth of, for example, *Pneumocystis*.
- Mechanical effects of large cysts (e.g. hydatid).

Exotoxins are a common cause of serious tissue damage, especially in bacterial infection

The parasite may actively secrete 'exotoxins' *(Fig. 12.3)*. In some cases these are clearly part of its strategy for entry, spread or defense against the host, but sometimes they seem to be of little or no benefit to the parasite.

Most exotoxins are proteins and are often coded not by the bacterial DNA, but in plasmids (e.g. *Escherichia coli*) or phages (e.g. botulism, diphtheria, scarlet fever). In some cases they consist of two or more subunits, one of which is required for binding and entry to the cell while the other switches on or inhibits some cellular function.

Inactivation of toxins without altering antigenicity results in successful vaccines

Toxins can often be inactivated (e.g. by formaldehyde) without altering their antigenicity and the resulting toxoids are among the most successful of all vaccines (see Chapter 31), the classic examples being diphtheria and tetanus toxoids. Toxins are generally more highly conserved in their structure than the surface antigens of the organism secreting them. This allows for more effective cross-immunity and explains, for example, why scarlet fever (caused by streptococcal erythrotoxin) usually occurs only once, while streptococcal infections recur almost indefinitely.

An interesting offshoot of the two subunit structure of toxins is that by changing the specificity of the part responsible for attachment, the specificity of the toxin for a particular cell type can be changed. An example is the plant toxin ricin – the A subunit can be attached to a monoclonal antibody to make it a specific poison for tumor cells. The same strategy could obviously be used against parasites if desired.

Mode of action of toxins and consequences

These can be be considered under five headings *(Fig. 12.4)*.

Bacteria may produce enzymes to promote their survival or spread

A number of bacteria release enzymes that break down the tissues or the intercellular substances of the host, allowing the infection to spread freely. Among these enzymes are hyaluronidase, collagenase, DNAase and streptokinase. Some staphylococci release a coagulase, which deposits a protective layer of fibrin onto and around the cells, thus localizing them.

Toxins may damage or destroy cells and are then known as hemolysins

Cell membranes can be damaged enzymatically by lecithinases or phospholipases, or by insertion of pore-forming molecules, which destroy the integrity of the cell. The collective term for such toxins is 'hemolysins', although many cells other than red blood cells can be affected. Both staphylococci and streptococci produce pore-forming toxins; pseudomonads release enzymatic hemolysins.

EXOTOXINS OF IMPORTANCE IN DISEASE				
organism	**exotoxin**	**tissue damaged**	**action**	**disease**
bacteria				
Clostridium tetani	tetanospasmin	neurones	spastic paralysis	tetanus
Clostridium perfringens	α-toxin	erythrocytes, platelets leukocytes, endothelium	cell lysis	gas gangrene
Clostridium botulinum	neurotoxin	nerve–muscle junction	flaccid paralysis	botulism
Corynebacterium diphtheriae	diphtheria toxin	throat, heart, peripheral nerve	inhibits protein synthesis	diphtheria
Shigella dysenteriae	enterotoxin	intestinal mucosa	—	dysentery
Escherichia coli	enterotoxin	intestinal epithelium	fluid loss from intestinal cells	gastroenteritis
Vibrio cholerae	enterotoxin	intestinal epithelium	fluid loss from intestinal cells	cholera
Staphylococcus aureus	α-toxin	red and white cells (via cytokines)	hemolysis	abscesses
	hemolysin	red and white cells (via cytokines)	hemolysis	abscesses
	leucocidin	leukocytes	destroys leukocytes	abscesses
	enterotoxin	intestinal cells	induces vomiting, diarrhea	food poisoning
	TSST1	—	release of cytotoxins	toxic shock syndrome
	epidermolytic	epidermis	—	scalded skin syndrome
Streptococcus pyogenes	streptolysin O and S	red and white cells	hemolysis	hemolysis, pyogenic lesion
	erythrogenic	skin capillaries	skin rash	scarlet fever
Bacillus anthracis	cytotoxin	lung	pulmonary edema	anthrax
Bordetella pertussis	pertussis toxin	trachea	kills epithelium	whooping cough
Legionella pneumophila	numerous	neutrophils	cell lysis	legionnaire's disease
Listeria monocytogenes	hemolysin	leukocytes, monocytes	cell lysis	listeriosis
Pseudomonas aeruginosa	exotoxin A	cell lysis	cell lysis	various infections
fungi				
Aspergillus fumigatus	aflatoxin	liver	carcinogenic	?liver damage/cancer
protozoa				
Entamoeba histolytica	enterotoxin	colonic epithelium	cell lysis	amebic dysentery

Fig. 12.3 Important exotoxins in disease. Many bacteria and a few other organisms damage host tissues by secreting exotoxins. Some bacterial exotoxins are among the most powerful toxins known. Vaccination, by inducing antibody, is often very effective in protection. (TSST1, toxic shock syndrome toxin.)

Toxins may enter cells and actively alter some of the metabolic machinery

Characteristically these toxin molecules have two subunits. The A subunit is the active component, while the B subunit is a binding component needed to interact with receptors on the cell membrane. When binding occurs the A subunit, or the whole toxin–receptor complex, is taken into the cell by endocytosis, and the A subunit becomes activated. Two well-studied toxins of this type are those of diphtheria (see Chapter 15) and cholera.

Diphtheria toxin blocks protein synthesis

Diphtheria toxin is synthesized as a single polypeptide (from bacteriophage *n* genes) and binds by the B subunit to target cells *(Fig. 12.4)*. The polypeptide is partially cleaved and then the entire toxin–receptor complex is internalized. The A subunit then splits off and passes into the cytosol, where it inactivates the transfer of amino acids from transfer RNA to the polypeptide chain during translation of mRNA by ribosomes. It does this by catalyzing attachment of adenosine diphosphate (ADP) ribose to the elongation protein (ADP ribosylation), effectively blocking protein synthesis.

Cholera toxin results in massive loss of water from intestinal epithelial cells

Cholera toxin is released as a complex of five B subunits surrounding the A subunit. The latter is cleaved into two fragments – Al and A2 – held by disulfide bonds. The B subunits bind to ganglioside receptors on intestinal epithelial cells

leading to internalization of the A subunits, which then separate from one another *(Fig. 12.4)*. The A1 portion then ADP-ribosylates one of the regulatory molecules involved in the production of cyclic adenosine monophosphate (cAMP). As a result the molecule is unable to turn off production. The increased levels of cAMP in the cell change the sodium/chloride flux across the cell membrane, resulting in a massive outflow of water and electrolytes from the cell and causing the profuse diarrhea of cholera. The exotoxins of

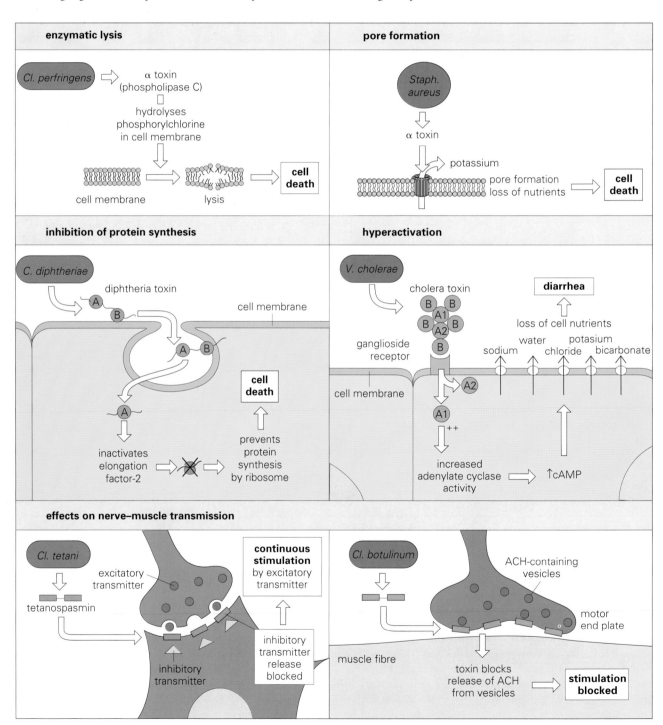

Fig. 12.4 The mode of action of some exotoxins. Bacterial toxins act in a variety of ways. Often the toxin is a two-chain molecule, one chain being concerned with entry into cells while the other has inhibitory activity against some vital function. (ACH, acetylcholine; cAMP, cyclic adenosine monophosphate; *C., Corynebacterium; Cl., Clostridium; Staph., Staphylococcus; V., Vibrio.*)

Escherichia coli and salmonella have similar actions, as does pertussis toxin.

Tetanus and botulinum toxins are among the most potent affecting nerve impulses

One gram of botulinum toxin is sufficient to kill 10 million people! Tetanus and botulinum toxins have the characteristic A + B structure, the B subunit binding to ganglioside receptors on nerve cells. The internalized A subunit of tetanus is carried by axonal transport from the point of production to the central nervous system (CNS), where it interferes with synaptic transmission in inhibitory neurones by blocking neurotransmitter release. This allows the excitatory transmitter to continuously stimulate the motor neurones, causing spastic paralysis. Botulinum toxin enters the body via the intestine, escaping digestion and crossing the gut wall. The toxin affects peripheral nerve endings at the neuromuscular junction, blocking presynaptic release of acetylcholine. This prevents muscle contraction, causing flaccid paralysis.

Diarrhea
Diarrhea is an almost invariable result of intestinal infections

Diarrhea is one of the major causes of death in children worldwide (see Chapter 20). It can be considered as:
- A means for the host to rid itself rapidly of the infectious organism.
- A means for the infection to spread to other hosts.

Diarrhea is a feature of a wide range of organisms, but in only a few cases is the exact mechanism understood. Damage to the intestinal epithelium is usually the underlying cause, and this may be due directly to infection of the cells (e.g. by rotaviruses) or the effect of toxins (e.g. cholera, shigellae). Many of the organisms causing diarrhea can be 'picked up' from food, but the term 'food poisoning' is usually reserved for those cases where toxins are already present in the food rather than being generated during the growth of organisms in the intestine. As would be expected, 'food poisoning' causes symptoms earlier – that is, hours after exposure rather than days (*Fig. 12.5*).

Pathologic Activation of Natural Immune Mechanisms

Overactivity can damage host tissues

The very potent natural immune mechanisms discussed in Chapter 9 have in-built safety as far as specificity is concerned. They have had to evolve in the constant presence of the host's 'self' antigens, which they do not therefore respond to. However, they are not so well controlled quantitatively, and there are many cases when overactivity not only damages an invading parasite, but also damages innocent host tissues.

INFECTIOUS CAUSES OF DIARRHEA		
food poisoning (due to pre-formed toxin in food)		
	onset	**source**
Staphylococcus aureus	1–6 hours	cream, meat, poultry
Clostridium perfringens	8–20 hours	reheated meat
Clostridium botulinum	12–36 hours	canned food
Bacillus cereus	1–20 hours	reheated foods
intestinal infections		
	onset	**source**
rotavirus	2–5 days	contact (fecal–oral)
salmonella	1–2 days	eggs
shigella	1–4 days	fecal–oral
campylobacter	1–4 days	poultry, domestic animals
Vibrio cholerae	2 days	fecal–oral
Escherichia coli	1–4 days	traveller's diarrhea
Yersinia enterocolitica	days–weeks	pets (e.g. dogs)
Giardia lamblia	1–2 weeks	contaminated water
Entamoeba histolytica	days–weeks	
Cryptosporidium	days–weeks	fecal–oral, opportunistic (e.g. in AIDS)
Isopora belli		

Fig. 12.5 Infectious causes of diarrhea. Worldwide infectious diarrhea is the major cause of infant mortality.

Endotoxins are typically lipopolysaccharides

'Endotoxins' of bacteria and other microorganisms have a deceptively similar name to exotoxins, but are profoundly different in their significance. Unlike exotoxins, these are integral parts of the microbial cell wall and are normally released only when the cell dies. Endotoxins are particularly characteristic of Gram-negative bacteria. A typical lipopolysaccharide (LPS) endotoxin is composed of:

- A lipid portion (lipid A) inserted into the cell wall.
- A conserved core polysaccharide.
- The highly variable O-polysaccharide, responsible for the serologic diversity which is a feature of organisms such as salmonellae and shigellae.

LPSs stimulate an extraordinary range of host responses – or perhaps one should say a wide range of responses have evolved to respond to LPSs. In the words of Lewis Thomas 'when we sense lipopolysaccharide, we are likely to turn on every defence at our disposal' *(Fig. 12.6)*. Evidently the body needs to be aware of invading Gram-negative bacteria at the earliest possible stage.

Clinically, the most important effects of LPS are:

- Fever.
- Vascular collapse (or shock).

As mentioned in Chapter 9, fever may benefit host or parasite or both, and is currently considered to be mainly due to the action of two cytokines – interleukin-1 (IL-1) and tumor necrosis factor (TNF) – on the hypothalamus. Both these cytokines are produced by macrophages in response to LPS (and to analogous molecules from other organisms, see below).

Endotoxin shock is usually associated with systemic spread of organisms

The commonest example of endotoxin (or 'septic') shock is septicemia with Gram-negative bacteria such as *E. coli* or *Neisseria meningitidis*. However, many other organisms also release molecules that stimulate TNF and/or IL-1

production *(Fig. 12.7)* and therefore function in part like LPS, although they are more or less unrelated in structure. For example, in the 'toxic shock syndrome' of young women with staphylococcal infections of the genital tract, toxic shock syndrome toxin (TSST1) is a protein.

The involvement of cytokines in the pathogenesis of shock is by no means a purely academic concern because it suggests the possibility of treatment by antagonists of a small number of cytokines (e.g. by monoclonal antibodies or inhibitors) rather than by antibodies to the toxins themselves, which are of enormous antigenic diversity. This idea is discussed further in Chapter 29.

The cytokine most closely linked to disease at present is TNF

Raised concentrations of TNF in the serum have been shown to correlate with severity in patients with meningococcal septicemia and with *Plasmodium falciparum* malaria. However, animal experiments indicate that in such cases TNF probably synergizes with other cytokines such as IL-1 and interferon-gamma (IFNγ) to produce its full effects. In meningococcal disease, TNF levels in blood and cerebrospinal fluid (CSF) can change independently, the former being raised in septicemia and the latter in meningitis; it therefore appears that the production and/or effects of TNF can be restricted to a particular body compartment.

Complement is involved in several tissue-damaging reactions

The activation of complement is a vital part of immunity to many bacteria, viruses and protozoa (see Chapter 9). Complement can, however, be involved in tissue-damaging reactions, for example immune complex disease, which also involves antibody and, usually, PMN. Complement also plays an important role in the acute inflammatory response by generating the chemotactic factors C3a and C5a (see Chapter 4).

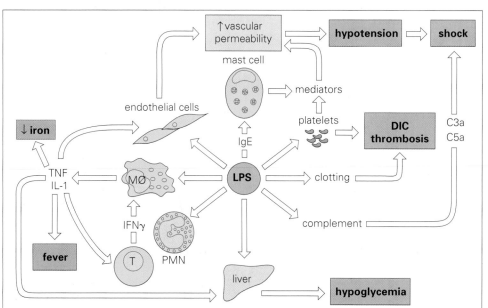

Fig. 12.6 The many activities of bacterial endotoxin. LPS activates almost every immune mechanism as well as the clotting pathway and as a result LPS is one of the most powerful immune stimuli known. (DIC, disseminated intravascular coagulation; IFN, interferon; IL, interleukin; LPS, lipopolysaccharide; MØ, macrophage; PMN, polymorphonuclear leukocyte; TNF, tumor necrosis factor.)

IMPORTANT ENDOTOXINS AND FUNCTIONALLY RELATED MOLECULES

organisms	toxin	cytokines induced
bacteria		
Gram-negative Salmonella Shigella Escherichia coli Neisseria meningitidis	LPS	TNF, IL-1
Gram-positive Staphylococcus aureus	TSST1	TNF
mycobacteria	lipoarabinomannan	TNF
Bordetella pertussis	endotoxin	TNF
fungi yeasts	zymosan	TNF
protozoa Plasmodium	phospholipids (exoantigens)	TNF

Fig. 12.7 Important endotoxins and functionally related molecules. Most endotoxins are lipopolysaccharides (LPS) and exert their main effects by stimulating cytokine release. (IL, interleukin; TNF, tumor necrosis factor; TSST1, toxic shock syndrome toxin.)

Direct activation of complement by LPS may contribute to the shock induced by toxic amounts of this endotoxin in which the levels of complement components (e.g. C3) drop profoundly; this response appears to involve both the classical and the alternative pathways, which are activated by the lipid and polysaccharide components, respectively. C3a and C5a are produced in large amounts and there is frequently a severe decrease in the number of polymorphonuclear leukocytes (PMNs) due to aggregation of these cells, adherence to vessel walls, and their activation to release toxic molecules, both oxidative and non-oxidative. When this occurs in the pulmonary capillaries, severe pulmonary edema may result – the 'adult respiratory distress syndrome' (ARDS).

Disseminated intravascular coagulation is a rare but serious feature of bacterial septicemia

Disseminated intravascular coagulation (DIC) can be a feature of bacterial (e.g. meningococcal) septicemia, but is also seen in some virus infections. The relative contributions of immune complexes, platelets, and direct activation of the clotting pathway via the effect of LPS on Hageman factor, remain controversial. For example, the hemorrhagic phenomena of yellow fever are probably secondary to coagulation defects due to the extensive liver damage, while in dengue ('hemorrhagic') fever it has been suggested that there is immune complex deposition in blood vessels. However, in all these hemorrhagic syndromes the role of cytokines such as TNF also needs to be considered.

Mast cell degranulation in response to LPS is thought to be secondary to IgE antibody formation

Some insect venoms, however, may be able to activate mast cells directly and reactions of this kind are called 'anaphylactoid'.

Pathologic Consequences of the Immune Response

Overreaction of the immune system is known as 'hypersensitivity'

Adaptive immune responses are vital to defense against infection, as witnessed by the increased susceptibility to infectious disease of immunodeficient patients (see Chapter 28). The antimicrobial effects of lymphocyte responses act mainly by specifically focusing or enhancing nonspecific effector mechanisms (see Chapter 5). This may, however, also enhance the pathologic effects outlined above. The tissue damaging effects of hypersensitivity are referred to as 'immunopathologic'.

The most widely used classification of hypersensitivity is that of Coombs and Gell, (types I to IV below) which is based on the immunologic mechanism underlying the tissue damaging reaction.

Each of the four main types of hypersensitivity can be of microbial or non-microbial origin

Hypersensitivity of microbial origin includes some of the most serious of these responses (Fig. 12.8). Organisms of many sorts can be involved, but one common feature is that the infection is prolonged, with continuous or repeated antigenic stimulation.

Type I hypersensitivity
Allergic reactions are a feature of worm infections

The most dramatic allergic (type I) reaction is that following the rupture of a hydatid cyst. Slow leakage of worm antigens ensures that the patient's mast cells are sensitized with specific IgE, and the massive flood of antigens on rupture may cause acute fatal anaphylaxis, with vascular collapse and pulmonary edema. Even the small amount of antigen used in diagnostic skin tests can have this effect.

Another worm associated with high levels of IgE is *Ascaris*, but here the pathologic consequences are mainly respiratory, with eosinophilic infiltrates and asthmatic episodes corresponding to passage of the parasite through the lung. The itching rashes characteristic of helminth infections when the worms die in the skin are probably also of this type, an example being 'swimmer's itch' due to animal or avian schistosomes.

Why allergic reactions are such a feature of worm infections is not really clear, but they may be due to some feature of the antigens; in addition, it has been suggested that IgE plays a role in protection against worms. One would hope so, as in all other respects this class of antibody appears to be nothing but a nuisance.

HYPERSENSITIVITY OF MICROBIAL ORIGIN		
Coombs and Gell classification	**principal mechanism**	**examples**
type I (allergic/anaphylactic)	IgE, mast cells	helminths *Ascaris* hydatid (ruptured cyst) ? viral skin rash ? upper respiratory tract viral infections
type II (cytotoxic)	IgG to surface complement cytotoxic cells	virus infected cells malaria infected erythrocytes autoantibodies in: *Mycoplasma* streptococci *Trypanasoma cruzi*
type III (immune complex-mediated)	immune complexes complement PMN	in tissues: allergic alveolitis actinomycosis in blood vessels: glomerulonephritis malaria streptococci hepatitis B syphilis
type IV (cell mediated)	T lymphocytes cytokines macrophages (and other non-specific cells)	granuloma tuberculosis leprosy (tuberculoid) schistosomiasis (eggs) *Histoplasma* mononuclear infiltration ± cell damage in many virus infections (i.e. tissue delayed-type hypersensitivity responses) with CD4, CD8, cytokines and macrophages playing roles viral rashes
autoimmunity	cross reaction with host polyclonal B cell activation	streptococcal myocarditis African trypanosomiasis

Fig. 12.8 Hypersensitivity of microbial origin. All four classic types of hypersensitivity can be induced by infectious organisms, types II and III being the most commonly encountered. Note that some mechanisms mediating hypersensitivity also take part in protective immunity. (PMN, polymorphonuclear leukocyte.)

Type II hypersensitivity
Type II reactions are mediated by antibodies to the infectious organism or autoantibodies

Strictly speaking, type II reactions are mediated by antibody (usually IgG) leading to cytotoxicity, either extracellular or intracellular (e.g. after phagocytosis). Cytotoxicity by T cells is considered under type IV reactions. An important distinction can be made between antibodies to the (foreign) infectious organism and autoantibodies; the former kill host cells because they display foreign antigens, whereas the latter bind to unaltered host antigens and both types of response occur in infectious disease *(Fig. 12.8)*. In the latter case, of course, the interesting question is why autoantibodies should be formed

during infection, and several mechanisms have been postulated for this. However the whole question of autoimmunity remains highly controversial.

In blood-stage malaria, microbial antigens attach themselves to host cells

It has been shown that the hemolytic anemia of blood-stage malaria is due not to autoantibody as previously thought, but to antibodies to parasite-derived antigen that have been picked up by red cells. In some cases it may be the antigen–antibody complex that binds to the cell. A similar reaction can occur following quinine treatment of *P. falciparum* malaria (blackwater fever). Viruses budding from cells are another good example of microbial and host antigens becoming closely associated.

Antimyocardial antibody of group A β-hemolytic streptococcal infection is the classic autoantibody triggered by infection

This reaction is due to the presence of the same cross-reacting carbohydrate antigen on the bacterium and the myocardium. However, as more protein sequences are obtained and compared, numerous other similar examples have come to light, and it is possible that cross-reaction between microbial and human antigens may underlie a number of diseases of currently unknown origin. Whether this mimicry of host antigens has any survival value to the microbe is discussed in Chapter 11.

Type III hypersensitivity
Immune complexes cause disease when they become lodged in tissues or blood vessels

Without the formation of immune complexes, antibody would have a very limited role in protective immunity. However, complications occur when the complexes escape removal by the phagocytes of the reticuloendothelial system and become lodged in the tissues or blood vessels, attracting complement and neutrophils. Release of lysosomal enzymes then results in local damage, which is particularly serious in small blood vessels, especially in the renal glomeruli. Immune complex disease is a major cause of both acute and chronic glomerulonephritis, and the majority of cases are probably the result of infection. There is also an important group in which autoantigen–autoantibody complexes are responsible (e.g. DNA/anti-DNA in systemic lupus erythematosus), but even these may ultimately be the consequence of a viral infection.

Like most other immunopathologic conditions, immune complex deposition is usually a feature of chronic infection (e.g. malaria). However, a persistent antigenic stimulus is not the only prerequisite, indicated by the fact that the most serious form of malarial nephropathy is found in *Plasmodium malariae* (quartan) malaria, which progresses despite successful treatment of the infection, while the nephropathy of *P. falciparum* (malignant tertian) malaria typically recovers after the infection has been cured. Predisposing factors may include a poor antibody response (in terms of amount or affinity), a particular tendency of the antigen itself to bind to vascular endothelium, or inhibition of the normal function of phagocytes or complement in removing circulating complexes.

Occupational diseases associated with inhalation of fungi are the classic examples of immune complex deposition in the tissues

Immune complex deposition in the tissues, made famous by the work of Arthus on antigens injected into the skin of animals with pre-existing antibody (mainly IgG), manifests as a combination of thrombosis in small blood vessels and necrosis in the tissues due to PMN degranulation *(Fig. 12.9)*. Perhaps the best-studied examples are the occupational diseases associated with inhalation of fungi (e.g. farmer's lung, pigeon-fancier's disease, maple bark stripper's disease) in which chronic inflammation of the lung can lead to a state of destruction and fibrosis known as 'extrinsic allergic alveolitis', an unfortunate name since classical (IgE-mediated) allergy does not seem to be involved.

Another well-known model of immune complex disease is serum sickness

Serum sickness follows repeated injections of foreign protein, leading to circulating complexes, which deposit in the kidneys *(Fig. 12.10)*, skin and joints. This was common in the pre-antibiotic days of passive serotherapy for infectious disease

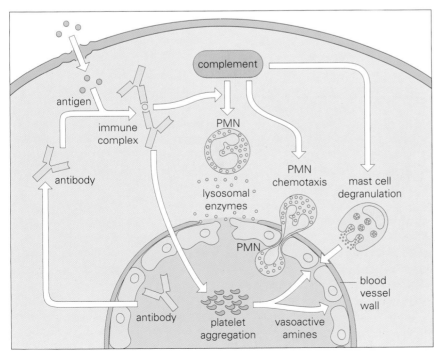

Fig. 12.9 The Arthus reaction. Microbial antigens that enter the tissues (e.g. fungal particles in the lung) encounter antibody and form immune complexes. These activate complement and initiate chemotaxis of polymorphonuclear leukocytes (PMNs), and degranulation of these and tissue mast cells. The resulting inflammatory response is further potentiated by damage induced by PMN-derived lysosomal enzymes.

(see Chapter 32). It is also a possible complication of treatment with monoclonal (usually murine) antibody, which is an increasingly attractive approach to many conditions, and this is one of the reasons why determined efforts are being made to produce monoclonal antibodies in which as much of the molecule as possible is of the human type.

Type IV hypersensitivity
Cell-mediated immune responses invariably cause some tissue destruction, which may be permanent

Despite the examples of antibody-mediated tissue damage discussed above, the antibody response generally achieves its purpose in eliminating invading organisms without any trace of damage to the host. Cell-mediated (type IV) responses are not quite so sure-footed, in that the activation of both cytotoxic T cells and macrophages invariably causes some tissue destruction, which may be reparable if not too prolonged, but can also lead to fibrosis and even calcification with serious permanent loss of tissue.

Confusion has occurred due to the use of a number of terms to describe and subdivide type IV responses. Some reflect actual pathologic conditions while others describe the results of diagnostic skin tests, and none correspond exactly to the processes by which cell-mediated immunity protects against infection (*Fig. 12.11*).

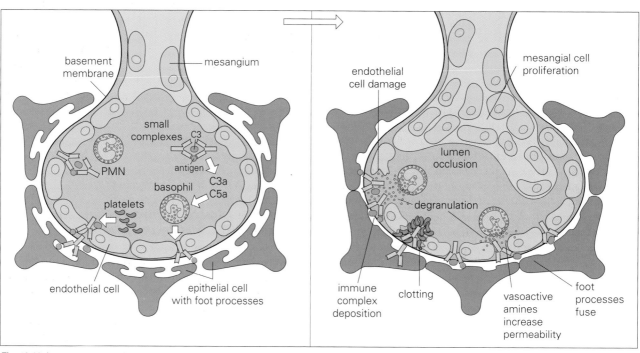

Fig. 12.10 Immune complex-mediated tissue damage. Type III hypersensitivity results in the deposition of immune complexes in the blood vessel walls, particularly at sites of high pressure, filtration or turbulence such as the kidney. (PMN, polymorphonuclear leukocyte.)

CELL-MEDIATED RESPONSES			
immune cells or molecules	protective effect against	pathologic effect	skin test
cytotoxic T cells (CD8)	virus infections *Theileria* ? mycobacteria	local tissue loss	–
basophils T cells	?	inflammation	24 h (Jones-Mote)
T cells macrophages cytokines giant cells epithelioid cells eosinophils	intracellular organisms viruses bacteria fungi protozoa worms	mononuclear cell infiltration granuloma fibrosis calcification (>14 days)	delayed/tuberculin type (>2 days)

Fig. 12.11 Cell-mediated immunity in protection and disease. The nomenclature of cell-mediated immune responses is complicated. Although often described in terms of skin tests, their real significance is related to protective and/or pathologic reactions in the tissues.

From the medical viewpoint granuloma formation is the most important type IV response

However, the complex involvement of the cytokine network in type IV responses is of major interest to the immunologist. For example, the tendency of some granulomas to undergo necrosis (e.g. caseation in tuberculosis) while others do not (e.g. leprosy, sarcoidosis) may be explained in terms of the different pattern of cytokines involved. TNF, often in association with some microbial products, is especially likely to cause necrosis through its effects on vascular endothelium, which probably accounts for much of its anti-tumor activity.

The clinical features of schistosomiasis are produced by cell-mediated immunity

The price paid for protective cell-mediated immunity is particularly well illustrated by the helminth disease schistosomiasis. *Schistosoma mansoni* (the blood fluke) lays eggs in the mesenteric venous system, some of which become lodged in small portal vessels in the liver. Strong cell-mediated reactions to secreted enzymes lead to granulomatous reactions around each egg, resulting in egg destruction and sparing of liver parenchyma from the toxic effects of the egg enzymes. However, the coalescent calcified granulomas ultimately cause portal cirrhosis, with portal hypertension, esophageal varices and hematemesis (see Chapter 20). An increased cell-mediated response would accelerate the cirrhosis, while a reduction would predispose to toxic parenchymatous liver failure, neither option being attractive. In such circumstances the conflict has gone too far for a 'perfect' solution, and the same is true for tuberculosis and many other persistent intracellular organisms, if the density of infection is comparable.

The rather unexpected effect of malnutrition in reducing the incidence and severity of certain diseases (e.g. typhus, malaria) may be attributable to a reduction in immunopathology, though in the majority of diseases (e.g. measles, meningococcal infection, tuberculosis) the reverse is true. Indeed, poor nutrition is regarded as a major factor predisposing to the greater severity of many common infections in tropical countries.

Skin Rashes

A variety of skin rashes have an immunologic origin

The ways in which infections can affect the skin are detailed in Chapter 23, but here it should be mentioned that some rashes are considered to be immunologically mediated. For example the characteristic skin rash of measles is absent in children with T cell deficiency (e.g. thymic aplasia or DiGeorge syndrome), who instead develop a fatal systemic infection, indicating that the skin lesions are T cell mediated and represent some form of successful cell-mediated immunity. In contrast, if children with T cell deficiency are infected with a vaccinia virus (i.e. vaccinated) they develop an inexorable spreading skin lesion, which is clearly a direct and not an immunopathologic effect.

Figure 12.12 lists the more common skin conditions of immunologic origin in which an infectious organism is thought to be involved. Further details can be found in Chapter 23.

Viruses and Cancer

A variety of RNA and DNA viruses can cause permanent malignant changes within cells (*Fig. 12.13*). Such malignant transformation by these 'tumor viruses' has been extensively studied. An account of proviruses and oncogenes (genes causing malignancy) is included in Chapter 3. However, only a small number of human cancers have been shown to be associated with such tumor viruses (*Fig. 12.14*).

Human T cell lymphotropic viruses are associated with certain lymphomas and leukemias

Human T cell lymphotropic virus (HTLV)1 and HTLV2 are retroviruses that have no oncogenes (see Chapter 3). Their proviral DNA is detectable in the cellular DNA of certain malignant lymphomas and leukemias. HTLV1 is known to cause adult T cell leukemia and lymphoma, particularly in Southern Japan, the Caribbean islands and West Africa. Less is known about the geographic distribution of HTLV2, which can be isolated from hairy T cell leukemia. The carcinogenic nature of HTLV1 is not due to activation of a cellular oncogene, but is due to the *tat* gene product enhancing transcription of host genes involved in cell division. These infections are described in more detail in Chapter 23.

Epstein–Barr virus (EBV) is associated with nasopharyngeal carcinoma

EBV is closely linked with the development of nasopharyngeal carcinoma (NPC) (see Chapter 24), which is common in Southern China and other parts of Asia (12–30 cases/100 000 people/year), less common in parts of North Africa, and rare elsewhere in the world. The reason for this restricted geographic distribution is unknown. There is no convincing evidence for specific carcinogenic EBV strains, but these effects could be due to the presence locally of cocarcinogens such as nitrosamines in salted fish. EBV DNA can be demonstrated in the cancer cells, but the precise mechanism for tumorigenicity is unknown; cellular oncogenes have not been implicated. People at high risk of developing NPC show high IgA titers to EBV capsid antigen a year or more before clinical symptoms appear.

EBV is associated with Burkitt's lymphoma

Burkitt's lymphoma, a tumor of immature B cells, occurs in parts of East Africa (Uganda) and in Papua New Guinea in 6–14-year-old children, especially boys. EBV DNA is present in the tumor cells, but most of the many copies of the EBV gene are not integrated into the host cell DNA. The tumor is probably caused by the action of EBV on B cells, causing them to proliferate and making activation of cellular oncogenes more likely. The cellular oncogene c-*myc* is translocated from chromosome 8 to the immunoglobulin heavy chain locus on chromosome 14, where it is expressed. As a result of this, the B cell may be prevented from entering the resting stage. There is also downregulation of adhesion and HLA molecules, so that the EBV-containing cells, which are normally subject to immune control, develop into tumor cells. The Burkitt's lymphoma cells also show other chromosomal

SKIN RASHES AND THEIR IMMUNOLOGIC BASIS			
organism	**disease**	**character**	**pathogenic basis**
viruses measles rubella	measles german measles	maculopapular rash maculopapular rash	⎤ T cells; immune ⎦ complex; allergy
varicella–zoster	chickenpox/zoster	vesicular rash	viral cytopathic
hepatitis B	hepatitis B	urticarial	immune complexes
bacteria *Streptococcus pyogenes*	scarlet fever	erythematous rash	erythrogenic toxin
Treponema pallidum *Treponema pertenue*	syphilis yaws	⎤ disseminated infectious ⎦ rash in secondary stage	immune complexes
Salmonella typhi *Neisseria meningitidis*	typhoid, enteric fever meningitis, spotted fever	sparse rose spots petechial or maculopapular lesions	⎤ ⎦ immune complexes
Mycobacterium leprae	tuberculoid leprosy	blotchy skin lesions	T cells, macrophages
Rickettsia prowazekii and others	typhus	maculopapular or hemorrhagic rash	thrombosis
fungi dermatophytes	dermatophytoid or allergic rash	–	immune complexes? hypersensitivity to fungal antigens
Blastomyces dermatitidis	blastomycosis	papule or pustule developing into granuloma	T cells
protozoa *Leishmania tropica*	cutaneous leishmaniasis	papules ulcerating to form crusted infectious sores	T cells, macrophages

Fig. 12.12 Many skin rashes represent immunologic reactions occurring in the skin. It is suspected that several skin diseases of unknown origin are in fact caused by viruses, either directly or indirectly.

abnormalities, but their role in tumorigenesis is unclear.

The fact that EBV is a common worldwide infection, whereas Burkitt's lymphoma, like NPC, is strikingly localized geographically, points once again to the involvement of local cofactors. One hypothesis is that malaria acts as a cofactor, perhaps by decreasing the intensity of T cell surveillance or in some way priming cells for malignant transformation.

EBV does not appear to be associated with non-endemic Burkitt's lymphoma nor with the lymphomas seen in immunosuppressed (e.g. post-renal transplant) patients. It may, however, be involved in HIV-associated lymphomas. About 3% of patients with AIDS develop non-Hodgkin's lymphomas, 20% of these occurring in the brain. However, there is no good evidence to suggest that Hodgkin's lymphomas are of EBV origin.

Certain human papillomavirus infections are associated with cervical cancer

There are clear associations between infection with human papillomavirus (HPV) types 16, 18, 31 and 33 and the development of cervical cancer (see Chapters 3 and 19). Penile, vulval and rectal cancers are also associated with these types of HPV. HPV types 6 and 11 cause cervical lesions, but have a lower risk of progression to malignancy.

In most primary and metastatic cancer cells, the HPV genomes are present in integrated form (i.e. within the host genome), and certain viral genes (E6, E7) are transcribed and translated. Integration occurs at different chromosomal locations and the E6 and E7 open reading frames seem to be involved in transformation of epithelial cells and in maintenance of the transformed state, probably by binding to and inactivating cellular proteins concerned with regulation of the cell cycle. Cervical cancer is an uncommon sequel to infection with these strains of HPV, and cocarcinogens such as cigarette smoke and herpes simplex virus (HSV) have been implicated.

HPV infection is associated with squamous cell carcinoma of the skin

It is possible that ultraviolet light acts as a cocarcinogen, as is known to be the case with papillomaviruses and skin cancers

MALIGNANT TRANSFORMATION	
changes	details
morphology	loss of shape; rounding; decreased adhesion to surface
growth, contact	loss of contact inhibition of growth and movement; increased ability to grow from a single cell; increased ability to grow in suspension; capacity for continued growth (immortalization)
cellular properties	DNA synthesis induced; chromosomal changes; appearance of new antigens (viral or cellular in origin);
biochemical properties	loss of fibronectin; reduced cAMP

Fig. 12.13 Malignant transformation. These changes occur when tumor viruses cause transformation of cultured cells. Many of these changes are obviously relevant for tumor production *in vivo*. (cAMP, cyclic adenosine monophosphate.)

in sheep and cattle. People with the rare autosomal recessive disease epidermodysplasia verruciformis are infected with 10–20 different but less common types of HPV, and 35% of patients develop multiple squamous cell carcinomas of the skin. Of these tumors 90% contain HPV5 or HPV8 DNA.

HPVs may also play a role in the genesis of the skin cancers that appear in immunosuppressed patients (e.g. renal transplant recipients), and cutaneous warts are common in these patients. However, there is no evidence that skin cancers in healthy individuals are associated with HPV infection.

Hepatitis B virus is a major cause of hepatocellular carcinoma

Integrated hepatitis B virus (HBV) sequences are found in the tumor cells of hepatocellular carcinoma. The exact mechanism is unclear, but insertion of HBV sequences may activate cellular oncogenes (e.g. of the *myc* family) or alter cell growth control by transcriptional transactivation.

Hepatocellular carcinoma is more common in certain parts of the world (e.g. West Africa) and this may be due to the presence of cocarcinogens (e.g. aflatoxin). However, the closely related hepadnavirus of woodchucks (see Chapter 20) causes the same tumor in these animals in the apparent absence of cocarcinogens. Perhaps HBV-associated hepatocellular carcinoma in humans is a sequel to the continuous hepatocyte regeneration that occurs during persistent carriage of HBV.

HSV2 was once thought to be a possible cause of cervical carcinoma

HSV2 DNA and protein are detectable in cancer cells and HSV2 can transform certain cells *in vitro*. However, HSV2 has now been relegated to a possible cocarcinogenic role. Women with cervical cancer have a higher incidence of antibody to HSV2, but this merely reflects the association of cervical cancer with multiple sexual partners.

VIRUSES AND HUMAN CANCER				
viruses	cancer	strength of association	viral genome in cancer cells	cofactor
Epstein–Barr virus	Burkitt's lymphoma	+ +	+	malaria
	nasopharyngeal carcinoma	+ +	+	nitrosamines
	Hodgkin's disease	-	-	-
human papillomavirus	cervical cancer	+ +	+	?cigarettes ?HSV2
	skin cancer	+/-	+	?UV light
hepatitis B virus	liver cancer	+ +	+	?aflatoxin ?hepatocyte regeneration
HTLV1, HTLV2	T cell leukemia	+ +	+	-
HSV2	cervical cancer	+/-	+/-	-

Fig. 12.14 Many viruses transform cells in culture, but only a few are important in human cancer. The associations are strongly supported by studies of naturally occurring or experimentally induced cancers in animals. (HTLV, human T cell lymphotropic virus; HSV, herpes simplex virus; UV, ultraviolet.)

Several DNA viruses can transform cells in which they are unable to replicate

In addition the viral genome is sometimes integrated into the host cell genome. Extensive studies have been carried out with the conclusion that despite high oncogenicity *in vitro* and in laboratory animals, these viruses do not seem to be important in human cancer. For instance:

- Human adenoviruses transform cells in culture and cause sarcomas experimentally in hamsters. About 10% of the adenovirus genome integrates and the T antigen is expressed. However, adenoviruses are not associated with human cancer.
- Polyomavirus (Latin: poly, many; oma, tumors), a mouse papovavirus, and simian vacuolating virus 40 (SV40), a monkey papovavirus, both cause tumors in experimentally inoculated hamsters. The viral DNA is integrated into tumor cells and T antigens are expressed. However,

neither of these viruses, nor their human equivalents (BK and JC viruses), are linked with human cancers. This is illustrated by an incident that occurred about 30 years ago when thousands of children were accidentally inoculated with SV40 virus present in certain batches of poliovirus vaccine. The formalin inactivation procedure had failed to kill the SV40 virus present in the monkey kidney cells in which the polio vaccine had been grown. There was, however, no consequent increase in tumor incidence in the SV40-infected individuals.

Kaposi's sarcoma is probably caused by a virus

Kaposi's sarcoma is 300-times more common among patients with AIDS than among other immunosuppressed groups, but is seen almost entirely in those who acquired HIV by sexual contact. HHV8 appears to be sexually transmitted and is present in the tumors

- Tissue damage or disease can be caused by infectious organisms in several ways.
- Infectious organisms may destroy cells directly (e.g. cytopathic viruses), release toxins that destroy cells or their cellular function (e.g. staphylococcus or tetanus toxins), overstimulate normal defense systems (e.g. LPS) or stimulate excessive or prolonged adaptive responses.
- Such effects of infectious organisms on defense systems may be antibody- or T cell-mediated and are collectively known as 'hypersensitivity reactions' or 'immunopathology'.
- Some viruses have been shown to be involved in the initiation of tumors, with the viral genome in the cancer cells. The restricted geographic distribution of some of these tumors may be due to the local presence of cocarcinogens.

1. Distinguish between exotoxins and endotoxins.
2. What is 'septic shock' and how might it be prevented?
3. What is an immune complex and how can it cause disease?
4. Which types of skin rash have an immunologic origin?
5. Which viruses are suspected of causing cancer?

Further Reading

Arbuthnot JR. Host damage from bacterial toxins. *Phil Trans R Soc Lond B* 1983;**303**:149–165.

Dalgleish AG. Viruses and Cancer. *Brt Med Bull* 1991:**47**;21–46

Mims CA, Dimmock HJ Nash A, Stephen J. *Mims' Pathogenesis Of Infectious Disease*, 4th edition. London: Academic Press, 1995.

Parkes R. *Occupational Lung Disease.* Kent: Butterworths, 1982.

Rees AJ, Andres GA, Peters DK eds. Symposium on pathogenetic mechanisms in nephritis. *Kidney Int* 1989;**35**:921–1033.

Root RK, Saude MA eds. *Septic Shock.* New York: Churchill Livingstone, 1985.

3

diagnostic principles of clinical manifestations

Quality specimens are needed for reliable microbiological diagnoses

The precise identification of the causative organism in infection has become increasingly important now that therapeutic intervention is possible. The ability to achieve this depends upon a positive interaction between the clinician and the microbiologist; the clinician must be aware of the complexity of the tests and the time required to achieve a result. In turn, the microbiologist must appreciate the nature of the patient's condition and be able to assist the clinician in interpreting the laboratory report. A fundamental step in any diagnosis is the choice of an appropriate specimen, which ultimately depends upon an understanding of the pathogenesis of infections.

Although the issues of this chapter may at first seem mundane, it is of fundamental importance to recognize that a microbiological diagnosis is only as reliable as the quality of the specimen on which it is based.

The Aims of the Clinical Microbiology Laboratory

The aims of the microbiology laboratory are:

- To provide accurate information about the presence or absence of microorganisms in a specimen that may be involved in a patient's disease process.
- Where relevant, to provide information on the antimicrobial susceptibility of the microorganisms isolated.

Identification is achieved by detecting the microorganism or its products or the patient's immune response

Laboratory tests are carried out:

- To detect microorganisms or their products in specimens collected from the patient.
- To detect evidence of the patient's immune response (production of antibodies) to infection.

The tests fall into three main categories:

- Identification of microorganisms by isolation and culture. Microorganisms may grow in artificial media, or in the case of viruses, in cell cultures. In some instances, quantitation is important (e.g. more than 10^5 bacteria/ml of urine is indicative of infection whereas lower numbers are not, see Chapter 18). Once an organism has been isolated in culture, its susceptibility to antimicrobial agents can be determined.
- Identification of a specific microbial product. Non-cultural techniques that do not depend upon the growth and multiplication of microorganisms to detect microorganisms have the potential to yield more rapid results. These techniques include the detection of structural components of the cell (e.g. cell wall antigens) and extracellular products (e.g. toxins). Alternatively, specific gene sequences can be detected by the application of DNA probes to clinical specimens. These techniques are becoming more widely used, especially with the possibilities for amplification of DNA by the polymerase chain reaction (PCR; see Chapter 14). They are potentially applicable to all microorganisms but antimicrobial susceptibilities cannot be determined without culture (although the presence of resistance genes may be detectable by specific probes).

- Detection of specific antibodies to a pathogen. This may be the method of choice when the pathogen cannot be cultivated in laboratory media (e.g. *Treponema pallidum*, many viruses) or when culture would be particularly hazardous to laboratory staff (e.g. culture of *Francisella tularensis* the cause of tularemia, or the fungus *Coccidioides immitis*). The usual method is by detection of a rise (fourfold or greater) in antibody titer between 'paired' sera, collected in the acute phase of an infection and in convalescence. Such tests therefore tend to result in a delayed or retrospective diagnosis. However, detection of antibodies in a single serum collected during the acute phase of illness can be helpful in diagnosis, for example of rare diseases such as Lassa fever or if specific IgM is detected (e.g. in rubella infection).

The methods used in the laboratory for processing patients' specimens are given in detail in the Appendix.

Specimen Collection

Specimens must be relevant and of good quality

As it is usually impracticable to transport the patient to the laboratory, specimens are collected from the patient in the ward or clinic and sent to the laboratory. Obtaining the specimen is the clinician's responsibility but the laboratory must help by providing suitable containers and instructions *(Fig. 13.1)*. Specimen collection should be performed with care, avoiding harm or unnecessary discomfort to the patient. When the patient is asked to collect a specimen (e.g. of urine or sputum), clear instructions must be given. In order to be useful in the diagnosis and treatment of infection, specimens must be relevant (i.e. representative of the infectious process, see below), of good quality and adequate quantity. Whenever

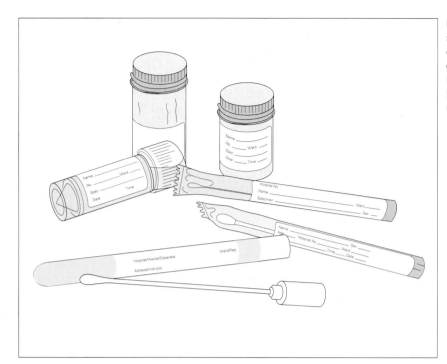

Fig. 13.1 Specimen containers should be a suitable size for ease of use. Instructions for collection of specimens should be clear and concise. Each specimen should be clearly labelled before it is despatched to the laboratory and should be accompanied by a request form.

possible, specimens should be collected before antimicrobial therapy is commenced.

Fluid or tissue is used for culture or for detecting microbial products

Specimens intended for isolation and cultivation of microorganisms can be divided into two main types:

- Fluid (including exudate and excreta).
- Tissue.

Swabs may be used to collect samples of fluids (e.g. wound exudate) or for sampling surfaces (e.g. skin), but whenever possible actual fluid should be collected as swabs absorb only a small quantity of sample and provide an arid unfriendly environment for transport to the laboratory. Many microbiological techniques are relatively insensitive so it is important to collect a large enough volume of sample and to maintain the viability of the organisms in the sample while in transit to the laboratory. Important specimens from various sites of infection are listed in *Figure 13.2*. Specimens for culture should be collected in sterile containers and should not be put into histologic fixatives such as formalin as such fixatives kill microorganisms.

The same specimens are used for detecting microbial products as for culture, but maintaining the viability of the organisms is not of prime importance because the detection of microbial products does not depend upon the presence of living organisms. However, it is important to minimize the risk of contamination by extraneous organisms.

Antibody responses are detectable in serum samples

'Paired' sera, collected in the acute and convalescent phases of the disease (ideally 10–14 days apart), are tested in parallel. Serum samples can be stored in the cold (–20°C) for months or years without loss of antibody titer. Sometimes cerebrospinal fluid (CSF) is used.

All specimens must be properly labelled and accompanied by an appropriate request form

The person collecting the specimen must label the specimen accurately as errors in specimen identification can have disastrous consequences. It is equally important that correct identification continues during the specimen's passage through the laboratory. The results of all tests on the specimen should be compiled into a report, which must also be suitably identified so that it is returned to the correct patient's records. In many hospitals, laboratory test requests and results are computerized.

In addition to the label, each specimen should be accompanied by a request form providing the necessary information about the patient, the clinical diagnosis and current antimicrobial therapy. An example is shown in *Figure 13.3*. The information on the request form allows the laboratory staff to process the specimen in the optimum manner.

All clinical specimens should be considered to be potentially infectious

It is sensible to assume that all clinical specimens (including serum samples for antibody detection) are potentially infectious and to handle them with suitable precautions, both while in transit and within the diagnostic laboratory. However specimens known to be of high risk (e.g. those from patients who are hepatitis B or HIV positive) should be clearly labelled as such, both on the specimen and on the request form.

Transport of Specimens

Specimens should be transported to the laboratory as quickly as possible

Some samples (e.g. urine, sputum) provide a good medium for growth of non-fastidious bacteria and fungi, so that organisms may multiply during the time between collection and cultivation in the laboratory, giving falsely high results in quantitative cultures (see Chapter 18). With time, the hardy species may overgrow the fastidious one, giving a

IMPORTANT SPECIMENS FROM VARIOUS SITES AND TYPES OF INFECTIONS				
site/type of infection	**type of specimen**			
	fluid	**tissue**	**swab**	**other**
urinary tract bladder kidney	urine urine	renal biopsy		
gastrointestinal tract intestine mouth liver biliary tract abdomen	washings bile pus peritoneal aspirate ascitic fluid	liver biopsy	rectal swab	feces
respiratory tract nose nasopharynx throat lung pleural space ear eye	washings (V) sputum alveolar lavage pleural fluid	lung biopsy	nasal swab pernasal swab throat swab ear swab eye swab	'cough plate' – patient coughs directly onto agar plate direct inoculation of culture plates at bedside
central nervous system meninges encephalitis (herpes) brain abscess	cerebrospinal fluid (CSF) pus; CSF	brain biopsy		
genital tract urethra vagina cervix endometrium		endometrial biopsy	urethral swab high vaginal swab cervical swab	direct microscopy and culture in clinic
skin and soft tissue skin wound	vesicle fluid (V) pus	skin biopsy (M) scrapings (F)	skin swab (carriage) wound swab	impression plates
bone and joint osteomyelitis joint	pus aspirate	bone*		
septicemia	blood			
pyrexia of unknown origin	blood			blood films for malarial parasites
endocarditis	blood	heart valve*		
* collected at operation (V) specimens for virology (F) specimens for fungi (M) specimens for mycobacterium				

Fig. 13.2 Important specimens from various sites and types of infection. Where possible specimens of fluid (e.g. pus, urine, feces) or tissue should be sent to the laboratory as swabs provide an unsatisfactory volume of specimen and a hostile environment for certain organisms.

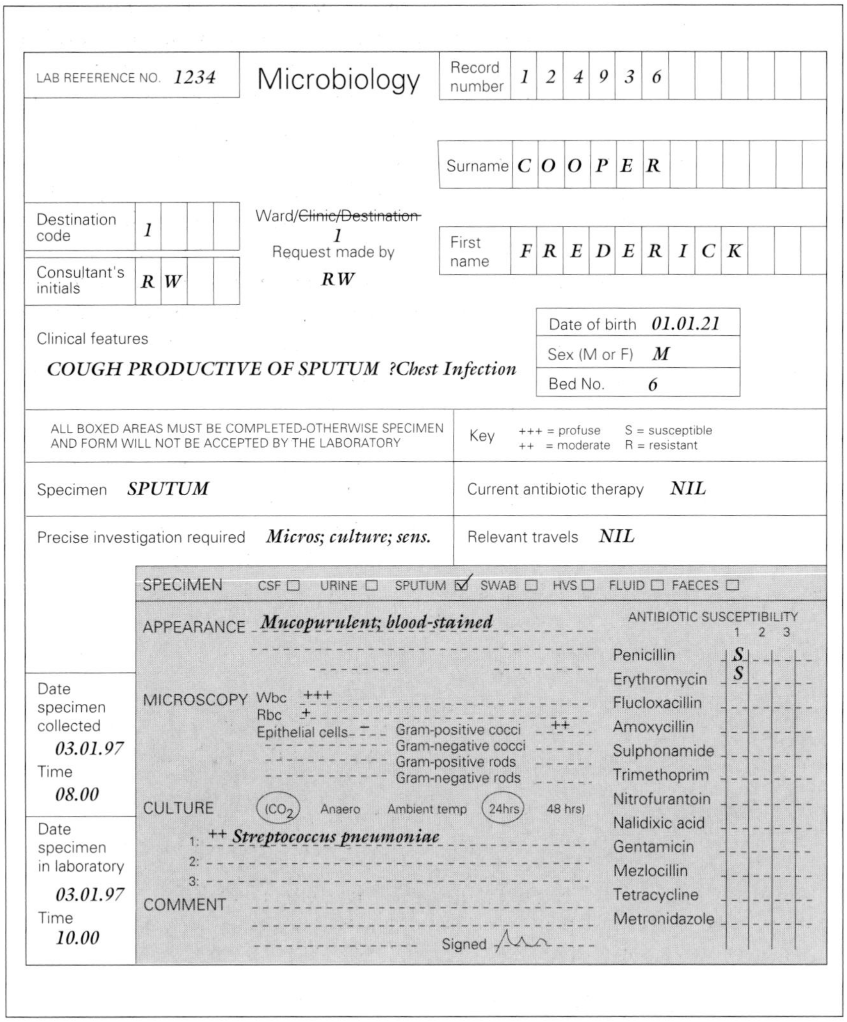
LAB REFERENCE NO. *1234* Microbiology Record number *1 2 4 9 3 6*

Surname *C O O P E R*

Destination code *1* Ward/~~Clinic/Destination~~ *1* Request made by *RW*

First name *F R E D E R I C K*

Consultant's initials *R W*

Date of birth *01.01.21*

Sex (M or F) *M*

Bed No. *6*

Clinical features *COUGH PRODUCTIVE OF SPUTUM ?Chest Infection*

ALL BOXED AREAS MUST BE COMPLETED-OTHERWISE SPECIMEN AND FORM WILL NOT BE ACCEPTED BY THE LABORATORY

Key +++ = profuse ++ = moderate S = susceptible R = resistant

Specimen *SPUTUM* Current antibiotic therapy *NIL*

Precise investigation required *Micros; culture; sens.* Relevant travels *NIL*

SPECIMEN CSF ☐ URINE ☐ SPUTUM ☑ SWAB ☐ HVS ☐ FLUID ☐ FAECES ☐

APPEARANCE *Mucopurulent; blood-stained*

MICROSCOPY Wbc *+++* Rbc *+* Epithelial cells *–* Gram-positive cocci *++* Gram-negative cocci Gram-positive rods Gram-negative rods

CULTURE (CO₂) Anaero Ambient temp (24hrs) 48 hrs)

1: *++ Streptococcus pneumoniae*

2:

3:

COMMENT

Signed

Date specimen collected *03.01.97* Time *08.00*

Date specimen in laboratory *03.01.97* Time *10.00*

ANTIBIOTIC SUSCEPTIBILITY 1 2 3

Penicillin *S*; Erythromycin *S*; Flucloxacillin; Amoxycillin; Sulphonamide; Trimethoprim; Nitrofurantoin; Nalidixic acid; Gentamicin; Mezlocillin; Tetracycline; Metronidazole

Fig. 13.3 Every specimen sent to the laboratory should be accompanied by a completed request form or identified so that it can be linked to a computer-generated request on arrival in the laboratory. Information about the patient, such as name, date of birth and bed number, will ensure that the report is directed back to the correct patient's notes. Age and sex are important for some infections, and the patient's clinical features and any current antibiotic therapy, which may make it difficult to isolate the pathogen, must be included. This latter information also directs the laboratory to test the appropriate antibiotic if the patient is already on treatment. Relevant travel details are also important to indicate possible exposure to pathogens in endemic areas. The precise investigation required indicates to the laboratory the type of test the clinician wants (e.g. microscopy, culture, antibiotic susceptibility of any pathogens isolated). Finally the date and time of specimen collection and of arrival in the laboratory indicate how long ago the specimen was taken. Once the form reaches the laboratory, the relevant tests are carried out and the report completed by the microbiologist (area in gray), including macro- and microscopic reports, antibiotic susceptibility and culture results, indicating what has grown and in what quantity.

false impression of the balance between species or in fact making it impossible to isolate and identify the less hardy species. In other specimens (e.g. throat swabs, urethral swabs) delicate organisms such as *Neisseria* species survive poorly. Specimens for the detection of viruses may be rendered useless if overgrown by bacteria and fungi, hence the inclusion of antibacterials and antifungals in viral transport media (see below).

Refrigeration for short periods may preserve the organisms in a urine specimen in roughly the same numbers as they occurred in the specimen when it was first collected, but similar conditions will kill certain fastidious organisms and greatly reduce the chances of isolating small numbers of bacteria, from blood cultures for example.

Transport media preserve microorganisms

Fluids and tissue specimens should be transported to the laboratory in sterile containers, without the addition of preservative. Swabs are better transported in a medium that helps to preserve the organisms in the specimen, but prevents them from multiplying, thereby maintaining the ratios of the various species. Transport media often contain a sloppy agar, which helps to prevent drying out of the organisms, and charcoal or other absorbent substances to remove toxic agents such as fatty acids. Examples of transport media suitable for swabs destined for bacterial culture are those of Stuart or Amies, or thioglycollate media. If anaerobic bacteria are suspected and a pus sample is obtainable, it should be aspirated into a syringe, the needle removed, the syringe tip capped and the specimen sent without delay to the laboratory to minimize exposure to air.

The optimal virus transport medium is one that preserves the virus in the specimen, prevents loss of the specimen due to bacterial or fungal contamination, is non-toxic to cell cultures, and can be used both for virus isolation and for direct tests to detect and identify virus antigens (e.g. immunofluorescence, enzyme immunoassays). Several such systems exist, including:

- Sucrose-based and broth-based liquid media.
- 'Transporters' containing a monolayer of human diploid fibroblast cells in buffered serum with added antibiotics. The addition of antibiotics to viral transport media helps to reduce bacterial contamination, but means that the same specimen cannot be used for isolation of viruses and bacteria.

Specimen Processing

Specimen handling and interpretation of results is based upon a knowledge of normal flora and contaminants

Specimens intended for cultivation of microorganisms can be divided into two types:

- Those from sites that are normally sterile.
- Those from sites that usually have a commensal flora (*Fig. 13.4*; see also Chapter 3).

A thorough knowledge of the microorganisms normally isolated from specimens from non-sterile sites, and the common contaminants of specimens collected from sterile sites is important to ensure that specimens are properly handled and the results are correctly interpreted. Some specimens from sites that should be sterile (e.g. bladder urine, sputum from the lower respiratory tract) are usually collected after passage through orifices that have a normal flora, which may contaminate the specimens. This needs to be considered when interpreting the culture results of these specimens.

Ideally each specimen arriving in the laboratory is considered in turn together with the information provided about the patient on the request form so that the microbiologist can assess which pathogens are likely to be present and can devise an 'individualized' processing plan. In reality this approach is not practicable because of constraints on time and money; specimens tend to be processed by type (e.g. urine, blood, feces) and the microbiologist looks for easily cultivated pathogens known to be associated with each sample type. However, if the laboratory is provided with suitable information, such as a statement of possible etiology, more fastidious or unusual pathogens can be sought and relevant antibiotic susceptibilities assessed. The schemes used for the basic processing of specimens are outlined in Chapter 14.

To obtain a test result that correctly identifies the infection, it is important to collect an appropriate specimen, to use the appropriate transport conditions and to deliver specimens rapidly to the laboratory. These conditions all affect the accuracy of the laboratory report, and therefore its value to the clinician and ultimately to the patient. The key points to remember about specimen collection are summarized in *Figure 13.5*.

SAMPLING SITES AND THE NORMAL FLORA

body sites that are normally sterile

blood and bone marrow
cerebrospinal fluid
serous fluids
tissues
lower respiratory tract
bladder

body sites that have a normal commensal flora

mouth, nose and upper respiratory tract
skin
gastrointestinal tract
female genital tract
urethra

Fig. 13.4 Sampling sites and interpretation of results. Some sites in the body are sterile in health so that growth of any organism is indicative of infection provided that the specimen has been properly collected and transported, and examined in the laboratory without delay. The significance of isolates from sites that have a commensal flora depends upon the identity of the isolate and the quantity, as well as the immune status of the patient.

AIDE-MEMOIRE FOR SPECIMEN COLLECTION

take the appropriate specimen;
e.g. blood and cerebrospinal fluid in suspected meningitis

collect the specimen at the appropriate time, during the acute phase of the disease;
e.g. malarial films, virus isolation

if possible collect specimen before patient receives antimicrobials

collect enough material and an adequate number of samples e.g. enough blood/serum for more than one set of blood cultures

avoid contamination
(a) from normal flora; e.g. midstream urine
(b) from non-sterile equipment

use the correct containers and appropriate transport media

label specimens properly

complete request form with enough clinical information and a statement of possible etiology

talk to the microbiologist and inform the laboratory if special tests are required

transport specimens rapidly to the laboratory

Fig. 13.5 Important steps in specimen collection and delivery to the laboratory. The responsibility of the clinician does not end with collection of the specimen and requesting tests. Good communication with the microbiologist is essential.

- Microbiologic confirmation of a clinical diagnosis of infection depends upon the collection of high quality specimens and their rapid despatch to the laboratory with all the necessary supporting information.
- Laboratory tests detect microorganisms or their products, or evidence of a patient's immune response to infection. Although new techniques such as the PCR are increasingly used to detect pathogens rapidly, antimicrobial susceptibility can only be determined and appropriate treatment information provided by isolating organisms in culture.
- Growth of bacteria requires at least 18 hours (isolation of viruses and of fungi may take much longer); culture results cannot therefore be expected in less than 24 hours.
- Interpretation of culture results depends upon the source of the specimen. From sites that are normally sterile, any isolated organism is significant. From sites colonized by a commensal flora, isolating and identifying the pathogen can be more difficult.
- Good communication between the clinician and the microbiologist is extremely important.

1. List three body sites that are sterile in health and three that have a normal commensal flora.
2. Which specimens would you collect to assist in the diagnosis of a) urinary tract infection, b) meningitis, c) osteomyelitis, d) malaria, and e) whooping cough?
3. What specimens would you collect to detect antibodies? What is important about the timing of these specimens?
4. What is the shortest time you would expect it to take to get a result from the laboratory for a) significant bacteriuria in a midstream urine specimen from a patient with dysuria, b) microscopic evidence of infection in the CSF of a young patient with a stiff neck, and c) antibiotic susceptibility of *Staphylococcus aureus* isolated from a blood culture of a febrile patient?

Further Reading

Brent Johnson F. Transport of viral specimens. *Clin Microbiol Rev* 1990;**3**:120–131.

Collins CH, Lyne PM, Grange JM eds. *Collins and Lyne's Microbiological Methods,* 6th edition. Oxford: Butterworth–Heinemann Ltd, 1989.

Hawkey PM, Lewis DA eds. *Medical Microbiology: A Practical Approach.* Oxford: IRL Press, 1989.

Diagnosis of Infection and Assessment of Host Defense Mechanisms

Introduction

In the previous chapter, we stressed the importance of the specimen in the laboratory diagnosis of infection and discussed types of specimens and their collection and transport to the laboratory. In this chapter we will examine methods for the microbiological diagnosis of disease and the processing of specimens in the laboratory, and outline briefly methods for the assessment of the individual components and functional activity of the host defense systems.

Microbiology differs from other clinical laboratory disciplines in the amount of interpretative input required. When a specimen is received, the microbiologist must decide on the appropriate processing pathway, and when the result is received it must be interpreted in relation to the specimen and the patient. Specimen analysis is less mechanized and automated than in the other disciplines.

Culture takes at least 18 hours to produce a result

Time is a key factor because the conventional methods of microbiological diagnosis depend upon growth and identification of the pathogen. Results of culture cannot be achieved in less than 18 hours and may take as long as six weeks for a minority of pathogens, such as the mycobacteria. Thus specimen processing can be categorized according to the time required to achieve a result and the method – cultural or non-cultural. An alternative route to the diagnosis of an infection is an immunologic one, relying on the detection of an antibody response to the putative pathogen in the patient's blood. These diagnostic routes are summarized in *Figure 14.1*, but we must expect major contributions from rapid technologies based on identification of microbial DNA using hybridization to microarrays of hundreds of thousands of oligonucleotide probes on small chips, in the near future.

Non-Cultural Techniques for the Laboratory Diagnosis of Infection

Non-cultural techniques do not require microorganism multiplication before detection

Although medical microbiology has long been synonymous with the cultivation of microorganisms from patients' specimens, these techniques are labor-intensive and slow to produce results (days rather than hours) because replication of organisms is a necessary, but rate-limiting, step. In addition, some microorganisms cannot be cultured in artificial media, and viable organisms may be difficult to recover from specimens of patients who have received antimicrobial therapy. Non-cultural techniques do not require multiplication of the microorganism before its detection. Some techniques, such as microscopy and detection of microbial antigens in specimens, can provide very rapid results (i.e. within two hours). Other non-cultural methods such as the use of DNA probes and amplification of DNA by the polymerase chain reaction (PCR) may require up to 1–2 days to complete.

Microscopy
Microscopy is an important first step in the examination of all specimens

Microscopy plays a fundamental role in microbiology. Although microorganisms show a wide range in size (see Chapters 1 and 3) they are too small to be seen individually by the naked eye and therefore a microscope is an essential tool in microbiology. The various types of microscopy are summarized in *Figure 14.2*. The light microscope magnifies objects and therefore improves the resolving power of the naked eye from 20 mm to about 0.2 mm; the electron microscope can improve this to about 0.001 mm.

Light microscopy
Bright field microscopy is used to examine specimens and cultures as wet or stained preparations

Wet preparations are used to demonstrate:
- Blood cells and microbes in fluid specimens such as urine, feces or cerebrospinal fluid (CSF).
- Cysts, eggs and parasites in feces.
- Fungi in skin.
- Protozoa in blood and tissues.
  Living organisms can be examined to detect motility.

Dyes are used to stain cells so that they can be seen more easily. Stains are usually applied to dried material that has been fixed (by heat or alcohol) onto the microscope slide. Samples from specimens themselves, or pure cultures can be stained. The slide can then be viewed in the light microscope with an oil immersion lens, which improves the resolving power of the microscope.

The most important differential staining technique in bacteriology is the 'Gram' stain

Differential staining procedures exploit the fact that cells with different properties stain differently and thus can be distinguished. Based on their reaction to Gram's stain *(Fig. 14.3)*, bacteria are divided into two broad groups:
- Gram positive (stain purple).
- Gram negative (stain pink).

This difference is related to differences in the structure of the cell walls of the two groups (see Chapter 3).

The Ziehl–Neelsen stain is used to detect mycobacteria

Some organisms, particularly mycobacteria, which have waxy cell walls, do not readily take up the Gram stain and special staining techniques are used to demonstrate their presence. The Ziehl–Neelsen stain (see Chapter 17, *Fig. 17.24*) is a differential staining procedure that uses heat to drive the fuchsin stain into the cells; mycobacteria stained with fuchsin withstand decolorization with acid and alcohol and are therefore known as 'acid-' and 'alcohol-fast' – other bacteria lose the stain after acid and alcohol treatment. Alternatively, the fluorescent dye auramine, which has a strong affinity for the waxy cell wall of mycobacteria, can be used to demonstrate these organisms by fluorescence microscopy *(Fig. 14.6)*.

Other staining techniques can be used to demonstrate particular features of cells

Examples of such features to aid identification include the volutin (polyphosphate) storage granules in *Corynebacterium*

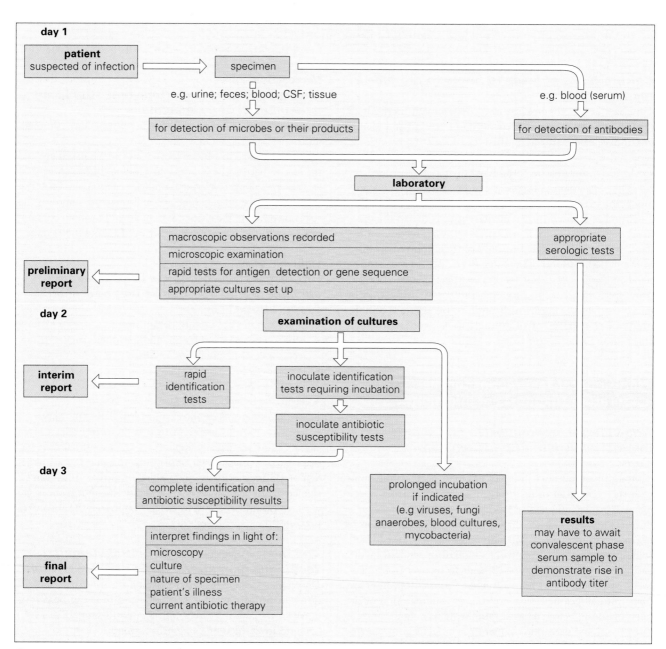

Fig. 14.1 Route from patient to microbiological diagnosis. This scheme shows the key steps in specimen processing. Some tests can be performed on the specimen immediately and yield 'same day' results. Culture of specimens involves a minimum of 18 hours' incubation before colonies are visible and can be identified. Antibiotic susceptibility tests involve a further incubation period. Alternatively the diagnosis may be based on the detection of specific antibodies in serum samples. (CSF, cerebrospinal fluid.)

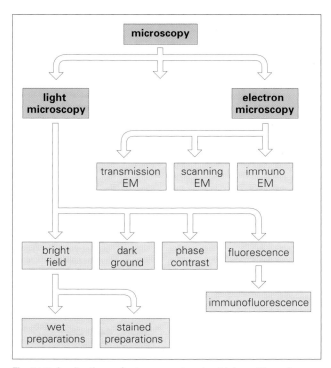

Fig. 14.2 Applications of microscopy to microbiology. The scheme shows the different uses of light and electron microscopy (EM) for looking at microbes.

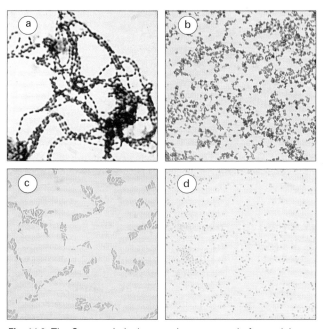

Fig. 14.3 The Gram stain is the most important stain for studying bacteria. The combination of the violet dye (crystal violet) and iodine (acting as a mordant) binds to the cell wall. Gram-positive cells retain the stain when challenged with acetone and remain purple. Gram-negative cells lose the purple stain and appear colorless until stained with a pink counterstain (neutral red or safranin). Examination of Gram-stained films also allows the shape of the cells to be noted. Some examples are shown: (a) Gram-positive cocci in chains (streptococci); (b) Gram-positive rods (*Listeria*); (c) Gram-negative rods (*Escherichia coli*); (d) Gram-negative cocci (*Neisseria*).

spp. and lipid in *Bacillus* spp. *(Fig. 14.4)*. Protocols for these staining methods are given in the Appendix.

Dark ground (dark field) microscopy is useful for observing motility and thin cells such as spirochetes

The light microscope may be adapted by modifying the condenser so that the object appears brightly lit against a dark background. Living organisms can be examined by dark ground microscopy and thus motility can be observed. The method is also used for visualizing very thin cells such as spirochetes because the light reflected from the surface of the cells makes them appear larger and therefore more easily visible than when examined by bright field microscopy *(Fig. 14.5)*.

Phase contrast microscopy increases the contrast of an image

This technique enhances the very small differences in refractive index and density between living cells and the fluid in

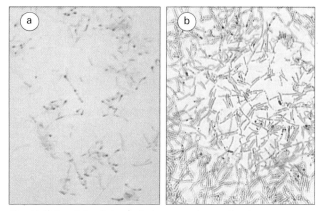

Fig. 14.4 Special staining techniques can be used to demonstrate particular features of bacterial cells. (a) Corynebacteria stained to demonstrate polymetaphosphate storage granules (volutin granules), which appear as dark spots in blue-green cells (Albert's stain). (b) Lipid storage granules in *Bacillus cereus* stained with Sudan black (black lipid against red cells).

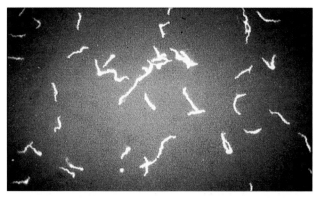

Fig. 14.5 Spirochetes visualized by dark ground microscopy. Spirochetes and leptospires are much thinner than most bacterial cells (approximately 0.1 mm in diameter compared with 1 mm for *Escherichia coli*), but they appear larger when viewed by dark ground illumination.

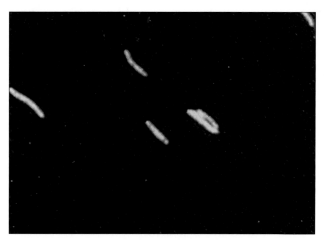

Fig. 14.6 Fluorochrome stain of *Mycobacterium tuberculosis* with a mixture of auramine O and rhodamine B. Mycobacteria appear fluorescent under ultraviolet light. (Courtesy of DK Banerjee.)

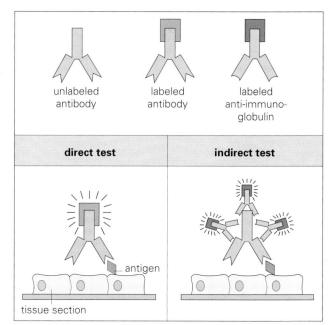

Fig. 14.7 The fluorescent antibody test for detection and identification of microbial (or tissue) antigens or antibodies directed against them.

which they are suspended and therefore produces an image with a higher degree of contrast than that achieved by bright field microscopy. However, phase contrast microscopy is now rarely used in the diagnostic laboratory.

Fluorescence microscopy is used for substances that are either naturally fluorescent or have been stained with fluorescent dyes

If light of one wavelength shines on a fluorescent object, it emits light of a different wavelength. Some biological substances are naturally fluorescent; others can be stained with fluorescent dyes and viewed in a microscope with an ultraviolet light source instead of white light *(Fig. 14.6)*.

Fluorescence microscopy is widely used in microbiology and immunology and has been developed to detect microbial antigens in specimens and tissues by 'staining' with specific antibodies tagged with fluorescent dyes (immunofluorescence). The method can be made more sensitive or can be adapted to the detection of antibody by labelling a second antibody in an indirect test *(Fig. 14.7)*.

Electron microscopy
The specimen needs to be cut into thin sections for electron microscopy

The electron microscope uses a beam of electrons instead of light, and magnets are used to focus the beam instead of the lenses used in a light microscope. The whole system is operated under a high vacuum. Electron beams penetrate poorly and a single microbial cell is too thick to be viewed directly. To overcome this the specimen is fixed and mounted in plastic and cut into thin sections, which are examined individually. Electron-dense stains such as osmium tetroxide, uranyl acetate or glutaraldehyde, are applied to the specimen to improve contrast. The electrons pass through the section and produce an image on a fluorescent screen. Images are photographed and enlarged so that the original specimen is magnified many thousandfold *(Fig. 14.8)*.

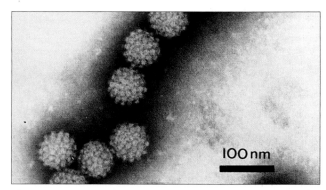

Fig. 14.8 Electron micrograph of papillomavirus, the human wart virus. (Courtesy of the Regional Virus Laboratory, Birmingham.)

Electron microscopy can be used to identify virus particles

Direct examination of specimens allows rapid identification of virus particles and detection of viruses that are difficult or impossible to cultivate (e.g. rotaviruses, hepatitis A virus). Fluid for examination is dried onto a copper grid and examined. About one million virus particles per ml are needed if they are to be detectable. The sensitivity can be increased by reacting the fluid with antiviral antibody so that clumps of virus particles are visible. This is known as immunoelectron microscopy, a technique analogous to immunofluorescence in light microscopy.

Detection of microbial antigens in specimens

Detection of specific microbial antigens can be a more rapid method for detecting the presence of an organism than attempting to grow and identify the microbe. The methods include:

NON-CULTURAL TECHNIQUES
non-specific techniques for detection of microbial products
fatty acid end-products of metabolism of anaerobes can be detected in fluid specimens (e.g. pus, blood) by gas liquid chromatography
antigen detection
detection of soluble carbohydrate antigens by agglutination of antibody-coated latex particles or red blood cells
e.g.
Streptococcus pneumoniae capsule *Haemophilus influenzae* type b capsule ⎤ in CSF *Neisseria meningitidis* capsule ⎦ and urine *Cryptococcus neoformans* capsule
Strep. pyogenes group antigen in throat swabs
detection of particular antigens by binding to antibodies labelled with:
radioisotope, enzyme or   e.g. ELISA for hepatitis B, fluorescent molecule   rotavirus
toxin detection
detection of exotoxins
Clostridium botulinum toxin by injection of patient's serum into mice (unprotected and protected with specific antiserum)
Clostridium difficile cytotoxin in feces by addition of suspension to cell culture
Clostridium perfringens and *Staphylococcus aureus* enterotoxins in feces by agglutination of antitoxin-coated latex particles
Escherichia coli toxin genes (LT, ST, vero) in feces by DNA probes
detection of endotoxin
endotoxin from cell walls of Gram-negative bacteria detected by *Limulus* lysate assay (clotting of extracts of amebocytes of the horseshoe (*Limulus*) crab)

Fig. 14.9 Non-cultural techniques for detection of microbial products. Identification of specific microbial products can be a more rapid method for detecting microorganisms than isolation and culture. The available techniques vary in their specificity. Toxins may be detected either by virtue of their antigenic properties or by demonstrating their action. (CSF, cerebrospinal fuid; ELISA, enzyme-linked immunosorbent assay.)

- Those that detect antigens by their interaction with specific antibodies.
- Those that detect microbial toxins.

They are summarized in *Figure 14.9*.

Specific antibody coated onto latex particles will react with the organism or its product, resulting in visible clumping

For example, the common causative agents of bacterial meningitis (*Streptococcus pneumoniae*, *Haemophilus influenzae* and *Neisseria meningitidis* types A and C) can be detected in CSF by mixing the specimen with specific antibody coated onto latex particles. If the antigen (i.e. the organism or its product) is present the particles will clump together (*Fig. 14.10*). These tests give results within minutes of receipt of the specimen, but their sensitivity is not significantly greater than that of the Gram stain and false positive results may occur due to cross-reacting antigens. However,

they can be a useful diagnostic aid when the patient has received antibiotics and organisms may appear morphologically unidentifiable in the CSF and fail to grow in culture.

Radioimmunoassay can be used to measure antigen concentration

The binding of radioactively labeled antigen to a limited but standard amount of antibody can be partially inhibited by addition of unlabeled antigen. The ratio of free antigen to that bound to antibody can be used as a measure of the unlabeled material that has been added. In practice, this is usually achieved by binding the antibody to a plastic surface to facilitate the separation of bound from free antigen. The principle of this form of saturation analysis is outlined in *Figure 14.11*. In another variation, unlabeled test antigen is added to solid phase antibody, and the percentage occupancy of antibody sites, which is proportional to antigen concentration, is determined by adding a labeled second antibody.

There is a tendency now to replace the radioisotope with:
- Enzymatic labels – as in the enzyme-linked immunosorbent assay (ELISA) *(Fig. 14.12)*.
- Chemiluminescent or time-resolved fluorescent labels, which give assays of very high sensitivity.

Monoclonal antibodies can distinguish between species and between strains of the same species on the basis of antigenic differences

Monoclonal antibodies *(Fig. 14.13)* are being used increasingly as diagnostic tools. Direct ELISA (see above) frequently

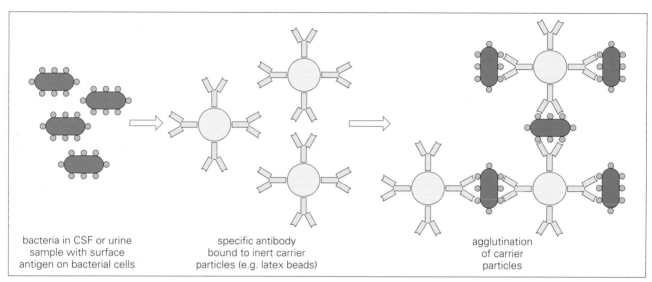

| bacteria in CSF or urine sample with surface antigen on bacterial cells | specific antibody bound to inert carrier particles (e.g. latex beads) | agglutination of carrier particles |

Fig. 14.10 When a specimen of cerebrospinal fluid (CSF) containing bacteria (e.g. *Haemophilus influenzae*) is mixed with a suspension of latex particles coated with specific antibody (e.g. *H. influenzae* anticapsular antibodies), the interaction between antigen and antibody causes an immediate agglutination of particles, which is visible to the naked eye.

◆ radioactive antigen ◇ unlabeled antigen	free antigen	bound antigen	ratio free:bound radioactivity
(a) baseline			
3 *Ag + 2 Ab ⟹	1 *Ag +	2 *Ag Ab	**1 : 2**
(b) unlabeled test Ag added			
3 *Ag / 3 Ag + 2 Ab ⟹	2 *Ag / 2 Ag +	1 *Ag Ab / 1 Ag Ab	**2 : 1**

Fig. 14.11 The principle of radioimmunoassay, simplified by assuming a very highly avid antibody and one combining site per antibody molecule. (a) If three molecules of radiolabeled antigen (Ag) are added to two molecules of antibody (Ab), one molecule of Ag will be free and two will be bound to Ab. The ratio of the free to bound radioactivity will be 1:2. (b) If three molecules of unlabeled Ag plus three molecules of labeled Ag are added to the Ab, again only two molecules of total Ag will be bound, but since the Ab cannot distinguish labeled from unlabeled Ag, half will be radioactive. The remaining antigen will be free and the ratio of free to bound radioactivity changes to 2:1. This ratio will vary with the amount of unlabeled Ag added, enabling the construction of a calibration curve.

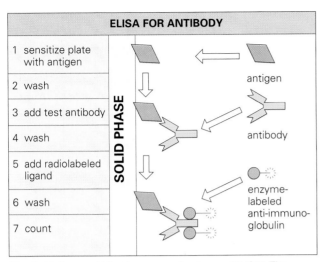

ELISA FOR ANTIBODY

	SOLID PHASE
1 sensitize plate with antigen	
2 wash	
3 add test antibody	
4 wash	
5 add radiolabeled ligand	
6 wash	
7 count	

antigen

antibody

enzyme-labeled anti-immuno-globulin

Fig. 14.12 Enzyme-linked immunosorbent assay (ELISA). The binding of antibody in the test serum to solid phase antigen is measured by the binding of a labeled second reagent, usually an anti-immunoglobulin (see indirect test in *Fig. 14.7*) labeled with an enzyme, which can be detected by a color reaction.

employ enzyme-conjugated monoclonal antibodies to detect antigens in specimens from patients. Rotaviruses, HIV, hepatitis B virus, herpes virus and respiratory syncytial virus (RSV) can all be detected directly with monoclonal antibodies in ELISAs. *Chlamydia trachomatis* infection can be diagnosed within a few hours by a direct fluorescent antibody test employing a monoclonal antibody labeled with fluorescein (see Chapter 19).

Detection of microbes by probing for their genes
Organisms carrying genes for virulence factors can be detected by nucleic acid probes for the virulence factors

A gene probe is a nucleic acid molecule that when in the single-stranded state and labeled, can be used to detect a complementary sequence of DNA by hybridizing to it. Polynucleotide probes are obtained from naturally occurring DNA by cloning DNA fragments into appropriate plasmid vectors and then isolating the cloned DNA. However, if the sequence of the gene of interest is known, oligonucleotide probes can be synthesized. Probes are labeled either with a radioactive isotope (e.g. ^{32}P) or

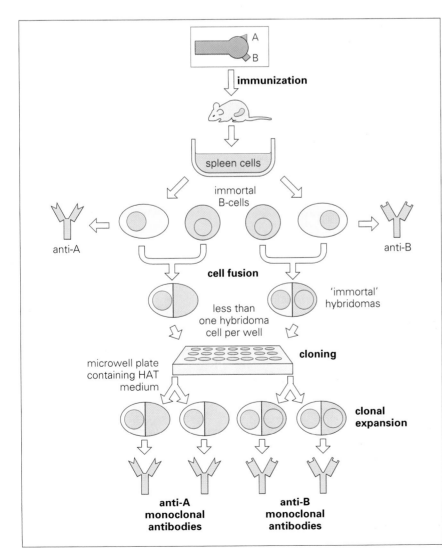

immunization

spleen cells

immortal B-cells

anti-A

anti-B

cell fusion

less than one hybridoma cell per well

'immortal' hybridomas

microwell plate containing HAT medium

cloning

clonal expansion

anti-A monoclonal antibodies

anti-B monoclonal antibodies

Fig. 14.13 Production of monoclonal antibodies. Mice immunized with an antigen bearing for example, two epitopes, A and B, develop spleen cells making anti-A and anti-B, which appear as antibodies in the serum. The spleen is removed and the individual cells fused in polyethylene glycol with constantly dividing (i.e. 'immortal') B tumor cells selected for a purine deficiency and often for their inability to secrete immunoglobulin. The resulting cells distributed into microwell plates in HAT (hypoxanthine, aminopterin, thymidine) medium, which kills off the perfusion partners, at such a high dilution that on average each well will contain less than one hybridoma cell. Each hybridoma is the fusion product of a single antibody-forming cell and a tumor cell and has the ability of the former to secrete a single species of antibody and the immortality of the latter enabling it to proliferate continuously, clonal progeny providing an unending supply of antibody with a single specificity – the monoclonal antibody. These monoclonal antibodies can be 'labeled' with enzymes or fluorescent molecules and can then be visualized when they bind to specific antigens (e.g. on virus particles).

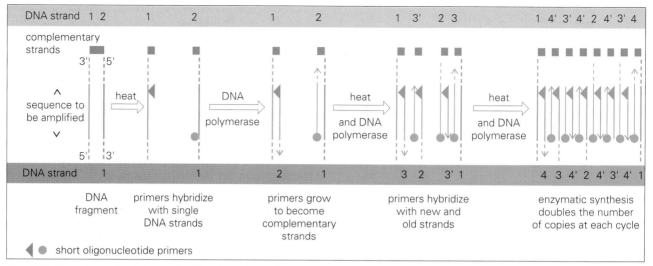

Fig. 14.14 The polymerase chain reaction. The short oligonucleotide primers hybridize with the nucleotide sequences on complementary strands at each end of the DNA fragment to be expanded. These, together with a heat-stable polymerase, produce rapidly increasing numbers of fragments consisting of the sequence to be amplified and after several cycles millions of copies can be obtained. The individual strands are numbered so that their fate can be followed with each succeeding cycle.

with compounds that give color reactions in suitable conditions (e.g. biotin streptavidin or alkaline phosphatase).

By constructing probes for virulence factors such as toxins, organisms carrying these genes can be detected in specimens without the need for culture (e.g. probes for enterotoxins of *Escherichia coli* or cholera toxin can be applied directly to feces). A commercially available ^{125}I-labeled DNA probe directed against sequences specific for *Mycoplasma pneumoniae* ribosomal RNA has been used successfully to detect the organism in sputum specimens.

Nucleic acid probes are of limited use for small numbers of organisms

There is no doubt that gene probes will be developed increasingly for diagnostic purposes, but detection of small numbers of organisms (i.e. few copies of the gene) can be a limiting factor and in these circumstances the combination of gene amplification by the polymerase chain reaction (PCR; see below) followed by hybridization with oligonucleotide probes may become the method of choice, especially for organisms that are slow or difficult to grow in the laboratory.

The PCR can be used to amplify a specific DNA sequence to produce millions of copies within a few hours

Although theoretically, PCR *(Fig. 14.14)* can detect a single gene sequence, such sensitivity is seldom achieved in clinical specimens, but bacteria present in numbers between 10–100 can be detected by standard PCR techniques and more sophisticated methods can detect one HIV proviral DNA sequence in 10^6 cells. A further advantage is the speed with which this can be achieved. Amplification takes only about five hours although confirmation of the identity of the product by probing or sequencing can add up to 36 hours, although this should speed up with the advent of micro-array technology.

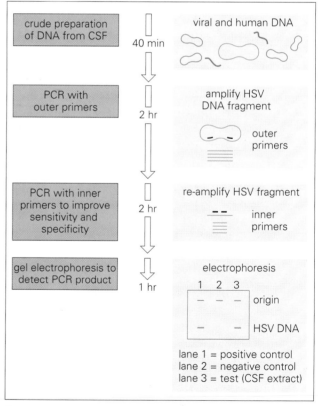

Fig. 14.15 Detection of herpes simplex virus (HSV) DNA in cerebrospinal fluid (CSF) from a patient with encephalitis by nested polymerase chain reaction (PCR). Nested PCR is a modification of the original PCR technique in which the DNA of interest is amplified first with two primers, which recognize sequences some distance apart, and then in a second reaction, with a further pair of primers, which recognize sequences within the length of the DNA amplified by the first pair. This technique improves the sensitivity and specificity of PCR.

The specificity of PCR is determined by careful choice of primers

These primers (oligonucleotides) are complementary to the target DNA – therefore in order to synthesize suitable primers, the sequence of the target DNA must be known. At the present time this is one of the limitations of PCR, but this versatile technique will undoubtedly be developed for wider clinical applications. Currently it is used in the research laboratory setting, but it seems only a matter of time before the methods become available for routine diagnostic use. Already PCR has been applied to a variety of specimens such as CSF, urine, sputum, blood, biopsies and paraffin-embedded specimens, to diagnose infections caused by bacteria, viruses, fungi and protozoa *(Fig. 14.15)*.

Cultivation (Culture) of Microorganisms

Bacteria and fungi can be cultured on solid nutrient or liquid media

Bacteria and fungi grow on the surface of solid nutrient media to produce colonies composed of thousands of cells derived from a single cell implanted on the agar surface. Colonies of different species often have characteristic appearances, which can give a clue to their likely identity *(Fig. 14.16)*. It takes 12–48 hours for colonies of most species to become macroscopically visible, but some organisms multiply much more slowly and may take several weeks to produce visible colonies. Cultures can also be made in liquid media (broth) and growth detected by observing the development of turbidity. However, it is not possible to tell whether there is more than one species present in a liquid culture or whether there are few or many organisms. Solid media are therefore more useful in diagnostic microbiology.

Different species of bacteria and fungi have different growth requirements

It is possible to grow the majority of species of bacteria and fungi of medical importance in artificial media in the laboratory, but there is no one universal culture medium that will support the growth of them all, and there are still some species that can only be grown in experimental animals (e.g. *Mycobacterium leprae* and *Treponema pallidum*). Some bacteria that cannot be cultivated on artificial media (e.g. chlamydia and rickettsia) can be grown in cell cultures (see below).

Many culture media are designed not only to support the growth of the desired organisms, but also to inhibit the growth of others (i.e. they are 'selective media'). Constituents common to all bacteriologic culture media are shown in *Figure 14.17*. The important media used in the diagnostic laboratory and schemes using these media for processing different clinical specimens are outlined in the Appendix.

Specimens collected from body sites that have a normal commensal flora will contain a mixture of organisms from which the pathogen has to be recognized. Specimens are 'plated out' on a carefully chosen range of nutrient and selective media to produce single colonies. These are subcultured

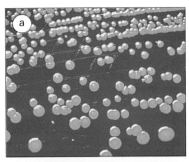
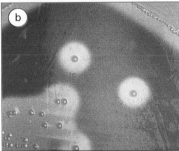
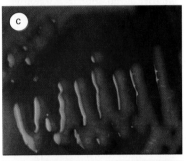
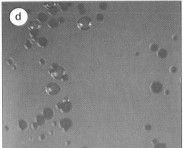

Fig. 14.16 Bacterial colonies. A bacterial cell implanted on a solid nutrient medium will multiply to produce a colony containing millions of cells. Different species produce characteristically different colonies and this feature can be used as a preliminary clue to the identity of the organism. (a) Golden colonies of *Staphylococcus aureus*. (b) Additional features such as the ability to lyse red blood cells can be demonstrated by culturing bacteria on blood-containing media. Here, β-hemolysis (complete hemolysis) is produced by *Streptococcus pyogenes* on horse blood agar. (c) Culture media can be made selective by including agents that are inhibitory to some species. For example, MacConkey agar contains bile salts so only those organisms tolerant to bile will grow. In addition it contains lactose and a pH indicator. Species that ferment lactose change the indicator to bright pink (c). Non-lactose fermenting species, such as *Salmonella* and *Shigella* form yellowish colonies (d).

to fresh media for identification and antibiotic susceptibility tests (see below). This procedure takes at least 48 hours, and sometimes longer, to yield results *(Fig. 14.1)*.

Parasites such as *Leishmania*, *Trypanosoma* and *Trichomonas* can be cultivated in liquid media to allow small numbers present in the original specimen (e.g. blood or vaginal secretions) to multiply and thus become easier to detect by microscopic examination. Parasites do not form colonies on solid media in the same way as bacteria and fungi.

Viruses, chlamydia and rickettsia must be grown in cell or tissue cultures

This is because these organisms are incapable of a free-living existence. Most cell cultures used in the diagnostic laboratory are continuous cell lines – human or animal cells adapted to growth *in vitro* that can be stored at –80°C until required. The specimen is introduced into the cell culture

CONSTITUENTS OF BACTERIOLOGIC CULTURE MEDIA	
amino-nitrogen base (digested protein)	e.g. peptone
growth factors	e.g. blood, serum, yeast extract
energy source	e.g. sugars, carbohydrates
buffer salts	e.g. phosphate, citrate
mineral salts	e.g. calcium, magnesium, iron
selective agents	e.g. chemicals, dyes, antimicrobials
indicators	e.g. phenol red
gelling agent (for solid media)	e.g. agar

Fig. 14.17 Constituents of bacteriologic culture media. All culture media share a number of common constituents, which are necessary to enable bacteria to grow *in vitro*. Hundreds of different media have been described.

medium and the presence of viruses detected by observing the cells for a 'cytopathic effect' (CPE).

Cell culture techniques are specialized and labor intensive, and some viruses either cause no CPE (e.g. rubella) or cause a CPE that takes a week or more to evolve (e.g. cytomegalovirus (CMV), although CMV antigens can be detected after 1–2 days in cells). Therefore alternative methods such as antigen detection (see above) or antibody detection (see below) are used to diagnose viral infections whenever possible.

Identification of Microorganisms Grown in Culture

Identification tests should always be performed on single colonies or pure cultures

A colony or a pure culture is one that consists of only one type of microorganism and is derived from a single cell. Aseptic techniques must be used to isolate and maintain pure cultures of microorganisms (*Fig. 14.18*).

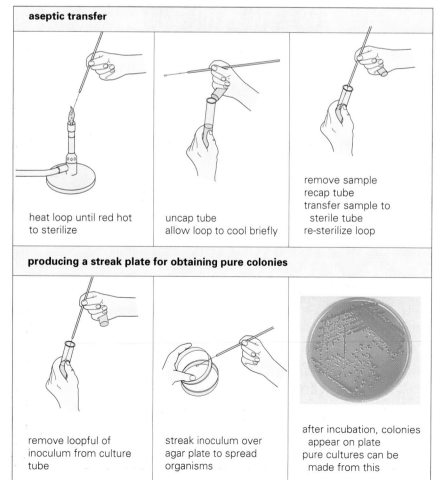

aseptic transfer

heat loop until red hot to sterilize

uncap tube
allow loop to cool briefly

remove sample
recap tube
transfer sample to
sterile tube
re-sterilize loop

producing a streak plate for obtaining pure colonies

remove loopful of
inoculum from culture
tube

streak inoculum over
agar plate to spread
organisms

after incubation, colonies
appear on plate
pure cultures can be
made from this

Fig. 14.18 Aseptic technique. As culture media provide excellent conditions for microbial growth, bacteria and fungi from the air and the environment that settle on the medium will grow and contaminate the cultures. It is vital to prevent this to ensure that the organisms growing in the cultures originate from the specimen. Therefore culture media are sterilized before use and handled with aseptic techniques. Likewise, aseptic techniques are an important part of patient care in operating theaters and wound dressing to prevent surgical wounds becoming contaminated (see Chapter 34).

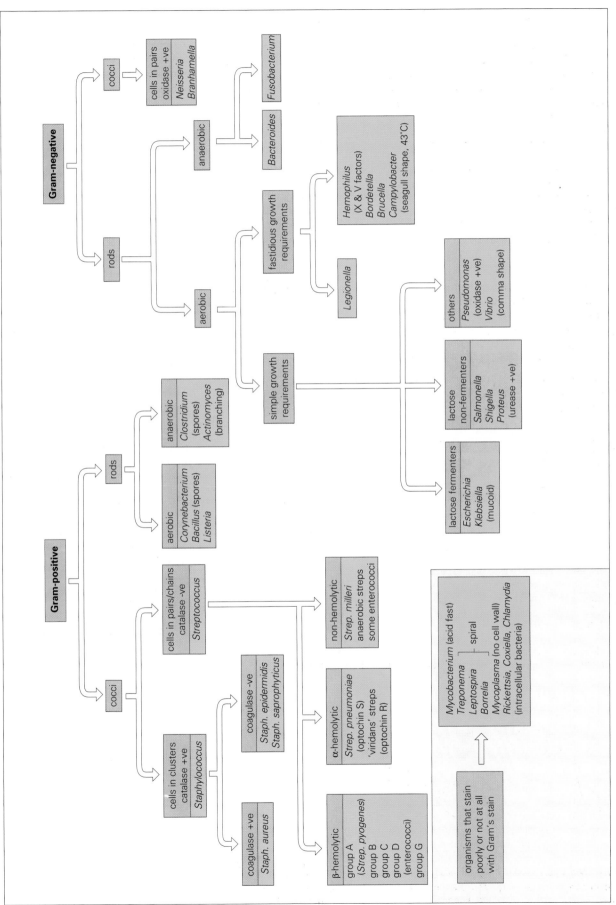

Fig. 14.19 Identifying bacteria. The preliminary investigation of the bacteria of medical importance can be made on the basis of a few key characteristics (see text). Further identification is made on the basis of biochemical and serologic tests.

Bacteria are identified by simple characteristics and biochemical properties

A preliminary identification of many of the bacteria of medical importance can be made on the basis of the following few simple characteristics of the cells (Fig. 14.19):

- Gram reaction.
- Cell morphology (e.g. rod or coccus) and arrangement (e.g. pairs or chains).
- Ability to grow under aerobic or anaerobic conditions.
- Growth requirements (simple or fastidious).

Further identification is made on the basis of biochemical properties such as:

- Ability to produce enzymes that can be detected by simple tests (e.g. coagulase, catalase, oxidase, lecithinase, *Fig. 14.20*).
- Ability to metabolize sugars oxidatively or fermentatively (e.g. the Hugh and Liefson oxidation/fermentation test, *Fig. 14.21*).
- Ability to use a range of substrates for growth (e.g. glucose, lactose, sucrose). These tests can be done individually (e.g.

in broth media containing the test sugar) or in commercial kits, which allow a range of different tests to be set up simultaneously on each organism (see *Fig. 34.17*).

Some species are identified on the basis of their antigens by reacting cell suspensions with specific antisera. The key tests for species of medical importance are given in the Appendix.

Antibiotic susceptibility can only be determined after the bacteria have been isolated in a pure culture

Bacterial antibiotic susceptibility can usually be tested by exposing a lawn of the test organism seeded on an agar plate to antibiotics contained in filter paper discs. During overnight incubation the organisms grow and multiply and the antibiotics diffuse out from the discs and inhibit growth around the disc. Therefore after isolation of bacteria from a specimen, a further overnight incubation period is required before antibiotic susceptibility results are available. Methods for antibiotic susceptibility tests are described in more detail in Chapter 30.

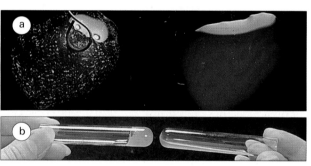

Fig. 14.20 Once bacteria have been isolated in pure cultures they can often be identified by their biochemical reactions. For example, the ability to produce certain enzymes can be easily demonstrated. The production of coagulase distinguishes *Staphylococcus aureus* from *Staph. epidermidis*. The slide test (a) demonstrates bound coagulase by its ability to cause staphylococcal cells to clump within a few seconds when mixed with plasma. The tube test (b) detects free coagulase by its ability to cause plasma to clot after incubation at 37°C for about four hours.

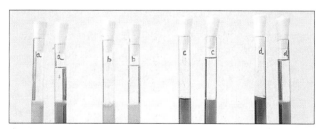

Fig. 14.21 Oxidation/fermentation test. The distinction between fermentative and non-fermentative bacteria is important in the identification of the Gram-negative rods. Some species can utilize sugars such as glucose and produce acid (shown by the indicator change from green to yellow) by both aerobic (oxidative) and anaerobic (fermentative) pathways (b). Others can only grow aerobically (a). Some species cannot metabolize glucose but break down the peptone (peptides) in the medium producing alkaline end-products as shown by the indicator turning blue (d). Other species are non-reactive in an oxidation/fermentation test and the green indicator remains unchanged (c).

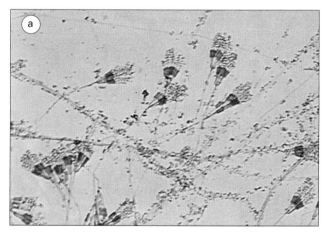

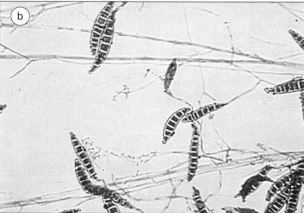

Fig. 14.22 Fungi under the microscope. Fungi can be grown on agar culture media in the same way as bacteria, but most species grow much more slowly than bacteria and it may take up to two weeks for a colony to form. Colonial characteristics (such as color) are helpful in the identification of fungi, but confirmation depends upon microscopic examination of the hyphae and sporing structures. (a) *Penicillium* in a wet preparation showing the conidiophores and free conidia. (b) Macroconidia of *Microsporum canis* stained with lactophenol cotton blue.

Fungi are identified by their colonial characteristics and cell morphology

Fungi are identified from colonies or pure cultures largely on the basis of colonial characteristics (e.g. color) and the morphology of the individual cells viewed under the microscope *(Fig. 14.22)*. Biochemical tests (substrate assimilation) can be used for detailed identification of yeasts of medical importance. In general, fungi grow more slowly than bacteria and final identification may take up to two weeks.

Protozoa and helminths are identified by direct examination

Many protozoa and parasites can be identified by direct examination of specimens without resort to culture and therefore the results can be obtained on the day of receipt of the specimen in the laboratory:

- Protozoa are identified on the basis of their morphologic characteristics – different stages of the life cycle may be visible in different specimens from the same patient and at different stages in the disease *(Fig. 14.23)*.
- Helminths are identified by the macroscopic appearance of the worm (e.g. *Ascaris* or *Enterobius*) or by microscopic examination of specimens (e.g. feces or urine) for eggs of, for example, schistosomes (see Chapter 20).

Viruses are usually identified using serologic tests

Viruses may be identifiable by their cytopathic effect in cell culture and their morphology in electron microscopic preparations *(Fig. 14.8)*, but diagnosis is more often made by detecting viral antigens or by testing for the presence of specific antibodies in the patient's serum (see below).

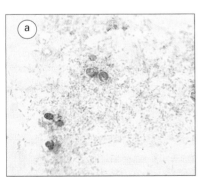

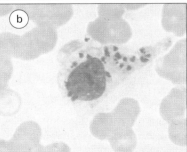

Fig. 14.23
Although some parasites can be cultivated in the laboratory, identification is usually based on microscopic appearances in the specimen. (a) Acid-fast stain of *Cryptosporidium* in feces. Like mycobacteria, this organism is able to retain the pink carbol fuchsin stain when challenged with acid alcohol. (b) *Leishmania donovani* (Donovan bodies) in a stained preparation from a specimen of bone marrow.

Antibody Detection Methods for the Diagnosis of Infection

Serologic tests (the study of antigen–antibody interactions) are used:
- To diagnose infections.
- To identify microorganisms (see above).
- To type blood for blood banks and tissues for transplantation.

Diagnoses based on detecting antibodies in patients' sera are retrospective

The major disadvantage of a diagnosis based on the detection of antibodies in a patient's serum is that it is retrospective as 2–4 weeks must elapse before IgG antibodies produced in response to the infection are detectable. What is more, a positive result indicates only that the patient has come into contact with the infection at some time in the past. IgM antibodies may be detected earlier in the infection (7–10 days) and are usually indicative of active, as opposed to past, infection. It is desirable to show that the patient has 'seroconverted' by demonstrating a fourfold or greater rise in antibody titer between sera collected in the acute and convalescent phases of the disease.

Antibody detection can be invaluable for identifying organisms that grow either slowly or with difficulty

Despite the drawbacks mentioned above, antibody detection is the main method for the laboratory diagnosis of viral infections. The techniques employed often allow several different infections to be screened for simultaneously (e.g. causes of atypical pneumonia, see Chapter 17). Sera should be collected during the acute phase of the disease and stored at –20°C until a convalescent phase serum is available; the two sera are then tested in parallel. Few diagnoses can be made with any confidence on the results of single serum samples, but sometimes early testing is justified if there is a clinical suspicion of a rare infection that the patient is unlikely to have encountered before (e.g. legionellosis). Previous immunization makes it difficult if not impossible to interpret some serologic tests because antibodies detected may be the result of immunization or infection (e.g. the Widal test for the serologic diagnosis of enteric fever, see Chapter 20).

Common serologic tests used in the laboratory to diagnose infection
Precipitation reactions are based on the precipitation of antigen–antibody aggregates

When antigen and antibody meet in solution at sufficiently high concentrations, their multivalency results in the formation of aggregates which usually precipitate. These precipitation reactions can be visualized more sensitively by allowing the antigen and antibody to diffuse towards each other through agar gels *(Fig. 14.24)*. Provided there is no immunochemical relationship (i.e. cross-reaction between the antigens), each antigen reacts with a corresponding set of antibodies present within the serum to form separate lines of precipitation in the gel. A practical example is the Elek test for the detection of diphtheria toxin from isolates of *Corynebacterium diphtheriae*.

antigen and antibody applied to holes punched in agar gel	leave to diffuse
	wash and stain
(a) precipitin band 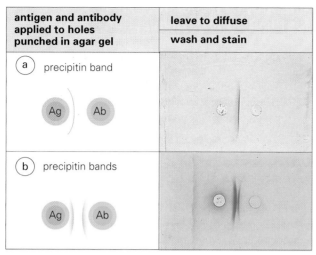	
(b) precipitin bands	

Fig. 14.24 Double diffusion and immunoprecipitation in agar gels. The opaque lines can be better visualized by staining. (a) Precipitin band formed with a single antigen. The two independent antigens in (b) give separate precipitation bands with their corresponding antibody sets (Abs), coexisting within the complex.

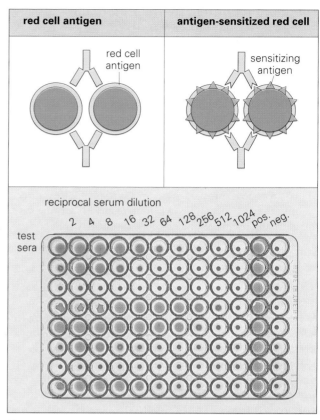

Fig. 14.25 The hemagglutination test for antibodies using red cells sensitized by antigen. Doubling dilutions of sera are made (horizontal row), with positive and negative controls in vertical rows 11 and 12 respectively. A tight button of cells indicates a negative reaction. Agglutinated cells form a carpet over the bottom of the well. A rapid microagglutination method is used for the detection of antibodies to *Legionella* in the patient's serum.

Hemagglutination can be used to detect antibodies against any antigen that can be linked to the surface of red cells

Antibodies directed against antigens on the surface of red cells cause cross-linking in such a way that when the cells are allowed to sediment in a microtiter agglutination tray, they form a mat on the bottom of the well rather than a tight button *(Fig. 14.25)*. This system can be used to detect antibodies against any antigen that can be linked, whether covalently or non-covalently, to the surface of the red cell or even to other particles such as latex. It can also be used to detect antigens (e.g. hepatitis B surface antigens) if specific antibody has been linked to the particle surface.

Antibodies can also mask viral molecules such as the influenza hemagglutinins, which are involved in specific adherence to cells allowing the development of a hemagglutination inhibition test *(Fig. 14.26)*.

Complement consumption can form the basis of a test for either antigen or antibody

Complement consumption can be used provided the immune complex is capable of activating the complement system. The complement fixation test (CFT) is carried out as shown in *Figure 14.27*. Serum to be tested for antibody is mixed with the known antigen. If antibodies are present, complexes will be formed, which will consume some or all of the complement subsequently added. The consumption of complement is measured by adding indicator red cells coated with a subagglutinating amount of erythrocyte antibody *(Fig. 14.27)*; any residual complement will lyse these indicator cells. Alternatively, with a standard antiserum the system can be used to look for antigen in a given sample.

ELISAs can be used to assay antibody in a given sample

These assays have been described previously. The amount of antibody binding to the solid phase antigen is a measure of the antibody content of the original sample, and can be detected by adding a second antibody conjugated with an enzyme (e.g. phosphatase or peroxidase) that produces a color reaction with a given substrate.

A variety of tests assess the ability of antibodies to inhibit microbial activity

A number of tests focus on the ability of antibodies in a patient's serum to inhibit some biologic faculty of the microorganism in question. An example is the anti-streptolysin O test, in which the streptolysin O toxin is neutralized by antibody. The extent to which the test serum can be diluted before it fails to prevent the toxin from lysing red cells provides a convenient titer *(Fig. 14.28)*. The ability of a patient's serum containing specific antibody to immobilize motile bacteria – for example the *Treponema pallidum* inhibition (TPI) test – is another example.

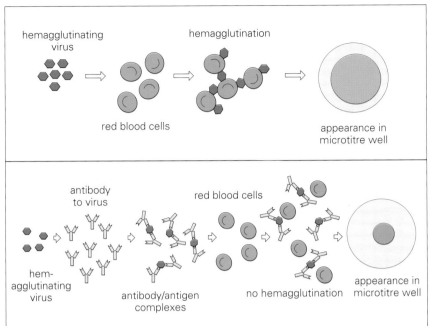

Fig. 14.26 Hemagglutination inhibition. Some viruses (e.g. influenza) have hemagglutinin molecules on their outer surface, and when virus particles are mixed with red blood cells they cause hemagglutination. In the presence of specific antibody, however, hemagglutination is inhibited. This test can therefore be used to detect the presence of antibodies to influenza virus in a patient's serum.

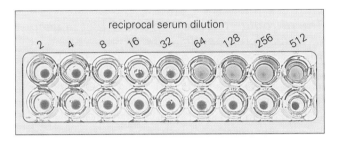

Fig. 14.27 Complement fixation tests (CFTs) are available for the serologic diagnosis of a range of infections. If antigen plus a source of complement (usually guinea pig serum) is added to a test serum, any antibodies present will bind the antigen and in most cases the complexes formed will 'fix' the complement, which is now unavailable to cause lysis of the antibody-coated red cells used as indicators. Therefore lysis of red cells is a negative reaction; no lysis is a positive test for antibodies. This figure shows a CFT for antibodies to *Coxiella burnetii* (a cause of atypical pneumonia). In the top row using dilutions of acute serum, complement has been fixed only in the first five wells (i.e. the antibody titer is 1/32), whereas with convalescent serum in the second row there is no lysis of the red blood cells at any dilution of serum and so the antibody titer is equal to or greater than 1/512. This demonstrates a fourfold rise in titer between acute and convalescent phase sera, indicating infection with *Coxiella burnetii*. CFTs are rather cumbersome and there is a tendency to replace them with other more modern tests such as enzyme-linked immunosorbent assays (ELISAs).

Antibodies to cytopathic viruses can be detected by the ability of the patient's serum to prevent virus infectivity

In the case of cytopathic viruses, antibodies can be detected by the ability of the patient's serum to prevent the development of a cytopathic effect. These antibodies are called neutralizing antibodies. The important applications of these methods are referred to in the appropriate systems chapters (see Chapters 15–28).

Assessment of Host Defense Systems

Innate immunity
Serum complement is assayed by lysis of antibody-sensitized red cells

The overall biologic activity of complement in serum can be assayed by its ability to lyse antibody-sensitized red cells through activation of the classical pathway and insertion of the terminal cytolytic complement components *(Fig.14.29)*. The relative hemolytic activity of a number of

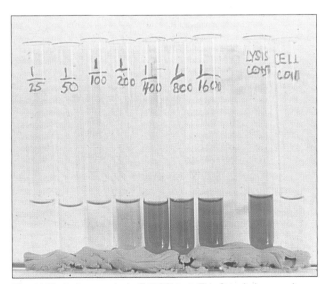

Fig. 14.28 Anti-streptolysin O (ASO) test. The O-toxin lyses red cells and test serum is diluted until it no longer inhibits lysis by a standard concentration of toxin. Positive and negative controls are included in the test (right).

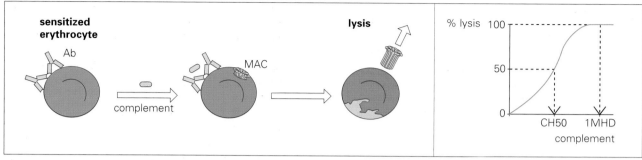

Fig. 14.29 The lysis of red cells sensitized by antibody (left) is used to assay the hemolytic complement activity of a serum sample. The curve (right) shows the lysis of antibody-sensitized red cells with increasing amounts of complement. Because of the sigmoid shape of the curve, the minimum hemolytic dose (MHD) cannot be measured as accurately as the amount giving 50% hemolysis (CH50) so the latter is preferred as a unit. (MAC, membrane attack complex.)

different serum samples can be assessed simultaneously by placing the sample in a well punched into agar gel that contains a suspension of antibody-coated red cells; the size of the clear plaque in the agar surrounding the well is a reflection of the overall lytic complement activity in that sample.

The opsonic activity and activities of individual components of complement can also be assessed

Additionally, it is sometimes of value to assess the opsonic activity of complement in the serum sample by looking at its ability to facilitate the uptake of a microbial particle by a phagocytic cell (Fig. `14.30).

The activities of individual components of the complement system can be evaluated either by:
- Their ability to be titrated into a complement-dependent lytic system in which the component to be tested is lacking.
- Direct immunochemical measurement, often using gel precipitation reactions.

The nitroblue tetrazolium (NBT) test is used to assess phagocytic activity

The ability of neutrophils to become phagocytic and to concurrently reduce molecular oxygen can be assayed by the nitroblue tetrazolium (NBT) test. When yellow NBT dye is added to blood, it forms complexes with heparin or fibrinogen in the sample. These complexes are then phagocytosed by neutrophils that have been activated by the addition of exogenous endotoxin. The dye complex is taken into the stimulated neutrophils and substitutes for oxygen by acting as a substrate for the reduction process, forming as a result a blue insoluble formazan.

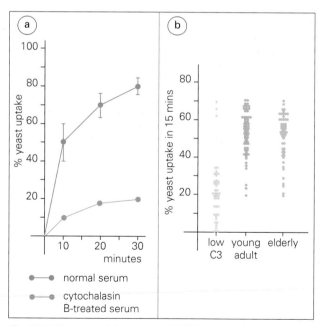

Fig. 14.30 Opsonic activity of serum. (a) Time course for the uptake of yeast opsonized with the same normal serum by polymorphonuclear neutrophil leukocytes (PMNs) from 12 healthy donors, and uptake of yeast by PMNs from one donor after treatment with cytochalasin B (40 mg/ml), which inhibits phagocytosis. (b) The distribution of opsonic activity for 150 sera from young healthy, elderly and pathologic sera. (Redrawn from Kerr et al. 1983.)

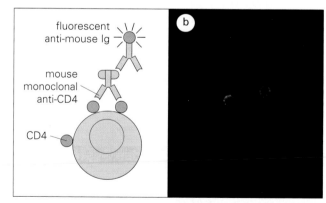

Fig. 14.31 Visualization of lymphocyte surface differentiation molecules by immunofluorescence. (a) The double antibody test using mouse monclonal antibodies to the required surface molecule. (b) Direct demonstration of antibody receptors on the surface of two B lymphocytes by fluorescent anti-immunoglobulin. Aggregation and capping of the surface receptors by the anti-immunoglobulin reagent is evident.

Lymphocytes

Lymphocytes are counted and classified by detecting their cell surface molecules

Lymphocyte differentiation is accompanied by the expression of related molecules on the cell surface. Detection of these molecules by immunofluorescent techniques allows their enumeration and, in addition, their classification into different subpopulations (*Fig. 14.31*). Monoclonal antibodies are widely used to define these differentiation molecules, and increasing use is being made of the technique of flow cytofluorimetry (*Fig. 14.32*), which is a more rapid and less laborious means of analyzing lymphocyte subpopulations than conventional fluorescent microscopy.

The development of T effector cells to an antigen can often be revealed by intradermal challenge with that antigen

Such an intradermal challenge usually gives rise to erythema and induration, peaking at around 48 hours (*Fig. 14.33*).

This time course has led to the reaction being described as 'delayed-type hypersensitivity'.

Overall responsiveness of the T cell population can be probed by using materials such as phytohemagglutinin or concanavalin A, which are polyclonal stimulators in the sense that they activate T cell populations independently of their precise antigen specificity. However, when peripheral blood cells are incubated with antigen *in vitro*, the specifically sensitized T cells, which represent only a very small fraction of the total, become activated and divide. Examination of the cultures will reveal blast cells and mitotic divisions, but the most convenient way of assessing the response is by the incorporation of radiolabeled thymidine, which provides a measure of cell proliferation (*Fig. 14.34*).

Cytokines can now be studied in great detail

Stimulated T cells also release cytokines. Originally, cytokines were recognized by their activity within a biologic assay, with specificity being confirmed by abrogation of activity with a

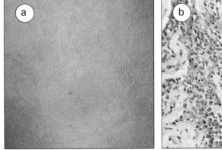
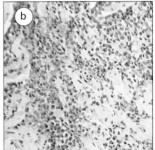

Fig. 14.32 Flow cytofluorimetry. Cells in the sample are stained with specific fluorescent reagents to detect surface molecules and then stream one at a time past a laser. Each cell is measured for size (forward light scatter) and granularity (90° light scatter), as well as for red and green fluorescence, to detect two different surface markers. The three-dimensional plots show a whole lymphocyte population (left) and a CD8+ population obtained by cell sorting (right), stained with anti-CD8.

Fig. 14.33 Tuberculin-type delayed sensitivity. The dermal response to antigens of leprosy bacillus in a sensitive subject (the Fernandez reaction) is characterized by (a) red induration maximal at 48–72 hours and (b) dense infiltration of the injection site with lymphocytes and macrophages. (Hematoxylin and eosin, × 80)

Fig. 14.34 Lymphocyte stimulation assessed by incorporation of radioactive thymidine. A high count indicates that lymphocytes have proliferated and confirms their sensitivity to the antigen.

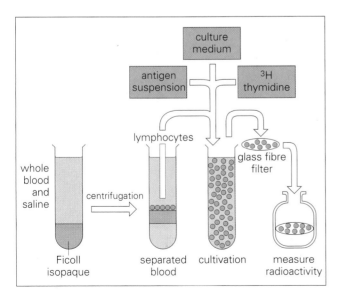

specific antibody. However, with the advent of cloned cytokines and monoclonal antibodies directed against them, there is a strong move towards immunoassay of the individual cytokines and cytokine receptors.

The ability of cytotoxic T cells to attack targets is conventionally assayed using a radioisotope

Cytotoxic T cells attack targets such as virally infected cells and this ability is conventionally assayed by prelabeling the target with a radioisotope such as ^{51}Cr, and then looking for release of the isotope into the supernatant from damaged cells *(Fig. 14.35)*.

Protocols for Specimen Processing

There are basic protocols used in the diagnostic laboratory for processing specimens of:
- Urine.
- Feces.

- Genital tract specimens.
- Skin and soft tissue specimens.
- Eye swabs.
- Respiratory tract specimens including nose, throat and ear swabs, and sputum.
- CSF.
- Pus.
- Other fluids such as pleural and pericardial fluids and joint aspirates.
- Blood.
- Bone marrow and other biopsy specimens.
- Autopsy and forensic specimens.
   These are detailed in the Appendix.

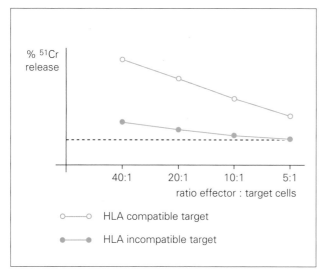

Fig. 14.35 Measurement of cytotoxic activity of human lymphocytes against influenza-infected target cells. Only those targets that share human leukocyte antigens (HLA) haplotype with the cytotoxic cell donor are attacked (haplotype restriction) with consequent release of ^{51}Cr. The dotted line indicates background release of isotype from target cells incubated in the absence of effector cells.

- In this chapter, we have outlined the techniques used for the laboratory diagnosis of infections.
- For many years confirmation of a clinical diagnosis of a bacterial or fungal infection has been based largely on isolating the pathogen from the patient's specimens. This allows complete identification of the organism and tests for susceptibility to antimicrobial agents.
- As cultural methods are time consuming and labor intensive, and are unavailable or hazardous for some organisms, serologic methods are also important.
- The application of molecular techniques to diagnostic microbiology has the potential of increasing the sensitivity, specificity and speed of laboratory diagnosis, but it will be a few years before the techniques will be sufficiently versatile to allow a hunt for all 'unknown' organisms in patients' specimens.

Further Reading

Collins CH, Lyne PM, Grange JM. *Microbiological Methods,* 6th edition. Oxford: Butterworths, 1989.

Hayden JD, Ho SA, Hawkey PM, Taylor GR, Quirke P. The promises and pitfalls of PCR. *Rev Med Microbiol* 1991;**2**:129–137.

Kerr MA, Falconer JS, Bashey A, Swanson Beck J, *et al*. The effect of C3 levels on yeast opsonization by normal and pathological sera; identification of a complement-dependent opsonin. *Clin Exp Immunol* 1983;**54**:793–800.

Lennette EH, Balows A, Hausler WJ, Shadomy J eds. *Manual of Clinical Microbiology*, 5th edition. Washington: American Society for Microbiology, 1990.

Sheehan C. *Clinical Immunology: Principles and Laboratory Diagnosis.* Philadelphia: JB Lippincott, 1990.

4

clinical manifestations and diagnosis of infections by body system

Introduction to Section 4
The Clinical Manifestations of Infection

As there are at least 150 different infectious diseases to describe, a system of classification is essential. In Chapters 15–23, infections are classified according to the body system primarily involved at the clinical level. For example, rhinoviruses specifically cause infection of the upper respiratory tract, and bacillary or amebic dysentery are gastrointestinal tract infections. Other infections characteristically cause damage predominantly to one part of the body, although other parts may be affected. Thus, tuberculosis is considered in Chapter 17 (lower respiratory tract infections) and typhoid in Chapter 20 (gastrointestinal tract infections), these being the sites primarily affected. Again, when microbes are transmitted as a result of certain states or activities, they can be grouped together with others acquired in the same way, even though more than one system may be involved. Hence syphilis and AIDS are dealt with in Chapter 19 (sexually transmitted diseases) and rubella in Chapter 21 (obstetric and perinatal infections).

The systems approach is useful because it includes infections caused by a wide variety of microbes on the basis of the clinical syndrome produced. As with any system of classification, however, there are gray areas and overlaps. Referral to the Appendix where definitive accounts of the most important infectious organisms are given, will help clarify any ambiguities.

Chapters 24–28 deal with those infections that cannot be readily pigeon-holed into systems. These include multisystem infections (i.e. infections that are not obviously localized to any one system of the body). Some of these are virus infections that occur worldwide and are exclusively human (e.g. measles, herpes simplex, Epstein–Barr virus infections; see Chapter 24). However, many multisystem infections are also multihost in that they can be transmitted:

- From person to person by an intermediate vector (usually an arthropod), their distribution depending upon climate, ecology, and the presence of adequate numbers of the required arthropod (see Chapter 25).
- Directly to humans from other vertebrates, in which case they are known as 'zoonoses' (see Chapter 26), with distributions ranging from highly restricted (Rocky Mountain spotted fever, Lassa fever) to widespread (Q fever, leptospirosis).

Finally there are two further disease groupings, founded on clinical presentation:

- Those presenting as 'pyrexias of unknown origin' (see Chapter 27).
- Those seen in the compromised host (see Chapter 28).

The latter category has become increasingly important because of the large number of patients whose defenses are impaired as a result of disease (cystic fibrosis, diabetes mellitus), infection (AIDS), immunosuppressive therapy (transplant patients) or other causes (e.g. burns, catheters).

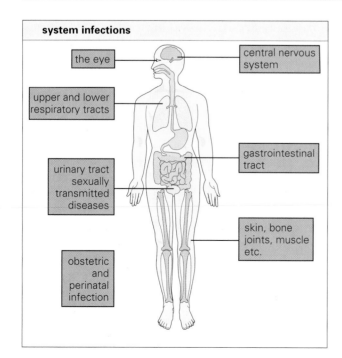

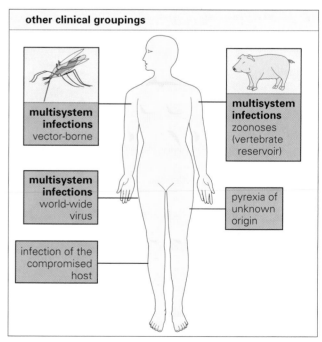

Introduction

The mucociliary system and the flushing action of saliva are defenses against upper respiratory tract infection

The air we inhale contains millions of suspended particles, including microorganisms. Nearly all these microorganisms are harmless, except in the vicinity of infected individuals where the air may contain large numbers of pathogenic microorganisms. Efficient cleansing mechanisms (see Chapters 4 and 8) are therefore vital components of the body's defense against infection of both the upper and lower respiratory tract. Infection takes place against the background of these natural defense mechanisms, and it is then appropriate to ask why the defenses have failed. For the upper respiratory tract, the mucociliary system is important in the nasopharynx and the flushing action of saliva in the oropharynx.

As on other surfaces of the body (see Chapter 2), a variety of microorganisms live harmlessly in the upper respiratory tract and oropharynx *(Fig. 15.1)*; they colonize the nose, mouth, throat and teeth and are well adapted to life in these sites. Normally they are well-behaved guests, not invading tissues and not causing disease. However, as in other parts of the body, resident microorganisms can cause trouble when host resistance is weakened.

The upper and lower respiratory tracts form a continuum for infectious agents

We distinguish between upper and lower respiratory tract infections, but the respiratory tract from the nose to the alveoli is a continuum as far as infectious agents are concerned *(Fig. 15.2)*. There may, however, be a preferred 'focus' of infection (e.g. nasopharynx for coronaviruses and rhinoviruses), but parainfluenza viruses, for instance, can infect the nasopharynx to give rise to a cold as well as the larynx and trachea (croup or laryngotracheitis), and occasionally the bronchi and bronchioles (bronchitis, bronchiolitis or pneumonia).

Two useful generalizations can be made about upper and lower respiratory tract infections

These are that:

- Many microorganisms are restricted to the surface epithelium, but others spread to other parts of the body, before returning to the respiratory tract, oropharynx, salivary glands *(Fig. 15.3)*.
- Two groups of microbes can be distinguished: 'professional' and 'secondary' invaders.

Professional invaders are those that successfully infect the normally healthy respiratory tract *(Fig. 15.4)*. They generally possess specific properties that enable them to evade local host defenses, such as the attachment mechanisms of respiratory viruses *(Fig. 15.5)* and the other devices shown in *Figure 15.4*. Secondary invaders only cause disease when host defenses are already impaired *(Fig. 15.4)*.

The Common Cold

Rhinoviruses and coronaviruses together cause more than 50% of colds

Viruses are the commonest invaders of the nasopharynx and a great variety of types *(Fig. 15.5)* are responsible for the

NORMAL FLORA OF THE RESPIRATORY TRACT	
type of resident*	**microorganism**
common residents (>50% of normal people)	oral streptococci *Neisseria* spp., *Branhamella* corynebacteria *Bacteroides* anaerobic cocci (*Veillonella*) fusiform bacteria** *Candida albicans*** *Streptococcus mutans* *Hemophilus influenzae*
occasional residents (<10% normal people)	*Streptococcus pyogenes* *Streptococcus pneumoniae* *Neisseria meningitidis*
uncommon residents (<1% normal people)	*Corynebacterium diphtheriae* *Klebsiella pneumoniae* *Pseudomonas* ⎤ especially after *Escherichia coli* ⊢ antibiotic *C. albicans* ⎦ treatment
residents in latent state in tissues:*** lung lymph nodes etc. sensory neurone/glands connected to mucosae	*Pneumocystis carinii*, *Mycobacterium tuberculosis*, Cytomegalovirus (CMV) herpes simplex virus Epstein-Barr virus

  * all except tissue residents are present in the oronasopharynx or on teeth
  ** present in mouth; also *Entamoeba gingivalis*, *Trichomonas tenax*, micrococci, *Actinomyces* spp.
  *** all except *M. tuberculosis* are present in most humans

Fig. 15.1 The normal flora of the respiratory tract.

common cold. They induce a flow of virus-rich fluid from the nasopharynx, and when the sneezing reflex is triggered, large

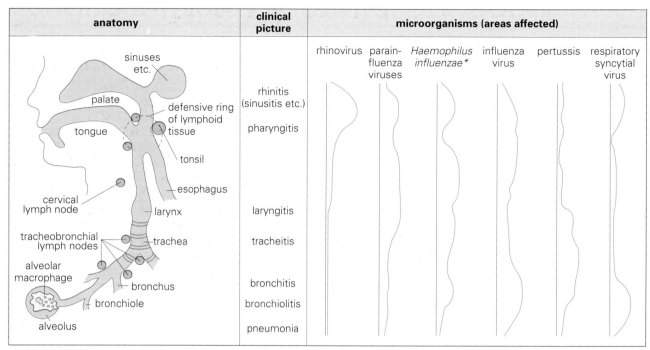

Fig. 15.2 The respiratory tract as a continuum. (*Asymptomatic nasopharyngeal colonization is common.)

TWO TYPES OF RESPIRATORY INFECTION		
type	**examples**	**consequences**
restricted to surface	common cold viruses influenza streptococci in throat chlamydia (conjunctivitis) diphtheria pertussis *Candida albicans* (thrush)	local spread local (mucosal) defenses important adaptive (immune) response sometimes too late to be important in recovery short incubation period (days)

spread through body	measles, mumps, rubella
	EBV, CMV
	Chlamydia psittaci
	Q fever
	cryptococcosis
		little or no lesion at entry site
		microbe spreads through body, returns to surface for
		  final multiplication and shedding e.g. salivary gland
		  (mumps, CMV, EBV), respiratory tract (measles)
		adaptive immune response important in recovery
		longer incubation period (weeks)

Fig. 15.3 After entry via the respiratory tract, microbes either stay on the surface epithelium or spread through the body. (CMV, cytomegalovirus; EBV, Epstein–Barr virus.)

numbers of virus particles are discharged into the air. Transmission is therefore by aerosol and also by virus-contaminated hands (see Chapter 8). Most of these viruses possess surface molecules that bind them firmly to host cells or to cilia or microvilli protruding from these cells. As a result, they are not washed away in secretions and are able to initiate infection in the normally healthy individual. Virus progeny from the first infected cell then spread to neighboring cells and via surface secretions to new sites on the mucosal surface. After a few days, damage to epithelial cells and the secretion of fluid containing inflammatory mediators such as bradykinin lead to common cold-type symptoms (*Fig. 15.6*).

RESPIRATORY INVADERS – PROFESSIONAL OR SECONDARY

type	requirement	examples
professional invaders (infect healthy respiratory tract)	adhesion to normal mucosa (in spite of mucociliary system)	respiratory viruses (influenza, rhinoviruses) *Streptococcus pyogenes (throat)* *Strep. pneumoniae* *Mycoplasma pneumoniae* chlamydia (psittacosis, chlamydial conjunctivitis and pneumonia, trachoma)
	ability to interfere with cilia	*Bordetella pertussis, M. pneumoniae* *Strep. pneumoniae* (pneumolysin)
	ability to resist destruction in alveolar macrophage	*Legionella, Mycobacterium tuberculosis*
	ability to damage local (mucosal, submucosal) tissues	*Corynebacterium diphtheriae* (toxin) *Strep. pneumoniae* (pneumolysin)
secondary invaders (infect when host defenses impaired)	initial infection and damage by respiratory virus (e.g. influenza virus)	*Staphylococcus aureus; Strep. pneumoniae* pneumonia complicating influenza
	local defenses impaired (e.g. cystic fibrosis)	*Staph. aureus, Pseudomonas*
	chronic bronchitis local foreign body or tumor	*Hemophilus. influenzae, Strep. pneumoniae*
	depressed immune responses (e.g. AIDS, neoplastic disease)	*Pneumocystis carinii*, cytomegalovirus, *M. tuberculosis*
	depressed resistance (e.g. elderly, alcoholism, renal or hepatic disease)	*Strep. pneumoniae, Staph. aureus, H. influenzae*

Fig. 15.4 The two types of respiratory invader.

VIRUSES CAUSING COMMON COLDS

virus	types involved	attachment mechanism	disease
rhinoviruses (>100 types)*	several at any given time in the community	capsid protein binds to ICAM-1 type molecule on cell**	common cold
coxsackie virus A (24 types)	especially A21	capsid protein binds to ICAM-1 type molecule on cell**	common cold; also oropharyngeal vesicles (herpangina) and hand, foot and mouth disease (A16)
influenza viruses	several	hemagglutinin binds to neuraminic acid-containing glycoprotein on cell	may also invade lower respiratory tract
parainfluenza virus (4 types)	1,2,3,4	viral envelope protein binds to glycoside on cell	may also invade larynx
respiratory syncytial virus	(1 type)	—	may also invade lower respiratory tract
coronaviruses (several types)	all	viral envelope protein binds to glycoprotein receptors on cell	common cold
adenovirus (41 types)	5–10 types	penton fiber binds to cell receptor	mainly pharyngitis; also conjunctivitis, bronchitis
echoviruses (34 types)	11, 20	—	common cold

* a given type shows little or no neutralization by antibody against other types
** ICAM-1: intercellular adhesion molecule expressed on a wide variety of normal cells; member of immunoglobulin superfamily, coded on chromosome 19

Fig. 15.5 Common cold viruses and their mechanisms of attachment.

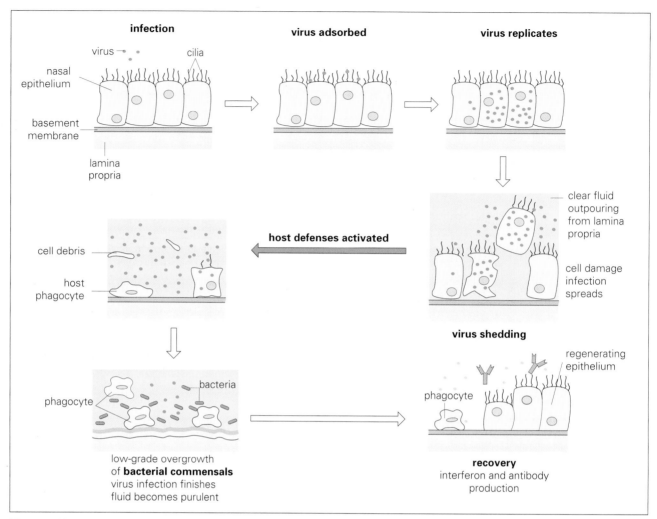

Fig. 15.6 The pathogenesis of the common cold. For simplification, the epithelium is represented as one cell thick.

Common cold virus infections are diagnosed by clinical appearance

In view of the large variety of viruses and because common colds are generally mild and self-limiting with no systemic spread, laboratory tests are not worthwhile. Diagnosis becomes important when the lower respiratory tract is involved, as for instance with influenza viruses or in children with respiratory syncytial virus (RSV) infection. The antigens of these viruses can be detected in exfoliated cells in the nasopharyngeal aspirates from children (see *Fig. 17.4*), and a rise in virus-specific antibodies will confirm the diagnosis, which is generally retrospective. Virus isolation is tedious and can be difficult, but is usually carried out for public health purposes by central laboratories when, for instance, there is a new pandemic strain of influenza virus.

Treatment of the common cold is symptomatic

It is often said that a common cold will resolve in 48 hours if vigorous treatment with anticongestants, analgesics and antibiotics is undertaken, while untreated it will take two days!

There are no worthwhile vaccines for the common cold viruses and treatment is for the most part symptomatic. There are, however, vaccines for influenza virus.

Pharyngitis and Tonsillitis

About 70% of acute sore throats are caused by viruses

Microorganisms that cause acute pharyngitis are listed in *Figure 15.7*. Common cold and other upper respiratory tract viruses inevitably encounter the submucosal lymphoid tissues that form a defensive ring around the oropharynx (*Fig. 15.2*). The throat becomes sore (pharyngitis) either because the overlying mucosa is infected or because of inflammatory and immune responses in the lymphoid tissues themselves. Adenoviruses are common causes, often infecting the conjunctiva as well as the pharynx to cause pharyngoconjunctival fever. Epstein–Barr virus (EBV) multiplies locally in the pharynx to produce a characteristic type of sore throat (*Fig. 15.8*), while herpes simplex virus (HSV) and certain coxsackie A

CAUSE OF ACUTE PHARYNGITIS		
organisms	examples	comments
viruses	rhinoviruses, coronaviruses	a mild symptom in the common cold
	adenoviruses (types 3, 4, 7, 14, 21)	pharyngoconjunctival fever
	parainfluenza viruses	more severe than common cold
	influenza viruses	not always present
	coxsackie A and other enteroviruses	small vesicles (herpangina)
	Epstein–Barr virus	occurs in 70–90% of glandular fever patients
	herpes simplex virus type 1	can be severe, with palatal vesicles or ulcers
bacteria	*Streptococcus pyogenes*	causes 10–20% of cases of acute pharyngitis; sudden onset; mostly in 5–10-year-old children
	Neisseria gonorrhoeae	often asymptomatic; usually via orogenital contact
	Corynebacterium diphtheriae	pharyngitis often mild, but toxic illness can be severe
	Haemophilius influenzae	epiglottitis
	Borrelia vincenti plus fusiform bacilli	Vincent's angina; commonest in adolescents and adults

Fig. 15.7 Microorganisms that cause acute pharyngitis.

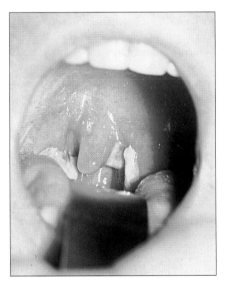

Fig. 15.8 Infectious mononucleosis caused by Epstein–Barr virus. The tonsils and uvula are swollen and covered in white exudate. There are petechiae on the soft palate. (Courtesy of JA Innes.)

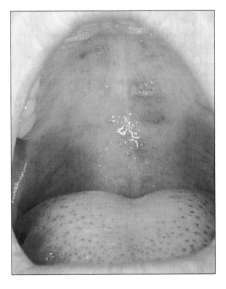

Fig. 15.9 Ulcers on the hard palate and tongue in hand, foot and mouth disease due to coxsackie A virus. (Courtesy of JA Innes.)

viruses multiply in the oral mucosa to produce a painful local lesion or ulcer. Certain enteroviruses (e.g. coxsackie A16) can cause additional vesicles on the hands and feet and in the mouth (hand, foot and mouth disease, *Fig. 15.9*).

Bacteria responsible for pharyngitis include:
- *Strep. pyogenes* (group A β-hemolytic, *Fig. 15.10*), the commonest and most important to diagnose because it can lead to complications (see below), but can be readily treated with penicillin.
- *Corynebacterium diphtheriae* (see page 15)
- *Haemophilius influenzae* (type B), which occasionally causes severe epiglottitis with obstruction of the airways, especially in young children.

- *Borrelia vincenti* together with certain fusiform bacilli, which can cause throat or gingival ulcers.
- *Neisseria gonorrhoeae*.

Each of these bacteria attach to the mucosal surface, sometimes invading local tissues.

Generally a laboratory diagnosis is not necessary for pharyngitis and tonsillitis

There are many possible viral causes of pharyngitis and tonsillitis and, generally, the clinical condition is not serious enough to seek laboratory help. EBV infection is diagnosed by the presence of lymphocytosis, atypical lymphocytes, and heterophil antibodies (detected by the Paul–Bunnell test). HSV is readily

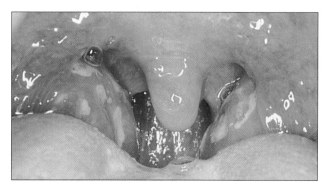

Fig. 15.10 Streptococcal tonsillitis due to group A β-hemolytic *Streptococcus pyogenes* with intense erythema of the tonsils and a creamy-yellow exudate. (Courtesy of JA Innes.)

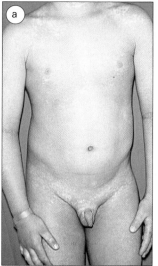
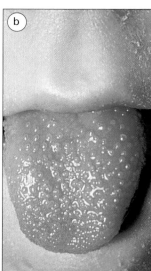

Fig. 15.11 Scarlet fever. (a) Punctate erythema is followed by peeling for 2–3 weeks. (b) The tongue is furred at first and then becomes raw with prominent papillae. (Courtesy of WE Farrar.)

isolated in the laboratory, but clinical diagnosis is usually adequate. Bacteria are identified by culturing throat swabs (see Chapter 14). It is especially important to diagnose *Strep. pyogenes* infection because of the possible complications (see below), and because, unlike *Strep. pneumoniae*, it remains susceptible to penicillin. Resistance to erythromycin and tetracycline, however, is increasing. Although during the winter months up to 16% of schoolchildren carry group A streptococci in the throat without symptoms, treatment is recommended.

Complications of Strep pyogenes throat infection include quinsy, scarlet fever, rheumatic fever, rheumatic heart disease and glomerulonephritis

These complications are important enough to be listed separately, although most are uncommon in developed countries where there is good access to medical care and probably less exposure to streptococci. The complications include:

- Peritonsillar abscess ('quinsy'), an uncommon complication of untreated streptococcal sore throat.
- Otitis media, sinusitis, mastoiditis (see below), caused by local spread of *Strep. pyogenes.*
- Scarlet fever. Certain strains of *Strep. pyogenes* produce an erythrogenic toxin coded for by a lysogenic phage. The toxin spreads through the body and localizes in the skin to induce a punctate erythematous rash (scarlet fever; *Fig. 15.11*). The tongue is initially furred, but later red. The rash begins as facial erythema and then spreads to involve most of the body except the palms and soles. The face is generally flushed with circumoral pallor. The rash fades over the course of a week and is followed by extensive desquamation. The skin lesions themselves are not serious, but they signal infection by a potentially harmful streptococcus, which in pre-antibiotic days could sometimes spread through the body to cause cellulitis and septicemia.
- Rheumatic fever. This is an indirect complication. Antibodies formed to antigens in the streptococcal cell wall cross-react with the sarcolemma of human heart, and with tissues elsewhere. Granulomas are formed in the heart (Aschoff's nodules) and 2–4 weeks after the sore throat the patient (usually a child) develops myocarditis or pericarditis, which may be associated with subcutaneous

nodules, polyarthritis and, rarely, chorea. Chorea is a disease of the central nervous system resulting from anti-streptococcal antibodies reacting with neurones.
- Rheumatic heart disease. Repeated attacks of *Strep. pyogenes* with different M types (see Appendix) can lead to damage to the heart valves. Certain children have a genetic predisposition to this immune-mediated disease. If a primary attack is accompanied by rising or high antistreptolysin O (ASO) antibody levels (see Appendix), future attacks must be prevented by penicillin prophylaxis throughout childhood. In many developing countries, rheumatic heart disease is the commonest type of heart disease.
- Acute glomerulonephritis. Antibodies to streptococcal components combine with these components to form circulating immune complexes, which are then deposited in glomeruli. Here, the complement and coagulation systems are activated, resulting in local inflammation. Blood appears in the urine (red cells, protein) and there are signs of an acute nephritis syndrome (edema, hypertension) 1–2 weeks after the sore throat. ASO antibodies are usually elevated. Only four to five of the 65 M types of Strep. pyogenes give rise to this condition and repeated infection with different 'nephritogenic' types is unlikely. Penicillin prophylaxis is therefore is not given. In contrast to rheumatic fever, second attacks are rare.

Otitis and Sinusitis

Otitis and sinusitis can be caused by many viruses and a range of secondary bacterial invaders

Many viruses are capable of invading the air spaces associated with the upper respiratory tract (sinuses, middle ear, mastoid). Mumps virus or RSV for instance, can cause vestibulitis or deafness, which is generally temporary. The range of secondary bacterial invaders is the same as for other upper respiratory tract infections, that is *Strep. pneumoniae* and *H. influenzae* and sometimes anaerobes such as *Bacteroides fragilis*. Brain abscess is a major complication (see Chapter 22). Blockage of the eustachian (auditory) tube or the opening of sinuses due to allergic swelling of the mucosa prevents mucociliary clearance of infection and the local accumulation of inflammatory bacterial products causes further swelling and blockage.

Acute otitis media
Common causes of acute otitis media are viruses, Strep. pneumoniae and H. influenzae
This condition is extremely common in infants and small children, partly because the eustachian (auditory) tube is open more widely at this age. A study in Boston showed that 83% of three year olds had had at least one episode, and 46% had had three or more episodes since birth. At least 50% of the attacks are viral in origin and the bacterial invaders are nasopharyngeal residents, most commonly *Strep. pneumoniae* or *H. influenzae*, and sometimes *Strep. pyogenes* or *Staph. aureus*. There may be general symptoms, and acute otitis media should be considered in any child with unexplained fever, diarrhea or vomiting. The ear drum shows dilated vessels with bulging of the drum at a later stage *(Fig. 15.12)*. Fluid often persists in the middle ear for weeks or months ('glue ear') regardless of therapy, and contributes to impaired hearing and learning difficulties in infants and small children.

If acute attacks are inadequately treated there may be continued infection with a chronic discharge through a perforated drum and impaired hearing. This is 'chronic suppurative otitis media'.

Otitis externa
Causes of otitis externa are Staph. aureus, Candida albicans and Gram-negative opportunists
Infections of the outer ear can cause irritation and pain, and must be distinguished from otitis media. In contrast to the middle ear, the external canal has a bacterial flora similar to that of the skin (staphylococci, corynebacteria and, to a lesser extent, propionibacteria), and the pathogens responsible for otitis media are rarely found in otitis externa. The warm moist environment favors *Staph. aureus*, *Candida albicans* and Gram-negative opportunists such as *Proteus* and *Pseudomonas aeruginosa*.

Ear drops containing polymyxin or other antibiotics are usually an effective treatment.

Acute sinusitis
The etiology and pathogenesis of acute sinusitis are similar to those of otitis media. Clinical features include facial pain and localized tenderness. It may be possible to identify the causative bacteria by microscopy and culture of pus aspirated from the sinus, but sinus puncture is not often carried out. In addition, as is the case for otitis media, the patient can be treated empirically with ampicillin or amoxycillin, or with the newer oral cephalosporins (e.g. cefixime) to deal with beta-lactamase-producing organisms.

Acute Epiglottitis

Acute epiglottitis is generally due to H. influenzae capsular type B infection
Acute epiglottitis is most often seen in young children. For unknown reasons, *H. influenzae* capsular type B spreads from the nasopharynx to the epiglottis, causing severe inflammation and edema. There is usually a bacteremia.

Acute epiglottitis is an emergency and necessitates intubation and treatment with antibiotics
Acute epiglottitis is characterized by difficulty breathing because of respiratory obstruction and, until the airway has been secured (intubation), extreme care must be taken when examining the throat in case the swollen epiglottis is sucked into the edematous airway and causes total obstruction. Treatment is begun immediately with antibiotics effective against *H. influenzae* (cefotaxime, chloramphenicol). The clinical diagnosis is confirmed by isolating bacteria from the blood and possibly the epiglottis. The *H. influenzae* type B (Hib) vaccine is likely to greatly reduce the frequency of this and other infections due to *H influenzae* type B.

Respiratory obstruction due to diphtheria (see below) is rare in developed countries, but the characteristic false membrane and local swelling can extend from the pharynx to involve the uvula.

Oral Cavity Infections

Saliva flushes the mouth and contains a variety of antibacterial substances
The oral cavity is continuous with the pharynx, but is dealt with separately because of the presence of teeth, which are subject to a particular set of microbiological problems. The normal mouth contains commensal microorganisms, some of which are, to a large extent restricted to the mouth *(Fig. 15.1)*. Most of them make specific attachments to teeth or mucosal surfaces and are shed into the saliva as they multiply. The liter or so of saliva secreted each day mechanically flushes the mouth. It also contains secretory antibodies, polymorphs, desquamated

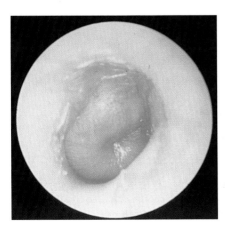

Fig. 15.12 Acute otitis media with bulging ear drum. (Courtesy of M Chaput de Saintonge.)

mucosal cells and antibacterial substances such as lysozyme and lactoperoxidase. When salivary flow is decreased for a few hours, as between meals, there is a four-fold increase in the number of bacteria in saliva, and in dehydrated patients or in severe illnesses such as typhoid or pneumonia, the mouth becomes foul because of microbial overgrowth.

Oral candidiasis
Changes in the oral flora produced by broad-spectrum antibiotics and impaired immunity predispose to thrush

The presence of commensal bacteria in the mouth makes it difficult for invading microorganisms to become established, but changes in oral flora upset this balance. For instance, prolonged administration of broad-spectrum antibiotics allows the normally harmless *C. albicans* to flourish, penetrating the epithelium with its pseudomycelia, and causing thrush. Oral thrush (candidiasis, *Fig. 15.13*) is also seen when immunity is impaired, as in HIV infection and malignancy, and occasionally in newborn infants and the elderly. It sometimes spreads to involve the esophagus. The diagnosis is readily confirmed by Gram stain and culture of scraped material, which shows large Gram-positive budding yeasts.

Topical antifungal agents such as nystatin are effective treatments for thrush, together with attention to any predisposing factors.

Another example of the shifting boundary between harmless coexistence and tissue invasion by resident microbes is seen with vitamin C deficiency, which reduces mucosal resistance and allows residents to cause gum infections.

Caries
In the USA and western Europe 80–90% of people are colonized by Streptococcus mutans, which causes dental caries

The microorganisms specifically adapted for life on teeth form a film called dental plaque on the tooth surface. This is a complex mass containing about 10^9 bacteria/g embedded in a polysaccharide matrix *(Fig. 15.14)*. The film, visible as a red layer when a dye such as erythrocin is taken into the mouth, is largely removed by thorough brushing, but re-establishes itself within a few hours. The clean teeth become covered with salivary glycoproteins to which certain streptococci (especially *Strep. mutans* and *Strep. sobrinus*) become attached and multiply. In the USA and western Europe, 80–90% of people are colonized by *Strep. mutans*. *Strep. mutans* itself synthesizes glucan (a sticky high molecular weight polysaccharide) from sucrose and this forms a matrix between these streptococci. Certain other bacteria, including anaerobic filamentous fusobacteria and actinomycetes, are also present. When the teeth are not cleaned for several days, plaque becomes thicker and more extensive – a tangled forest of microorganisms.

The bacteria in plaque use dietary sugar and form lactic acid, which decalcifies the tooth locally. Proteolytic enzymes from the bacteria help to break down other components of the enamel to give rise to a painful cavity in the tooth (caries).

The pH in an active caries lesion may be as low as 4.0

Therefore caries usually develops in crevices on the tooth when suitable bacteria (*Strep. mutans*) are in the plaque and there is a regular supply of sucrose. It may legitimately be regarded as an infectious disease – one of the most prevalent infectious diseases in developed countries due to closely placed bacteria-coated teeth and a sugary, often fluoride-deficient, diet.

Periodontal disease
Actinomyces viscosus, Actinobacillus and Bacteroides spp. are commonly involved in periodontal disease

A space (the gingival crevice) readily forms between the gums and tooth margin, and it may be considered as an oral backwater. It contains polymorphs, complement, IgG and IgM antibodies, and easily becomes infected. Gingival crevices normally contain an average of 2.7×10^{11} microbes/g, and 75% of them are anaerobes. Bacteria such as *Actinomyces viscosus*, *Actinobacillus* and *Bacteroides* spp. are commonly

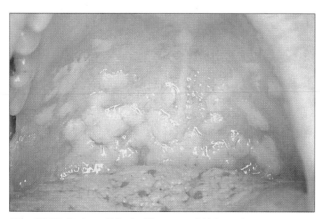
Fig. 15.13 Oral candidiasis. (Courtesy of JA Innes.)

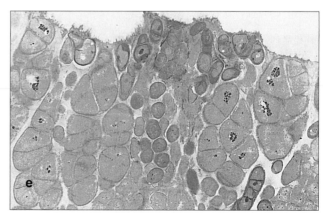
Fig. 15.14 Dental plaque on the deep surface of a child's tooth. ×20 000. (e, enamel.) (Courtesy of HN Newman.)

involved. In periodontal disease, the space enlarges to become a 'pocket', with local inflammation, an increasing number of polymorphs and a serum exudate. The inflamed gum bleeds readily and later recedes, while the multiplying bacteria cause halitosis. Finally, the structures supporting the teeth are affected, with reabsorption of ligaments and weakening of bone, causing the teeth to loosen. Periodontal disease with gingivitis is almost universal, although its severity varies greatly. It is a major cause of tooth loss in adults.

Laryngitis and Tracheitis

Parainfluenza viruses are common causes of laryngitis

Viral infections of the upper respiratory tract may spread downwards to involve the larynx and the trachea. Usually the cause is a parainfluenza virus, but sometimes RSV or influenza virus. Diphtheria (see below) may involve the larynx or trachea.

In adults, laryngeal infection (laryngitis) and tracheitis causes hoarseness and a burning retrosternal pain on breathing in and out. The larynx and trachea have non-expandable rings of cartilage in the wall, which are easily obstructed in children due to their narrowness. Swelling of the mucous membrane may lead to croup, which consists of a dry cough and inspiratory stridor ('crowing'). Difficulty with respiration may lead to hospital admission.

Diphtheria

Diphtheria is caused by toxin-producing strains of C. diphtheriae and can cause life-threatening respiratory obstruction

Diphtheria is now rare in developed countries due to widespread immunization with toxoid (see Chapter 29), but it is still common in developing countries. Non-toxigenic strains occur in the normal pharynx, but toxigenic bacteria must be present to cause disease. They can colonize the pharynx (especially the tonsillar regions), the larynx, the nose, and occasionally the genital tract, and in the tropics or in indigent people with poor skin hygiene, the skin.

Adhesion mechanisms are not understood, but the bacteria multiply locally without invading deeper tissues or spreading through the body. The toxin destroys epithelial cells and polymorphs and an ulcer forms, which is covered with a necrotic exudate forming a 'false membrane'. This soon becomes dark and malodorous, and bleeding occurs on attempting to remove it. There is extensive inflammation and swelling (Fig. 15.15) and the cervical lymph nodes may be enlarged to give a 'bull neck' appearance.

Nasopharyngeal diphtheria is the most severe form of the disease. When the larynx is involved it can result in life-threatening respiratory obstruction. Anterior nasal diphtheria is a mild form of the disease if it occurs on its own, because the toxin is less well absorbed from this site and a nasal discharge may be the main symptom. The patient will, however, be highly infectious.

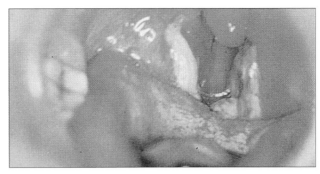

Fig. 15.15 Pharyngeal diphtheria with dirty-white exudate over the tonsils and severe local inflammation and swelling. (Courtesy of K Nye.)

Diphtheria toxin can cause fatal heart failure and a polyneuritis

The toxin (see panel and Fig. 15.16) is absorbed into the lymphatics and blood, and has several effects:
- Constitutional upset, with fever, pallor, exhaustion.
- Myocarditis, usually within the first two weeks. electrocardiographic changes are common and cardiac failure can occur. If this is not lethal, complete recovery is usual.
- Polyneuritis, which may occur, after the onset of illness due to demyelination. It may, for instance, affect the ninth cranial nerve resulting in paralysis of the soft palate and regurgitation of fluids.

Diphtheria is managed by immediate treatment with antitoxin and antibiotic

Diphtheria is a life-threatening disease and clinical diagnosis is a matter of urgency. As soon as the diagnosis is suspected clinically the patient is isolated to reduce the risk of the toxigenic strain spreading to other susceptible individuals, and treatment is begun with antitoxin. The antitoxin is produced in horses and tests for hypersensitivity to horse serum should be carried out. Penicillin or erythromycin is given as an adjunct. Laryngeal diphtheria may require tracheotomy.

The diagnosis is confirmed in the laboratory by isolation and identification of the organism (see Appendix, and Chapter 14) and demonstrating toxin production by a gel-diffusion precipitin reaction (Elek test).

Contacts may need chemoprophylaxis or immunization

Contacts of diphtheria patients should be tested for carriage of toxigenic C. diphtheriae and if necessary be given chemoprophylaxis or immunization. Toxigenic bacteria may be carried and transmitted by asymptomatic convalescents or by apparently healthy individuals.

Diphtheria is prevented by immunization

Diphtheria has almost disappeared from developed countries due to the immunization of children with a safe effective toxoid vaccine (see Chapter 31). However, the disease reappears when immunization is neglected. In 1990, epidemics began in the Russian Federation and have spread to 15 eastern European countries. Worldwide, there are still 100 000 cases and up to 8000 deaths per year.

Diphtheria toxin

The genes encoding toxin production are carried by a temperate bacteriophage which, during the lysogenic phase, is integrated into the bacterial chromosome. The toxin is synthesized as a single polypeptide (molecular weight 62 000; 535 amino acids) consisting of:

- Fragment B (binding) at the carboxy terminal end, which attaches the toxin to the host cells (or to any eukaryotic cell).
- Fragment A (active) at the amino terminal end, which is the toxic fragment.

Toxic fragment A is only formed by protease cleavage and reduction of disulphide bonds after uptake of the toxin into the cell. Fragment A inactivates elongation factor-2 (EF-2) by adenosine diphosphate (ADP) ribosylation and thereby inhibits protein synthesis *(Fig. 15.16)*. Prokaryotic and mitochondrial protein synthesis are not affected because a different EF is involved. A single bacterium can produce 5000 toxin molecules per hour and the toxic fragment is so stable within the cell that a single molecule can kill a cell. For unknown reasons myocardial and peripheral nerve cells are particularly susceptible.

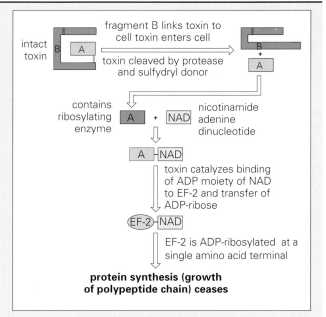

Fig. 15.16 Mechanism of action of diphtheria toxin.

- The respiratory tract from the nose to alveoli is a continuum, and any given microbe can cause disease in more than one segment.
- Some respiratory infections are restricted to the surface epithelium (influenza, diphtheria, pertussis), while others spread throughout the body (measles, rubella).
- 'Professional' invaders infect the healthy respiratory tract (e.g. common cold viruses, influenza viruses, *M. tuberculosis*), whereas 'secondary' invaders cause disease when host defenses are impaired (e.g. *Staph. aureus, P. carinii, Pseudomonas*).
- Common diseases of the teeth and neighboring structures – caries, periodontal disease are of microbial etiology.
- Diphtheria is a life-threatening disease caused by a biochemically defined bacterial toxin, and is completely preventable by vaccination.

An 18-month-old girl presents to the accident and emergency department in the early hours of the morning having woken up screaming with a fever. Her parents are unable to console her. She has a three-day history of cold and snuffles. On examination she is flushed and irritable and her ear drums are bright red and bulging.

1. What is the diagnosis?
2. What are the most likely pathogens?
3. How would you treat her?
4. What are the possible complications of this condition?

Further Reading

Efstratiou A, George RC. Microbiology and epidemiology of diphtheria. *Rev Med Microbiol* 1996;**7**:31–42.

Fischetti VA. Streptococcal M protein: molecular design and biological behaviour. *Clin Microb Revs* 1989;**2**:285–314.

Henderson FW, Collier AM, Sanyal MA *et al.* A longitudinal study of respiratory viruses and bacteria in the etiology of acute otitis media with effusion. *N Engl J Med* 1982;**366**:1377.

McMillan JA, Sandstrom C, Weiner LB *et al.* Viral and bacterial organisms associated with acute pharyngitis in a school-aged population. *J Pediatr* 1986;**109**:747–752.

Shaw JH. Causes and control of dental caries. *N Engl J Med* 1987;**317** 996.

Turner RB, Hendley JO, Gwaltney JM. Shedding of infected ciliated epithelial cells in rhinovirus colds. *J Infect Dis* 1982;**145**:849.

Introduction

The outer surface of the eye is exposed to the external world and therefore easily accessible for infective organisms
The conjunctiva is particularly susceptible. Not only is it a vulnerable epithelial surface, but it is covered by the eyelids, which create a warm moist enclosed environment in which contaminating organisms can quickly establish and set up a focus of infection. The eyelids and tears protect the external surfaces of the eye, both mechanically and biologically; any interference with their function increases the chance of a pathogen becoming established.

Eyelid infections are generally due to *Staphylococcus aureus*, with involvement of the lid margins causing blepharitis, or eyelid glands and follicles causing styes or hordeolums.

The conjunctiva can be invaded by other routes, such as the blood or nervous system *(Fig. 16.1)*. The deeper tissues of the eye can also be invaded from within, particularly by protozoan and worm parasites *(Fig. 16.2)*.

Conjunctivitis

Chlamydial infections
Different serotypes of Chlamydia trachomatis cause inclusion conjunctivitis and trachoma
To establish infection on the conjunctiva, microorganisms must avoid being rinsed and wiped away in tears. The best way of achieving this is to have a specific mechanism of attachment to conjunctival cells. Chlamydia, for example, have surface molecules that bind specifically to receptors on host cells. This is one of the reasons that of all the organisms infecting the conjunctiva *(Fig. 16.1)*, they are among the most successful. There are eight different serotypes of *Chlamydia trachomatis* responsible for inclusion conjunctivitis *(Fig. 16.3)* and another four serotypes responsible for trachoma, which is the most important eye infection in the world.

Five million people worldwide are blind due to trachoma
About 500 million people have trachoma and five million are blinded by it, while many others suffer visual impairment. Trachoma was known in ancient Egypt 4000 years ago and tweezers to remove interned eyelashes *(Fig. 16.4)* have been found in royal tombs. Transmission of *C. trachomatis* is by contact, for example by contaminated flies, fingers and towels.

Trachoma itself is the result of chronic repeated infections *(Fig. 16.4)*, which are especially prevalent when there is poor access to water preventing regular washing of the hands and face. Under these circumstances, chlamydial infection is frequently spread from one conjunctiva to another and this can be referred to as 'ocular promiscuity', comparable with the spread of genital secretions in non-specific urethritis (see Chapter 19). Some chlamydial serotypes can infect the urinogenital tract (see Chapter 19) as well as the conjunctiva, and the conjunctiva or lungs of a newborn infant may become infected after passage down an infected birth canal (see Chapter 21). In this situation, systemic treatment with erythromycin is generally needed.

Chlamydial infections are treated with antibiotic and prevented by face washing
Laboratory diagnosis of chlamydial infections (see Appendix) can be carried out using conjunctival fluid or scrapings. Treatment is with oral or topical antibiotic – tetracycline or doxycycline. Because infection and reinfection are facilitated by overcrowding, shortage of water and abundant fly populations, the disease can be prevented by improvements in standards of hygiene. For example, a study in Mexico showed that a daily face wash reduced the incidence of trachoma in children from 48% to 10%.

MICROBIAL INFECTIONS OF THE CONJUNCTIVA	
organism	**comments**
adenovirus	especially types 3,7,8,19
measles virus	infection of conjunctiva via blood
herpes simplex virus	virus reactivating in ophthalmic division of trigeminal ganglia causes corneal lesion (dendritic ulcer)
varicella zoster virus	may involve conjunctiva
enterovirus 70 coxsackie virus A 24	acute hemorrhagic conjunctivitis
Chlamydia trachomatis (types A–C)	cause of trachoma and commonly blindness
(types D–K)	cause of inclusion conjunctivitis; infection via fingers etc. or in newborn via birth canal
Neisseria gonorrhoeae	infection of newborn via birth canal
Staphylococcus aureus	cause of eyelid infection (styes) and 'sticky eye' in neonates

Fig. 16.1 Microbial infections of the conjunctiva.

INFECTIONS OF THE DEEPER LAYERS OF THE EYE		
organism	disease	route of infection
rubella	cataracts, microphthalmia	infection *in utero*
cytomegalovirus	chorioretinitis	infection *in utero*; may occur in AIDS*
Pseudomonas aeruginosa	serious inner eye infection	after trauma foreign bodies in eye eye operations bacteria can contaminate eye drops
Toxoplasma gondii (toxoplasmosis)	chorioretinitis	infection *in utero*
Echinococcus granulosus (hydatid disease)	distortion of the eye by growth of larval tapeworm in hydatid cyst	transmission by eggs passed by dogs
Toxocara canis (ocular toxocariasis)	chorioretinitis, blindness	transmission by eggs passed by dogs
Onchocerca volvulus (river blindness)	sclerosing keratitis chorioretinitis	larvae transmitted by blood-feeding *Simulium* flies

Fig. 16.2 Infections of the deeper layers of the eye. (*25% of patients with AIDS develop cytomegalovirus retinitis.)

In spite of many decades of research there are still no vaccines for chlamydial infections. This is partly because immunopathology itself makes a major contribution to the disease and vaccine-induced immune responses could be harmful.

Other conjunctival infections
In developed countries, chlamydia account for only 20% of cases of conjunctivitis
Several bacteria (e.g. *Streptococcus pneumoniae*, *Haemophilus influenzae* and *Leptospira*) can cause conjunctivitis *(Fig. 16.5)*. A clone of *H. influenzae* biotype *aegyptius* causes Brazilian purpuric fever (BPF), which occurs up to several weeks after an acute attack of conjunctivitis with this strain. BPF is characterized by fever, purpura and massive vascular collapse, and is rapidly fatal. The pathogenesis is not clear. Originally described in Brazil, cases have now occurred in most parts of the world.

Infection by *Neisseria gonorrhoeae* is a hazard of birth, through an infected birth canal, and can result in a severe purulent condition. It is seen on the first or second day of life (ophthalmia neonatorum) and requires urgent treatment with ceftriaxone (penicillin resistance is widespread), but can be prevented by applying erythromycin ointment shortly after birth. *Staph. aureus* also produces infections in

newborns as well as in adults. The eyes of infants may be invaded by this organism if the organism is transferred from the child's own body or from an infected adult.

Direct infection of the eye may be associated with wearing contact lenses
Excessive wearing of contact lenses can lead to a reduction in the effectiveness of the eye's defense mechanisms, allowing pathogens to become established, but more likely

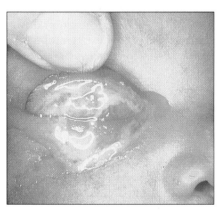

Fig. 16.3
Chlamydial conjunctivitis is the commonest form of neonatal conjunctivitis. (Courtesy of G Ridgway.)

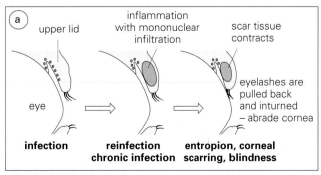

a
upper lid — inflammation with mononuclear infiltration — scar tissue contracts
eye
eyelashes are pulled back and inturned – abrade cornea
infection — **reinfection chronic infection** — **entropion, corneal scarring, blindness**

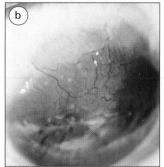

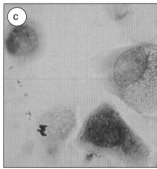

Fig. 16.4 *Chlamydia trachomatis* and blindness. The pathogenesis is outlined in (a). Scarring of the cornea (b) results from long-standing ocular trachoma. (Courtesy of RC Barnes.) Giemsa stain of an ocular scraping from trachoma (c) shows *C. trachomatis* as an intracellular inclusion. (Courtesy of G Ridgway.)

hazards are the use of contaminated eye drops or cleaning solutions and the insertion of contaminated lenses. A number of bacteria can be transmitted directly in this way. The free-living ameba *Acanthamoeba* can multiply in unchanged lens cleaning fluids and be transferred when the lens is inserted, causing corneal damage.

Conjunctival infection may be transmitted by the blood or nervous system

Several organisms invade the superficial tissues of the eye after transport through the blood or, in the case of herpes simplex virus (HSV), by movement along the trigeminal nerve. Reactivation of this virus can result in the development of a keratitis with the formation of dendritic ulcers *(Fig. 16.6)*. Inadvertent use of topical steroids may aggravate this condition, and the resultant severe ulceration can lead to corneal destruction.

Infection of the Deeper Layers of the Eye

Trauma to the eye may result in the establishment of a *Pseudomonas aeruginosa* infection, giving rise to serious inner eye infection. This organism may also be introduced via contaminated eye drops. Rubella and cytomegalovirus (CMV) may invade the fetal eye *in utero*, the former causing cataracts and microphthalmia, the latter a severe chorioretinitis. Congenital syphilis produces a retinopathy with quiescent lesions, and keratitis may appear in later life. Secondary syphilis is also associated with ocular inflammation.

Toxoplasmosis
Toxoplasma gondii infection can cause chorioretinitis leading to blindness

Chorioretinitis also occurs with toxoplasmosis. Although infection with this protozoan *(Toxoplasma gondii)* is widespread (see Chapter 3) it is not serious unless:

- Acquired *in utero* when the organism invades all tissues, especially the central nervous system (CNS).
- Acquired (or reactivated) under immunosuppression.

Infection occurs by swallowing oocysts released by infected cats (the primary host) or by eating meat containing tissue cysts. Women who become infected in pregnancy may transmit the infection to the fetus as tachyzoites can cross the placenta. Tissue cysts can form in the retina of the fetus and undergo continuous proliferation, producing progressive lesions, particularly when levels of immunity are low. These lesions may also involve the choroid *(Fig. 16.7)* and lead ultimately to blindness.

Parasitic worm infections
Toxocara canis larvae cause an intense inflammatory response and can lead to retinal detachment

Larval tapeworms (e.g. the hydatid cyst stage of *Echinococcus granulosus* transmitted by eggs passed from infected dogs) occasionally enter the eye, with growth of the cysts causing severe mechanical damage. Invasion by migratory larvae of the nematode *Toxocara canis* is more common. This parasite occurs naturally in the intestines of dogs, releasing thick-shelled resistant eggs into the environment. The eggs can hatch if swallowed by humans, the larvae initiating, but failing to complete, their customary migration through the tissues. In the canine host, migration results in the worms re-entering the intestine where they mature. In humans, larvae can enter almost any organ, often the CNS or eye *(Fig. 16.8)*, triggering an intense inflammatory response. In the eye, localized lesions in the retina may cause detachment. The misdiagnosis of such ocular lesions as retinoblastoma has led to enucleation. Anthelmintic treatment is beneficial.

Onchocerca volvulus infection causes 'river blindness' and is transmitted by Simulium flies

The other major worm infection associated with ocular damage is *Onchocerca volvulus* infection, the cause of river blindness in Africa and Central America. This infection is transmitted by the bites of *Simulium* flies, which take up microfilariae, larvae from the skin of infected hosts and reintroduce the larvae after they have become infective, when next feeding. Adult worms live in

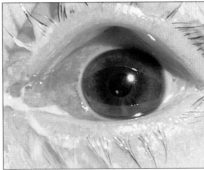

Fig. 16.5 Purulent discharge in bacterial conjunctivitis is often associated with infections by *Streptococcus pneumoniae*, *Haemophilus influenzae* or *Staphylococcus aureus*. (Courtesy of M Tapert.)

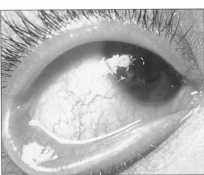

Fig. 16.6 Herpes simplex virus (HSV) keratitis. Dendritic ulcers, seen here on the cornea, are common in recurrent HSV infections. (Courtesy of MJ Wood.)

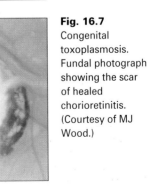

Fig. 16.7 Congenital toxoplasmosis. Fundal photograph showing the scar of healed chorioretinitis. (Courtesy of MJ Wood.)

subcutaneous nodules, and are comparatively harmless. The microfilariae, released by the females in enormous numbers for uptake by other flies, induce intense inflammatory reactions in the skin. This causes severe itching and eventually degenerative changes; lymphadenitis, lymphedema and elephantiasis may also occur. The larvae migrate through the subcutaneous tissue, and invasion of the eye is particularly common in certain regions of Africa as well as Central America.

The inflammatory responses in the eye cause a number of pathologic changes, which may affect both the anterior and posterior chambers *(Fig. 16.9)*. These include:

- Punctate and sclerosing keratitis.
- Iridocyclitis.
- Chorioretinitis.
- Optic atrophy.

The disease is called 'river blindness' because the *Simulium* flies develop in rivers and people living near rivers are most affected. Blindness rates may reach 40% of the adult population in endemic areas and, worldwide, 300 000 people are afflicted. Microfilariae can be seen in biopsies of affected skin. Anthelmintic treatment (ivermectin) may reduce microfilarial levels and block transmission, but the blindness is irreversible.

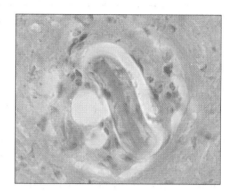

Fig. 16.8
Toxocara canis. Granuloma in the posterior pole of an infected eye. The larval nematode is clearly visible in the center of the granuloma. (Courtesy of D Spalton.)

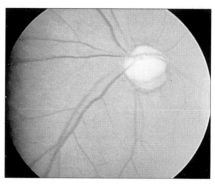

Fig. 16.9
Onchocerciasis. Sclerosis of the choroidal vessels caused by invading microfilaria of *Onchocerca volvulus.* (Courtesy of J Anderson.)

- The eye is particularly vulnerable to infectious organisms but is well protected against external invasion.
- The consequences of infection are always potentially serious given that sight is dependent upon the presence of an intact transparent cornea.
- Microbes infecting the conjunctiva have specific attachment mechanisms.
- Inflammatory responses, though 'designed' to limit invasion and repair damage, can irreversibly damage conjunctival and corneal surfaces.
- Relatively few organisms invade the retina, and those that do are potentially sight-threatening.
- Some of the most serious infection-related diseases of the eye involve invasion by protozoan or helminth parasites. The diagnosis then often follows rather than precedes the development of visual impairment.

A 42-year-old homosexual man with AIDS complains of blurred vision. He has noticed that he has floaters and a visual field loss, which he describes as black patches in his vision. His last CD4 count was very low at 20 cells/mm^3 and he has been admitted to hospital for treatment of *Pneumocystis carinii* pneumonia and Kaposi's sarcoma. Fundoscopy reveals areas of white infiltrates and hemorrhages consistent with a diagnosis of retinitis. Examination of his visual fields reveals a single scotoma (a blind spot) in the inferotemporal part of his retina.

1. What infections are associated with a choroidoretinitis?
2. How would you make the diagnosis?
3. How would you treat a patient with CMV retinitis?

Further Reading

D'Angelo LJ, Hierholzer JC, Holman RC *et al.* Epidemic keratoconjunctivitis caused by adenovirus type 8. Epidemiology and laboratory aspects of a large outbreak. *Am J Epidemiol* 1981;**113**:44.

Harding SP. Viral infections of the eye. *Rev Med Virol* 1993;**3**:161–171.

Holmes KK. The chlamydia epidemic. *J Am Med Assoc* 1981;**245**:1718.

Levin RM, Ticknor W, Jordan C *et al.* Etiology of conjunctivitis. *J Pediatr* 1981;**99**:831.

Weiss A, Brinser JH, Nazar–Stewart V. Acute conjunctivitis in children. *J Pediatr* 1993;**122**:10.

Wilcox ADP, Stapleton F. Ocular bacteriology. *Rev Med Microbiol* 1996;**7**:123–131.

Introduction

Although the respiratory tract is continuous from the nose to the alveoli, it is convenient to distinguish between infections of the upper and lower respiratory tract, even though the same microorganisms might be implicated in infections of both. Infections of the upper respiratory tract and associated structures are the subject of the Chapter 15. Here, we discuss infections of the lower respiratory tract. These infections tend to be more severe than infections of the upper respiratory tract and the choice of appropriate antimicrobial therapy is important and may be life saving.

Lower respiratory tract infections can be broadly divided into acute and chronic

Among the acute infections, four major syndromes can be identified:

- Acute bronchitis.
- Acute exacerbations of chronic bronchitis.
- Acute bronchiolitis.
- Pneumonia.

Influenza is a specific infection that if severe may proceed to bronchitis or pneumonia. Whooping cough will be considered in this chapter as a serious and acute infection of the lower respiratory tract.

The latter part of this chapter deals with chronic infections, including:

- Specific infections such as tuberculosis and aspergillosis.
- Conditions such as lung abscesses and empyema.
- Infections in cystic fibrosis patients.

Acute Infections of the Lower Respiratory Tract

Whooping cough
Whooping cough is caused by the bacterium *Bordetella pertussis*

Whooping cough or pertussis is a severe disease of childhood. *Bordetella pertussis* is confined to humans and is spread from person to person by airborne droplets. The organisms attach to, and multiply in, the ciliated respiratory mucosa, but do not invade deeper. Surface components such as filamentous hemagglutinin and fimbrial agglutinogens play an important role in specific attachment to respiratory epithelium.

B. pertussis infection is associated with the production of a variety of toxic factors

Some of these toxic factors affect inflammatory processes, while others damage ciliary epithelium. They are:

- Pertussis toxin, which resembles diphtheria and other toxins (see Chapter 12) in being a subunit toxin with an active (A) unit and a binding (B) unit. The A unit is an adenosine diphosphate (ADP)–ribosyl transferase, which catalyzes the transfer of ADP–ribose from nicotinamide adenine dinucleotide (NAD) to host cell proteins. The functional consequence of this is a disruption of signal transduction to the affected cell, but the toxin probably has other effects on the cell surface as well.

- Adenylate cyclase toxin, which is a single peptide that can enter host cells and cause them to increase their cyclic adenosine monophosphate (cAMP) to supraphysiologic levels. In neutrophils this results in an inhibition of defense functions such as chemotaxis, phagocytosis and bactericidal killing. This toxin may also be responsible for the hemolytic properties of *B. pertussis*.

- Tracheal cytotoxin, which is a cell wall component derived from the peptidoglycan of *B. pertussis* that specifically kills tracheal epithelial cells (see chapter 3).

- Endotoxin, which differs from the classic endotoxin of other Gram-negative rods, but has functional similarities and may play a role in the pathogenesis of infection.

B. pertussis infection is characterized by paroxysms of coughs followed by a 'whoop'

After an incubation period of 1–3 weeks, *B. pertussis* infection is manifest first as a catarrhal illness with little to distinguish it from other upper respiratory tract infections. This is followed up to one week later by a dry non-productive cough, which becomes paroxysmal. A paroxysm is characterized by a series of short coughs producing copious mucus, followed by a 'whoop', which is a characteristic sound produced by an inspiratory gasp of air. Despite the severity of the cough, the symptoms are confined to the respiratory tract and lobar or segmental collapse of the lungs can occur (*Fig. 17.1*).

Complications include central nervous system (CNS) anoxia, exhaustion and secondary pneumonia due to invasion of the damaged respiratory tract by other pathogens.

The early clinical picture is non-specific and the true diagnosis may not be suspected until the paroxysmal phase. The organisms can be isolated on suitable media from throat swabs or on 'cough plates' (see Chapter 14 and Appendix, p. 000), but they are fastidious and do not survive well outside the host's environment.

Whooping cough is managed with supportive care and erythromycin

Supportive care is of prime importance. Infants are at greatest risk of complications, and admission to hospital should be considered for children under one year of age. For specific

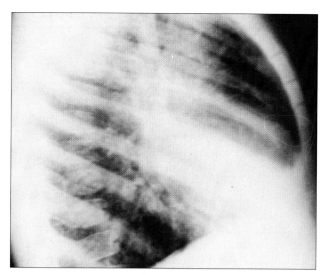

Fig. 17.1 Chest radiograph showing patchy consolidation and collapse of the right middle lobe in whooping cough. (Courtesy of JA Innes.)

antibacterial treatment to be effective it must penetrate the respiratory mucosa and inhibit or kill the infecting organism. Erythromycin is the drug of choice. Although the treatment is often not begun until the disease is recognized in the paroxysmal phase, it does appear to reduce its severity and duration. It also reduces the risk of organisms in the throat (thereby helping to reduce the infectivity of the patient) and helps to reduce the risk of secondary infections.

Erythromycin prophylaxis of close contacts of active cases is helpful in controlling the spread of infection.

Whooping cough can be prevented by active immunization

For many years a whole cell vaccine comprising a killed suspension of *B. pertussis* cells has been used. It is usually combined with purified diphtheria and tetanus toxoids and administered as 'DPT' or 'triple' vaccine. The efficacy of pertussis vaccine is generally high, but variable, and recent years have seen major concerns about side effects. These take the form of:

- Fever, malaise and pain at the site of administration, which may occur in up to 20% of infants and are not serious.
- Convulsions, thought to be associated with the vaccine in about 0.5% of vaccinees.
- Encephalopathy and permanent neurologic sequelae associated with vaccination, with an estimated rate of 1 in 100 000 vaccinations (< 0.001%).

Concern about side effects led to a marked fall in uptake of the vaccine and subsequently to a marked increase in the incidence of whooping cough (see Chapter 31). Efforts are now concentrated on the production of subunit vaccines containing only the 'protective' antigens. The difficulty has been in identifying these antigens, but combinations of inactivated pertussis toxin and filamentous hemagglutinin appear to be promising and such vaccines are already in use in Japan and some other countries.

Acute bronchitis
Acute bronchitis is an inflammatory condition of the tracheobronchial tree, usually due to infection

Causative agents include viruses (rhinoviruses, coronaviruses), which are also found infecting the upper respiratory tract, and lower tract pathogens such as influenza virus, adenoviruses and *Mycoplasma pneumoniae*. Secondary bacterial infection with *Streptococcus pneumoniae* and *Haemophilus influenzae* may also play a role in pathogenesis. The degree of damage to the respiratory epithelium varies with the infecting agent:

- With influenza virus infection it may be extensive and leave the host prone to secondary bacterial invasion (post-influenza pneumonia; see below).
- With *Mycoplasma pneumoniae* infection, specific attachment of the organism to receptors on the bronchial mucosal epithelium *(Fig. 17.2)* and the release of toxic substances by the organism results in sloughing of affected cells.

A cough is the most prominent presentation and treatment is largely symptomatic. The value of antibiotics is uncertain, but they are usually recommended.

Acute exacerbations of chronic bronchitis
Infection is only one component of chronic bronchitis

Chronic bronchitis is a condition characterized by cough and excessive mucus secretion in the tracheobronchial tree that are not attributable to specific diseases such as bronchiectasis, asthma or tuberculosis. Infection appears to be only one component of the syndrome, the others being cigarette smoking and inhalation of dust or fumes from the workplace. Bacterial infection does not appear to initiate the disease, but is probably significant in perpetuating it and in producing the characteristic acute exacerbations. *Strep. pneumoniae* and unencapsulated strains of *H. influenzae* are the organisms

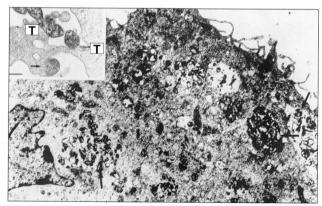

Fig. 17.2 Osponized *Mycoplasma pneumoniae* cells (arrowed) phagocytosed by an alveolar macrophage (bar, 2 μm). The insert shows *M. pneumoniae* cells adhering with the tip organelle (T) to macrophage surfaces. (Reproduced from E Jacobs, 1991; with permission from Churchill Livingstone Medical Journals.)

most frequently isolated, but interpretation of the significance of their presence in sputum is difficult because they are also commonly found in the normal throat flora and can therefore contaminate expectorated sputum. Other bacteria such as *Staphylococcus aureus* and *Mycoplasma pneumoniae* are less commonly associated with infection and exacerbation. Viruses are frequent causes of acute infection.

Antibiotic therapy may be helpful in the treatment of acute exacerbations although their efficacy is difficult to assess.

Bronchiolitis
75% of bronchiolitis infections are caused by respiratory syncytial virus
Bronchiolitis is a disease restricted to childhood, and usually to children under two years of age. The bronchioles of a young child have such a fine bore that if their lining cells are swollen by inflammation the passage of air to and from the alveoli can be severely restricted. Infection results in necrosis of the epithelial cells lining the bronchioles and leads to peribronchial infiltration, which may spread into the lung fields to give an interstitial pneumonia (see below). As many as 75% of these infections are caused by respiratory syncytial virus (RSV) and most of the remaining 25% are also of viral etiology, although *M. pneumoniae* is implicated occasionally.

RSV infection
RSV is the most important cause of bronchiolitis and pneumonia in infants
RSV is a typical paramyxovirus and there is only one antigenic type. Its surface spikes bear G protein (not hemagglutinin or neuraminidase) for attachment to the cell, and fusion (F) protein. The latter initiates viral entry by fusing the viral envelope to the cell membrane, and also fuses host cells to form syncytia.

RSV infection is transmitted by droplets and to some extent by hands. Outbreaks occur each winter *(Fig. 17.3)*, and during the RSV season infection can spread in hospitals as well as in the community. Nearly all individuals have been infected by two years of age. About one in every 100 infants with RSV bronchiolitis or pneumonia requires admission to hospital.

RSV infection can be particularly severe in young infants
After inhalation, the virus establishes infection in the nasopharynx and lower respiratory tract. Clinical illness appears after an incubation period of 4–5 days. The illness can be particularly severe in young infants (peak mortality at three months of age), the virus invading the lower respiratory tract by direct surface spread to cause bronchiolitis or pneumonia. In young children and adults, however, the virus is restricted to the upper respiratory tract, causing a less severe common cold-type illness. Young infants develop a cough, rapid respiratory rate and cyanosis. Otitis media is quite common. Secondary bacterial infection is rare.

The manifestations of RSV infection appear to have an immunopathologic basis
Maternal antibodies in the infant react with virus antigens, perhaps with the liberation of histamine and other mediators from the host's cells. In early trials a killed vaccine was used and often resulted in more severe disease, supporting the idea of immunopathology.

Neutralizing antibodies are formed (lower levels in younger infants), but cell-mediated immunity is needed to terminate the infection. The virus continues to be shed from the lungs of children lacking cell-mediated immunity for many months. Apparently healthy children may continue to show depressed pulmonary function or wheeze even 1–2 years after apparent recovery.

Recurrent infections are common, but are less severe. The reason for recurrence, which is also a feature of parainfluenza virus infection, is unknown.

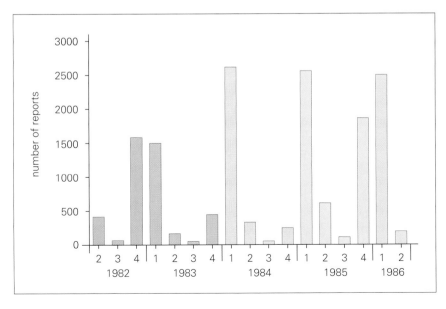

Fig. 17.3 Acute bronchiolitis in respiratory syncytial virus (RSV) infection. Seasonal variation is evident in quarterly reports of RSV infection in England and Wales. (Redrawn from Communicable Disease Surveillance Centre.)

RSV-specific antigens are detectable in smears of exfoliated cells and ribavirin is indicated for severe disease

RSV-specific antigens are detectable by immunofluorescence (*Fig. 17.4*) or enzyme-linked immunosorbent assay (ELISA) methods (see Chapter 14) in smears of exfoliated cells obtained by nasopharyngeal lavage. Virus isolation is less commonly useful and success depends on inoculating respiratory secretions as soon as possible into cell cultures.

The antiviral agent ribavirin used as an aerosol has occasionally been used successfully for severe disease. At present there is no vaccine.

Hantavirus pulmonary disease

A hantavirus present in wild rodents (see also Chapter 31), caused severe pulmonary disease in 1996 when it infected people in south-west USA. Viral invasion of the pulmonary capillary endothelium led to fluid outpouring into the lungs and at least 26 deaths were reported.

Pneumonia

Pneumonia has long been known as 'the old man's friend' as it is the most common cause of infection-related death in the USA and UK. It is caused by a wide range of microorganisms giving rise to indistinguishable symptoms. The challenge lies not in the clinical diagnosis of pneumonia, except perhaps in children in whom it may be more difficult to diagnose, but in the laboratory identification of the microbial cause (see Appendix, p. 000). In the absence of such identification, the choice of antimicrobial therapy may not be optimal.

Microorganisms reach the lungs by inhalation, aspiration or via the blood

Microorganisms gain access to the lower respiratory tract by inhalation of aerosolized material or by aspiration of the normal flora of the upper respiratory tract. The size of inhaled particles is important in determining how far they travel down the respiratory tract; only those less than about 5μm diameter reach the alveoli. Less frequently, the lungs become seeded with organisms as a result of spread via the blood from other infected sites. Healthy individuals are susceptible to infection by a range of pathogens possessing adhesins, which allow the pathogens to attach specifically to the respiratory epithelium (see Chapter 7). In addition, people with impaired defenses (e.g. immunocompromise, preceding viral damage, cystic fibrosis) may develop infections with organisms that do not cause infections in health (e.g. *Pneumocystis carinii* is an important cause of pneumonia in people with AIDS).

The respiratory tract has a limited number of ways in which it can respond to infection

The host's response can be defined by the pathologic and radiologic findings, but the terms can be confusing because they are applied differently in different situations. However four descriptive terms are in common use (*Fig. 17.5*):

- Lobar pneumonia refers to involvement of a distinct region of the lung. The polymorph exudate formed in response to infection, clots in the alveoli and renders

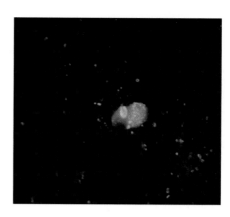

Fig. 17.4 Immunofluorescent preparation from the nasopharynx showing respiratory syncytial virus-infected cells (bright green). (Courtesy of H Stern.)

them solid. Infection may spread to adjacent alveoli until constrained by anatomic barriers between segments or lobes of the lung. Thus one lobe may show complete consolidation.

- Bronchopneumonia refers to a more diffuse patchy consolidation, which may spread throughout the lung as a result of the original pathologic process in the small airways.
- Interstitial pneumonia involves invasion of the lung interstitium and is particularly characteristic of viral infections of the lungs.
- Lung abscess, sometimes referred to as necrotizing pneumonia, is a condition in which there is cavitation and destruction of the lung parenchyma.

The outcomes common to all these conditions are respiratory distress resulting from the interference with air exchange in the lungs, and systemic effects as result from infection in any part of the body.

A wide range of microorganisms can cause pneumonia

Age is an important determinant (*Fig. 17.6*):

- Most childhood pneumonia is caused either by viruses or by bacteria invading the respiratory tract secondary to viral infection (e.g. after measles infection). Neonates born to mothers with genital *Chlamydia trachomatis* infection may develop a chlamydial interstitial pneumonitis (see Chapter 19) resulting from colonization of the respiratory tract during birth.
- In the absence of an underlying disorder such as cystic fibrosis, pneumonia is unusual in older children. Children and young adults with cystic fibrosis are very prone to lower respiratory tract infection, caused characteristically by *Staph. aureus*, *H. influenzae* and *Pseudomonas aeruginosa*.
- The cause of pneumonia in adults depends upon a number of risk factors such as age, underlying disease and exposure to pathogens through occupation, travel or contact with animals.

Pneumonia acquired in hospital tends to be caused by a different spectrum of organisms, particularly Gram-negative bacteria. The causative agents of adult pneumonia are summarized in *Figure 17.7*. Although clinical and epidemiologic clues help to suggest the likely cause, microbiological investigations are essential to confirm the diagnosis and ensure optimal antimicrobial therapy.

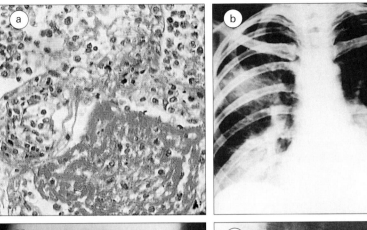

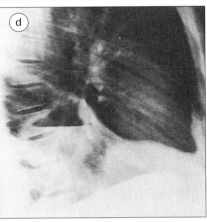

Fig. 17.5 Four types of pneumonia. (a) Pneumococcal lobar pneumonia, showing consolidated alveoli filled with neutrophils and fibrin. (Hematoxylin and eosin stain) (Courtesy of ID Starke and ME Hodson.) (b) *Mycoplasma* bronchopneumonia, with patchy consolidation in several areas of both lungs. (Courtesy of JA Innes.) (c) Interstitial pneumonia due to influenza virus. (Courtesy of ID Starke and ME Hodson.) (d) Lung abscess, showing an abscess cavity in the lower lobe of the right lung. (Courtesy of JA Innes.)

CAUSES OF PNEUMONIA RELATED TO AGE	
children	**adults**
mainly viral (e.g. respiratory syncytial virus, parainfluenza) or bacterial secondary to viral respiratory infection (e.g. after measles)	bacterial causes more common than viral
neonates may develop interstitial pneumonitis caused by *Chlamydia trachomatis* acquired from the mother at birth	etiology varies with age, underlying disease, occupational and geographic risk factors

Fig. 17.6 Pneumonia in children is more often viral in origin or bacterial secondary to a viral respiratory infection. In adults, bacterial pneumonia is more common.

It is often difficult to distinguish between bacterial and viral pneumonias clinically

Viral pneumonias show a characteristic interstitial pneumonia on chest radiography more often than bacterial pneumonias *(Fig. 17.5c)*, and for the sake of clarity are described separately below. Infections with RSV have been described earlier in this chapter and opportunist pathogens (such as *P. carinii*) associated specifically with pneumonia in the immunocompromised are described in Chapter 28.

Bacterial pneumonia
Strep. pneumoniae is the classic bacterial cause of acute community-acquired pneumonia

In the past, 50–90% of pneumonias were caused by *Strep. pneumoniae* (the 'pneumococcus'), but in recent years the relative importance of this pathogen has decreased and it now causes only 25–60% of cases *(Fig. 17.8)*. *H. influenzae* is estimated to be the cause of 5–15% of cases, but the true incidence is difficult to determine because this organism frequently colonizes the upper respiratory tract of bronchitic patients (see above).

A variety of bacteria cause primary atypical pneumonia

When effective antibiotic treatment (penicillin) for the pneumococcus became widely available, a significant proportion of cases of pneumonia failed to respond to this treatment and were labeled 'primary atypical pneumonia'. 'Primary' refers to pneumonia occurring as a new event (not secondary to influenza for example) and 'atypical' because *Strep. pneumoniae* is not isolated from sputum from such patients, the symptoms are often general as well as respiratory, and because of the failure to respond to penicillin or ampicillin. The causes of atypical pneumonia include *M. pneumoniae*, *Chlamydia pneumoniae* and *Chalmydia psittaci*, *Legionella pneumophila* and *Coxiella burnetii*. The relative importance of these pathogens varies in different studies *(Fig. 17.8)*. Infection with *C. pneumoniae* is common. About 50% of adults have antibodies, and in the

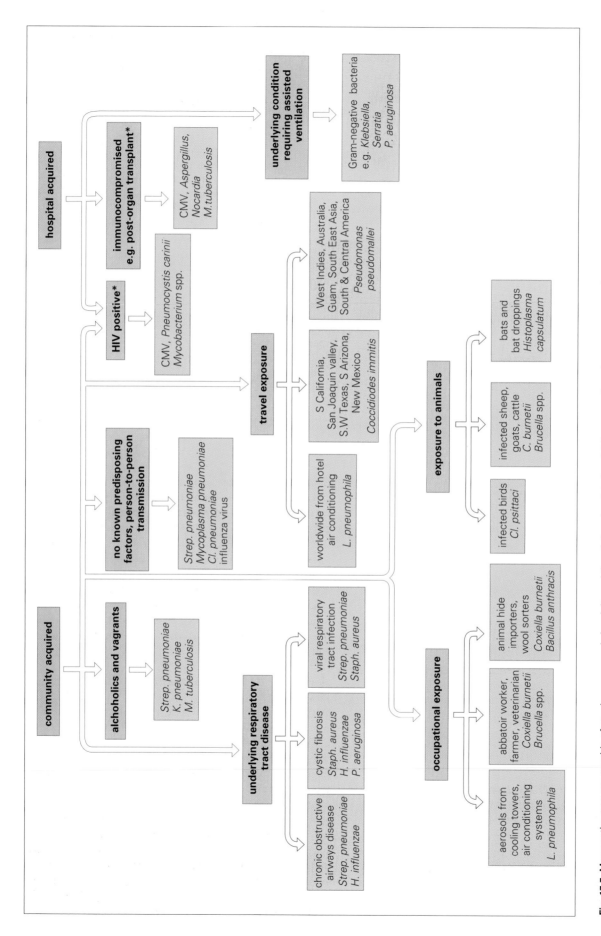

Fig. 17.7 Many pathogens are capable of causing pneumonia in adults and the etiology is related to risk factors such as the exposure to pathogens through occupation, travel and contact with animals. The elderly are more likely to be infected and tend to have a more severe illness than young adults. (*These infections are often reactivating endogenous infections rather than community or hospital acquired.) (*B., Brucella; Cl., Chlamydia; CMV, cytomegalovirus; H., Haemophilus; K., Klebsiella; L., Legionella; M., Mycobacterium; P., Pseudomonas; Staph., Staphylococcus; Strep., Streptococcus.)

USA it causes up to 300,000 cases of pneumonia each year in adults. *Mycoplasma pneumoniae* and *Chlamydia pneumoniae* appear to be solely human pathogens, whereas *C. psittaci* and *Coxiella burnetii* are acquired from infected animals, and *Legionella pneumophila* is acquired from contaminated environmental sources *(Fig. 17.7)*.

Moraxella catarrhalis (previously *Branhamella catarrhalis*) is increasingly recognized as a cause of pneumonia, particularly in patients with carcinoma of the lung or other underlying lung disease. Other etiologic agents of pneumonia associated with particular underlying diseases, occupations or exposure to animals and travel are summarized in *Figure 17.7* and described in other chapters. It is important to note that a causative organism is not isolated in as many as 35% of lower respiratory tract infections.

Patients with pneumonia usually present feeling unwell and with a fever

Signs and symptoms of a chest infection include:
- Chest pain, which may be pleuritic.
- A cough, which may produce sputum.
- Shortness of breath.
- Difficulty and pain on breathing.

Some infections result in symptoms confined mainly to the chest, whereas others such as Legionnaire's disease caused by *L. pneumophila* have a much wider systemic involvement and the patient may present with mental confusion, diarrhea and

COMMON CAUSES OF PNEUMONIA IN COMMUNITY-BASED STUDIES IN THREE COUNTRIES			
pathogen	percentage* of cases for which a pathogen was identified		
	Sweden	Denmark	Canada
Streptococcus pneumoniae	66	26	11
Legionella pneumophila	4	30	5
Mycoplasma Chlamydia	9	8	10
Haemophilus influenzae	13	32	8
Moraxella catarrhalis	3	0	1
Staphylococcus aureus	0	7	6
viral cause (not specified)	15	13	21

*note that more than one possible cause was isolated from some patients, therefore accounting for totals greater than 100%

Fig. 17.8 Despite the numerous possible pathogens, the vast majority of infections are caused by just a few. *Streptococcus pneumoniae* is the classic cause of lobar pneumonia, but its incidence has been declining in recent years in comparison with the incidence of the so-called atypical causes of pneumonia such as *Mycoplasma* and *Legionella*. (Data from TJ Marrie *et al*, 1987 and SS Pedersen, 1989.)

evidence of renal or liver dysfunction. However, the distinction between localized and systemic symptoms is not usually reliable enough for an accurate diagnosis.

Chest examination may reveal 'rales' (abnormal crackling sounds) and evidence of consolidation, even before changes become evident on radiography.

Patients with pneumonia usually have shadows in one or more areas of the lung

The chest radiograph is an important adjunct to the clinical diagnosis. Patients with pneumonia usually have shadows indicating consolidation (see above for descriptions of lobar, broncho- and interstitial pneumonia). However, careful interpretation is required to differentiate between infection and non-infective processes such as tumors.

Pneumonia is the most common cause of death from infection in the elderly

It is also an important cause of death in the young and previously healthy. Complications of infection include spread of the infecting organisms:
- Directly to extrapulmonary sites such as the pleural space, giving rise to empyema (see below).
- Indirectly via the blood to other parts of the body.

For example, the majority of patients with pneumococcal pneumonia have positive blood cultures, and pneumococcal meningitis not infrequently follows pneumonia in the elderly.

Sputum samples are best collected in the morning and before breakfast

Microscopic examination and culture of expectorated sputum remain the mainstays of respiratory bacteriology, despite doubts about the value of these procedures. Collection of sputum is non-invasive, but more invasive techniques, such as transtracheal aspiration, bronchoscopy and bronchoalveolar lavage, and open lung biopsy, may yield more useful results.

Sputum samples are best collected in the morning because sputum tends to accumulate while the patient is lying in bed, and before breakfast to reduce contamination by food particles and bacteria from food. It is important that the specimen submitted for examination is truly sputum and not simply saliva. A physiotherapist can be of great assistance to ill patients who may be unable to cough unaided.

The usual laboratory procedures on sputum specimens from patients with pneumonia are Gram stain and culture

Examination of the Gram-stained sputum (see Chapter 14) can give a presumptive diagnosis within minutes if the film reveals a host response in the form of abundant polymorphs and the putative pathogen (e.g. Gram-positive diplococci characteristic of *Strep. pneumoniae*, *Fig. 17.9*). The presence of organisms in the absence of polymorphs is suggestive of contamination of the specimen rather than infection, but it is important to remember that immunocompromised patients may not be able to mount a polymorph leukocyte response. Also remember that the causative agents of atypical pneumonia, with the exception of *L. pneumophila* (*Fig. 17.10*), will not be seen in Gram-stained smears.

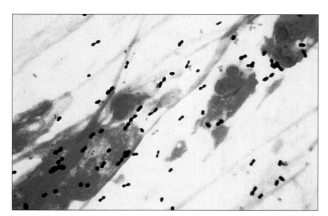

Fig. 17.9 Gram-stained smears of sputum can help the physician make a rapid diagnosis if, like this, they contain abundant Gram-positive diplococci characteristic of pneumococci, as well as polymorphs. However, many of the important causes of pneumonia will not be stained by Gram's stain.

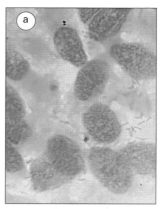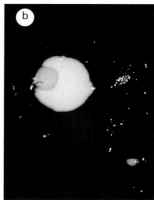

Fig. 17.10 *Legionella pneumophila.* (a) Gram stain of a specimen from bronchial biopsy in a patient with fulminant Legionnaire's disease. (Courtesy of S Fisher–Hoch.) (b) Culture plate showing white colonies on buffered charcoal yeast extract medium. (Courtesy of I Farrell.)

Standard culture techniques will allow the growth of the bacterial pathogens such as *Strep. pneumoniae*, *Staph. aureus*, *H. influenzae* and *Klebsiella pneumoniae* and other non-fastidious Gram-negative rods. Special media or conditions are required for the causative agents of atypical pneumonia, including *L. pneumophila* (*Fig. 17.10*, see Appendix, p. 000).

Rapid non-cultural techniques have been applied successfully to the diagnosis of pneumococcal pneumonia. Detection of pneumococcal antigen by agglutination of antibody-coated latex particles (see Chapter 14) can be used with both sputum and urine specimens (antigen is excreted in the urine). Use of this technique means the result is available within one hour of receipt of the specimen, but antibiotic susceptibility tests cannot be performed unless the organisms are isolated.

Microbiological diagnosis of atypical pneumonia is usually confirmed serologically

As mentioned above, several important causes of pneumonia will not be revealed in Gram-stained sputum smears and cannot be grown on simple routine culture media. For these reasons the diagnosis is usually confirmed by serologic tests rather than by culture. A single high titer of specific antibodies, or preferably demonstration of a rising titer between the acute and convalescent phase of the disease, is required; therefore serologic diagnosis is often retrospective. The important serologic tests are shown in *Figure 17.11*.

Pneumonia is treated with appropriate antimicrobial therapy

Once the cause of the pneumonia has been identified, selection of the appropriate antimicrobial therapy is relatively straightforward (*Fig. 17.12*), though there is increasing incidence of penicillin (and ampicillin) resistance in pneumococci in some countries.

The choice of treatment is more difficult when sputum is not produced or does not reveal the pathogen. It is there-

fore important to take a full history and use invasive diagnostic techniques if appropriate to help establish the cause.

Prevention of pneumonia involves measures to minimize exposure, and pneumococcal immunization post-splenectomy and for those with sickle cell disease

Respiratory infections are usually transmitted by airborne droplets so person to person spread is virtually impossible to prevent, although less crowding and better ventilation help to reduce the chances of acquiring infection. Infections acquired from sources other than humans may be more amenable to prevention – for example by avoiding contact with sick animals (Q fever) or birds (psittacosis). The contamination of cooling systems and hot water supplies by legionellae has been the subject of intense study, and regulations are now in force in UK and elsewhere to provide guidance for maintenance engineers.

Immunization is available for a few respiratory pathogens. A pneumococcal vaccine incorporating the polysaccharide capsular antigens of the most common types of *Strep. pneumoniae* is recommended for those at particular risk (e.g. post-splenectomy or individuals with sickle cell disease who are unable to deal effectively with capsulate organisms).

Viral pneumonia
Viruses can invade the lung from the bloodstream as well as directly from the respiratory tract

Many viruses cause pneumonia *(Fig. 17.13)* and, as with viral infections of the upper respiratory tract, generally accomplish infection in the face of normal host defenses. Perfectly healthy individuals are susceptible, and most of these viruses have surface molecules that attach specifically to the respiratory epithelium. RSV can cause pneumonia in infants and is described earlier in this chapter.

Even when viruses of this group do not themselves cause pneumonia they may damage respiratory defenses, laying the

SEROLOGIC DIAGNOSIS OF 'ATYPICAL' PNEUMONIA

pathogen	test	significant titer
Mycoplasma pneumoniae	complement fixation test (CFT)	1/16
	IgM by latex agglutination or ELISA	positive*
Legionella pneumophila	rapid microagglutination test	1/16
Chlamydia pneumoniae Chlamydia psittaci	microimmunofluorescence or ELISA using species-specific antigens	positive*
Coxiella burnetii	CFT (phase I and phase II antigens)	1/200
*any positive reaction is considered indicative of infection		

Fig. 17.11 Several of the bacterial causes of pneumonia are difficult to grow in the laboratory so examination of the patient's serum for specific antibodies is the usual method of diagnosis. It is always better to demonstrate a rising titer between acute and convalescent phase sera than to rely on a single sample, but the titers shown here give an indication of infection. (ELISA, enzyme-linked immunsorbent assay.)

ANTIBACTERIAL AGENTS FOR PNEUMONIA

initial treatment of community acquired pneumonia

first choice	ampicillin+erythromycin
unless clinical picture clearly indicates lobar pneumonia; if so	ampicillin
pneumonia secondary to viral respiratory tract infection	ampicillin+flucloxacillin
pneumonia in chronic bronchitic	augmentin or cefuroxime
pneumonia in vagrant, alchoholic, drug addict or a patient who may have aspirated	ampicillin+gentamicin

treatment of choice when pathogen has been identified

Streptococcus pneumoniae	ampicillin or penicillin (erythromycin if allergic to beta-lactams)
Mycoplasma pneumoniae Legionella pneumophila Chlamydia pneumoniae Chlamydia psittaci Coxiella burnetii	erythromycin
Staphylococcus aureus	flucloxacillin
Hemophilus influenzae	ampicillin*, augmentin or cefuroxime
Klebsiella pneumoniae	gentamicin, chloramphenicol or ciprofloxacin
*if non-beta-lactamase producer	

Fig. 17.12 Penicillin (or ampicillin) remains the agent of choice for pneumococcal infections as long as the isolates are susceptible. Penicillin-resistant pneumococci now occur in many countries and in some it is no longer safe to assume susceptibility to penicillin (or ampicillin). Many of the resistant strains are still susceptible to cephalosporins and in countries with a high incidence of resistance these agents may replace penicillin, at least until the results of antibiotic susceptibility are known. It is important to recognize that penicillin (and ampicillin and cephalosporins) are not active against the other common causes of pneumonia. Therefore a combination is often recommended for initial therapy.

ground for secondary bacterial pneumonia.Sometimes the virus fails to spread significantly to air spaces, but remains in interstitial tissues to cause interstitial pneumonia (e.g. cytomegalovirus (CMV) in immunodeficient patients).

Parainfluenza virus infection
As with RSV, parainfluenza viruses are most likely to cause lower respiratory tract disease (croup and pneumonia) in children.

VIRAL PNEUMONIA		
virus	**clinical condition**	**comments**
influenza A or B	primary viral pneumonia or pneumonia associated with secondary bacterial infection	pandemics (type A) and epidemics (type A or B); increased susceptibility in elderly or in certain chronic diseases
parainfluenza (types 1–4)	croup, pneumonia in children less than five years of age; upper respiratory illness (often subclinical) in older children and adults	antivirals and vaccines not available
measles	secondary bacterial pneumonia common; primary viral (giant cell) pneumonia in those with immunodeficiency	adult infection rare but severe; King and Queen of Hawaii both died of measles when they visited London in 1824
respiratory syncytial virus	pneumonitis pneumonia (infants); common cold syndrome (adults)	peak mortality in 3–4-month-old infants; secondary bacterial infection rare
adenovirus	pharyngoconjunctival fever, pharyngitis, atypical pneumonia (military recruits)	no antivirals; vaccines not generally available
cytomegalovirus	interstitial pneumonia	in immunodeficient patients (e.g. AIDS)
varicella-zoster virus	pneumonia in young adults suffering primary infection	uncommon; recognized 1–6 days after rash; lung lesions may eventually calcify

Fig. 17.13 Several different groups of viruses cause infection of the lower respiratory tract, particularly in children. Some, such as influenza and measles, leave the patient particularly prone to secondary bacterial infection.

There are four types of parainfluenza viruses (1–4) with differing clinical effects

The surface spikes of parainfluenza viruses are composed of hemagglutinin plus neuraminidase on one type of spike and fusion proteins on another. The four types of virus have different clinical effects and antigens. After infection by respiratory droplets these viruses spread locally on respiratory epithelium.

Parainfluenza viruses 1–3 cause pharyngitis, croup, otitis media, bronchiolitis and pneumonia. Croup is seen in children under five years of age, and consists of acute laryngotracheobronchitis with a harsh cough and hoarseness. Parainfluenza virus 4 is less common and generally causes a common cold-type illness.

Virus-specific antigens can often be detected in cells from respiratory washings. The virus can be isolated, and rises in antibody titer demonstrated. There are no effective antivirals and no vaccine.

Adenovirus infection
Adenoviruses cause about 5% of acute respiratory tract illness overall

There are 41 antigenic types of adenovirus, some of which cause upper respiratory tract infections such as pharyngoconjunctival fever and sore throat (see Chapter 15) and lower respiratory tract infections. Adenovirus respiratory tract infections generally cause non-specific symptoms in children under five years of age. As maternal antibody fades, lower respiratory tract illnesses become more frequent, especially with adenovirus 7.

Types 3, 4 and 7 have caused outbreaks of respiratory illness ranging from pharyngitis to atypical pneumonia in military recruits, with crowding and stress as possible cofactors.

Recovery is generally uneventful, but adenoviruses may persist in the body because they can be recovered from at least 50% of surgically removed tonsils. An enteric-coated vaccine for types 4 and 7 has been used to prevent infection in military recruits.

Influenza virus infection

Influenza viruses are classic respiratory viruses, and cause endemic, epidemic and pandemic influenza.

The structure of a typical myxovirus – single-stranded RNA – is shown in *Figure 17.14*, and the budding process in *Figure 17.15*.

There are three types of influenza virus – A, B and C

The internal ribonucleoprotein (RNP) is a group-specific antigen that distinguishes influenza A, B and C viruses:

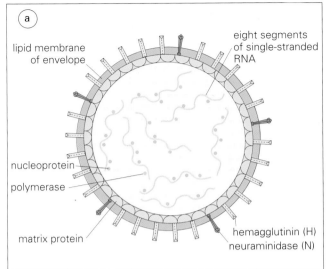

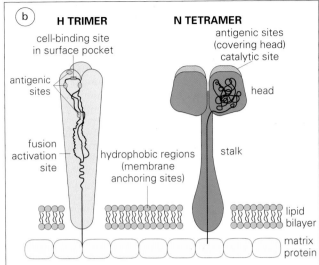

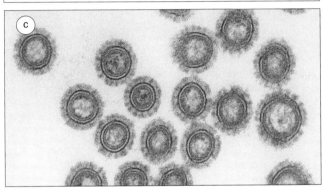

Fig. 17.14 The influenza A virus particle (a), with detail enlarged (b) to show surface hemagglutinin (H) and neuraminidase (N). Each particle has approximately 500 H spikes, which bind to the host cell and fuse the viral envelope to the cell's plasma membrane to initiate infection, and approximately 100 N spikes, which release the virus from the cell surface. Nucleoprotein and polymerase proteins are closely associated with RNA segments to form ribonucleoprotein (RNP). The N tetramer is propeller-shaped as viewed from the end. Detail of only one unit of H trimer and N tetramer is shown. The three-dimensional structure is known from X-ray crystallographic analysis. Electron micrograph (c) shows sectioned influenza virus particles. ×300 000. (Courtesy of D Hockley.)

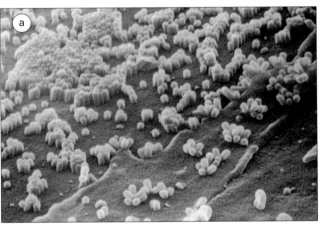

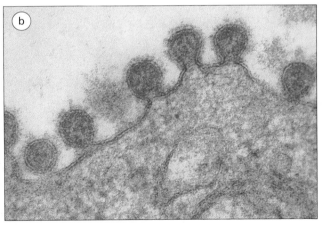

Fig. 17.15 Influenza virus budding from the surface of an infected cell. (a) Scanning electron micrograph. ×27 000. (b) In section. ×350 000. (Courtesy of D Hockley.)

- Influenza A viruses cause epidemics and occasionally pandemics, and there is an animal reservoir, notably in birds.
- Influenza B viruses only cause epidemics and do not involve animal hosts.
- Influenza C viruses do not cause epidemics and give rise to only minor respiratory illness.

The influenza virus envelope has hemagglutinin and neuraminidase spikes

These are shown in *Figure 17.14*. In the case of influenza A, the hemagglutinin (H) and neuramindase (N) are type-specific antigens and are used to characterize different strains of influenza A virus *(Fig. 17.16)*. Current strains are H3N2 and H1N1. In giving the full nomenclature, the influenza group,

HUMAN INFLUENZA VIRUSES				
type	subtype*	year	clinical severity	prototype virus
A	H3N2 (?) H1N1 (swine) H1N1 H2N2 (Asian) H3N2 (Hong Kong)**	1889 1918 1977 1957 1968	moderate severe mild severe moderate	designation based on serologic studies, viruses not isolated A/USSR/77 A/Japan/57/H2N2 A/Hong Kong/68/H3N2
B	none	1940	moderate	B/Lee/40
C	none	1947	very mild	C/Taylor/47

* antigenic shift in influenza A virus is shown by the appearance of novel combination of H and N antigens
** amino acid and base sequence analysis suggests that recombination between H3N8 (from ducks) and H2N2 gave rise to H3N2

Fig. 17.16 Human influenza viruses. Novel strains of virus arising in one continent spread rapidly to other continents, causing outbreaks during appropriate times of the year (winter months in temperate climates). There is a World Health Organization global surveillance system for influenza involving more than 100 laboratories in 79 different countries.

the location and year of isolation is also included (for example A/Phillipines/82/H3N2).

The single-stranded RNA genome is segmented and when virus particles of more than one strain infect a cell simultaneously, these segments can be reassorted during virus replication to give a progeny virus with a novel combination of H and N antigens.

Influenza viruses undergo genetic change as they spread through the host species

These changes are of two types:

- Antigenic drift. Small mutations affecting the H and N antigens occur constantly. When changes in these antigens enable the virus to multiply significantly in individuals with immunity to preceding strains, the new subtype can reinfect the community. Antigenic drift is seen with all types of influenza.
- Antigenic shift. Less commonly, and only with influenza A, there is a sudden major change (shift) in the antigenicity of the H or N antigens. This is based on recombination between different virus strains when they infect the same cell. The major change in H or N means that the new strain can spread through populations immune to preexisting strains and the stage is set for a new pandemic (Fig. 17.16). Associated with the change in H and N are other genetic changes, which may or may not confer increased pathogenicity or change the ability to spread rapidly from person to person.

There are 13 types of H and nine types of N, most of them occurring in birds. This gives 117 possible combinations of H and N, and 71 combinations have been found in birds – especially in ducks, sometimes leading to severe epidemics in chickens and turkeys – but so far only three combinations have been found in man. Evidently only some of the combinations are successful in man, from the virus's point of view. H3N2 has been with us since 1968; are we due for another pandemic strain? Influenza A viruses also infect pigs, horses, seals and other mammals, but it seems less likely that these species are sources of human infection.

Epidemics and pandemics are due to the appearance of new strains of viruses so that a given individual is regularly reinfected with different strains. This is in contrast to viruses that undergo minimal antigenic variation (monotypic viruses) such as measles or mumps, for which one infection confers life-long immunity.

Transmission of influenza is by droplet inhalation

Influenza occurs throughout the world and almost everyone in a given society is affected by it. Except in the tropics, the infection is almost entirely restricted to the coldest months of the year. This is largely because, during cold weather, people spend more time inside buildings with limited air space, which favors transmission, and perhaps also because of decreased host resistance (diet, depressed mucociliary activity). Influenza activity within a community is reflected not only in the numbers of people becoming ill and consulting doctors, but also in excess mortality due to acute respiratory disease (pneumonia), which particularly affects the elderly (Fig. 17.17).

The initial symptoms of influenza are due to direct viral damage and associated inflammatory responses

The virus enters the respiratory tract in droplets and attaches to sialic acid receptors on epithelial cells via the H components of the virus envelope. Fewer virus particles are needed to infect the lower respiratory tract than the upper respiratory tract. Just 1–3 days after infection the cytokines liberated from damaged cells and from infiltrating leukocytes cause symptoms such as chills, malaise, fever and muscular aches. There are also respiratory symptoms such as a runny nose and cough. The virus remains restricted to the respiratory tract and there is no viremia. Most people feel better within one week. The direct viral damage and associated inflammatory responses can be severe enough to cause bronchitis and interstitial pneumonia.

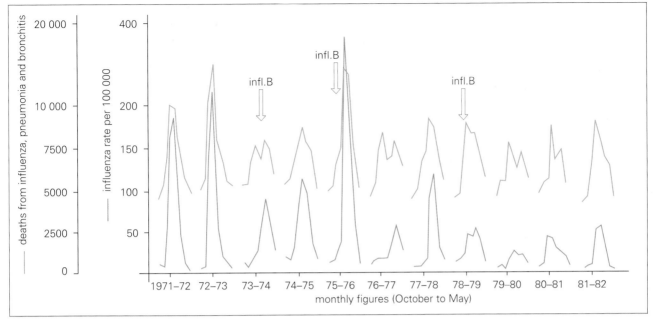

Fig. 17.17 Outbreaks of influenza within a community are reflected by a general increase in deaths from acute respiratory disease. Notifications of new cases of clinical influenza are paralleled by an increase in deaths attributed to influenza, pneumonia and bronchitis. Monthly figures from October to May for England and Wales (1971–83) are shown. The peaks are due to the spread of different strains of influenza A (H3N2 and H1N1) and influenza B (arrows) viruses in the community. (Data from the Office of Population, Censuses and Surveys.)

Influenzal damage to the respiratory epithelium predisposes to secondary bacterial infection

Secondary bacterial invaders include staphylococci, pneumococci and *H. influenzae*. Life-threatening influenza is often due to secondary bacterial infection, especially with *Staph. aureus*, the viral infection being brought under control by antibody and cell-mediated immune (CMI) responses to the infecting virus. Interferon probably plays a part during the early stages of the infection. Although antiviral antibodies may not be detected within the serum for 1–2 weeks, they are produced at an earlier stage, but are complexed with viral antigens in the respiratory tract.

Mortality due to secondary bacterial pneumonia is higher in apparently healthy individuals over 60 years of age and in those with impaired resistance due to, for example, chronic cardiorespiratory disease (e.g. emphysema) or renal disease. Pregnant women are also more vulnerable.

Rarely, influenza causes CNS complications

CNS complications include encephalomyelitis and polyneuritis (Guillain–Barré syndrome). These appear to be indirect immunopathologic complications rather then due to CNS invasion by the virus. The Guillain–Barré syndrome occurred as a significant but rare (1/100 000) sequel to the widespread vaccination of citizens in the USA with inactivated H3N2 influenza virus in 1976.

During influenza epidemics a diagnosis can generally be made clinically

Influenza-infected cells are seen after fluorescent antibody or immunoperoxidase staining of cells obtained from nasal aspirates. A rise in specific antibodies can be detected [by hemagglutination inhibition, complement fixation test or ELISA (see chapter 14)] in paired serum samples taken within a few days of illness and 7–10 days later. The virus can also be isolated from throat washings taken within 1–2 days of onset after inoculation into eggs or into certain cell cultures. This takes several days and is more important for public health authorities following infection with new virus strains rather than for diagnosis in individual patients.

Rimantadine (or amantadine) and vaccines can be used to prevent influenza

Rimantadine (or amantadine) inhibits the replication of influenza A viruses. They can reduce the severity of the infection, but only if given within 1–2 days of disease onset. They are more valuable when used for prophylaxis. Individuals at high risk can be protected if given 100 mg/day during epidemics.

Influenza virus vaccines in regular use are:
- Those consisting of egg-grown virus, which are then purified, formalin-inactivated and extracted with ether.
- The less reactogenic purified H and N antigens prepared from virus that has been disrupted ('split') by lipid solvents.

Influenza A (currently H3N2 and H1N1) and influenza B are included in the vaccine. The exact virus strains are reviewed annually in relation to the viruses circulating the previous year. The vaccines are given by parenteral injection, and provide protection against disease in up to 70% of individuals for about one year. Vaccination of individuals at high-risk, especially those over 65 years of age and those with chronic cardiopulmonary disease, is recommended. It might be expected that the respiratory route would be a better way of inducing respiratory immunity, and trials with live attenuated virus vaccines administered intranasally are in progress.

Measles
Secondary bacterial pneumonia is a frequent complication of measles in developing countries

Measles is dealt with in detail as a multisystem infection in Chapter 24. It is mentioned here because:

- It can cause 'giant cell' pneumonia in those with impaired immune responses.
- The virus replicates in the lower respiratory tract and, under certain circumstances, causes sufficient damage to lead to secondary bacterial pneumonia.

Secondary bacterial pneumonia is now uncommon in developed countries, but is a frequent complication among children in developing countries, and measles remains a major cause of death in childhood. Depressed immune responsiveness, inadequate vaccination programs, malnutrition (especially vitamin A) and poor medical care to deal with complications, tip the host–parasite balance markedly in favor of the virus.

After an incubation period of 10–14 days, there is fever, a runny nose, conjunctivitis and cough. Koplik's spots and then the characteristic rash appear 1–2 days later. The virus replicates in the epithelium of the nasopharynx, middle ear and lung, interfering with host defenses and enabling bacteria such as pneumococci, staphylococci and meningococci to establish infection. Pneumonia is what generally brings measles cases to hospital, but otitis media is also common. In children with severely impaired CMI responses virus replication continues unchecked to give rise to a giant cell pneumonia, which is a rare and usually fatal manifestation *(Fig. 17.18)*. Other complications are referred to in Chapter 24, and the neurologic complications in Chapter 22.

Measles is diagnosed on clinical grounds and measles virus isolation and detection of specific antibody responses are rarely necessary.

Antibiotics are needed for secondary bacterial complications of measles, but the disease can be prevented by immunization

No antiviral treatment is available, but antibiotics are needed for bacterial complications. Children with severe measles generally have very low levels of serum retinol; recovery is hastened and death is made less likely when they are given 400 000 IU vitamin A.

Measles is prevented by a highly effective, live, attenuated vaccine, given with mumps and rubella vaccines (MMR, see Chapter 31). Since immunization began, the number of cases has declined by 70%. In the USA, after a rise to nearly 30,000 cases in 1990, the number has fallen to 488 (47 of them imported) in 1996. It is planned to eliminate the disease in the Americas by the year 2000, and the WHO are thinking of global eradication by 2010–2015. Before the

vaccine was available in the 1960s, there were 135 million cases and 7–8 million deaths each year worldwide. Measles is still a killer, but deaths had already been reduced to one million a year by 1996.

CMV infection
CMV infection can cause an interstitial pneumonia in immunocompromised patients

This multisystem virus is described in Chapter 24. The virus does not normally replicate on respiratory epithelium or cause respiratory illness, but in immunocompromised patients (bone marrow transplant recipients, AIDS patients) it can give rise to an interstitial pneumonia. In AIDS, for instance, pneumonia is associated with reactivation of persistent CMV infection. The virus can be isolated and characteristic inclusions demonstrated in lung tissue *(Fig. 17.19)*, but *P. carinii* is also commonly present, contributing to the pathologic picture.

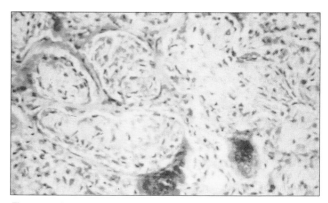

Fig. 17.18 Lung biopsy in measles pneumonia showing inflammatory cell infiltrate, proliferation of the alveolar lining cells and large, darkly staining, multinucleate giant cells. (Hematoxylin and eosin stain) (Courtesy of ID Starke and ME Hodson.)

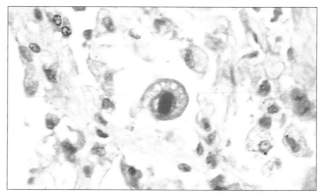

Fig. 17.19 Owl's eye inclusion body in cytomegalovirus infection. Large numbers of virus particles accumulate in the nucleus of the enlarged infected cell to produce a single dense inclusion. (Hematoxylin and eosin stain) (Courtesy of ID Starke and ME Hodson.)

Chronic Infections of the Lower Respiratory Tract

Tuberculosis is one of the most serious infectious diseases of the developing world

Tuberculosis kills about three million people and infects almost nine million others every year wherever poverty, malnutrition and poor housing prevail. It affects the apparently healthy as well as being a serious disease of the immunocompromised, as has become particularly obvious in patients with AIDS. Tuberculosis is primarily a disease of the lungs, but may spread to other sites or proceed to a generalized infection ('miliary' tuberculosis). It is also referred to in Chapters 18, 22 and 23.

Tuberculosis is caused by Mycobacterium tuberculosis

Other species of mycobacteria – so-called atypical mycobacteria, mycobacteria other than tuberculosis (MOTT) or non-tuberculous mycobacteria (NTM) – also cause infection in the lungs (Fig. 17.20).

Infection is acquired by inhalation of *M. tuberculosis* in aerosols and dust. Airborne transmission of tuberculosis is efficient because infected people cough up enormous numbers of mycobacteria, projecting them into the environment, where their waxy outer coat (see Chapter 3) allows them to withstand drying and therefore survive for long periods of time in air and house dust.

The pathogenesis of tuberculosis depends upon the history of previous exposure to the organism

In primary infection (i.e. infection in individuals encountering *M. tuberculosis* for the first time), the organisms are engulfed by the alveolar macrophages in which they can both survive and multiply. Non-resident macrophages are attracted to the site, ingest the mycobacteria and carry them via the lymphatics to the local (hilar) lymph nodes. In the lymph nodes the immune response – predominantly a CMI response – is stimulated. The CMI response is detectable 4–6 weeks after infection by introducing purified protein derivative (PPD) of *M. tuberculosis* into the skin. A positive result is shown by local induration and erythema, 48–72 hours later.

The CMI response helps to curb further spread of M. tuberculosis

However, some *M. tuberculosis* organisms may have already escaped to set up foci of infection in other body sites. Sensitized T cells release lymphokines that activate macrophages and increase their ability to destroy the mycobacteria. The body reacts to contain the organisms within 'tubercles', which are small granulomas consisting of epithelioid cells and giant cells (Fig. 17.21). The lung lesion plus the enlarged lymph nodes is often called the Ghon (or primary) complex. After a time the material within the granulomas becomes necrotic and caseous (cheesy).

The tubercles may heal spontaneously, become fibrotic or calcified, and persist as such for a lifetime in people who are otherwise healthy. They will show up on a chest radiograph

MYCOBACTERIA ASSOCIATED WITH HUMAN DISEASE	
species	**clinical disease**
*****slow growers** M. tuberculosis M. bovis M. leprae	tuberculosis bovine tuberculosis leprosy
M. avium M. intracellulare]**	disseminated infection in AIDS patients
M. kansasii	lung infections
M. marinum	skin infections and deeper infections (e.g. arthritis, osteomyelitis) associated with aquatic activity
M. scrofulaceum M. simiae M. szulgai M. ulcerans M. xenopi M. paratuberculosis	cervical adenitis in children lung, bone and kidney infections lung, skin and bone infections skin infections lung infections ? association with Crohn's disease
*****rapid growers** M. fortuitum M. chelonae	opportunist infections with introduction of organisms into deep subcutaneous tissues; usually associated with trauma or invasive procedures.

*slow growers require >7 days for visible growth from a dilute inoculum; rapid growers require <7 days for visible growth from a dilute inoculum

**M. avium complex; recent studies show that the two species are distinct. Of the M. avium complex, serotypes 1–6 and 8–11 are assigned to M. avium, serotypes 7, 12–17, 19, 20 and 25 assigned to M. intracellulare

Fig. 17.20 Many species of mycobacteria are associated with occasional disease, but the major pathogens of the genus are *M. tuberculosis, M. bovis* and *M. leprae.*

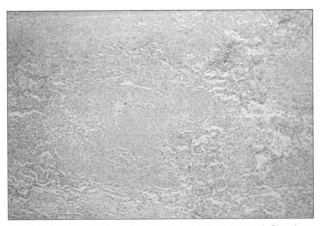

Fig. 17.21 Histopathology showing dense inflammatory infiltration, granuloma formation and caseous necrosis in pulmonary tuberculosis. (Courtesy of R Bryan.)

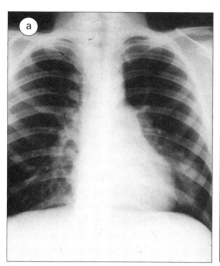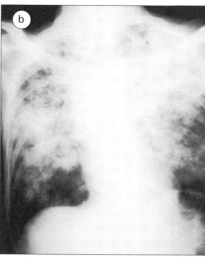

Fig. 17.22 Chest radiographs of (a) primary tuberculosis, showing the Ghon focus (arrow) in the lower left lung, and (b) post-primary pulmonary tuberculosis showing advanced disease. (Courtesy of JA Innes.)

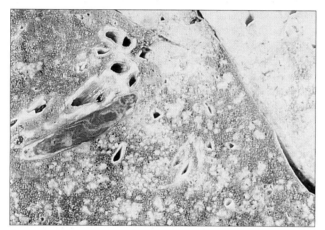

Fig. 17.23 Miliary tuberculosis. Gross specimen of lung showing the cut surface covered with white nodules, which are the miliary foci of tuberculosis. (Courtesy of JA Innes.)

as radio-opaque nodules *(Fig. 17.22)*. However, in a small percentage of people with primary infection, and particularly in the immunocompromised, the mycobacteria are not contained within the tubercles, but invade the bloodstream and cause disseminated disease ('miliary' tuberculosis, *Fig. 17.23*).

Secondary tuberculosis is due to reactivation of dormant mycobacteria, and is usually a consequence of impaired immune function resulting from some other cause such as malnutrition, infection (e.g. AIDS), chemotherapy for treatment of malignancy, or corticosteroids for the treatment of inflammatory diseases.

Tuberculosis illustrates the dual role of the immune response in infectious disease

On the one hand, the CMI response controls the infection and, when it is inadequate, the infection disseminates or reactivates. On the other hand, nearly all the pathology and disease is a consequence of this CMI response, as *M. tuberculosis* causes little or no direct or toxin-mediated damage.

Reactivation occurs most commonly in the apex of the lungs. This site is more highly oxygenated than elsewhere, allowing the mycobacteria to multiply more rapidly to produce caseous necrotic lesions, which spill over into other sites in the lung, and from where organisms spread to more distant sites in the body.

Primary tuberculosis is often asymptomatic

In contrast to pneumonia, which is usually an acute infection, the onset of tuberculosis is insidious, the infection proceeding for some time before the patient becomes sufficiently ill to seek medical attention. Primary tuberculosis is usually mild and asymptomatic and in 90% of cases does not proceed further. However, in the remaining 10% clinical disease develops.

Mycobacteria have the ability to colonize almost any site in the body. The clinical manifestations are variable: fatigue, weight loss, weakness and fever are all associated with tuberculosis. Infection in the lungs characteristically causes a chronic productive cough and the sputum may be blood-stained as a result of tissue destruction. Necrosis may erode blood vessels, which can rupture and cause death through hemorrhage.

Complications of M. tuberculosis infection arise from local spread or dissemination

The organism may disseminate via the lymphatics and bloodstream to other parts of the body. This usually occurs at the time of primary infection, and in this way chronic foci are established, which may proceed to necrosis and destruction in, for example, the kidney. Alternatively, spread may be by extension to a neighboring part of the lung – for instance when a tubercle erodes into a bronchus and discharges its contents, or into the pleural cavity, resulting in a pleural effusion.

Although the number of cases of pulmonary tuberculosis has been declining in developed countries since the beginning of the twentieth century, hastened by the advent of specific chemotherapy, the incidence of extrapulmonary tuberculosis has stayed roughly constant for many years and therefore makes up a greater proportion of the tuberculosis caseload in developed countries than in developing countries.

The Ziehl–Neelsen stain of sputum can provide a diagnosis of tuberculosis within one hour, while culture can take six weeks

A diagnosis of tuberculosis is suggested by the clinical signs and symptoms referred to above, supported by characteristic changes on chest radiography *(Fig. 17.22)* and positive skin test reactivity in the tuberculin (Mantoux) test. These tests are confirmed by microscopic demonstration of acid-fast rods and culture of *M. tuberculosis*. Microscopic examination of a smear of sputum stained by Ziehl–Neelsen's method or by auramine (see Chapter 14 and Appendix) often reveals acid-fast rods *(Fig. 17.24)*. This result can be obtained within one hour of receipt of the specimen in the laboratory. This is important because *M. tuberculosis* can take up to six weeks to grow in culture (although radiometric methods may reduce the time required for detection, see Appendix) and therefore confirmation of the diagnosis is necessarily delayed. Rapid non-culture tests to detect mycobacteria – for example using the polymerase chain reaction (PCR, see chapter 14) – are becoming increasingly available. Further tests are required to identify the species of *Mycobacterium* and to establish susceptibility to antituberculous drugs.

Specific antituberculous drugs and prolonged therapy are needed to treat tuberculosis

Mycobacteria are innately resistant to most antibacterial agents and specific antituberculous drugs have to be used and are reviewed in Chapter 30. The key features of treatment are the use of:

- Combination therapy – usually three drugs (e.g. isoniazid, rifampin, ethambutol) to prevent emergence of resistance.
- Prolonged therapy – minimum six months – which is necessary to eradicate these slow-growing intracellular organisms.

The number of strains resistant to the first-line antituberculous drugs has increased and has stimulated health agencies to monitor treatment more carefully (e.g. DOTS – directly observed treatment, short-course) and rekindled research interest in finding new agents.

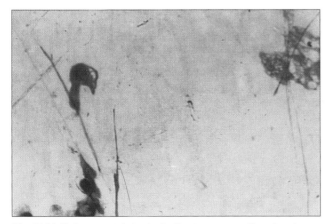

Fig. 17.24 Pulmonary tuberculosis. Sputum preparation showing pink-stained, acid-fast tubercle bacilli. (Ziehl–Neelsen stain) (Courtesy of JA Innes.)

Tuberculosis is prevented by improved social conditions, immunization and chemoprophylaxis

The steady decline in incidence of tuberculosis since the beginning of the twentieth century, and before specific preventive measures were available, underlines the importance of improvements in social conditions in the prevention of this and many other infectious diseases. However, recent years have seen an increase in the number of cases associated with AIDS and, in some countries in the developing world, HIV infection and AIDS are threatening to overwhelm tuberculosis control programs; an estimated one-third of AIDS-related deaths in 1995 were thought to be due to tuberculosis.

Immunization with a live attenuated vaccine, the so-called BCG (bacille Calmette-Guérin) vaccine, has been used effectively in situations where tuberculosis is prevalent. Immunization, which confers positive skin test reactivity, does not prevent infection, but it allows the body to react quickly to limit proliferation of the organisms. In areas where there is a low prevalence of disease, immunization has been largely replaced by chemoprophylaxis.

Prophylaxis with isoniazid for one year is recommended for people who have had close contact with a case of tuberculosis. It is also advocated for individuals who show recent conversion to skin test positivity, when it is essentially early treatment of subclinical infection rather than prophylaxis.

Aspergillosis

Aspergillus fumigatus can cause allergic bronchopulmonary aspergillosis, aspergilloma or disseminated aspergillosis

The genus *Aspergillus* contains many species of fungi, which are ubiquitous in the environment. They do not form part of the normal flora of man, but some species, notably *A. fumigatus*, are able to cause a range of diseases, including:

- Allergic bronchopulmonary aspergillosis, which is, as its name suggests, an allergic response to the presence of *Aspergillus* antigen in the lungs and occurs in patients with asthma.
- Aspergilloma in patients with pre-existing lung cavities or chronic pulmonary disorders. *Aspergillus* colonizes a cavity and grows to produce a fungal ball, a mass of entangled hyphae – the aspergilloma *(Fig. 17.25)*. The fungi do not invade the lung tissue, but the presence of a large aspergilloma can cause respiratory problems.
- Disseminated disease in the immunosuppressed patient when the fungus invades from the lungs.

Treatment of invasive aspergillosis is very difficult due to the limited number and toxic nature of antifungal agents active against *Aspergillus* (see Chapter 30) and the lack of functional host defenses.

Cystic fibrosis

Cystic fibrosis is the most common lethal inherited disorder among Caucasians, with an incidence of approximately 1 in 2500 live births. The disease is characterized by pancreatic insufficiency, abnormal sweat electrolyte concentrations and production of very viscid bronchial secretions. The latter tend to lead to stasis in the lungs and this predisposes to infection.

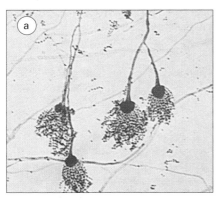
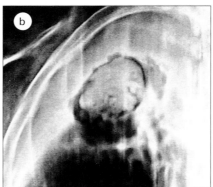
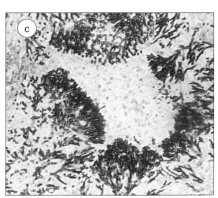

Fig. 17.25 *Aspergillus fumigatus.* (a) Lactophenol cotton blue stained preparation showing the characteristic conidiophores. (b) Aspergilloma. Tomogram showing fungus ball contained within the lung cavity, outlined by air space. (Courtesy of JA Innes.) (c) Invasive aspergillosis. Histologic section showing fungal hyphae invading the lung parenchyma and blood vessels. (Grocott stain) (Courtesy of C Kibbler.)

Ps. aeruginosa colonizes the lungs of almost all 15–20-year-olds with cystic fibrosis

The respiratory mucosa of individuals with cystic fibrosis presents a different environment for potential pathogens to that found in healthy individuals without cystic fibrosis, and the common infecting organisms and the nature of infections differ from other lung infections. These invaders include:

- *Staph. aureus,* which causes respiratory distress and lung damage, but can be well controlled by specific antistaphylococcal chemotherapy.
- *Pseudomonas aeruginosa,* which is the pathogen of paramount importance (see below).
- In recent years *Ps. cepacia,* another member of the genus *Pseudomonas,* which has become an increasing problem.
- *H. influenzae,* typically non-encapsulated strains, which may be found in association with *Staph. aureus* and *Ps. aeruginosa*; their pathogenic significance is unclear, but they appear to contribute to respiratory exacerbations.

Ps. aeruginosa infection is uncommon in those under five years of age, but colonizes the lungs of almost all patients aged 15–20 years, often encouraged by its intrinsic resistance to antistaphylococcal agents. Early in the course of infection normal colony types are grown from sputum cultures, but as infection progresses the organism changes to a highly mucoid form, almost mimicking the mucoid secretions of the patient *(Fig. 17.26).* These mucoid forms are thought to grow in microcolonies in the lung, but most of the lung damage is due to immunologic responses to the organisms and to the alginate, which forms the mucoid material *(Fig. 17.27). Ps. aeruginosa* rarely invades beyond the lung even in the most severely infected individuals.

Although specific antibacterial chemotherapy can reduce the symptoms of infection and improve the quality of life, infections, particularly with *Ps. aeruginosa* and *Ps. cepacia,* are impossible to eradicate and are frequently a cause of death. Heart–lung transplantation is a successful alternative treatment for some patients.

Lung abscess
Lung abscesses usually contain a mixture of bacteria including anaerobes

This is a suppurative infection of the lung, sometimes referred to as 'necrotizing pneumonia'. The most common predisposing cause is aspiration of respiratory or gastric secretions as a result of altered consciousness. The infection is therefore endogenous in origin and cultures often reveal a mixture of bacteria, with anaerobes such as *Bacteroides* and *Fusobacterium* playing an important role *(Fig. 17.28).*

Patients with lung abscesses may be ill for at least two weeks before presentation and usually produce large amounts of sputum, which, if foul-smelling, gives a strong hint of the presence of anaerobes and often suggests the diagnosis. Most diagnoses are made from chest radiographs *(Fig. 17.5d)* and the cause confirmed by microbiologic investigation.

Treatment of lung abscess should include an anti-anaerobic drug and last 2–4 months

Because of the likely presence of anaerobes, a suitable anti-anaerobic agent such as metronidazole should be part of the treatment regimen, and treatment may needed for 2–4 months to prevent relapse. If diagnosis and treatment are delayed, infection may spread to the pleural space, giving rise to empyema (see below).

Pleural effusion and empyema
Up to 50% of patients with pneumonia have a pleural effusion

Pleural effusions arise in a variety of different diseases. Sometimes the organisms infecting the lung spread to the pleural space and give rise to a purulent exudate or 'empyema'.

Pleural effusions can be demonstrated radiologically, but

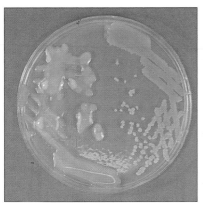

Fig. 17.26
Pseudomonas aeruginosa isolated from the sputum of patients with cystic fibrosis characteristically grows in a very mucoid colonial form, shown here on the left of the picture, with the normal colonial form on the right for comparison.

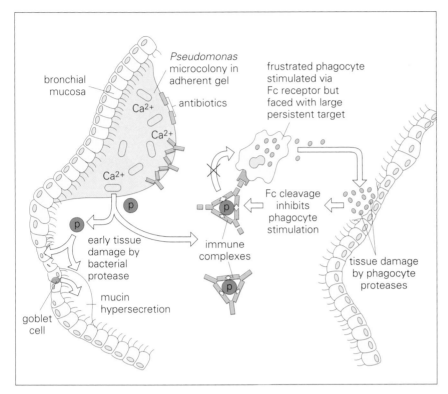

Fig. 17.27 *Pseudomonas* infection in the lung of cystic fibrotics is chronic, but rarely invasive beyond the bronchial mucosa. The organisms are thought to grow in microcolonies embedded in a calcium (Ca^{2+})-dependent mucoid alginate gel, which contains DNA and tracheobronchial mucin, and attaches to the bronchial mucosa. This protects the organisms from the host defenses and provides a physical and electrolyte barrier to antibiotics. Much of the damage to tissue is thought to be due to the slow release of bacterial proteases (which disrupt the mucosa and cause mucin hypersecretion), immunopathologic mechanisms exacerbated by the size, antigenicity and persistence of the alginate matrix, and the indirect action of immune complexes associated with *Pseudomonas* antigens (P). Tissue damage is also caused by phagocyte proteases. Intermittent exacerbations can be explained by the cleavage of the Fc of immune complexes by these proteases and consequent inhibition of further phagocyte stimulation. (Redrawn from Govan and Glass, 1990.)

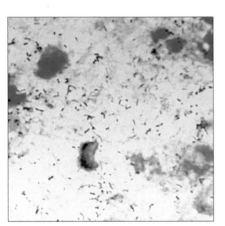

Fig. 17.28 Gram-stain of pus from a lung abscess showing Gram-positive cocci and both Gram-negative and Gram-positive rods. (Courtesy of JR Cantey.)

detection of empyema can be difficult, particularly in a patient with extensive pneumonia.

Aspiration of pleural fluid provides material for microbiologic examination and *Staph. aureus*, Gram-negative rods and anaerobes are commonly involved.

Treatment should be directed at drainage of pus, eradication of infection and expansion of the lung.

Parasitic Infections of the Lower Respiratory Tract

A variety of parasites localize to the lung or involve the lung at some stage in their development

Such parasites include:

- Nematodes such as *Ascaris* and the hookworms (see Chapter 20), which migrate through the lungs as they move to the small intestine, breaking out of the capillaries around the alveoli to enter the bronchioles. The damage caused by this process, and the development of inflammatory responses, can lead to a transient pneumonitis.
- Schistosome larvae, which may cause mild respiratory symptoms as they migrate through the lungs (see Chapter 25).
- The microfilarae of filarial nematodes such as *Wuchereria* or *Brugia*, which appear in the peripheral circulation with a regular diurnal or nocturnal periodicity, their appearance coinciding with the time at which the vector blood-sucking insects are likely to feed. Outside these periods the larvae become sequestered in the capillaries of the lung. Under certain conditions, as yet undefined, and in certain individuals, the presence of the larvae triggers a condition known as 'tropical pulmonary eosinophilia' (TPE or Weingarten's syndrome). This is characterized by cough, respiratory distress and marked eosinophilia; microfilariae are usually absent from the blood.
- *Ascaris* and *Strongyloides* infections, which may also trigger a pulmonary eosinophilia, although the condition is distinct from TPE.
- *Echinococcus granulosus* infection, which leads to the development of hydatid cysts in a proportion (20–30%) of cases due to localization of the larvae of the tapeworm in the lungs (see Chapter 12). These cysts may reach a considerable size, causing respiratory distress, largely as a consequence of the mechanical pressure exerted on lung tissue.
- *Entamoeba histolytica* infection, which may rarely involve the lung.
- *Paragonimus westermani*, the oriental lung fluke, which is the most important example of one of the very few adult parasites that live in the lung. Infection is acquired by eating crustaceans containing the infective metacercariae. These migrate from the intestine across the body cavity

and penetrate into the lungs. The adults develop within fibrous cysts, which connect with the bronchi to provide an exit for the eggs *(Fig. 17.29)*. Infections cause chest pain and difficulty in breathing, and can cause bronchopneumonia when large numbers of parasites are present. Praziquantel is an efficient anthelmintic for this infection.

Summary

Respiratory tract infections are among the most common infections seen in people attending their family doctor, and account for considerable morbidity and absence from school and work. Infections of the upper respiratory tract, covered in Chapter 15, are usually mild and self-limiting. In contrast, infections lower in the respiratory tract, which are sometimes caused by the same pathogens, tend to be severe and may be life-threatening. Respiratory disease (mostly bacterial) is the single largest cause of death in childhood worldwide, especially in the first year of life.

The spectrum of pathogens is wide, but the most common causes of lower respiratory tract infection tend to be viral in children and bacterial in adults. Precise identification of the etiology is important to ensure optimal therapy. Many of the infectious agents are spread from person to person in aerosols and therefore prevention of infection is difficult to achieve, although improvements in living conditions and avoiding overcrowding undoubtedly play impor-

tant roles. The recognition of the risk of *Legionella* infection associated with aerosols from cooling towers and air conditioning systems has led to recommendations for the maintenance of such systems. The associations between exposure to particular animals or travel in certain areas of the world and specific pathogens are well-documented and stress the importance of taking a full history whenever possible.

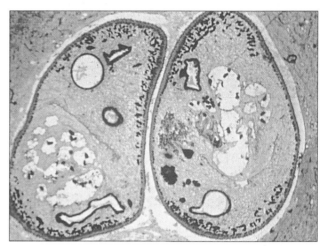

Fig. 17.29 Two adult *Paragonimus* contained within a fibrous cyst in the lung. (Courtesy of H Zaiman.)

A 30-year-old man presents with a 10-day history of tiredness, headache, fever and dry cough. He smokes 20 cigarettes a day, his past medical history is unremarkable, and there is nothing else of note on systems review. Relevant findings on examination include a temperature of 38°C, dyspnea and a skin rash consistent with erythema multiforme. Auscultation of his chest reveals a few scattered crepitations and is otherwise unremarkable. The results of investigations are: hemoglobin 10 g/dl; white cell count 6 x 109/l; erythrocyte sedimentation rate 45 mm/h; urea and electrolytes normal; chest radiograph, patchy shadowing.

1. What is the differential diagnosis?
2. Which questions particularly relevant to the differential diagnosis have not been asked?
3. What further investigations would you perform?
4. The results of some of these investigations are *Mycoplasma* particle agglutination test titer 1024; *Mycoplasma* CFT acute serum titer 160; *Mycoplasma* CFT convalescent serum titer 2560; cold agglutinins, positive. What is the diagnosis?
5. How would you treat this patient?

- Although continous from nose to alveoli, the respiratory tract is divided into 'upper' and 'lower' from the viewpoint of infection.
- Infections in the lower respiratory tract are spread by the airborne route (except parasites), are acute or chronic, tend to be severe and may be fatal without correct treatment. They are caused by a wide range of organisms – usually bacteria or viruses, but also fungi and parasites.
- Bronchitis, an inflammatory condition of the tracheobronchial tree, is usually chronic with acute exacerbations associated with infection by viruses and bacteria. The disease is characterized by cough and excessive mucus production and the diagnosis is clinical. Antibiotics are often given, but their efficacy is uncertain.
- Bronchiolitis, usually caused by RSV, is acute and severe in young children. RSV causes outbreaks in the community and in hospitals. The disease has an immunopathologic basis and specific treatment (ribavirin) is difficult. No vaccine is available.
- Pneumonia is caused by a variety of pathogens depending upon the patients' age, previous or underlying disease, and occupational and geographic factors. Correct microbiologic diagnosis is essential to optimize therapy. Mortality from pneumonia remains significant.
- *B. pertussis* colonizes the ciliated respiratory epithelium causing the specifically human infection whooping cough. Pertussis toxin and other toxic factors are important for virulence. Diagnosis is clinical, alerted by the characteristic paroxysmal cough. Supportive care is paramount; antibiotics play a peripheral role. Prevention by immunization is effective, and new safer vaccines are becoming available.
- Influenza viruses cause endemic, epidemic and pandemic infections as a result of the capacity of the virus for antigenic drift and shift. The disease is acute in onset and can be clinically severe. Viral damage to the respiratory mucosa predisposes to secondary bacterial pneumonia. Antiviral agents are available, but of limited efficacy. Immunization is important, but needs to be kept up to date due to the frequent antigenic changes in the circulating virus.
- Tuberculosis, a major killer, is becoming more common due to its association with AIDS. Infection is usually chronic. Primary infection with *M. tuberculosis* results in a localized pulmonary lesion, while secondary disease is due to reactivation as a result of an impairment of immune function. Clinical diagnosis is supported by demonstrating the acid-fast *M. tuberculosis* in sputum. Effective treatment is available, but long courses of drug combinations are essential. Chemoprophylaxis and BCG immunoprophylaxis are important in prevention.
- *A. fumigatus* causes disease in the lung ranging from invasive disease in the immunocompromised to allergic conditions in the otherwise healthy. Effective treatment is difficult due to the limited number of active antifungals and lack of host defenses.
- Cystic fibrosis is an inherited disease that predisposes to a particular pattern of lung disease characterized by infection with *Ps. aeruginosa*. Infection can be controlled by antibacterials, but rarely eradicated.
- Various species of parasites pass through or localize in the lungs at some stage in their life cycle. Damage is limited unless the parasite load is high, and is usually immunopathologic in nature.

Further Reading

Alonzo de Velasco E, Verheul AF, Verhoef J, Snipple H. Streptococcus pneumoniae: virulence factors, pathogenesis, and vaccines. Microbiol Rev 1995;**59**:591–603.

Couch RB, Kasel JA, Glezen WP et al. Influenza: Its control in persons and populations. J Infect Dis 1986;**153**:431–447.

Department of Health and Welsh Office. The control of legionellae in health care premises. London: HMSO, 1988.

Govan JRW, Glass S. The microbiology and therapy of cystic fibrosis lung infections. Rev Med Microbiol 1990;**1**:19–28.

Hutchinson DN. Nosocomial legionellosis. Rev Med Microbiol 1990;**1**:108–115.

Jacobs E. Mycoplasma pneumoniae virulence factors and the immune response. Rev Med Microbiol 1991;**2**:83–90.

Kawaoka Y, Webster RG. Molecular mechanisms of acquisition of virulence in influenza virus in nature. Microb Pathogenesis 1988;**5**:311–318.

La Via WV, Marks MI, Stutman HR. Respiratory syncytial virus puzzles. Clinical features, pathophysiology, treatment and prevention. J Pediatr 1992;**121**:503–510.

Marrie TJ, Grayston JT, Wang P, Kuo C–C. Pneumonia associated with the TWAR strain of Chlamydia. Ann Intern Med 1987;**106**:507–511.

Moser MR, Bender TR, Marelolis NS et al. An outbreak of influenza aboard a commercial airliner. Am J Epidemiol 1979;**110**:1–7.

Pedersen SS. Clinical efficacy of ciprofloxacin in lower respiratory tract infections. Scand J Infect Dis 1989;Suppl.**60**:89–97.

Sudre P, ten Dam G, Kochi A. Tuberculosis: a global overview of the situation today. Bull WHO 1992;**70**:149–159.

Webster RG, Bean WJ, Gorman OT et al. Evolution and ecology of influenza viruses. Microbiol Rev 1992;**56**:152–179.

Introduction

Urinary tract infections are common, especially among women
The urinary tract is one of the most common sites of bacterial infection, particularly in females; 10–20% of women have a urinary tract infection (UTI) at some time in their life and a significant number have recurrent infections. Although the majority of infections are acute and short-lived, they contribute to a significant amount of morbidity in the population. Severe infections result in a loss of renal function and serious long-term sequelae. In females, a distinction is made between cystitis, urethritis and vaginitis, but the genitourinary tract is a continuum and the symptoms often overlap.

Acquisition and Etiology

Bacterial infection is usually acquired by the ascending route from the urethra to the bladder

The infection may then proceed to the kidney. Occasionally, bacteria infecting the urinary tract invade the bloodstream to cause septicemia. Less commonly, infection may result from hematogenous spread of an organism to the kidney, with the renal tissue being the first part of the tract to be infected.

The Gram-negative rod Escherichia coli is the commonest cause of ascending UTI

Other members of the Enterobacteriaceae are also implicated *(Fig. 18.1)*. *Proteus mirabilis* is often associated with urinary stones (calculi), probably because this organism produces a potent urease, which acts on urea to produce ammonia, rendering the urine alkaline. *Klebsiella, Enterobacter, Serratia* spp. and *Pseudomonas aeruginosa* are more frequently found in hospital-acquired UTI because their resistance to antibiotics favors their selection in hospital patients (see Chapter 34).

Among the Gram-positive species, *Staphylococcus saprophyticus* seems to have a particular propensity for causing infections in young sexually active women. *Staphylococcus epidermidis* and *Enterococcus* species are more often associated with UTI in hospitalized patients, where their multiple antibiotic resistance can cause treatment difficulties. More recently, capnophilic species (organisms that grow better in air enriched with carbon dioxide), including corynebacteria and lactobacilli, have been implicated as possible causes of UTI. Obligate anaerobes are very rarely involved.

When there has been hematogenous spread to the urinary tract, other species may be found e.g. *Salmonella typhi, Staphylococcus aureus* and *Mycobacterium tuberculosis* (renal tuberculosis).

Viral causes of UTI appear to be rare

Certain viruses may be recovered from the urine in the absence of urinary tract disease and include:
- The human polyomaviruses, JC and BK, enter the body via the respiratory tract, spread through the body and infect epithelial cells in the kidney tubules and ureter, where they establish latency with persistence of the viral genome, but not infectious virus. About 35% of kidneys from healthy individuals contain polyomavirus DNA sequences. However, during normal pregnancy the viruses may reactivate asymptomatically, with the appearance of large amounts of virus in the urine. Reactivation also occurs in immunocompromised patients (see Chapter 28).
- High titers of cytomegalovirus (CMV) may be shed asymptomatically in the urine of congenitally-infected infants (see Chapter 21).

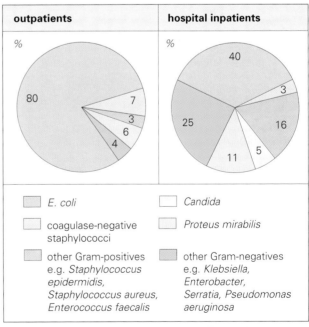

Fig. 18.1 Common causes of urinary tract infection. The percentages of infections caused by different bacteria in outpatients and hospital inpatients are shown. *Escherichia coli* is by far the most common isolate in both groups of patients, but note the difference in the percentage of infections caused by other Gram-negative rods. These isolates often carry multiple antibiotic resistance and colonize patients in hospital, especially those receiving antibiotics.

- In contrast to asymptomatic shedding, some serotypes of adenovirus have been implicated as a cause of hemorrhagic cystitis.
- Finally, the rodent-borne hantavirus responsible for Korean hemorrhagic fever, infects capillary blood vessels in the kidney and can cause a renal syndrome with proteinuria.

Very few parasites cause UTIs

Other causes of UTI include:

- The fungi *Candida* spp. and *Histoplasma capsulatum*.
- The protozoan *Trichomonas vaginalis* (see Chapter 19), which can cause urethritis in both males and females, but is most often considered as a cause of vaginitis.
- Infections with *Schistosoma haematobium* (see Chapter 25), which result in inflammation of the bladder and commonly hematuria. The eggs penetrate the bladder wall, and in severe infections large granulomatous reactions can occur and the eggs may become calcified. Bladder cancer is associated with chronic infections, although the mechanism is uncertain. Obstruction of the ureter as a result of egg-induced inflammatory changes can also lead to hydronephrosis.

Pathogenesis of UTIs

A variety of mechanical factors predispose to UTI

Anything that disrupts normal urine flow or complete emptying of the bladder or facilitates access of organisms to the bladder will predispose an individual to infection *(Fig. 18.2)*. The shorter female urethra is a less effective deterrent to infection than the male urethra (see Chapter 8). Sexual intercourse facilitates the movement of organisms up the urethra, particularly in females, so the incidence of UTI is higher among sexually active women than among celibate women. Preceding bacterial colonization of the periurethral area of the vagina is perhaps important (see below).

In male infants, UTIs are more common in the uncircumcised and this is associated with colonization of the inside of the prepuce and urethra with fecal organisms.

Pregnancy, prostatic hypertrophy, renal calculi, tumors and strictures are the main causes of obstruction to complete bladder emptying

When there is a residual urine of more than 2–3 ml, infection is more likely. Infection, superimposed on urinary tract obstruction, may lead to ascent of infection to the kidney and rapid destruction of renal tissue.

Loss of neurologic control of the bladder and sphincters (e.g. in spina bifida, paraplegia or multiple sclerosis), and the resultant large residual volume of urine in the bladder, causes a functional obstruction to urine flow and such patients are particularly prone to recurrent infections.

Vesicoureteral reflux (reflux of urine from the bladder cavity up the ureters, sometimes into the renal pelvis or parenchyma) is common in children with anatomic abnormalities of the urinary tract and may predispose to ascending infection and kidney damage. Reflux may also occur in association with infection in children without underlying abnormalities, but tends to disappear with age.

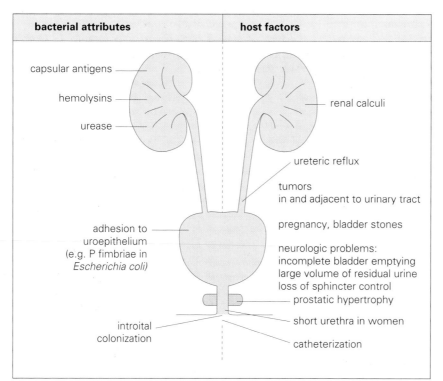

bacterial attributes	host factors
capsular antigens	renal calculi
hemolysins	ureteric reflux
urease	tumors in and adjacent to urinary tract
adhesion to uroepithelium (e.g. P fimbriae in *Escherichia coli*)	pregnancy, bladder stones
introital colonization	neurologic problems: incomplete bladder emptying large volume of residual urine loss of sphincter control
	prostatic hypertrophy
	short urethra in women
	catheterization

Fig. 18.2 Bacterial attributes and host factors favoring urinary tract infection (UTI). Abnormalities of the urinary tract tend to predispose to infection. Bacterial adherence factors have been studied in detail, but relatively little is known about other bacterial virulence factors in UTI.

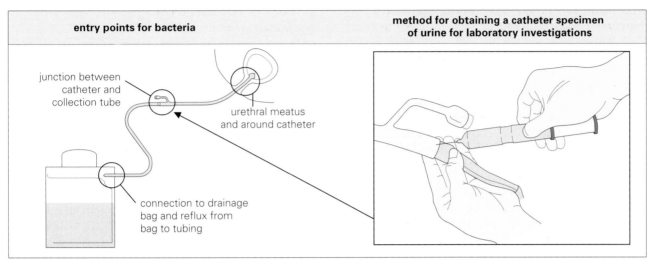

| entry points for bacteria | method for obtaining a catheter specimen of urine for laboratory investigations |

junction between catheter and collection tube

urethral meatus and around catheter

connection to drainage bag and reflux from bag to tubing

Fig. 18.3 The urinary catheter. Catheterization is an important predisposing factor for infection. Bacteria can be pushed into the bladder as the catheter is inserted and, while the catheter is in place, bacteria reach the bladder by tracking up between the outside of the catheter and the urethra. Contamination of the catheter drainage system by bacteria from other sources can also result in infection.

Specimens of bladder urine for laboratory investigations can be collected from catheterized patients as shown. The second port (above) is for putting fluids into the bladder. Urine from the drainage bag should not be tested because it may have been standing for several hours.

Despite reports that pyelonephritis (infection of the kidney) is a common finding in people with diabetes mellitus at postmortem, clinical surveys have failed to produce convincing evidence that there is a significant difference in the prevalence of UTI between people of the same age with and without diabetes mellitus. However, people with diabetes mellitus may have more severe UTIs, and if diabetic neuropathy interferes with normal bladder function, persistent UTIs are common.

Catheterization is a major predisposing factor for UTI

During insertion of the catheter, bacteria may be carried directly into the bladder and, while *in situ*, the catheter facilitates bacterial access to the bladder either via the lumen of the catheter or by tracking up between the outside of the catheter and the urethral wall *(Fig. 18.3)*. The catheter disrupts the normal bladder's protective function action and allows bacteria to get a foothold.

Relatively little is known about the virulence factors of the causative organisms (Fig. 18.2)

The conflict between host and parasite in the urinary tract has been discussed in Chapter 7. Most urinary tract pathogens originate in the fecal flora, but only the aerobic and facultative species such as *E. coli* possess the attributes required to colonize and infect the urinary tract. The ability to cause infection of the urinary tract is limited to certain serogroups of *E. coli* (e.g. 01, 02, 04, 06, 07 and 075) and these serotypes differ from those associated with gastrointestinal tract infection (see Chapter 20). The success of these strains may be attributable in part to their ability to colonize the periurethral areas. Some *E. coli* have been shown to have particular types of fimbriae (pili), which enable them to adhere to urethral and bladder epithelium. Studies

with other species of urinary tract pathogens have confirmed the presence of adhesins for uroepithelial cells *(Fig. 18.4)*.

Other features of *E. coli* appear to assist in the localization of organisms in the kidney and in renal damage:
- The capsular acid polysaccharide (K) antigens are associated with the ability to cause pyelonephritis and are known to enable *E. coli* strains to resist host defenses by inhibiting phagocytosis.
- Hemolysin production by *E. coli* is linked with the capacity to cause kidney damage; many hemolysins act more generally as membrane-damaging toxins.

The production of urease by organisms such as *Proteus* spp. has been correlated with their ability to cause pyelonephritis and stones.

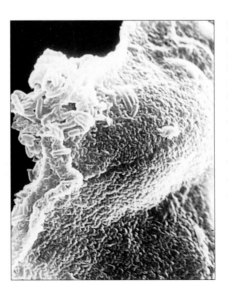

Fig. 18.4 Scanning electron micrograph showing bacteria attached to an exfoliated uroepithelial cell from a patient with acute cystitis. (Courtesy of Dr TSJ Elliot and the editor of *British Journal of Urology.*)

The healthy urinary tract is resistant to bacterial colonization

With the exception of the urethral mucosa, the urinary tract usually eliminates microorganisms rapidly and efficiently (see Chapter 7). The pH, chemical content and flushing mechanism of urine help to dispose of organisms in the urethra. Although urine is a good culture medium for most bacteria, it is inhibitory to some, and anaerobes and other species (non-hemolytic streptococci, corynebacteria and staphylococci), which comprise most of the normal urethral flora do not readily multiply in urine.

The role of humoral immunity in the host's defense against infection of the urinary tract is poorly understood. After infection of the kidney, IgG and secretory IgA antibodies can be detected in urine, but the protective role of these antibodies against subsequent infection is unclear. Infection of the lower urinary tract is usually associated with a low or undetectable serologic response reflecting the superficial nature of the infection; the bladder and urethral mucosa are rarely invaded in UTIs.

Clinical Features and Complications

Acute lower UTIs cause dysuria, urgency and frequency

Acute infections of the lower urinary tract are characterized by a rapid onset of:
- Dysuria (burning pain on passing urine).
- Urgency (the urgent need to pass urine).
- Frequency of micturition.

However, UTIs in the elderly and those with indwelling catheters are usually asymptomatic.

The urine is cloudy due to the presence of pus cells (pyuria) and bacteria (bacteriuria), and may contain blood (hematuria). Examination of urine specimens in the laboratory is essential to confirm the diagnosis. Patients with genital tract infections such as vaginal thrush or chlamydial urethritis may present with similar symptoms (see Chapter 19).

Pyuria in the absence of positive urine cultures can be due to chlamydiae or tuberculosis and is also seen in patients receiving antibacterial therapy for UTI, as the bacteria are inhibited or killed by the antibacterial agent before the inflammatory response dies away.

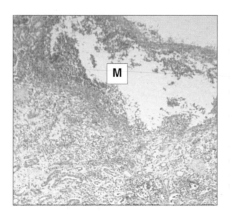

Fig. 18.5 Histologic appearance of the kidney in acute pyelonephritis showing the intense inflammatory reaction and microabscesses(M). (Hematoxylin and eosin stain) (Courtesy of MJ Wood.)

Recurrent infections of the lower urinary tract occur in a significant proportion of patients. They may be:
- Relapses, caused by the same strain of organism.
- Reinfections by different organisms.

Recurrent infections can result in chronic inflammatory changes in the bladder, prostate and periurethral glands.

Acute bacterial prostatitis causes systemic symptoms (fever) and local symptoms (perineal and low back pain, dysuria and frequency)

Acute bacterial prostatitis may arise from ascending or hematogenous infection, and people lacking the antibacterial substances normally present in prostatic fluid are perhaps more susceptible. Chronic bacterial prostatitis, however, although usually caused by *E. coli*, is difficult to cure and can be a source of relapsing infection within the urinary tract.

Upper UTIs

Although it may be important to know whether an infection is restricted to the bladder (lower urinary tract) or has ascended to the upper urinary tract and kidney, there are no satisfactory methods for distinguishing the two other than by examining urine directly from the ureter by ureteric catheterization.

Pyelonephritis causes a fever and lower urinary tract symptoms

Patients with pyelonephritis (infection of the kidney, *Fig. 18.5*) present with lower urinary tract symptoms and usually have a fever. Staphylococci are a common cause and renal abscesses are generally present. Recurrent episodes of pyelonephritis result in a loss of function of renal tissue, which may in turn cause hypertension, itself a cause of renal damage. Infection associated with stone formation can result in obstruction of the renal tract and septicemia.

Hematuria is a feature of endocarditis and a manifestation of immune complex disease, as well as a result of infections of the kidney, and its presence warrants careful investigation. Pyuria may be associated with kidney infection with *M. tuberculosis*. This organism cannot be grown by normal urine culture methods (see Appendix) and therefore the patient may appear to have a sterile pyuria.

Asymptomatic infection (i.e. significant numbers of bacteria in the urine in the absence of symptoms, see below) can be detected only by screening urine samples in the laboratory. It is important in:
- Pregnant women and young children, where failure to treat may result in chronic renal damage.
- People undergoing instrumentation of the urinary tract in whom bacteriuria may proceed to bacteremia.

Laboratory Diagnosis of UTIs

Methods for processing urine specimens in the laboratory are summarized in the Appendix. A key feature is the detection of significant bacteriuria.

Infection can be distinguished from contamination by quantitative culture methods

In health the urinary tract is sterile, though the distal region of the urethra is colonized with commensal organisms, which may include periurethral and fecal organisms. As urine specimens are usually collected by voiding a specimen into a sterile container they become contaminated with the periurethral flora during collection. Infection can be distinguished from contamination by quantitative culture methods. Bacteriuria is defined as 'significant' when a properly collected midstream urine (MSU) specimen is shown to contain over 10^5 organisms/ml. Infected urine usually contains only a single bacterial species. Contaminated urine usually has less than 10^4 organisms/ml and often contains more than one bacterial species *(Fig. 18.6)*. Distinguishing infection from contamination when counts are 10^4–10^5 organisms/ml can be difficult. Careful collection and rapid transport of urine specimens to the laboratory are essential (see below and Chapter 13).

It is important to recognize that the criteria for 'significant bacteriuria' do not apply to urine specimens collected from catheters or nephrostomy tubes or by suprapubic aspiration directly from the bladder, in which any number of organisms may be significant because the specimen is not contaminated by periurethral flora. In addition, infection of sites in the urinary tract below the bladder, and by organisms that are not members of the normal fecal flora, may not lead to the presence of significant numbers in the urine.

The usual urine specimen for microbiological examination is an MSU sample

An MSU sample should be collected into a sterile wide-mouthed container after careful cleansing of the labia or glans with soap (not antiseptic) and water, and after allowing the first part of the urine stream to be voided as this helps to wash out contaminants in the lower urethra. After suitable instruction the majority of adult patients can collect satisfactory samples with minimum supervision, though collection may be difficult for elderly and bedridden patients and consideration should be given to these difficulties when interpreting results.

Collection of MSU samples from babies and young children is obviously difficult. 'Bag urine' may be collected by sticking a plastic bag to the perineum in girls or to the penis in boys, but such specimens are frequently heavily contaminated with fecal organisms. These problems can be overcome by suprapubic aspiration of urine directly from the bladder *(Fig. 18.7)*.

Urine specimens should be transported to the laboratory with minimum delay because urine is a good growth medium for many bacteria and multiplication of organisms in the specimen between collection and culture will distort the results (see Chapter 13).

Ideally, samples should be collected before antimicrobial therapy is started. If the patient is receiving, or has received, therapy within the past 48 hours, this should be stated clearly on the request form.

For patients with a catheter, a catheter specimen of urine is used for microbiological examination

Patients should not be catheterized simply to obtain a urine sample. Urine is obtained from patients who have a catheter *in situ* by withdrawing a sample with a syringe and needle from the catheter tube as shown in *Figure 18.3*. Urine that has been standing in the catheter drainage bag for hours is unsuitable for testing because the organisms may have multiplied to give much greater numbers than those present in the patient.

Special urine samples are required to detect M. tuberculosis and S. haematobium

These include:

* Three early morning urine samples on consecutive days for *M. tuberculosis*. These do not require the same precautions during collection as an MSU sample because the culture technique prohibits the growth of organisms other than mycobacteria.
* The last few millilitres of a morning urine sample collected after exercise for detection of *S. haematobium*.

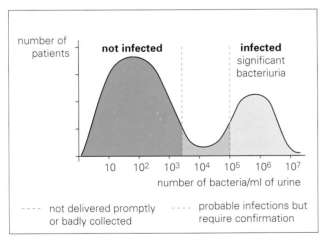

Fig. 18.6 Significant bacteriuria. Voided specimens of urine are rarely sterile because the urine is contaminated with organisms from the periurethral area during collection. Even well-collected specimens from healthy individuals may contain up to 10^3 bacteria/ml of urine. Studies by Kass (1956, see Further Reading) suggested that a count of 10^5 bacteria/ml was a reliable indicator of infection. However, there are various reasons why lower counts may sometimes be significant, as discussed in the text.

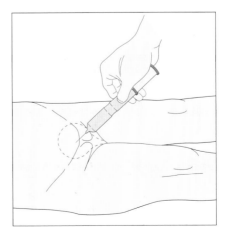

Fig. 18.7 Suprapubic aspiration of bladder urine. Urine samples can be collected directly from the bladder by insertion of a needle. This method is useful in young children from whom it is difficult to obtain uncontaminated midstream urine specimens.

Laboratory investigations

Urine specimens should be examined macroscopically and microscopically and should be cultured by quantitative or semiquantitative methods, as summarized in Chapter 14.

Microscopic examination of urine allows a rapid preliminary report

Bacteria may be seen on microscopy when present in the specimen in large numbers. However, they are not necessarily indicative of infection, but may indicate that the specimen has been poorly collected or left at room temperature for a prolonged period of time.

The presence of red and white blood cells, although abnormal, is not necessarily indicative of UTI. Hematuria may be present in association with:

- Infection of the urinary tract and elsewhere (e.g. bacterial endocarditis).
- Renal trauma.
- Calculi.
- Urinary tract carcinomas.
- Clotting disorders.
- Thrombocytopenia.

Occasionally, red blood cells may contaminate urine specimens of menstruating women.

White blood cells are present in the urine in very small numbers (e.g. < 10/ml) in health; a count of over 10/ml is considered abnormal, but is not always associated with bacteriuria. Sterile pyuria is an important finding and may reflect:

- Concurrent antibiotic therapy.
- Other diseases such as neoplasms or urinary calculi.
- Infection with organisms not detected by routine urine culture methods (see Appendix).

Renal tubular cells, seen in the urine of aspirin-misusers, may be confused with white blood cells. Urinary casts are also indicative of renal tubular damage.

A laboratory diagnosis of significant bacteriuria requires quantification of the bacteria

Culture media and methods are outlined in the Appendix. Conventional methods produce results within 18–24 hours, but rapid methods based on bioluminescence, turbidimetry and flow cytometry are also available. In some laboratories, direct antibiotic susceptibility tests are set up on detecting abnormal numbers of white blood cells or bacteria on microscopy so that both culture and susceptibility results are available within 24 hours.

Interpretation of the significance of bacterial culture results depends upon a variety of factors

These factors relate to:

- Collection – specimen collection must be carried out properly.
- Storage – the urine must be cultured within one hour of collection or held at 4°C for not more than 18 hours before culture.
- Antibiotic treatment – in a patient receiving antibiotics, smaller numbers of organisms may be significant and may represent an emerging resistant population. Simple laboratory methods are available to detect antibacterial substances.
- Fluid intake – the patient may be taking more or less fluid than usual and this will clearly influence the quantitative result.
- The specimen – the quantitative guidelines are valid for MSU specimens; they do not apply to catheter specimens, suprapubic aspirates or nephrostomy samples.

Treatment of UTIs

Uncomplicated UTI is treated with an oral antibacterial as a single dose or for three days

Uncomplicated UTI (cystitis) should be treated with antibacterial agents taken by mouth as a single dose or for three days depending upon the drug. The commonly prescribed agents are shown in *Figure 18.8*. The choice of agent should be based on the results of susceptibility tests. However, for uncomplicated UTIs in patients in the community, therapy is often 'best guess', at least until laboratory results are available. This requires a knowledge of the likely pathogens and their antibiotic susceptibility patterns in the locality. Follow-up cultures should be carried out after treatment has been completed (at least two days later) to confirm eradication of the infecting organism. In addition to antibacterial therapy, the patient should be advised to drink large volumes of fluid to help the normal flushing out process.

Children and pregnant women with asymptomatic bacteriuria should be treated with antibacterials and followed up to check for eradication of the infection. Instrumentation of the urinary tract should be delayed in patients with significant bacteriuria until appropriate treatment has rendered the urine sterile.

Complicated UTI (pyelonephritis) should be treated with a systemic antibacterial agent

The organism should be known to be susceptible to the antibacterial, and systemic treatment should continue until the signs and symptoms subside. It can then be replaced by oral therapy. The usual length of treatment is 10 days, but longer treatment may be necessary to sterilize the kidney.

Hospital-acquired infections or recurrent infections, particularly in catheterized patients, may be caused by antibiotic-resistant organisms and the agent of choice will depend upon the antibacterial susceptibility pattern. If possible, the catheter should be removed as eradication of infection is extremely difficult to achieve in catheterized patients and some would advocate treatment only when the patient complains of symptoms or before invasive procedures. Guidelines for catheter care and for the prevention of catheter-associated UTIs are shown in *Figure 18.9*.

Infections acquired by hematogenous spread require specific antibacterial therapy, as described in Chapter 30 for tuberculosis, Chapter 20 for *S. typhi*, Chapter 23 for *Staph. aureus* and Chapter 25 for schistosomiasis.

ORAL ANTIBACTERIALS FOR URINARY TRACT INFECTIONS		
antibacterial	**class of agent***	**comments**
ampicillin amoxycillin	beta-lactam beta-lactam	note that >50% of Gram-negative rods causing UTI are beta-lactamase producers and are therefore resistant
augmentin	beta-lactam + beta-lactamase inhibitor	active against most Gram-negative rods, resistant to ampicillin by virtue of beta-lactamase production
cephalexin cefaclor	beta-lactam beta-lactam	relatively beta-lactamase stable, therefore wider spectrum than ampicillin not active against enterococci
trimethoprim	nucleic-acid synthesis inhibitor	incidence of resistant strains increasing
cotrimoxazole	combination of trimethoprim with sulfamethoxazole (also nucleic-acid synthesis inhibitor)	may be useful in 'blind' treatment but more toxic than trimethoprim alone
nitrofurantoin	urinary antiseptic	for uncomplicated UTI only not active in alkaline pH (therefore not useful for *Proteus* infections)
nalidixic acid	quinolone	for uncomplicated UTI Gram-negative infections only not active against Gram-positive
ciprofloxacin	quinolone	very broad spectrum only oral agent active against *Pseudonomas aeruginosa* not active against enterococci

Fig. 18.8 Oral antibacterials for urinary tract infections (UTIs). Several different classes of antibacterial are available in oral formulations and suitable for treatment of UTI. Nitrofurantoin and nalidixic acid are useful only for lower UTIs as they do not achieve adequate serum and tissue concentrations to treat upper UTIs. Ciprofloxacin is an example of the new generation of quinolones; others may be preferred in different countries. (*For details see Chapter 30.)

GUIDELINES FOR CATHETER CARE
avoid catheterization whenever possible
keep duration of catheterization to a minimum
use intermittent rather than continuous catheterization when feasible
insert catheters with good aseptic technique
use a closed sterile drainage system
maintain a gravity drain
use topical antiseptics around the meatus in women
wash hands before and after inserting catheters and collecting specimens, and after emptying drainage bags

Fig. 18.9 Guidelines for catheter care. Catheters that drain into open collecting vessels are particularly conducive to infection. Virtually every patient who has such a catheter in place for more than four days becomes infected. Closed drainage systems are therefore now used in most hospitals, but even then bacteriuria occurs in 10–25% of patients. Hospitals with active catheter care programs can keep this rate below 10%.

Prevention of Urinary Tract Infections

Many of the features of the pathogenesis of UTI and host predispositions are not clearly understood.

Recurrent infections in otherwise healthy women can be prevented by regularly emptying the bladder. This washes bacteria out of the urinary tract and is particularly important following intercourse. The prophylactic use of antibiotics may also prevent recurrent infections, but in the presence of underlying abnormalities there is a tendency to select antibiotic-resistant strains, which subsequently cause infections that are more difficult to treat.

Infection in catheterized patients is very common, but can be reduced by good catheter care procedures (*Fig. 18.9*, see Chapter 34). Catheterization should be avoided if possible or kept to a minimum duration.

Summary

UTIs are the cause of a considerable amount of morbidity, especially in the female population. They are important and often asymptomatic in pregnancy, and some studies have shown a correlation between UTI in pregnancy and low birth weight babies. Antibacterial agents play an important role in the treatment and prevention of UTI, but in the absence of laboratory investigations to confirm infection, treatment may be inappropriate or unnecessary. When associated with underlying structural or neurologic abnormalities, a UTI is difficult to treat effectively.

- UTIs are among the most common bacterial infections, especially in women.
- Most UTIs are acute episodes without sequelae.
- UTIs are usually endogenously acquired, with colonizing bacteria ascending the urinary tract from the periurethral area. *E. coli* is the predominant pathogen; other Gram-negative rods are also responsible, especially in hospitalized patients. Viruses are not important causes of UTI.
- Structural or mechanical factors in the host or catheterization predispose to infection.
- Bacterial attributes such as adhesions and capsular polysaccharides may be important in the development of UTI. Specific toxins are not implicated, but hemolysins (cytotoxins) may be.
- Lower UTI usually presents with acute frequency and dysuria. Asymptomatic infection is common in pregnancy and in children. Infection is recurrent in a significant proportion of people.
- Pyelonephritis (upper UTI) has a more severe presentation than lower UTI, with fever and loin pain; recurrent infection results in renal damage.
- Bacteriologic confirmation of the diagnosis requires quantitative methods. Pyuria also implies infection.
- Short-course treatment with oral antibacterials is effective for lower UTI; pyelonephritis needs longer treatment, often commencing with systemically administered drugs.
- Hospital-acquired UTI is often caused by multiple-resistant Gram-negative bacteria, and treatment should be based on the results of antibiotic susceptibility tests.

An eight-month pregnant 22-year-old teacher presents to her doctor with a 48-hour history of dysuria and lower abdominal pain. This is her first pregnancy and it has previously been unremarkable. On examination she is apyrexial and her uterus is normal size for dates. There is some lower abdominal tenderness, but her renal angles are not tender. A dipstick test of her urine in the surgery reveals the presence of protein, but no glucose or blood. Her urine is sent for culture in the laboratory and grows more than 10^5 coliforms/ml.

1. What is the significance of the bacterial count in this patient's urine specimen?
2. Why is urine screened for infection in pregnancy?
3. List, in rank order, the three most likely causes of this woman's infection.
4. Which antimicrobials would be suitable for treating this infection in pregnancy?

Further Reading

Kass EH. Asymptomatic infections of the urinary tract. *Trans Assoc Am Phys* 1956;**69**:56–64.

Komeroff AL, Friedland G. The dysuria–pyuria syndrome. *N Engl J Med* 1980;**303**:452–453.

Kunin CM. Natural history of lower urinary tract infections. *Infection* 1990;**18**(Suppl. 2):s44–s49.

Measley RE, Levison ME. Host defence mechanisms in the pathogenesis of urinary tract infection. *Med Clin North Am* 1991;**75**:275–286.

Introduction

Sexually transmitted infections usually cause diseases

Sexually transmitted infections (STIs) that do not cause sexually transmitted diseases (STDs) include asymptomatic gonorrhea in females and the early stages of HIV infection. STDs are of major medical importance throughout the world, and HIV infection/AIDS has the greatest global impact, affecting an estimated 20 million adults. In 1995, in addition to HIV, there were at least 333 million new cases of other STDs.

The incidence of most STDs is increasing

The reasons for this increase include:

- Increasing density and mobility of human populations.
- The difficulty of engineering changes in human sexual behavior.
- The absence of vaccines for almost all STI.

The last two factors may change. There is already evidence of changes in male homosexual behavior leading to decreased transmission of STDs in this group, and eventually there will be vaccines for certain infections – herpes simplex, gonorrhea, HIV.

The emergence of HIV infection and AIDS has overshadowed other STDs. Nevertheless, despite its immense impact as a new and highly lethal infectious disease for which there is so far no satisfactory treatment or vaccine, it is still uncommon in developed countries compared with other STDs.

The 'top ten' STDs are listed in *Figure 19.1*, while those that are less common are listed in *Figure 19.2*; *Figure 19.3* gives examples of the strategies used by the microorganisms to overcome host defenses.

STDs and Sexual Behavior

The general principles of entry, exit and transmission of the microorganisms that cause STDs are set out in Chapter 8.

The spread of STDs is inextricably linked with sexual behavior

There are therefore many more opportunities for controlling STIs than, for instance, respiratory infections. Infected but asymptomatic individuals play an important role, and important determinants are promiscuity and sexual practices involving contact between different orifices and mucosal surfaces (see Chapter 8):

- Transmission between heterosexuals or male homosexuals can take place following oral or anal intercourse. The gonococcus, for instance, causes pharyngitis and proctitis, although it infects stratified squamous epithelium less readily than columnar epithelium.
- Condom usage is another major determinant. Condoms have been shown to retain gonococci, herpes simplex virus (HSV), HIV and chlamydia in simulated coital tests of the syringe and plunger type (even when the 'infected' plunger

was left in place for an extra eight hours!).

Further discussion of the control of STDs is included in Chapter 33.

Various host factors influence the risk of acquiring an STD

It is not surprising that the type of sexual activity is important or that genital lesions or ulcers increase the risk of acquiring infections such as HIV. Other factors are less well understood, such as the numerous observations that uncircumcised men have a higher risk of infection.

STDs do not necessarily occur singly, and the possibility of multiple infection must always be borne in mind. For instance, syphilis can accompany gonorrhea, and there is evidence that genital herpes may be reactivated during an attack of gonorrhea.

Syphilis

Syphilis is caused by the spirochete Treponema pallidum and is less common than other STDs

Treponema pallidum (see Appendix), is closely related to the treponemes that cause the non-venereal infections of pinta and yaws *(Figs 19.4, 19.5)*. *T. pallidum* has a worldwide distribution, (the World Health Organization estimates that there are 12 million new cases of syphilis worldwide each year) but syphilis is now uncommon in the UK (approximately 1000 new cases/year) and is much less prevalent than other STDs. Despite this, syphilis remains a problem, especially in developing countries, because of the serious sequelae and the risk of congenital infection.

T. pallidum enters the body through minute abrasions on the skin or mucous membranes. Transmission of *T. pallidum* requires close personal contact because the organism does not survive well outside the body and is very sensitive to drying, heat and disinfectants. Horizontal spread (see Chapter 8) occurs through sexual contact and vertical spread via transplacental infection of the fetus (see Chapter 21).

Local multiplication leads to plasma cell, polymorph and macrophage infiltration, with later endarteritis. The bacteria multiply very slowly, and the average incubation period is three weeks.

THE TOP TEN SEXUALLY TRANSMITTED DISEASES				
organism	disease	comment	treatment	new cases (millions) per year worldwide*
papillomaviruses (six of the 70 types)	genital warts, dysplasias	the commonest of all STDs; associated with cancer of cervix, penis, etc.	podophyllin, surgical removal	32
Chlamydia trachomatis (D–K serotypes)	non-specific urethritis,	increasing incidence	+ doxycycline, azithromycin	97
C. trachomatis (L1, L2, L3 serotypes)	lymphogranuloma venereum	mainly tropical countries	+ (doxycycline, tetracycline, erythromycin)	
Candida albicans	vaginal thrush, balanitis	very common; predisposing factors	+ (nystatin, fluconazole)	
Trichomonas vaginalis	vaginitis, urethritis	very common	+ (metronidazole)	94
herpes simplex virus types 1 and 2	genital herpes	? increasing; problem of latency and reactivation	± (acyclovir)	21
Neisseria gonorrhoeae	gonorrhea	decreasing incidence in developed countries	++ (penicillin, ceftriaxone, cefixime, ciprofloxacin spectinomycin, azithromycin)*	78
HIV	AIDS	highly lethal; incidence increasing worldwide	± (zidovudine)	2
Treponema pallidum	syphilis	decreasing incidence in developed countries	++ (penicillin)	19
Hepatitis B virus	hepatitis	especially male homosexuals (? decreasing incidence)	–	
Haemophilus ducreyi	chancroid	mainly tropical 9 million infected individuals	+ (erythromycin, ceftriaxone, cotrimoxazole)	

Fig. 19.1 The 'top ten' sexually transmitted diseases (STDs). Vaccine is available only for hepatitis B. *Current recommendations for uncomplicated gonorrhea in adults are for a single dose of cefixime or ciprofloxacin orally, followed by doxycycline or azithromycin for possible concurrent infection with chlamydia. (*WHO figures up to December 1995.)

OTHER SEXUALLY TRANSMITTED DISEASES			
organism	disease	comment	treatment
Calymmato-bacterium granulomatis	granuloma inguinale	tropical	+ (tetracycline)
Sarcoptes scabiei	genital scabies	common	+ (benzyl benzoate)
Phthirus pubis	pediculosis pubis	common	+ (malathion)
Mycoplasma (T strains)	non-specific urethritis	less important than chlamydia	+ (tetracycline)
Gardnerella vaginalis	vaginitis	acts together with anaerobes	+ (metronidazole)

Fig. 19.2 Other sexually transmitted diseases. No vaccines available.

STRATEGIES ADOPTED BY SEXUALLY TRANSMITTED MICROORGANISMS TO COMBAT HOST DEFENSES		
host defenses	**microbial strategies**	**examples**
integrity of mucosal surface	specific attachment mechanism	gonococcus or chlamydia to urethral epithelium
urine flow (for urethral infection)	specific attachment; induce own uptake and transport across urethral epithelial surface in phagocytic vacuole	gonococcus
	infection of urethral epithelial or subepithelial cells	herpes simplex virus (HSV), chlamydia
phagocytes (especially polymorphs)	induce negligible inflammation	*Treponema pallidum*; mechanism unclear, perhaps poorly activates alternative complement pathway due to sialic acid coating
	resist phagocytosis	gonococcus (capsule) *T. pallidum* (absorbed fibronectin)
complement	C3d receptor on microbe binds C3b/d and reduces C3b/d-mediated polymorph phagocytosis	*Candida albicans*
inflammation	induce strong inflammatory response, yet evade consequences	gonococcus, *C. albicans*, HSV, chlamydia; mechanism unknown
antibodies (especially IgA)	produce IgA protease	gonococcus
cell-mediated immune response (T cells, lymphokines, natural killer cells etc.)	antigenic variation; allows re-infection of a given individual with an antigenic variant	gonococcus, chlamydia, papillomaviruses (not HSV or *T. pallidum*)
	antigenic variation within a given individual	HIV
	poorly understood factors cause ineffective cell-mediated immune response	*T. pallidum*, HIV

Fig. 19.3 Strategies adopted by sexually transmitted microorganisms to combat host defenses.

SPIRAL ORGANISMS OF MEDICAL IMPORTANCE				
family	**genus**	**species**	**subspecies**	**disease**
Spirochaetales	*Treponema*	*pallidum*	*pallidum*	syphilis
		pallidum	*pertenue*	yaws
		carateum	–	pinta
	Borrelia	*recurrentis*	–	relapsing fever
		burgdorferi	–	Lyme disease
Leptospiraceae	*Leptospira*	*icterohaemorrhagiae*	–	leptospirosis
		hardjo	–	(Weil's disease)

Fig. 19.4 Spiral organisms of medical importance.

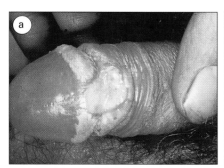 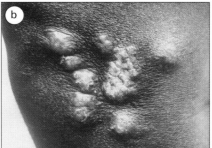 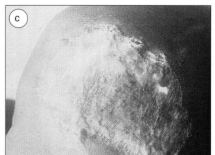

Fig. 19.5 (a) Typical penile chancre of primary syphilis. (Courtesy of RD Catterall.) Yaws (b) and pinta (c) are endemic in tropical and subtropical countries and are spread by direct contact. (Courtesy of PJ Cooper and G Griffin.)

Classically, T. pallidum infection is divided into three stages

The three classical stages of syphilis are primary, secondary and tertiary syphilis *(Fig. 19.6)*. However, not all patients go through all three stages; a substantial proportion remains permanently free of disease after suffering the primary or secondary stages of infection. The lesion of primary syphilis is illustrated in *Fig. 19.5*. The secondary stage may be followed by a latent period of some 3–30 years, after which the disease may recur – the tertiary stage. Unlike most bacterial pathogens, *T. pallidum* can survive in the body for many years despite a vigorous immune response. It has been suggested that the healthy treponeme evades recognition and elimination by the host by maintaining a cell surface rich in lipid. This layer is antigenically unreactive and the antigens are only uncovered in dead and dying organisms when the host is then able to respond. Tissue damage is mostly due to the host response.

Despite many years of effort, *T. pallidum* still cannot be cultivated in the laboratory in artificial media. It has therefore been difficult to study possible virulence factors at a molecular level, although genes have been cloned in *Escherichia coli* and major proteins have been characterized.

An infected woman can transmit T. pallidum to her baby in utero

Congenital syphilis is acquired after the first three months of pregnancy. The disease may manifest as:

- Serious infection resulting in intrauterine death.
- Congenital abnormalities, which may be obvious at birth.
- Silent infection, which may not be apparent until about two years of age (facial and tooth deformities).

PATHOGENESIS OF SYPHILIS		
stage of disease	**signs and symptoms**	**pathogenesis**
initial contact ⇩ 2–10 weeks (depends on inoculum size)	primary chancre* at site of infection	multiplication of treponemes at site of infection; associated host response
primary syphilis ⇩ 1–3 months	enlarged inguinal nodes spontaneous healing	proliferation of treponemes in regional lymph nodes
secondary syphilis ⇩ 2–6 weeks	flu-like illness myalgia, headache, fever mucocutaneous rash* spontaneous resolution	multiplication and production of lesions in lymph nodes, liver joints, muscles, skin and mucous membranes
latent syphilis ⇩ 3–30 years		treponemes dormant in ?liver and spleen re-awakening and multiplication of treponemes
tertiary syphilis	neurosyphilis; general paralysis of the insane, tabes dorsalis cardiovascular syphilis; aortic lesions, heart failure progressive destructive disease	further dissemination and invasion and host response (cell-mediated hypersensitivity) gummas in skin, bone, testis

*chancre: Initially a papule; forms a painless ulcer; heals without treatment within two months. Live treponemes can be seen in dark-ground microscopy of fluid from lesions; patient highly infectious.

Fig. 19.6 The pathogenesis of syphilis. A feature of *Treponema pallidum* infection is its chronic nature, which seems to involve a delicately balanced relationship between pathogen and host.

Laboratory diagnosis of syphilis

As *T. pallidum* cannot be grown *in vitro*, laboratory diagnosis hinges on microscopy and serology.

Microscopy

Exudate from the primary chancre should be examined by either:

- Dark-ground microscopy immediately after collection.
- Ultraviolet (UV) microscopy after staining with fluorescein-labelled anti-treponemal antibodies.

The organisms have tightly wound, slender coils with pointed ends and are sluggishly motile in unstained preparations. *T. pallidum* is very thin (about 0.2 mm in diameter, compared with *E. coli*, which is about 1 mm) and cannot be seen in Gram-stained preparations. Silver impregnation stains can be used to demonstrate the organisms in biopsy material.

Serology

Serologic tests for syphilis are the mainstay of diagnosis. They are divided into non-specific and specific tests for the detection of antibodies in patients' serum.

Non-specific tests (non-treponemal tests) for syphilis are the VDRL and RPR tests

The term non-specific is used because the antigens are not treponemal in origin, but are from extracts of normal mammalian tissues. Cardiolipin, from beef heart, allows the detection of anti-lipid IgG and IgM formed in the patient in response to lipoidal material released from cells damaged by the infection, as well as to lipids in the surface of *T. pallidum*. The two tests in common use today are:

- The Venereal Disease Research Lab (VDRL) test.
- The rapid plasma reagin (RPR) test.

  Both are available in kit form.

Non-specific tests show up as positive within 4–6 weeks of infection (or 1–2 weeks after the primary chancre appears) and decline in positivity in tertiary syphilis or after effective antibiotic treatment of primary or secondary disease. Therefore, these tests are useful for screening. However, they are non-specific and may give positive results in conditions other than syphilis (biologic false positives, *Fig. 19.7*). All positive results should therefore be confirmed by a specific test.

Commonly used specific tests for syphilis are the FTA-ABS test and the TPHA

These tests use treponemal antigens extracted from *T. pallidum*. Two tests are in common use:

- The fluorescent treponemal antibody absorption (FTA-ABS, *Fig. 19.8*) test in which the patient's serum is first absorbed with non-pathogenic treponemes to remove cross-reacting antibodies before reaction with *T. pallidum* antigens.
- The *T. pallidum* hemagglutination assay (TPHA).

These tests should be used to confirm that a positive result with a non-specific test is truly due to syphilis. Also, because they become positive earlier in the course of the disease, they can be used for confirmation when the clinical picture is strongly indicative of syphilis. They tend to remain positive for many years and may be the only positive test in patients with late syphilis. However, they remain positive after appropriate antibiotic treatment and cannot therefore be used as indicators of therapeutic response. They can also give false positive reactions *(Fig. 19.7)*.

Confirmation of a diagnosis of syphilis depends upon several serologic tests

Positive serologic test results for babies born to infected mothers may represent passive transfer of maternal antibody or the baby's own response to infection. These two possibilities can be distinguished by testing for IgM and retesting at six months of age, by which time maternal antibody levels have waned. Antibody titers remain elevated in babies with congenital syphilis.

At present several serologic tests are needed to confirm a diagnosis of syphilis. None of these tests distinguish syphilis from the non-sexually transmitted treponematoses, yaws and

FALSE POSITIVES IN SYPHILIS SEROLOGY	
test	**conditions associated with false positive results**
non-specific (non-treponemal) VDRL RPR	viral infection, collagen vascular disease, acute febrile disease, post-immunization, pregnancy, leprosy, malaria
specific (treponemal) FTA-ABS TPHA	diseases associated with increased or abnormal globulins, lupus erythematosus, skin diseases, antinuclear antibodies, drug misuse, pregnancy

Fig. 19.7 Serologic tests for syphilis and conditions associated with false-positive results. (FTA-ABS, fluorescent treponemal antibody absorbtion test; RPR, rapid plasma reagin test; TPHA, *Treponema pallidum* hemagglutination assay; VDRL, Venereal Disease Research Lab test.)

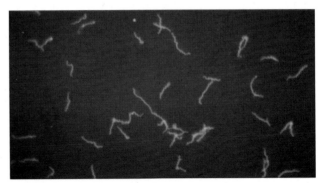

Fig. 19.8 The fluorescent treponemal antibody absorption test for syphilis. Antibody in the patient's serum binds to bacteria and is visualized by a fluorescent dye.

pinta. In future, monoclonal antibodies may be useful in detecting specific treponemal protein antigens and in the development of competition assays for the host's antibody.

Penicillin is the drug of choice for treating people with syphilis and their contacts

Penicillin is very active against *T. pallidum* (*Fig. 19.1*). For patients who are allergic to penicillin, treatment with tetracycline, doxycycline or erythromycin should be given. Only penicillin therapy reliably treats the fetus when administered to a pregnant mother.

Prevention of secondary and tertiary disease depends upon early diagnosis and adequate treatment. Contact tracing with screening and treatment is also important. Several STDs may be present in one patient concurrently, and patients with other STDs should be screened for syphilis.

Congenital syphilis is completely preventable if women are screened serologically early in pregnancy (less than three months) and those who are positive are treated with penicillin.

Gonorrhea

Gonorrhea is caused by the Gram-negative coccus Neisseria gonorrhoeae (the 'gonococcus')

This bacterium is a human pathogen and does not cause natural infection in other animals. Therefore its reservoir is human and transmission is direct, usually through sexual contact, from person to person. The organism is sensitive to drying and does not survive well outside the human host, so intimate contact is required for transmission. It is thought that a woman has a 50% chance of becoming infected after a single sexual intercourse with an infected man, while a man has a 20% chance of acquiring infection from an infected woman.

Asymptomatically infected individuals (almost always

women, see below) form the major reservoir of infection. Infection may also be transmitted vertically from an infected mother to her baby during childbirth. Infection in babies is usually manifest as ophthalmia neonatorum (see Chapter 16).

The gonococcus has special mechanisms to attach itself to mucosal cells

The usual site of entry of gonococci into the body is via the vagina or the urethral mucosa of the penis, but other sexual practices may result in the deposition of organisms in the throat or on the rectal mucosa. Special adhesive mechanisms (*Fig. 19.9*) prevent the bacteria from being washed away by urine or vaginal discharges. Following attachment, the gonococci rapidly multiply and spread through the cervix in women, and up the urethra in men. Spread is facilitated by various virulence factors (*Fig. 19.9*), although the organisms do not possess flagella and are non-motile. Production of an IgA protease helps to protect them from the host's secretory antibodies.

Host damage in gonorrhea results from gonococcal-induced inflammatory responses

The gonococci invade non-ciliated epithelial cells, which internalize the bacteria and allow them to multiply within intracellular vacuoles, protected from phagocytes and antibodies. These vacuoles move down through the cell and fuse with the basement membrane, discharging their bacterial contents into the subepithelial connective tissues. *Neisseria gonorrhoeae* does not produce a recognized exotoxin. Damage to the host results from inflammatory responses elicited by the organism. Persistent untreated infection can result in chronic inflammation and fibrosis.

Infection is usually localized, but the bacteria can invade the bloodstream and so spread to other parts of the body. Strains of *N. gonorrhoeae* that are associated with disseminated disease have particular characteristics, including resistance to the bactericidal action of serum (*Fig. 19.10*).

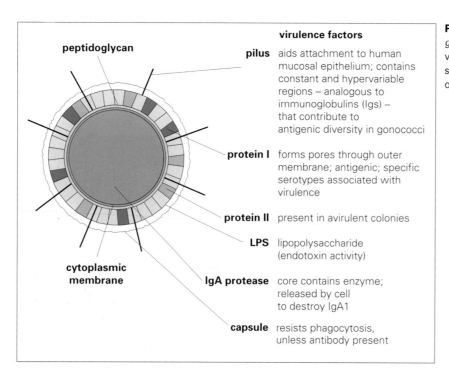

virulence factors

pilus aids attachment to human mucosal epithelium; contains constant and hypervariable regions – analogous to immunoglobulins (Igs) – that contribute to antigenic diversity in gonococci

protein I forms pores through outer membrane; antigenic; specific serotypes associated with virulence

protein II present in avirulent colonies

LPS lipopolysaccharide (endotoxin activity)

IgA protease core contains enzyme; released by cell to destroy IgA1

capsule resists phagocytosis, unless antibody present

peptidoglycan

cytoplasmic membrane

Fig. 19.9 The spread of *Neisseria gonorrhoeae* is facilitated by various virulence factors. Changes in the surface structure of the gonococcus render the organism avirulent.

Gonorrhea is initially asymptomatic in many women, but can later cause infertility

Symptoms develop within 2–7 days of infection and are characterized:

- In the male by urethral discharge (Fig. 19.11) and pain on passing urine (dysuria).
- In the female by vaginal discharge.

At least 50% of all infected women have only mild symptoms or are completely asymptomatic. They do not therefore seek treatment and will continue to infect others. Asymptomatic infection, however, is not the usual course of events in men. Women may not be alerted to their infection unless or until complications arise such as:

- Pelvic inflammatory disease (PID).
- Chronic pelvic pain.
- Infertility resulting from damage to the fallopian tubes.

Ophthalmia neonatorum is characterized by a sticky discharge (see Fig. 21.10).

Gonococcal infection of the throat may result in a sore throat (see Chapter 17) and infection of the rectum also results in a purulent discharge.

In men, local complications of urethral infection are rare (Fig. 19.12). Invasive gonococcal disease is much more common in infected women than in men, but prompt treatment is important in containing local infection. The common occurrence of asymptomatic infection in women is an important factor in the occurence of complications (i.e. it is unrecognised and untreated). In 10–20% of untreated women, infection spreads up the genital tract to cause PID and damage to the fallopian tubes.

Disseminated infection occurs in 1–3% of women, but is less common in men (see above and Fig. 19.13). It is a function not only of the strain of gonococcus (see above and Fig. 19.10), but also of ill-understood host factors. About 5% of people with disseminated infection have deficiencies in the late-acting components of complement (C5–C8).

A diagnosis of gonorrhea is made from microscopy and culture of appropriate specimens

Urethral and vaginal discharges and other specimens where indicated are used for microscopy and culture. Although a purulent discharge is characteristic of local gonococcal infection, it is not possible to distinguish reliably between gonococcal discharge and that caused by other pathogens such as Chlamydia trachomatis on clinical examination.

With experience, the finding of Gram-negative intracellular diplococci in a smear of urethral discharge from a symptomatic male patient is a highly sensitive and specific test for the diagnosis of gonorrhea.

Culture is essential in the investigation of infection in women and asymptomatic men, and for specimens taken from sites other than the urethra. Specimens from symptomatic men should also be cultured:

- To confirm the identity of the isolate; misinterpretation of microscopy or culture results can cause severe distress and may result in litigation.
- To perform antibiotic susceptibility tests (see Chapter 14).
- To aid in the distinction between treatment failure and reinfection.

BACTERIAL FEATURES OF *N. GONORRHOEAE* ASSOCIATED WITH DISSEMINATION
resistance to bactericidal action of serum
marked susceptibility to penicillin
require arginine, uracil and hypoxanthine for growth in laboratory

Fig. 19.10 Characteristics of *Neisseria gonorrhoeae* strains associated with disseminated disease.

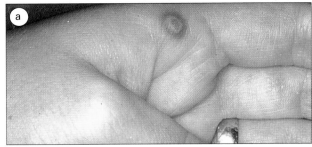
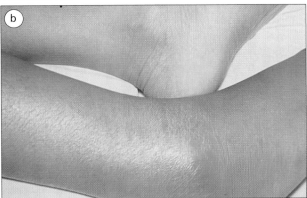

Fig. 19.12 Local and systemic complications of gonococcal infection. (a) Skin lesions start as erythematous papules, which often become pustular and hemorrhagic with necrotic centers. (Courtesy of JS Bingham.) (b) Septic arthritis of the ankle with marked erythema and swelling of the ankle and leg. (Courtesy of TF Sellers, Jr.)

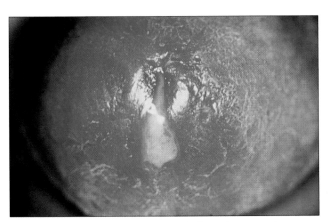

Fig. 19.11 Gonococcal urethritis. Typical purulent meatal discharge with inflammation of the glans. (Courtesy of J Clay.)

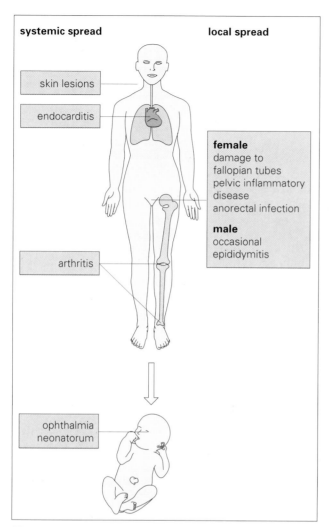

systemic spread   local spread

skin lesions

endocarditis

female
damage to
fallopian tubes
pelvic inflammatory
disease
anorectal infection

male
occasional
epididymitis

arthritis

ophthalmia
neonatorum

Fig. 19.13 Local and systemic spread of gonococcal infection and complications.

Because of the organism's sensitivity to drying, cultures should be made on to warmed media in the clinic or at the bedside and transported to the laboratory without delay. Blood cultures should be collected if disseminated disease is suspected, and joint aspirates may yield positive cultures.

Serologic tests are unsatisfactory. Recently, kits have become available to detect bacterial nucleic acids in specimens. They appear to be reliable, and give a result within 1–2 hours.

Antibacterials used to treat gonorrhea are penicillin, ceftriazone, ciprofloxacin and spectinomycin, but resistance is increasing

The antibacterial agents of choice are shown in *Figure 19.1.* The incidence of resistance is increasing and has severely compromised the effective treatment of gonorrhea in some parts of the world such as Southeast Asia. Early treatment of a significant proportion of sexually promiscuous patients achieves a striking reduction in the duration of infectiousness and transmission rates. Prophylactic use of antibacterials has no effect in preventing sexually-acquired gonorrhea, but the

application of antibacterial eye drops to babies born to mothers with gonorrhea or suspected gonorrhea is effective. Infection can be prevented by the use of condoms.

Follow-up of patients and contact tracing are vital to control the spread of gonorrhea. At present effective vaccines are not available, but the possibility of using some of the pilus proteins or other outer membrane components of the gonococcal cell as antigens is under investigation. However, immunization may prevent symptomatic disease without preventing infection, and the dangers of asymptomatic infection have been discussed above.

Repeated infections can occur with strains of bacteria with different pilin proteins.

Chlamydial Infection

C. trachomatis serotypes D–K cause sexually transmitted genital infections

The chlamydiae are very small bacteria that are obligate intracellular parasites. They have a more complicated life cycle than free-living bacteria because they can exist in different forms:
- The elementary body (EB) is adapted for extracellular survival and for initiation of infection.
- The reticulate body (RB) is adapted for intracellular multiplication *(Fig. 19.14).*

Three species of *Chlamydia* are currently recognized: *C. trachomatis, C. psittaci* and *C. pneumoniae (Fig. 19.15). C. psittaci* and *C. pneumoniae* infect the respiratory tract and have been discussed in Chapter 22. The species *C. trachomatis* can be subdivided into different serotypes (also known as serovars) and these have been shown to be linked characteristically with different infections:
- Serotypes A, B and C are the causes of the serious eye infection trachoma (see Chapter 16).
- Serotypes D–K are the cause of genital infection and associated ocular and respiratory infections *(Fig. 19.16).*
- Serotypes L1, L2 and L3 cause the systemic disease lymphogranuloma venereum (LGV) (see p.238).

C. trachomatis serotypes D–K have a worldwide distribution whereas the distribution of LGV serotypes is more restricted.

The majority of infections are genital and are acquired during sexual intercourse. Asymptomatic infection is common, especially in women. Ocular infections in adults are probably acquired by autoinoculation from infected genitalia or by ocular–genital contact. Ocular infections in neonates are acquired during passage through an infected maternal birth canal and the infant is also at risk of developing *C. trachomatis* pneumonia (see Chapter 17).

Chlamydiae enter the host through minute abrasions in the mucosal surface

They bind to specific receptors on the host cells and enter the cells by 'parasite-induced' endocytosis (see Chapter 8). Once inside the cell, fusion of the chlamydia-containing vesicle with lysozomes is inhibited by an unknown mechanism and the EB begins its developmental cycle *(Fig. 19.14).*

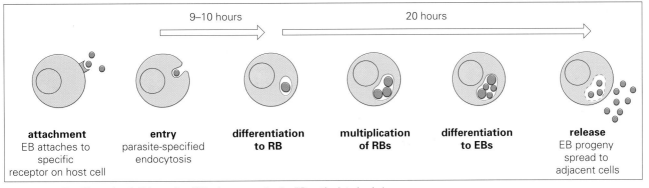

Fig. 19.14 The life cycle of *Chlamydia*. (EB, elementary body; RB, reticulate body.)

MEDICALLY IMPORTANT SPECIES OF CHLAMYDIA			
species	serotype	natural host	disease in humans
C. trachomatis	A,B,C	humans	trachoma
	D–K	humans	cervicitis urethritis proctitis conjunctivitis pneumonia (in neonates)
	L1,L2,L3	humans	lymphogranuloma venereum
C. psittaci	?	birds and non-human mammals	pneumonia
C. pneumoniae	1	humans	acute respiratory disease

Fig. 19.15 Medically important species of chlamydia. *Chlamydia trachomatis* is the species associated with sexually transmitted disease.

Within 9–10 hours of cell invasion the EBs differentiate into metabolically active RBs, which divide by binary fission and produce fresh EB progeny. These are then released into the extracellular environment within a further 20 hours.

The clinical effects of *C. trachomatis* infection appear to result from cell destruction and the host's inflammatory response

It is not yet clear, however, whether release of the EB progeny involves host cell rupture or exocytosis. The released EBs invade adjacent cells or cells distant from the site of infection if carried in lymph or blood.

Growth of *C. trachomatis* serotypes D–K seems to be restricted to columnar and transitional epithelial cells, but serotypes L1, L2 and L3 cause systemic disease (LGV). The site of infection determines the nature of clinical disease *(Fig. 19.16)*. Genital tract infection with serotypes D-K is locally asymptomatic in most women, but usually symptomatic in men.

CHLAMYDIA TRACHOMATIS: CLINICAL SYNDROMES AND THEIR COMPLICATIONS		
infection in:	clinical syndromes	complications
men	urethritis epididymitis proctitis conjunctivitis	systemic spread Reiter's syndrome*
women	urethritis cervicitis bartholinitis salpingitis conjunctivitis	ectopic pregnancy infertility systemic spread: perihepatitis arthritis dermatitis
neonates	conjunctivitis	interstitial pneumonitis
*Urethritis, conjunctivitis, polyarthritis, mucocutaneous lesions		

Fig. 19.16 Clinical syndromes and complications caused by *C. trachomatis*, serotypes D–K.

Laboratory tests are essential to diagnose chlamydial urethritis and cervicitis

Chlamydial urethritis and cervicitis cannot be reliably distinguished from other causes of these conditions on clinical grounds alone. The methods available include:
- Cell culture.
- Direct antigen detection.

Most infected patients develop antibodies, but serology is unreliable for diagnostic purposes. As chlamydiae are obligate intracellular parasites, isolation must be performed in cell cultures. The specimen is suspended in fluid and centrifuged on to a monolayer of tissue culture (McCoy) cells pretreated with cycloheximide, which enhances the uptake of chlamydiae. After 48–72 hours, *C. trachomatis* forms characteristic cytoplasmic inclusions, which stain with iodine because they contain glycogen *(Fig. 19.17)* or can be visualized with immunofluorescent stains.

C. trachomatis can be detected directly on microscopy using the direct fluorescent antibody test

C. trachomatis can be detected directly in smears of clinical specimens made on microscope slides stained with fluorescein-

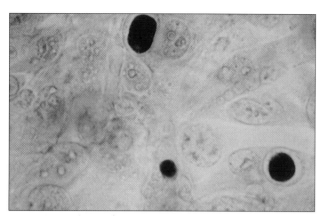

Fig. 19.17 Chlamydial inclusion bodies stained dark brown with iodine.

conjugated monoclonal antibodies and viewed by UV microscopy – the direct fluorescent antibody (DFA) test. The EBs stain as bright yellow-green dots *(Fig. 19.18)*. Results can be obtained within a few hours. Compared with culture, this method is extremely specific, but often not sensitive enough for asymptomatic infections. Chlamydial antigens can also be detected in specimens using an enzyme-linked immunosorbent assay (ELISA), but this test also suffers from reduced sensitivity in asymptomatic patients.

Nucleic acid probes to detect chlamydial nucleic acid (e.g. in urine samples) are being developed and will probably replace the methods descibed above.

Chlamydial infection is treated or prevented with doxycycline or tetracycline

It is important to remember that chlamydiae are not susceptible to the beta-lactam antibiotics, which are the drugs of choice for the treatment of gonorrhea and syphilis. It is recommended that patients receiving treatment for gonorrhea are also treated with doxycycline for possible concurrent chlamydial infection *(Fig. 19.1)*. In addition, patients with clinically-diagnosed chlamydial genital infections, their sexual contacts and babies born to infected mothers should be treated. Erythromycin should be used for babies.

Prevention depends upon recognizing the importance of asymptomatic infections. Early diagnosis and treatment of cases and of their sexual partners is important in order to avoid complications and reduce opportunities for transmission. Remember that STDs are not mutually exclusive and patients may have concurrent infections with quite different pathogens.

Other Causes of Inguinal Lymphadenopathy

Genital infections are common causes of inguinal lymphadenopathy (swelling of lymph nodes in the groin) among sexually active people. Syphilis and gonorrhea have been discussed above. LGV, chancroid and donovanosis are rare in Europe and the USA, but are much more common in tropical and subtropical countries, and may be imported by travellers who have acquired the disease through sexual contact in these areas.

LGV

LGV is caused by C. trachomatis serotypes L1, L2 and L3

LGV is a serious disease and is common in Africa, Asia and South America. It occurs sporadically in Europe, Australia and North America, particularly among homosexual males. The prevalence appears to be higher among males than females probably because symptomatic infection is more common in men.

LGV is a systemic infection involving lymphoid tissue and is treated with tetracycline or doxycycline

The clinical picture can be contrasted with the more restricted infection seen with *C. trachomatis* serotypes D–K (see above). The primary lesion is an ulcerating papule at the site of inoculation (after an incubation period of 1–4 weeks) and may be accompanied by fever, headache and myalgia. The lesion heals rapidly, but the chlamydiae proceed to infect the draining lymph nodes, causing characteristic inguinal buboes *(Fig. 19.19)*, which gradually enlarge.

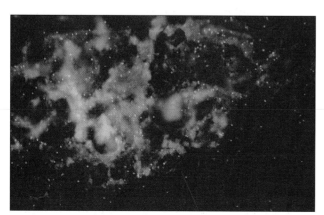

Fig. 19.18 Direct fluorescent antibody test for *Chlamydia trachomatis*. Elementary bodies can be seen as bright yellow-green dots under the ultraviolet microscope. (Courtesy of JD Treharne.)

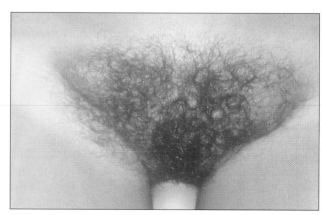

Fig. 19.19 Lymphogranuloma venereum. Bilateral enlargement of inguinal glands. (Courtesy of JS Bingham.)

Chlamydiae may disseminate from the lymph nodes via the lymphatics to the tissues of the rectum to cause proctitis. Other systemic complications include fever, hepatitis, pneumonitis and meningo-encephalitis. The infection may resolve untreated, but:

- Abscesses may form in lymph nodes, which suppurate and discharge through the skin.
- Chronic granulomatous reactions in lymphatics and neighboring tissues can eventually give rise to fistula in ano or genital elephantiasis.

Cell culture methods are available (see above), but the chlamydial isolation rate is reported to be low (24–30%). Classically, the 'Frei' skin test was used in diagnosis. This involves intradermal injection of the LGV antigen, but it is unreliable, lacking sensitivity in early disease and lacking specificity because the Frei antigen is only genus specific. Treatment with tetracycline or doxycycline (*Fig. 19.1*) is recommended.

Chancroid (soft chancre)
Chancroid is caused by Haemophilus ducreyi and is characterized by painful genital ulcers
Infection by the Gram-negative bacterium *Haemophilus ducreyi* is manifest as painful non-indurated genital ulcers and local lymphadenitis (*Fig. 19.20*). Note the difference between this and the chancre of primary syphilis, which is painless, but the ulcers may be confused with those of genital herpes, though they are usually larger and have a more ragged appearance. In the USA there are a few thousand cases each year, but in Africa and Asia chancroid is the commonest cause of genital ulcers. Epidemiologic information is important because the diagnosis is usually clinical as the organism is difficult to grow in the laboratory. Chancroid may also be confused with donovanosis (see below).

Chancroid is diagnosed by microscopy and culture and treated with erythromycin, ceftriaxone or cotrimoxazole
Gram-stained smears of aspirates from the ulcer margin or enlarged lymph node characteristically show large numbers of short Gram-negative rods and chains, often described as having a 'school of fish' appearance, within or outside

polymorphs. Aspirates should be cultured on a rich medium (chocolate agar with 1% isovitalex) at 30–34°C. *H. ducreyi* will not tolerate higher temperatures. Growth is slow and it may take 2–9 days for colonies to appear. Treatment with erythromycin, ceftriaxone or cotrimoxazole (*Fig. 19.1*) is recommended.

Donovanosis
Donovanosis is caused by Calymmatobacterium granulomatis and is characterized by genital nodules and ulcers
Donovanosis (granuloma inguinale or granuloma venereum) is rare in temperate climates, but common in tropical and subtropical regions such as the Caribbean, New Guinea, India and central Australia. The infection is characterized by nodules, almost always on the genitalia, which erode to form granulomatous ulcers that bleed readily on contact. The infection may extend and the ulcers may become secondarily infected. The pathogen is a Gram-negative rod called *Calymmatobacterium granulomatis* (*Fig. 19.2*). The bacteria invade and multiply within mononuclear cells and are liberated when the cells rupture.

Donovanosis is diagnosed by microscopy and treated with tetracycline
The diagnosis of donovanosis is made by examining a smear from the lesion stained with Wright's or Giemsa stain. 'Donovan bodies' appear as clusters of blue- or black-stained organisms in the cytoplasm of mononuclear cells. Treatment with tetracyclines is recommended (*Fig. 19.2*).

The role of sexual transmission of this infection is still controversial. The disease is often absent in sexual contacts of infected individuals and in a study in New Guinea was present in young children and adults, but not in 5 to 15-year-old children.

Mycoplasmas and Non-Gonococcal Urethritis

Mycoplasma hominis and Ureaplasma urealyticum may be causes of genital tract infection
Although *Mycoplasma pneumoniae* has a proven role in the causation of pneumonia (see Chapter 17), the role of *M. hominis* in non-gonococcal urethritis is uncertain. *M. hominis* and the related organism *Ureaplasma urealyticum* (which metabolizes urea; also called 'T strains') are frequently found colonizing the genital tracts of healthy sexually active men and women. They are less common in sexually inactive populations, which supports the view that they may be sexually transmitted. It is difficult to prove that they cause infection of the genital tract, but *M. hominis* may cause PID and postabortal and postpartum fevers. *U. urealyticum* has been associated with urethritis in men and prostatitis.

Fortunately, both *M. hominis* and *U. urealyticum* are susceptible to tetracyclines, which are also the treatment of choice for chlamydial infections.

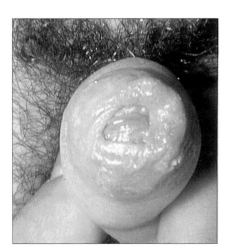

Fig. 19.20
Chancroid. Several irregular ulcers on the prepuce. (Courtesy of L Parish.)

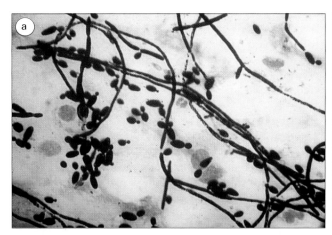

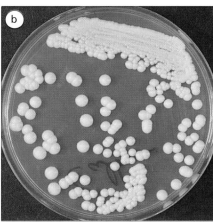

Fig. 19.21
Candida albicans.
(a) Light
microscopic
appearance and (b)
culture of vaginal
discharge.

Other Causes of Vaginitis and Urethritis

Candida infection

Candida albicans causes a range of genital tract diseases, which are treated with oral or topical antifungals

These vary from mild superficial, localized infections in an otherwise healthy individual to disseminated often fatal infections in the immunocompromised. This yeast is a normal inhabitant of the female vagina, but in some women and in circumstances which are not clearly understood, the candidal load increases and causes an intensely irritant vaginitis with a cheesy vaginal discharge. This may be accompanied by urethritis and dysuria and may present as a urinary tract infection (see Chapter 18). The diagnosis can be confirmed by microscopy and culture of the discharge *(Fig. 19.21)*.

Treatment with an oral antifungal such as fluconazole or a topical preparation such as nystatin is recommended, but recurrence is frequent in a small proportion of women. Balanitis is seen in up to 10% of male partners of females with vulvovaginal candidiasis, but urethritis is uncommon in men and rarely symptomatic.

Trichomonas infection

Trichomonas vaginalis is a protozoan parasite and causes vaginitis with copious discharge

Trichomonas vaginalis inhabits:

- The vagina in women.
- The urethra (and sometimes the prostate) in men.

It is transmitted during sexual intercourse. In women, heavy infections cause vaginitis with a characteristic copious foul-smelling discharge. There is an associated increase in the vaginal pH. The infection should be distinguished from bacterial vaginosis (see below) by microscopic examination of the discharge, which shows actively motile trophozoites *(Fig. 19.22)*.

Metronidazole is recommended for symptomatic T. vaginalis infections

In men, *Trichomonas vaginalis* is rarely symptomatic, but sometimes causes a mild urethritis; however, regular sexual partners of symptomatic women should be treated to prevent reinfection.

Bacterial vaginosis

Bacterial vaginosis is associated with Gardnerella vaginalis plus anaerobic infection and a fishy-smelling vaginal discharge

This non-specific vaginitis is a syndrome in women characterized by at least three of the following signs and symptoms:

- Excessive malodorous vaginal discharge.
- Vaginal pH greater than 4.5.
- Presence of clue cells (vaginal epithelial cells coated with bacteria, *Fig. 19.23*).
- A fishy amine-like odor.

There is a significant increase in the numbers of *G. vaginalis* in the vaginal flora and a concomitant increase in the

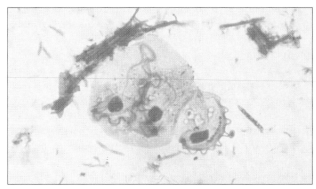

Fig. 19.22 Motile trophozoites in vaginal discharge in *T. vaginalis* infection. (Giemsa stain) (Courtesy of R Muller.)

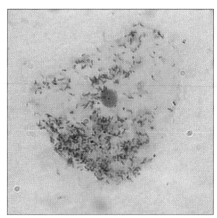

Fig. 19.23 Clue cells in bacterial vaginosis.

numbers of obligate anaerobes such as *Bacteroides (Fig. 19.2)*.

G. vaginalis is consistently found in association with vaginosis, but is also found in 20–40% of healthy women. It is generally present in the urethra of male partners of women with vaginosis, indicating that it can be sexually transmitted. *G. vaginalis* has also been isolated from blood cultures from women with postpartum fever.

G. vaginalis has had a chequered taxonomic history, being first classified as a haemophilus, then as a corynebacterium, reflecting the fact that it tends to be Gram-variable (sometimes appearing Gram-negative, sometimes Grampositive). It grows in the laboratory on human blood agar in a moist atmosphere enriched with carbon dioxide.

The pathogenesis of bacterial vaginosis is still unclear, but appears to be related to factors that disrupt the normal acidity of the vagina and the equilibrium between the different constituents of the normal vaginal flora. Whether any of these or other unknown factors are sexually transmissible is unclear. Symtomatic infections can be treated with metronidazole

Genital Herpes

HSV2 is the 'genital strain' of HSV, but both HSV1 and HSV2 may be recovered from genital sites

HSV1 is generally transmitted via saliva causing primary oropharyngeal infection in children and, later in life, after reactivation, cold sores. However, a separate virus strain, HSV2, has emerged as a result of independent transmission by the venereal route. HSV2 shows biologic and antigenic differences from the original HSV1 strain, but special laboratory techniques are needed to distinguish them. There is little cross-immunity. Although originally recovered from separate sites, orogenital sexual practices have become prevalent enough to obscure the topographic difference between the strains, so that HSV1 and HSV2 can be recovered from oral and genital sites.

Genital herpes is characterized by ulcerating vesicles that take up to two weeks to heal

The primary genital lesion (e.g. on the penis or vulva) is seen 3–7 days after infection. It consists of vesicles that soon break down to form painful shallow ulcers *(Fig. 19.24)*. Local lymph nodes are swollen, and there may be constitutional symptoms (fever, headache, malaise). Occasionally the lesions are on the urethra, causing dysuria. Healing takes up to two weeks, but the virus in the lesion travels up sensory nerve endings to establish latent infection in dorsal root ganglion neurones (see Chapter 22). From this site it can reactivate, travel down nerves to the same area, and cause recurrent lesions ('genital cold sores').

Aseptic meningitis or encephalitis occurs in adults as a rare complication, and spread of infection from mother to infant at the time of delivery can give rise to neonatal disseminated herpes or encephalitis.

Genital herpes is generally diagnosed from the clinical appearance, and acyclovir can be used for treatment

Virus can be isolated from vesicle fluid or ulcer swabs, and viral antigens detected by the ELISA method. Topical acyclovir can be used for treatment of severe or early lesions, and this drug may need to be given intravenously if there are systemic complications. Recurrent attacks are troublesome and longer courses (1–3 years) of low-dose (e.g. 400 mg twice daily) acyclovir by mouth reduce the frequency of recurrences.

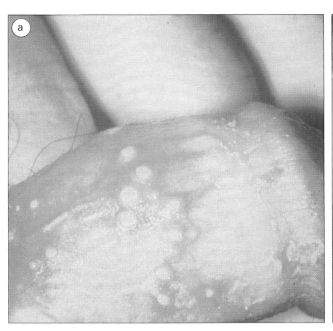

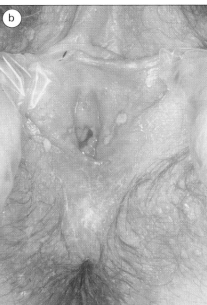

Fig. 19.24 Genital herpes. Vesicles on (a) the penis in male and (b) in the perianal area and vulva in female. Those on the labia minora and fourchette have ruptured to reveal characteristic herpetic erosions. (Courtesy of JS Bingham.)

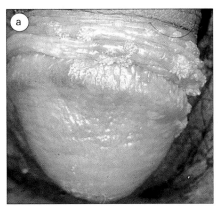
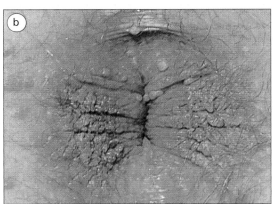
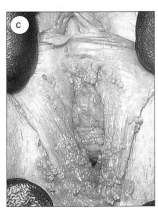

Fig. 19.25 Genital warts. (a) Warts on the penis are usually multiple, and on the shaft are often flat and keratinized. (b) Warts in the perianal area often extend into the anal canal. (c) Warts in the vulvoperineal area can enlarge dramatically and extend into the vagina. (Courtesy of JS Bingham.)

Human Papillomavirus Infection

There are now about 70 distinct types of human papillomaviruses, all infecting skin or mucosal surfaces, and the DNA of each showing less than 50% cross-hybridization with that of others. These are evidently ancient viral associates of man that have evolved extensively, and many of the different types are adapted to specific regions of the body.

Papillomavirus types 6, 11, 12, 16, 18 and 31 are transmitted sexually and cause genital warts

Warts (condylomata acuminata) appear on the penis, vulva and perianal regions *(Fig. 19.25)* after an incubation period of 1–6 months (see Chapter 22). They may not regress for many months and can be treated with podophyllin. On the cervix the lesion is a flat area of dysplasia visible by colposcopy as a white plaque *(Fig. 19.26)* after the local application of 5% acetic acid. Because of their association with cervical cancer (especially types 16 and 18), cervical lesions are best removed by laser.

Human Immunodeficiency Virus Infection

HIV is a retrovirus *(Fig. 19.27)*, so-called because this single-stranded RNA virus contains a pol gene that codes for a reverse transcriptase (Latin: retro, backwards).

AIDS was first recognized in 1981 in the USA

In 1981, the Communicable Disease Center, Atlanta, USA noted an increase in requests to use pentamidine for *Pneumocystis carinii* infection in previously well individuals who also suffered severe infections by other normally harmless microorganisms. These included *C. albicans* esophagitis, mucocutaneous HSV, toxoplasma CNS infection or pneumonia, and cryptosporidial enteritis; Kaposi's sarcoma was also often present. Patients had evidence of impaired immune function, as shown by skin test anergies, and depletion of CD4-positive T helper (TH) lymphocytes. This immunodeficiency syndrome appearing in an individual without a known cause such as treatment with immunosuppressive drugs was referred to as 'acquired immune deficiency syndrome' (AIDS). An internationally agreed definition of AIDS soon followed. Epidemics subsequently occurred in San Francisco, New York and other cities in the USA, and in the UK and Europe a few years later (see Chapter 33).

HIV, the causative virus of AIDS, was isolated from blood lymphocytes in 1983

It was recognized as belonging to the lentivirus (slow virus) group of retroviruses and related to similar agents in monkeys and to visnavirus in sheep and goats. The structure of the viral particle and its genome are illustrated in *Figure 19.28* and its replication mechanism in *Figures 19.29* and *19.30*.

Virus replication is regulated by the products of six genes. The replication cycle is often halted after integration of the provirus so that the infection remains latent in the cell. The *tat* and *rev* genes function as transactivating factors, and can increase production of viral RNAs and proteins when latently infected cells are:

- Stimulated to differentiate (e.g. TH cells by antigen).
- Stimulated by infection with certain other viruses such as HSV, cytomegalovirus (CMV).

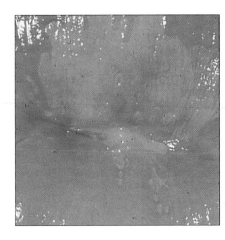

Fig. 19.26 Cervical dysplasia caused by papillomavirus should be removed by laser. (Courtesy of A Goodman.)

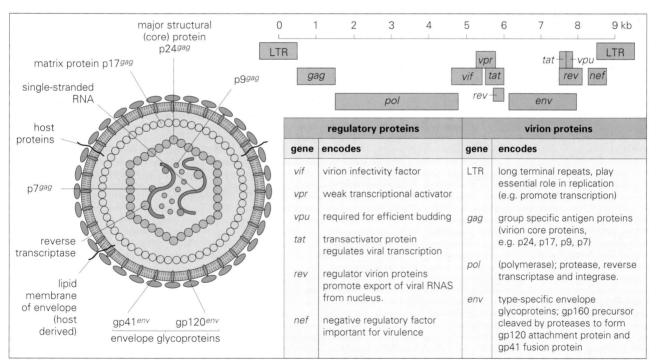

HUMAN RETROVIRUSES

virus	comment
HTLV1	endemic in West Indies and SW Japan; transmission via blood, human milk; can cause adult T cell leukemia, and HTLV1– associated myelopathy and tropical spastic paraparesis
HTLV2	uncommon, sporadic occurrence; transmission via blood; can cause hairy T cell leukemia
HIV1, HIV2	transmission via blood, sexual intercourse; responsible for ARC, AIDS, AIDS dementia etc.; HIV2 West African in origin, closely related to HIV1 but antigenically distinct
human foamy virus	causes foamy vacuolation in infected cells; little is known of its occurrence or pathogenic potential
human placental virus(es)	detected in placental tissue by electron microscopy and by presence of reverse transcriptase
human genome viruses	nucleic acid sequences representing endogenous retroviruses are common in the vertebrate genome, often in well-defined genetic loci; acquired during evolutionary history; not expressed as infectious virus; function unknown; perhaps should be regarded as mere parasitic DNA

Fig. 19.27 Human retroviruses. Human T cell lymphotropic virus (HTLV)1, HTLV2, HIV1 and HIV2 have been cultivated in human T cells *in vitro*. The human placental and genome viruses are not known as infectious agents. Retroviruses are also common in cats (FAIDS), monkeys (MAIDS), mice (mouse leukemia), and other vertebrates. (ARC,=AIDS related complex.)

Fig. 19.28 The structure and genetic map of HIV. The *rev* and *tat* genes are divided into non-contiguous pieces and the gene segments spliced together in the RNA transcript. Occasional host proteins such as major histocompatibility complex (MHC) molecules are present in the envelope. (p) is protein and (gp) is glycoprotein. About 10⁹ HIV1 particles are produced each day at the peak of infection and this, together with the low fidelity of reverse transcriptase, means that new virus variants are always appearing. Mutations are seen especially in *env* and *nef* genes. Any one patient contains many variants and drug resistant and immune resistant mutants emerge. There are also macrophage-tropic and T cell-tropic populations of virus and syncytium-inducing and non syncytium-inducing populations, with effects on disease progression. By genetic analysis HIV1 strains are subdivided into group M (most HIV1 isolates), which contains at least 10 subtypes (A–J) differing in geographic distribution, and group O (African). The degree of cross-immunity between these strains is not clear.

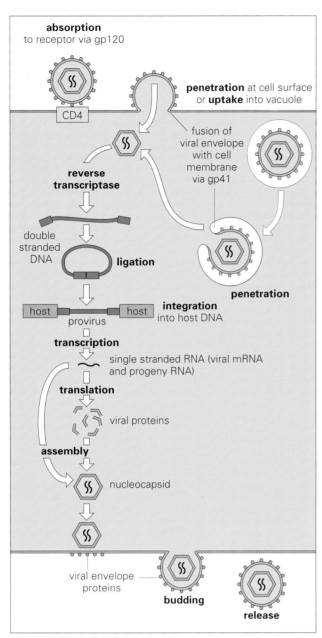

Fig. 19.29 The HIV replication cycle. The virus enters the cell either by fusion with the cell membrane at the cell surface or via uptake into a vacuole and release within the cell.

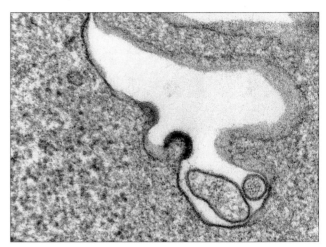

Fig. 19.30 Electron micrograph showing HIV budding from the cell surface before release. (Courtesy of D Hockley.)

HIV infection probably started in Africa in the 1950s, but has now infected 17 million people worldwide

The molecular biologic evidence (in terms of nucleic acid sequence) indicates that both HIV1 and the closely related HIV2 seen in West Africa probably arose from closely related primate viruses. HIV1 may have been present in humans in Central Africa for many years, but in the late 1970s it began to spread rapidly (*Fig. 19.31*), possibly with changed biologic properties as a result of increased transmission following major socioeconomic upheavals and migrations of people from Central to East Africa. Female prostitutes and mobile male soldiers and workers played a major part. The disease soon appeared in Haiti and the USA, followed by Europe and Australasia.

In the late 1980s, HIV began to appear in Asian countries, beginning with Thailand, and by 1995 there were more

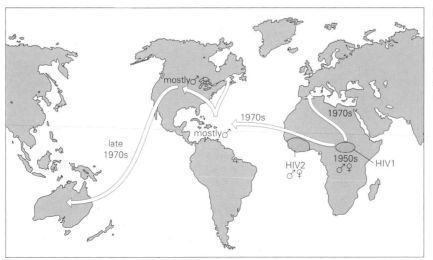

Fig. 19.31 Early spread of HIV infection (now worldwide). HIV1 may have been present in Central Africa for many years before increased migration and socioeconomic upheaval caused it to begin spreading in the late 1970s. Outside Africa, most infections occurred in men.

infections in Asia than in the rest of the world put together. Explosive spread was based on heterosexual transmission, with high infection rates in female sex workers and transmission among users of injected drugs. The next chapter in the HIV pandemic will be in China.

It is estimated that worldwide, until the end of 1995, about 17 million have been infected with HIV:

- 16 million in Africa.
- Four million in Asia.
- Two million in Latin America/Caribbean.
- 1.3 million in North America.
- 0.65 million in Europe.

So far six million people have developed AIDS and five million of these have died. Extrapolation to the year 2000 indicates that total infections could reach 40 million, and by then the incidence of new infections in females will equal that in males (nine million of the 25 million people already infected have been female); 5–10 million children will have been orphaned by the death of infected parents.

HIV infects cells bearing the CD4 antigen

These include TH cells, monocytes and dendritic cells (Figs 19.32, 19.33). The CD4 molecule acts as a binding site for the gp120 envelope glycoprotein of the virus. Productive replication and cell destruction does not occur until the TH cell is activated. TH cell activation is greatly enhanced not only in attempts to respond to HIV antigens, but also as a result of the secondary microbial infections seen in patients. Monocytes and macrophages, Langerhans' cells and follicular dendritic cells also express the CD4 molecule and are infected, but are not generally destroyed. Langerhans' cells (dendritic cells in the skin and genital mucosa) may be the first cells infected. Later in the disease there is a remarkable disruption of histologic pattern in lymphoid follicles due to the breakdown of follicular dendritic cells.

Infected cells bear the fusion protein gp41 and may therefore fuse with other infected or uninfected cells. This helps the virus to spread and accounts for the multinucleated cells seen especially in the brain.

At first the immune system fights back against HIV infection, but then begins to fail

During the first few months virus-specific CD8-positive T cells are formed and reduce the viremia. This is followed by the appearance of neutralizing antibodies. Then the immune system begins to suffer gradual damage, and the number of circulating CD4-positive T cells steadily falls. Nearly all infected CD4-positive T cells are in lymph nodes. The cell-mediated immune responses to viral antigens, as judged by lymphoproliferation, weakens, whereas responses to other antigens are normal. Perhaps the virus initially engineers a specific suppression of protective responses to itself. Eventually the patient loses the battle to replace lost T cells, and the number falls more rapidly. Skin test delayed type hypersensitivity (DTH) responses are absent, natural killer (NK) cell and cytotoxic T (TC) cell activity are reduced, and there are various other immunologic abnormalities, including polyclonal activation of B cells. Functional changes in T lymphocytes – reduced responses to mitogens, reduced interleukin-2 (IL-2) and interferon-gamma (IFNγ) production – are also seen. As AIDS develops, responses to HIV and

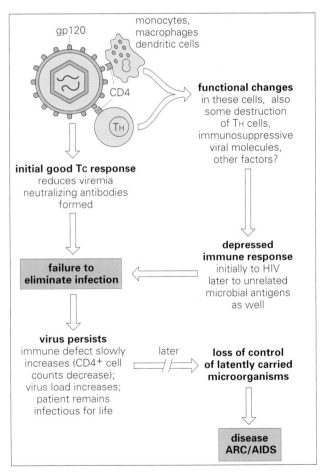

Fig. 19.33 The pathogenesis of AIDS. Although CD4 is the first receptor, there is secondary binding of the virus to chemokine receptors (not shown) on host cells, and this increases the efficiency of infection. Genetic defects in chemokine receptors may account for the failure of certain sex workers in Africa to become infected despite repeated exposure to HIV. (ARC, AIDS-related complex; TC, cytotoxic T cell; TH; T helper lymphocyte.)

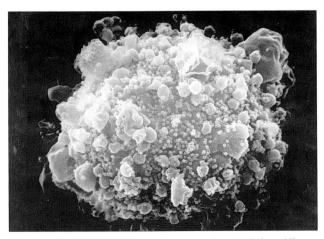

Fig. 19.32 Scanning electron micrograph of an HIV-infected TH cell. ×20 000. (Courtesy of D Hockley.)

unrelated antigens are further depressed. The immune system has lost control.

The exact mechanism of the immuno-suppression in HIV infection is still unclear

The following factors need to be considered:

- TH cells directly killed by virus.
- TH cells induced to commit suicide (apoptosis, programmed cell death) by virus.
- TH cells made vulnerable to immune attack by Tc cells.
- T cell replenishment impaired by damage to the thymus and lymph nodes and by infection of stem cells.
- Defects in antigen presentation associated with infection of dendritic cells.
- Immunosuppressive virus-coded molecules (gp120, gp41).

The host response is further handicapped by antigenic variation in the 'hypervariable' region of gp120. This occurs during infection and as a result different antigenic variants can be isolated from a given individual. Some of the variants show resistance to currently circulating Tcs (i.e. are immune escape variants). Others show increased pathogenicity.

The immunosuppression is permanent, the patient remains infectious and the virus persists in the body. The eventual mortality due to opportunist infections and tumors approaches 100%.

Studies of pathogenicity of HIV2 are in progress. It appears to be transmitted less easily than HIV1, probably because less virus is formed in the patient and the progression to AIDS is slower.

A subacute encephalitis, often with dementia, is a feature of HIV infection

Viral invasion of the CNS and CNS disease occurs independently of AIDS. Multiple small nodules of inflammatory cells are seen, and most of the infected cells appear to be microglia or infiltrating macrophages. These cells express the CD4 antigen, and it has been suggested that infected monocytes carry the virus into the brain. Most AIDS patients develop neurologic disease, and the picture is complicated by the various persistent infections that are activated and give rise to their own CNS pathology. These include infections by HSV, varicella-zoster virus (VZV), *Toxoplasma gondii*, JC virus (progressive multifocal leukoencephalopathy – PML) and *Cryptococcus neoformans*.

Kaposi's sarcoma in AIDS patients is associated with human herpesvirus 8 (HHV8)

Although 21% of homosexual or bisexual males with AIDS develop the Kaposi's sarcoma, it is seen in only 10% of hemophiliacs who have been infected by contaminated blood (Factor VIII) products. Some of the B cell lymphomas are attributable to reactivating Epstein–Barr virus (EBV).

HIV is present in peripheral blood mononuclear cells, which are the major source of transmitted virus

HIV titers are, however, quite low – about 10 000 infectious doses/ml of blood, so the blood is much less infectious than in hepatitis B virus infections. The amount present falls after seroconversion and rises again during the development of AIDS related complex (ARC) and AIDS. Smaller amounts of virus are also present in semen and saliva, and probably even smaller amounts in colostrum, the human cervix and tears. Infection is reported in CD4-positive submucosal cells in the rectum and large bowel and could be a route for entry in homosexuals.

In developed countries, homosexual men have so far been the group most vulnerable to HIV infection and AIDS, especially the passive partner in anal intercourse. Hemophiliacs who have received contaminated blood products have also been contaminated, though less commonly, as well as intravenous drug misusers. Infection is transmitted primarily from male to male and from male to female *(Fig. 19.34)*, although not very efficiently compared with other STDs. Transmission from female to male, however, is a common and well-established

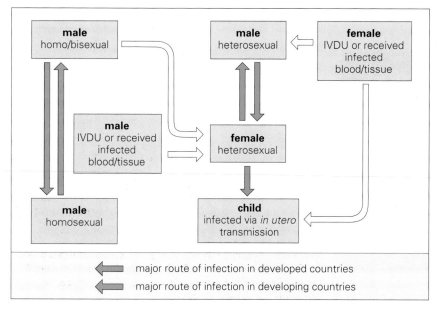

Fig. 19.34 Major routes of transmission of HIV. Although the heterosexual route of transmission has so far been well established only in developing countries, there is evidence that this route is becoming more important in the developed countries. (IVDU, intravenous drug user.)

feature of HIV in Africa and Asia. In randomly selected rural communities in parts of Central and East Africa, seropositivity rates of up to 40% are encountered, mostly in young adults.

Heterosexual transmission has not so far been as important in developed countries as in developing countries

One explanation for the greater heterosexual spread in developing countries is that other STIs are more common, causing ulcers and discharges, which are sources of infected lymphocytes and monocytes. Genital ulcers are associated with a fourfold increase in the risk of infection. Also, viral strains from Asia and sub-Saharan Africa have been shown to infect Langerhans' cells in genital mucosa more easily than other strains. It is not clear whether HIV can infect males by the urethra or whether pre-existing genital skin breaks are necessary. As with other STDs, uncircumcised males are more likely to be infected.

HIV can also be transmitted vertically from infected mother to offspring. This occurs in about 20% of cases, especially *in utero*, but also peri- and postnatally. At least 50% of the infected offspring develop AIDS within the first year of life, but at this age there are fewer latent infections available for reactivation.

As infection in Africa does not generally occur until after the onset of sexual maturity, it is probable that arthropod transmission does not occur. Transmission by close contact, aerosols, kissing and coughing is virtually unknown.

Initial HIV infection may be accompanied by a mild mononucleosis-type illness

Symptoms of the mild mononucleosis-type illness associated with HIV infection include fever and malaise *(Fig. 19.35)*. Antibodies often take many months to become detectable, and Tc cells are formed. Viral replication is reduced, and the individual remains well. Infected cells are, however, still present, and at a later stage the infected individual may develop weight loss, fever, persistent lymphadenopathy, oral candidiasis and diarrhea (i.e. ARC). Further viral replication takes place until finally, some years after initial infection, full-blown AIDS develops *(Fig. 19.35)*.

Factors causing progression from seropositivity to ARC and AIDS are not well understood

HIV exercises complex control over its own replication *(Fig. 19.29)*. Replication is also affected by responses to other infections, which act as antigenic stimuli, and some of them directly as transactivating agents.

A subacute encephalitis, sometimes with dementia, may occur, and also a variety of reactivating infections of the CNS *(Fig. 19.35)* (see Chapter 22). In infants, the CNS picture may include arrested CNS development with microcephaly. Some patients, especially in Africa, develop a wasting disease ('slim' disease), possibly due to unknown intestinal infections or infestations, and perhaps also to the direct effects of the virus infecting cells of the intestinal wall.

The disease AIDS consists of the microbial diseases acquired or reactivated as a result of the underlying immunosuppression due to HIV *(Fig. 19.36)*. The disease picture of

AIDS is an indirect result of infection with HIV, which by itself causes only a minor clinical illness. The neurologic disease, however, is an independent and direct result of neural invasion by HIV, although complicated by reactivation or infection with other infectious agents.

In one study in New York, 80% of patients were dead five years after the onset of the disease and the average survival time after hospital admission was 242 days.

Laboratory tests for HIV infection depend upon the demonstration of specific antibodies

AIDS itself is a clinical definition and in the presence of antibodies to HIV any of the conditions listed in *Figure 19.37*, regardless of the presence of other causes of immunodeficiency, indicate AIDS.

Initially, an ELISA is carried out (see Chapter 14). A positive result is confirmed on a further blood sample by either

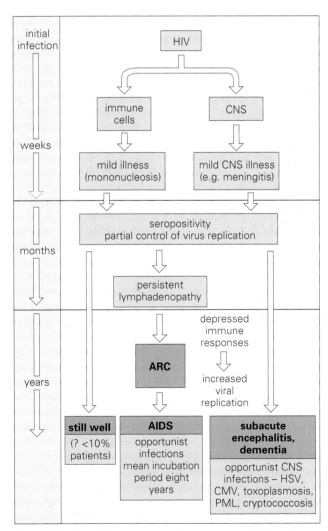

Fig. 19.35 The clinical features and progression of HIV infection. (ARC, AIDS-related complex; CMV, cytomegalovirus; CNS, central nervous system; HSV, herpes simplex virus; PML, progressive multifocal leukoencephalopathy.)

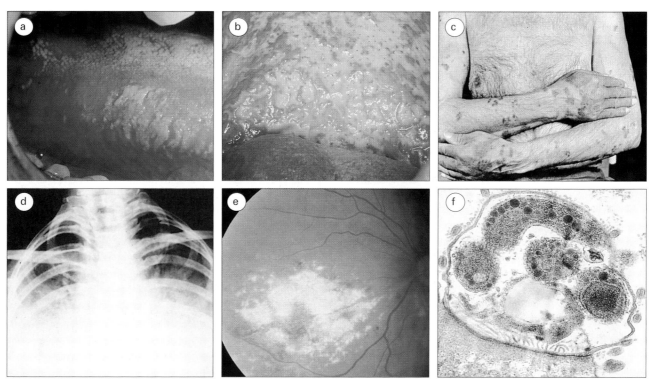

Fig. 19.36 Opportunist infections and tumors associated with HIV infection. (a) Hairy leukoplakia – raised white lesions of oral mucosa, predominently along the lateral aspect of the tongue, due to Epstein-Barr virus infection. (Courtesy of HP Holley.) (b) Extensive oral candidiasis. (Courtesy WE Farrar.) (c) Kaposi's sarcoma – brown pigmented lesions on the upper extremities. (Courtesy of E Sahn.) (d) *Pneumocystis* pneumonia, with extensive infiltrates in both lungs. (Courtesy of JA Innes.) (e) Cytomegalovirus retinitis showing scattered exudates and hemorrhages, with sheathing of vessels. (Courtesy of CJ Ellis.) (f) Cryptosporidiosis – electron micrograph showing mature schizont with several merozoites attached to intestinal epithelium. (Courtesy of WE Farrar.)

Western blotting, radioimmunoassay or immunofluorescence testing. This is done because:

- The ELISA very occasionally gives a false positive report.
- To eliminate possible clerical errors in the clinic or laboratory.

Tests for the infectious virus, for viral antigens or for viral nucleic acids are not routinely available, requiring specialized and expensive technology. Tests to distinguish between antibodies to HIV1 and HIV2 are also available only in specialized laboratories.

Diagnosis of HIV infection in newborn infants is a problem. If IgG antibodies are present they are presumably of maternal origin, but tests for virus-specific IgM antibodies, which would signify *in utero* infection (see Chapter 21), are not yet available. Hopefully reliable tests for HIV antigens or nucleic acid sequences will soon be developed.

Many developed countries have taken measures to reduce the spread of HIV

In developed countries, unlike in Africa and Asia, most cases so far have been in male homosexuals or bisexuals (*Fig. 19.38*), though the picture is changing. All blood donors are tested for antibodies and are discouraged from volunteering if they belong to high-risk HIV groups. Also, all donors of blood for Factor VIII and other blood products are screened for HIV antibody. Heat treatment of Factor VIII is carried out as a fur-

ther precaution before this product is used to treat hemophiliac patients. HIV has a delicate outer envelope and is highly susceptible to heat and chemical agents – much more susceptible than hepatitis B. HIV is inactivated under pasteurization conditions and also by hypochlorites, even at concentrations as low as 1 in 10 000 ppm; 2.5% glutaraldehyde and ethyl alcohol are also effective against the virus.

The main effort in the prevention of HIV infection concerns mass public education programs. These involve inducements to change sexual behavior, particularly a reduction in promiscuous behavior, and the use of barrier contraceptives (condoms). In developed countries there are signs that gay communities are controlling the spread of STDs by altering their behavior in these ways. Infection rates for gonorrhea, syphilis and hepatitis B have been falling. The problem of transmission between intravenous drug users is being tackled in some areas by measures that were originally controversial, such as the free distribution of clean needles and syringes.

The importance of reducing transmission rates is discussed in Chapter 33. The biggest risk for the future in developed countries is that heterosexual transmission becomes more common, following the African and Asian pattern. Unfortunately, the determinants of heterosexual transmission are not understood, but the means for prevention are nevertheless clear – condoms and decreased promiscuity. So far it has proved difficult to induce changes in sexual behavior of

OPPORTUNIST INFECTIONS AND TUMORS IN AIDS	
viruses	disseminated CMV (including lungs, retina, brain) HSV (lungs, gastrointestinal tract, CNS, skin) JC papovavirus (brain – PML) EBV (hairy leukoplakia)
bacteria*	mycobacteria, (e.g. *Mycoplasma avium*, *M. tuberculosis* – disseminated, extrapulmonary) *Salmonella* (recurrent, disseminated) septicemia
protozoa	*Toxoplasma gondii* (disseminated, including CNS) *Cryptosporidium* (chronic diarrhea) *Isospora* (with diarrhea, persisting more than one month)
fungi	*Pneumocystis carinii* (pneumonia) *Candida albicans* (esophagitis, lung infection) *Cryptococcus neoformans* (CNS) histoplasmosis (disseminated, extrapulmonary) *Coccidioides* (disseminated, extrapulmonary)
tumors	Kaposi's sarcoma** B cell lymphoma (e.g. in brain, some are EBV induced)
other	wasting disease (cause unknown) HIV encephalopathy (AIDS dementia complex)

  * also pyogenic bacteria (e.g. *Haemophilus, Streptococcus, Pneumococcus*) causing septicemia, pneumonia, meningitis, osteomyelitis, arthritis, abscesses etc.; multiple or recurrent infections, especially in children
 ** associated with HHV8, an independently-transmitted agent; 300-times as frequent in AIDS as in other immunodeficiencies

Fig. 19.37 Opportunist infections and tumors in AIDS. AIDS is defined as the presence of antibodies to HIV plus one of the conditions in this table. (CMV, cytomegalovirus; CNS, central nervous system; EBV, Epstein-Barr virus; HSV, herpes simplex virus; PML, progressive multifocal leukoencephalopathy.)

AIDS AND ITS CONTROL IN THE UK					
risk group	male		female		control
	to 1992	to 1996	to 1992	to 1996	
homosexual	4421	9120	-	-	+
heterosexual	297	977	184	835	±
intravenous drug users (IVDU)	187	550	76	232	±
haemophiliacs	304	578	4	6	+
blood/tissue transfer	32	50	47	76	++
mother to child	24	96	34	100	±
IVDU and homosexual	88	224	-	-	
other (undetermined)	64	113	10	19	±

Fig. 19.38 Total numbers of AIDS cases reported in the UK up to March 1992 and to June 1996. More than twice as many people are infected (HIV-seropositive) and infectious. (Data courtesy of PHLS Communicable Disease Surveillance Centre, London.)

heterosexuals by means of public health educational programs via the press and television. If these changes in heterosexual behavior can take place, a dramatic reduction in the incidence of all STDs would be assured.

HIV transmission following a needle stick injury involving a patient with HIV is less than 1%

Protection of healthcare staff has been thoroughly investigated. The risk of transmission is much less than with hepatitis B and extensive studies have shown that there is less than a 1% chance of becoming infected with HIV following a needle stick injury involving an HIV-infected patient. Regular precautions such as the wearing of gloves, especially by dentists, will minimize the chances of infection.

The prospects for a successful vaccine against HIV infection are limited, but hopeful

The prospects are limited partly because of antigenic variation of the virus in a given infected patient. Intensive work is in progress and various subunit envelope glycoprotein and whole virus vaccines are being developed and tested. Trials are being carried out in animal (monkey) models and also preliminary trials in humans. Good virus-specific responses are probably needed. The danger of inducing antibodies that enhance infectivity has been noted. Enhancing antibodies are known to be important in the hemorrhagic shock syndrome caused by dengue virus. They combine with the virus without neutralizing it, and the complex then attaches to the Fc receptor present on monocytes, which ingest the complex and thus become infected. In other words, the antibody not only fails to protect, but is responsible for carrying the virus into the susceptible cell! The fact that there is a successful killed virus vaccine for a feline retrovirus (feline leukemia), and that a similar vaccine protects monkeys from simian AIDS does, however, give some hope for the development of an HIV vaccine.

To prevent sexual transmission mucosal immunity is needed, and this is likely to come from a mucosally-administered vaccine. Peptide vaccines at present seem less likely because of the general problem of immunogenicity (e.g. carrier proteins, adjuvants, see Chapter 31) and because numerous T cell epitopes would have to be included in view of the extensive class II MHC antigen variations in human populations.

Treatment of AIDS involves treatment of opportunist infections and antiretrovirals

The opportunist infections are treated appropriately (e.g. cotrimoxazole and pentamidine for *P. carinii*; ganciclovir for CMV).

Zidovudine – azidothymidine (AZT), see Chapter 30 – was the first anti-HIV drug licensed for AIDS and with it:

- The frequency of opportunist infections is reduced.
- Survival is increased.
- There are increases in TH cells.
- It prevents infection of the fetus when given to pregnant women.

However, when used in symptom-free HIV-infected people the drug does not prevent the progression from HIV seropositivity to AIDS and the neurologic disease. In addition, 90% of deaths from AIDS are in parts of the world with no access to antiretroviral treatments.

Four other nucleoside analogues have now been licensed, and combination therapy is best, but the search continues for more effective or cheaper antiviral agents. Possibilities have included inhibitors of HIV protease (e.g. retonavir). The protease is needed to cleave viral proteins from precursors (e.g. gp120 and gp41 from gp160); without it the virus is non-infectious. Other anti-HIV strategies are mentioned in Chapter 30. Numerous trials are in progress.

Opportunist STDs

Opportunist STDs include salmonellae, shigellae, hepatitis A, Giardia lamblia and Entamoeba histolytica infections

Although STDs are classically transmitted during regular heterosexual intercourse, they can also be transmitted whenever two mucosal surfaces are brought together. Anal intercourse allows the transfer of microorganisms from penis to rectal mucosa or to anal and perianal regions. Gonococcal or papillomavirus lesions, for instance, may occur in any of these sites. A few microorganisms (hepatitis B, HIV) are transmitted more often across rectal mucosa. If there is oro-anal contact, a variety of intestinal pathogens are given the opportunity to spread as STDs and can then be regarded as 'opportunist STDs'. These include salmonellae, shigellae, hepatitis A virus, *Giardia lamblia* and *Entamoeba histolytica* (see Chapter 20). Together with persistent infections such as CMV and cryptosporidiosis, they contribute to intestinal symptoms and diarrhea in AIDS patients.

Hepatitis B virus is often transmitted sexually

Such transmission of hepatitis B (see Chapter 20) is especially common among male homosexuals. The virus and its surface antigen, HBs, are detectable in semen, saliva and vaginal secretions, although infectivity titers in these fluids are probably low. Hepatitis B virus transmission among male homosexuals parallels the transmission of HIV, with passive anal intercourse as a high-risk factor. Infection rates have fallen as a result of the reduction in promiscuous condom-free sexual activity in this group of individuals. Hepatitis C and D viruses can also be transmitted sexually.

Arthropod Infestations

Infection with the pubic or crab louse causes itching and is treated with malathion

The 'crab louse', *Phthirus pubis*, is distinct from the other human lice, *Pediculosis humanus corporis* and *Pediculosis humanus capitis*. The crab louse is well adapted for life in the genital region, clinging tightly to the pubic hairs (see Chapter 3). Occasionally hairs on the eyebrows or in the axilla are colonized. It takes up to 10 blood feeds a day and this causes itching at the site of the bites. Eggs called 'nits' are seen attached to the pubic hairs and the characteristic lice, up to 2 mm long, are visible (often at the base of a hair) under a hand lens or by microscopy. Infestation is common, for example there are more than 10 000 cases/year in the UK.

Treatment is by the application of malathion to all affected hair sites.

Genital scabies is treated with benzyl benzoate or benzene hexachloride

Sarcoptes scabiei (see Chapter 23) may cause local lesions on the genitalia, and can be spread as an STD. Patients may have evidence of scabies elsewhere on the body, with burrows between the fingers or toes. Genital scabies is treated with 10% benzyl benzoate or 1% benzene hexachloride.

- Microorganisms transmitted by the sexual route in humans include representatives from all groups apart from the rickettsia and helminths.
- STDs are becoming more widespread in the community rather than remaining confined to high-risk groups.
- Genital warts and chlamydial urethritis are by far the most common of all the STDs, but HIV infection has had a major impact, eclipsing all the other well-known STDs such as gonorrhea and HSV because it is usually eventually lethal.

- Except for hepatitis B there are no vaccines for these infections, but chemotherapy is often available.
- At present, the best method of control is prevention.
- Transmission depends upon human behavior, which is notoriously difficult to influence.
- The longer the interval between the onset of infectiousness and disease and the less incapacitating the disease, the greater the chances of transmission.

A 24-year-old art critic presents with a fever, dry cough, and shortness of breath for 10 days, which have been getting worse. She seems very anxious, but otherwise nothing can be found either in the medical history or on physical examination. A blood sample is collected for an atypical pneumonia screen and her doctor gives her amoxycillin and erythromycin. Five days later she feels much worse and calls her doctor, who arranges for her admission to hospital. The results of the blood tests taken after she had been ill for 10 days are as follows: hemoglobin 13 g/dl; white cell count 2.3×10^9/l; *Mycoplasma* latex agglutination test < 8; complement fixation test for antibodies to chlamydia group < 40, influenza A and B < 40, adenoviruses < 40, *Mycoplasma pneumoniae* < 40, *Coxiella burnetii* < 40.

The patient later admits to weight loss and night sweats, and says that she has been worried because four years ago she had intimate contact over a few months with a boyfriend who was later diagnosed as HIV1 seropositive. On examination the relevant findings are a temperature of 37.8°C, dyspnea, and tachypnea. There are no other findings in the respiratory system. A chest radiograph shows bilateral shadowing and a ground-glass appearance, sparing the upper zones. After appropriate counselling she consents to an HIV antibody screening test.

1. What is the most likely diagnosis?
2. What further investigations would you perform?
3. How would you manage her?
4. She improves over the next two weeks. What is her prognosis and how would you follow her up?

Further Reading

Coates TJ *et al*. HIV prevention in developed countries. *Lancet* 1996;**348**:1143–1148.

d'Cruz–Grote D. Prevention of HIV infection in developing countries. *Lancet* 1996;**348**:1071–1074.

Greene WC. The molecular biology of human immunodeficiency virus type 1 infection. *N Eng J Med* 1991;**324**:308–317.

Hook EW, Holmes KK. Gonococcal infections. *Ann Intern Med* 1985;**102**:229–243.

Kelly GE, Stanley BS, Weller IVD. The natural history of human immunodeficiency virus infection; a five year study in a London cohort of homosexual men. *Genitourin Med* 1990;**2**:238–243.

Levy JA. Pathogenesis of human immunodeficiency virus infection. *Microbiol Revs* 1993;**57**:183–289.

Mindell A, ed. Sexually transmitted diseases. *Curr Opin Infect Dis* 1990;**3**:1–38.

Morrison PRP, Belland RJ, Lyng K *et al*. Chlamydial disease pathogenesis. *J Exp Med* 1989;**170**:1271–1283.

Peckham C, Gibb D. Mother-to-child transmission of the human immunodeficiency virus. *N Engl J Med* 1995;**333**:298–302.

Plummer FA, Brunham RC. Gonococcal recidivism, diversity and ecology. *Rev Inf Dis* 1987;**9**:846.

Quinn TC. Global burden of the HIV pandemic. *Lancet* 1996;**348**:99–106.

Treharne JD, Ballard RC. The expanding spectrum of the *Chlamydia* – a microbiological and clinical appraisal. *Rev Med Microbiol* 1990;**1**:10–18.

Introduction

Ingested pathogens may cause disease confined to the gut or involving other parts of the body

Ingestion of pathogens can cause many different infections. These may be confined to the gastrointestinal tract or initiated in the gut before spreading to other parts of the body. In this chapter we consider the important bacterial causes of diarrheal disease and summarize the other bacterial causes of food-associated infection and food poisoning. Viral and parasitic causes of diarrheal disease are discussed, as well as infections acquired via the gastrointestinal tract and causing disease in other body systems, including typhoid and paratyphoid fevers, listeriosis, and some forms of viral hepatitis. For clarity, all types of viral hepatitis are included in this chapter. Infections of the liver can also result in liver abscesses, and several parasitic infections cause liver disease. Peritonitis and intra-abdominal abscesses can arise from seeding of the abdominal cavity by organisms from the gastrointestinal tract. Several different terms are used to describe infections of the gastrointestinal tract; those in common use are shown in *Figure 20.1*.

A wide range of microbial pathogens is capable of infecting the gastrointestinal tract and the important bacterial and viral pathogens are listed in *Figure 20.2*. They are acquired by the fecal–oral route, from fecally-contaminated food, fluids or fingers.

For an infection to occur, the pathogen must be ingested in sufficient numbers or possess attributes to elude the host defenses of the upper gastrointestinal tract and reach the intestine (*Fig. 20.3*; see also Chapter 7). Here they remain localized and cause disease as a result of multiplication and/or toxin production, or they may invade through the intestinal mucosa to reach the lymphatics or the bloodstream *(Fig. 20.4)*. The damaging effects resulting from infection of the gastrointestinal tract are summarized in *Figure 20.5*.

Food-associated infection versus food poisoning

Infection associated with consumption of contaminated food is often termed 'food poisoning', but 'food-associated infection' is a better term. True food poisoning occurs after consumption of food containing toxins, which may be chemical (e.g. heavy metals) or bacterial in origin (e.g. from *Clostridium botulinum* or *Staphylococcus aureus*). The bacteria multiply and produce toxin within contaminated food. The organisms may be destroyed during food preparation, but the toxin is unaffected, consumed and acts within hours. In food-associated infections, the food may simply act as a vehicle for the pathogen (e.g. *Campylobacter*) or provide conditions in which the pathogen can multiply to produce numbers large enough to cause disease (e.g. *Salmonella*).

Diarrheal Diseases

Diarrhea is the most common outcome of gastrointestinal tract infection

Infections of the gastrointestinal tract range in their effects from a mild self-limiting attack of 'the runs' to severe, sometimes fatal, diarrhea. There may be associated vomiting, fever and malaise. Diarrhea is the result of an increase in fluid and

---

TERMS USED TO DESCRIBE GASTROINTESTINAL TRACT INFECTIONS

gastroenteritis
a syndrome characterized by gastrointestinal symptoms including nausea, vomiting, diarrhea and abdominal discomfort

diarrhea
abnormal fecal discharge characterized by frequent and/or fluid stool; usually resulting from disease of the small intestine and involving increased fluid and electrolyte loss

dysentery
an inflammatory disorder of the gastrointestinal tract often associated with blood and pus in the feces and accompanied by symptoms of pain, fever, abdominal cramps; usually resulting from disease of the large intestine

enterocolitis
inflammation involving the mucosa of both the small and large intestine

Fig. 20.1 As well as many colloquial expressions, several different clinical terms are used to describe infections of the gastrointestinal tract. Diarrhea without blood and pus is usually the result of enterotoxin production, whereas the presence of blood and/or pus cells in the feces indicates an invasive infection with mucosal destruction.

IMPORTANT BACTERIAL AND VIRAL PATHOGENS OF THE GASTROINTESTINAL TRACT			
pathogen	animal reservoir	foodborne	waterborne
Bacteria			
Escherichia coli	+?	+(EHEC)	+(ETEC)
Salmonella	+	+++	+
Campylobacter	+	+++	+
Vibrio cholerae	–	+	+++
Shigella	–	+	–
Clostridium perfringens	+	+++	–
Bacillus cereus	–	++	–
Vibrio parahaemolyticus	–	++	–
Yersinia enterocolitica	+	+	–
Viruses			
rotavirus	–	–	–
small round viruses	–	++	+

Fig. 20.2 Many different pathogens cause infections of the gastrointestinal tract. Some are found in both humans and animals while others are strictly human parasites. This difference has important implications for control and prevention. (EHEC, verotoxin-producing *Escherichia coli*; ETEC, enterotoxigenic *E. coli*.)

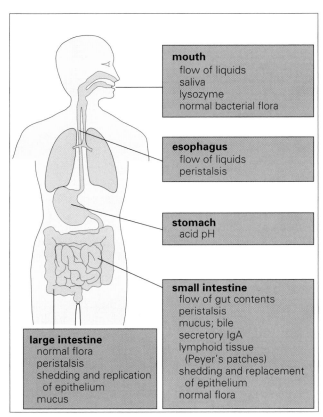

Fig. 20.3 Every day we swallow large numbers of microorganisms. Because of the body's defense mechanisms, however, they rarely succeed in surviving the passage to the intestine in sufficient numbers to cause infection.

electrolyte loss into the gut lumen, leading to the production of unformed or liquid feces and can be thought of as the method by which the host forcibly expels the pathogen (and in doing so, aids its dissemination). However, diarrhea also occurs in many non-infectious conditions, and an infectious cause should not be assumed.

In the developing world, diarrheal disease is a major cause of mortality in children

In the developing world, diarrheal disease is a major cause of morbidity and mortality, particularly in young children. In the developed world it remains a very common complaint, but is usually mild and self-limiting except in the very young, the elderly, and immunocompromised patients. Most of the pathogens listed in *Figure 20.2* are found throughout the world, but some such as *Vibrio cholerae*, have a more limited geographic distribution. However, such infections can be acquired by travellers to these areas and imported into their home countries.

Many cases of diarrheal disease are not diagnosed, either because they are mild and self-limiting and the patient does not seek medical attention, or because medical and laboratory facilities are unavailable, particularly in developing countries. It is generally impossible to distinguish on clinical grounds between infections caused by the different pathogens. However, information about the patient's recent food and travel history, and macroscopic and microscopic examination of the feces for blood and pus can provide helpful clues. A precise diagnosis can only be achieved by laboratory investigations. This is especially important in outbreaks, because of the need to instigate appropriate epidemiologic investigations and control measures.

Bacterial causes of diarrhea
Escherichia coli

This is one of the most versatile of all bacterial pathogens. Some strains are important members of the normal gut flora in man and animals (see Chapter 3), whereas others possess virulence factors that enable them to cause infections in the intestinal tract or at other sites, particularly the urinary tract (see Chapter 18). Strains that cause diarrheal disease do so by several distinct pathogenic mechanisms and differ in their epidemiology *(Fig. 20.6)*.

There are four distinct groups of E. coli with different pathogenetic mechanisms

Enterotoxic *Escherichia coli* (ETEC) *(Fig. 20.6)* possess colonization factors, which bind the bacteria to specific receptors

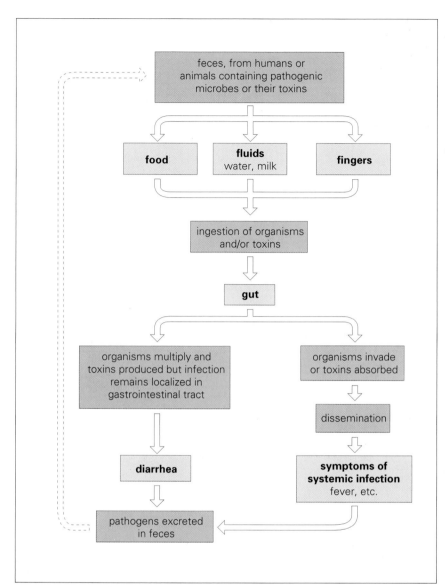

Fig. 20.4 Infections of the gastrointestinal tract can be grouped into those that remain localized in the gut and those that invade beyond the gut to cause infection in other sites in the body. In order to spread to a new host, pathogens are excreted in large numbers in the feces and must survive in the environment for long enough to infect another person directly or indirectly through contaminated food or fluids.

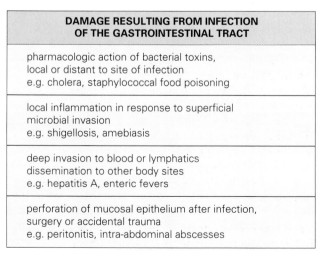

Fig. 20.5 Infection of the gastrointestinal tract can cause damage locally or at distant sites.

on the intestinal cell membrane *(Fig. 20.7)* where the organisms produce powerful enterotoxins:
- Heat-labile enterotoxin (LT) is very similar in structure and mode of action to cholera toxin produced by *V. cholerae*, and infections with strains producing LT can mimic cholera, particularly in young and malnourished children.
- Other ETEC strains produce heat-stable enterotoxins (STs) in addition to or instead of LT. STs have a similar but distinct mode of action to that of LT. ST_A activates guanylate cyclase activity causing an increase in cyclic guanosine monophosphate, which results in increased fluid secretion. The mechanism of action of ST_B is unknown. Unlike LT, the STs are not immunogenic and cannot therefore be detected by immunologic tests *(Fig. 20.6)*.

Other *E. coli* strains produce a verotoxin, so-called because it is toxic to tissue cultures of 'vero' cells. After attachment to the intestinal mucosa (by an 'attaching–effacing' mechanism), the organisms elaborate verotoxin, which has a direct effect on

CHARACTERISTICS OF *ESCHERICHIA COLI* STRAINS CAUSING GASTROINTESTINAL INFECTIONS		
pathogenic group	**epidemiology**	**laboratory diagnosis***
enterotoxigenic *E. coli* (ETEC)	most important bacterial cause of diarrhea in children in developing countries most common cause of travellers' diarrhea water contaminated by human or animal sewage may be important in spread	isolate organisms from feces test for production of LT (but not ST) by immunologic techniques e.g. ELISA *test for production of STs by detecting accumulation of fluid in ligated ileal loops of experimental animals (not in routine use)* *gene probes specific for LT and ST genes available for detection of ETEC in feces and in food and water samples*
enteroinvasive *E. coli* (EIEC)	important cause of diarrhea in areas of poor hygiene infections usually foodborne; no evidence of animal or environmental reservoir	isolate organisms from feces; *test for enteroinvasive potential in tissue culture cells*
verotoxin-producing *E. coli* (EHEC)	serotype 0157 most important EHEC in human infections outbreaks and sporadic cases occur worldwide food and unpasteurized milk important in spread	isolate organisms from feces proportion of EHEC in fecal sample may be very low (often <1% of *E. coli* colonies) usually sorbitol non-fermenters *EHEC-producing colonies can be identified with DNA probes in colony hybridization tests*
enteropathogenic *E. coli* (EPEC)	EPEC strains belong to particular O serotypes cause sporadic cases and outbreaks of infection in babies and young children importance in adults not known	isolate organisms from feces determine serotype of several colonies with polyvalent antisera for known EPEC types *adhesion to tissue culture cells can be demonstrated by a fluorescence actin staining test*

Fig. 20.6 *Escherichia coli* is a major cause of gastrointestinal infection, particularly in developing countries and in travellers. There is a range of pathogenic mechanisms within the species, resulting in more or less invasive disease. *Specialized tests are given in italics. (ELISA, enzyme-linked immunosorbent assay; LT, heat-labile enterotoxin; ST, heat-stable enterotoxin.)

intestinal epithelium resulting in diarrhea. These strains are referred to as verotoxin-producing *E. coli* (EHEC) *(Fig. 20.6)* because they cause hemorrhagic colitis (HC) and hemolytic–uremic syndrome (HUS). In HC there is destruction of the mucosa and consequent hemorrhage; this may be followed by HUS. Verotoxin receptors have been identified on renal epithelium and may account for the kidney involvement.

Enteropathogenic *E.coli* (EPEC) were the first group of *E. coli* intestinal pathogens to be described, but their mechanism of pathogenicity remains unclear. They do not appear to produce any toxins, but have a particular mechanism of adhesion ('attaching–effacing' as with EHEC) to enterocytes that appears to destroy the microvilli *(Fig. 20.8)*.

Enteroinvasive *E. coli* (EIEC) attach specifically to the mucosa of the large intestine and invade the cells by being taken in by endocytosis. Inside the cell they lyse the endocytic vacuole, multiply and spread to adjacent cells, causing tissue destruction and consequently inflammation.

ETEC is the most important bacterial cause of diarrhea in children in developing countries

The diarrhea produced by *E. coli* varies from mild to severe depending upon the strain and the underlying health of the host. ETEC diarrhea in children in developing countries may be clinically indistinguishable from cholera. EIEC and EHEC strains both cause bloody diarrhea. Following EHEC infection, HUS is characterized by acute renal failure *(Fig. 20.9)*, anemia and thrombocytopenia, and there may be neurologic complications. HUS is the most common cause of acute renal failure in children in the UK and USA.

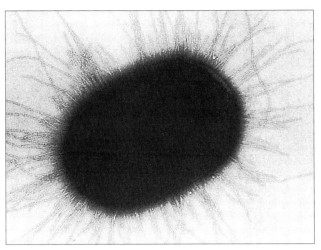

Fig. 20.7 Electron micrograph of enterotoxin *Escherichia coli*, showing pili necessary for adherence to mucosal epithelial cells. (Courtesy of S Knutton.)

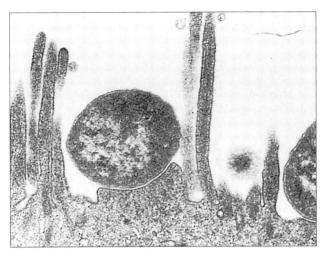

Fig. 20.8 Electron micrograph of enteropathogenic *Escherichia coli* adhering to the brush border of intestinal mucosal cells with localized destruction of microvilli. (Courtesy of S Knutton.)

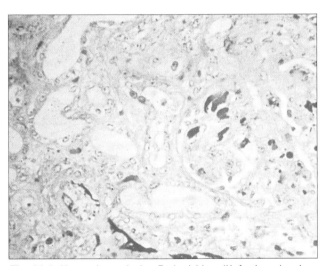

Fig. 20.9 Verotoxin-producing *Escherichia coli* infection, showing fibrin 'thrombi' in glomerular capillaries in hemolytic-uremic syndrome. Weigert stain. (Courtesy of HR Powell.)

Specific tests are needed to identify strains of pathogenic E. coli

Because *E. coli* is a member of the normal gastrointestinal flora, specific tests are required to identify strains that may be responsible for diarrheal disease. These are summarized in *Figure 20.6*. Infections are more common in children and are often travel-associated, and these factors should be considered when samples are received in the laboratory.

Antibacterial therapy is not indicated for E. coli diarrhea

Specific antibacterial therapy is not indicated. Fluid replacement may be necessary, especially in young children. Treatment of HUS is urgent and may involve dialysis.

Provision of a clean water supply and adequate systems for sewage disposal are fundamental to the prevention of diarrheal disease. Food and unpasteurized milk can be important vehicles of infection, especially for EIEC and EHEC, but there is no evidence of an animal or environmental reservoir.

Salmonella
Salmonellae are the most common cause of food-associated diarrhea in many developed countries

Until recently salmonellae were the most common cause of food-associated diarrhea in the developed world, but in some countries they have now been beaten into second place by campylobacter. Like *E. coli*, the salmonellae belong to the Enterobacteria and the genus *Salmonella* has been divided into more than 2000 species on the basis of differences in the cell wall (O) and flagellar (H) antigens (Kauffmann–White scheme). However, more recent studies indicate that there is a single species, or at most three species, and that serotypes should not be given species status (see Appendix). Nevertheless it is useful to be able to distinguish between serotypes for epidemiologic purposes, for example when tracing the source of an outbreak.

All salmonellae except for *Salmonella typhi* and *S. paratyphi* are found in animals as well as humans. There is a large animal reservoir of infection, which is transmitted to man via contaminated food, especially poultry and dairy products *(Fig. 20.10)*. Waterborne infection is less frequent. Salmonella infection is also transmitted from person to person and therefore secondary spread can occur, for example within a family after one member has become infected after consuming contaminated food.

Diarrhea is the most common manifestation of infection caused by Salmonella spp. other than S. typhi and S. paratyphi

Diarrhea is produced as a result of invasion by the salmonellae of epithelial cells in the terminal portion of the small intestine *(Fig. 20.11)*. Initial entry is probably through uptake by M cells (the 'antigenic samplers' of the bowel) with

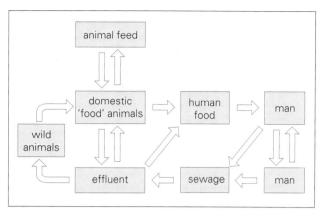

Fig. 20.10 The recycling of salmonellae. With the exception of *Salmonella typhi*, salmonellae are widely distributed in animals, providing a constant source of infection for man. Excretion of large numbers of salmonellae from infected individuals and carriers allows the organisms to be 'recycled'.

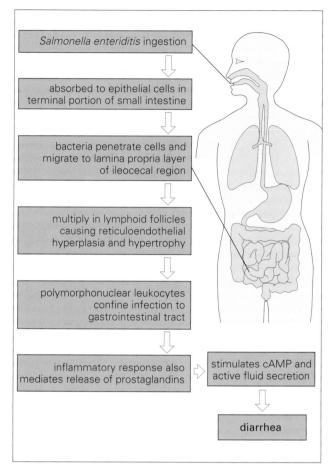

Fig. 20.11 The passage of salmonellae through the body to the gut. The vast majority of salmonellae cause infection localized to the gastrointestinal tract and do not invade beyond the gut mucosa. They do not produce enterotoxins. (cAMP, cyclic adenosine monophosphate.)

subsequent spread to epithelial cells. A similar route of invasion occurs in *Shigella*, *Yersinia* and reovirus infections. The bacteria migrate to the lamina propria layer of the ileocecal region, where their multiplication stimulates an inflammatory response, which both confines the infection to the gastrointestinal tract and mediates the release of prostaglandins. These in turn activate cyclic adenosine monophosphate (cAMP) and fluid secretion, resulting in diarrhea. Salmonellae do not appear to produce enterotoxins.

Species of *Salmonella* that normally cause diarrhea (e.g. *S. enteritidis*, *S. cholerae suis*) may become invasive in patients with particular predispositions (e.g. children and patients with cancer or sickle cell anemia). The organisms are not contained within the gastrointestinal tract, but invade the body to cause septicemia; consequently, many organs become seeded with salmonellae, sometimes leading to osteomyelitis, pneumonia or meningitis.

In the vast majority of cases, *Salmonella* spp. cause an acute but self-limiting diarrhea, though in the young and the elderly the symptoms may be more severe. Vomiting is rare and fever is usually a sign of invasive disease *(Fig. 20.12)*. In the UK there is a reported annual incidence of salmonella bacteremia of approximately 150 cases, with about 70 deaths. This should be set in context against the approximately 30 000 reported cases of diarrhea.

S. typhi and *S. paratyphi* invade the body from the gastrointestinal tract to cause systemic illness and are discussed in a later section.

Salmonella diarrhea can be diagnosed by culture on selective media

The methods for culturing fecal specimens on selective media are summarized in the Appendix. The organisms are not fastidious and can usually be isolated within 24 hours, although small numbers may require enrichment in selenite broth before culture. Preliminary identification can be made rapidly, but the complete result, including serotype, takes at least 48 hours.

Fluid and electrolyte replacement may be needed for salmonella diarrhea

Diarrhea is usually self-limiting and resolves without treatment. Fluid and electrolyte replacement may be required, particularly in the very young and the elderly. Unless there is evidence of invasion and septicemia, antibiotics should be positively discouraged because they do not reduce the symptoms or shorten the illness, and may prolong excretion of salmonellae in the feces. There is some evidence that symptomatic treatment with drugs that reduce diarrhea has the same adverse effect.

Salmonellae may be excreted in the feces for several weeks after a salmonella infection

Figure 20.10 illustrates the problems associated with the prevention of salmonella infections. The large animal reservoir makes it impossible to eliminate the organisms and therefore preventive measures must be aimed at 'breaking the chain' between animal and man, and person to person. Such measures include:

CLINICAL FEATURES OF BACTERIAL DIARRHEAL DISEASE						
pathogen	incubation period	duration	symptoms			
			diarrhea	vomiting	abdominal cramps	fever
Salmonella	6h–2 days	48h–7 days	+ +	+	–	+
Campylobacter	2–11 days	3 days–3 weeks	+ + +	–	+ +	+ +
Shigella	1–4 days	2–3 days	+ +/+ + +	–	+	+
Vibrio cholerae	2–3 days	up to 7 days	+ + + +	+	–	–
Vibrio parahaemolyticus	8h–2 days	3 days	+/+ +	+	+	+
Clostridium perfringens	8h–1 day	12h–1 day	+ +	–	+ +	–
Bacillus cereus diarrheal emetic	8h–12h 15min–4h	12h–1 day 12h–2 days	+ + +	– + +	+ +	–
Yersinia enterocolitica	4–7 days	1–2 weeks	+ +	–	+ +	+

Fig. 20.12 The clinical features of bacterial diarrhea infection. It is difficult, if not impossible, to determine the likely cause of a diarrheal illness on the basis of clinical features alone, and laboratory investigations are essential to identify the pathogen.

- Maintaining adequate standards of public health (clean drinking water and proper sewage disposal).
- Education programs on hygienic food preparation.

Following an episode of salmonella diarrhea, an individual can continue to carry and excrete organisms in the feces for several weeks. Although in the absence of symptoms the organisms will not be dispersed so liberally into the environment, thorough handwashing before food handling is essential. People employed as food handlers are excluded from work until three specimens of feces have failed to grow salmonella.

Campylobacter
Campylobacters are among the commonest causes of diarrhea

Campylobacter spp. are curved or S-shaped Gram-negative rods *(Fig. 20.13)*. They have long been known to cause diarrheal disease in animals, but are also one of the most common causes of diarrhea in humans. The delay in recognizing the importance of these organisms was due to their cultural requirements, which differ from those of the Enterobacteria as they are microaerophilic and thermophilic; they do not therefore grow on the media used for isolating *E. coli* and salmonellae. Several species of the genus *Campylobacter* are associated with human disease, but *Campylobacter jejuni* is by far the most common. *Campylobacter pylori*, now classified as *Helicobacter pylori* is an important cause of gastritis and gastric ulcers .

As with salmonellae, there is a large animal reservoir of campylobacter in cattle, sheep, rodents, poultry and wild birds. Infections are acquired by consumption of contaminated food, especially poultry, milk or water. Recent studies have shown an association between infection and consumption of milk from bottles with tops that have been pecked by wild birds. Household pets such as dogs and cats can become infected and provide a source for human infection, particularly for young children. Person to person spread by the fecal–oral route is rare, as is transmission from food handlers.

Campylobacter diarrhea is clinically indistinguishable from that of salmonella diarrhea

The pathogenesis of campylobacter diarrhea has not yet been elucidated. The gross pathology and histologic appearances of ulceration and inflamed bleeding mucosal surfaces in the jejunum, ileum and colon *(Fig. 20.14)* are compatible with invasion of the bacteria, but the production of cytotoxins by *C. jejuni* has also been demonstrated. Invasion and bacteremia are not uncommon, particularly in neonates and debilitated adults.

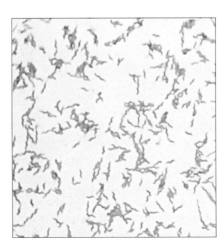

Fig. 20.13 *Campylobacter jejuni* infection. Gram stain showing Gram-negative, S-shaped bacilli. (Courtesy of I Farrell.)

The clinical presentation is indistinguishable from diarrhea caused by salmonellae although the disease may have a longer incubation period and a longer duration. The key features are summarized in *Figure 20.12.*

Cultures for campylobacter should be set up routinely in every investigation of a diarrheal illness

The methods are described in the Appendix, but it is important to note that the media and conditions for growth differ from those required for the Enterobacteria. Growth is often somewhat slow compared with that of the Enterobacteria, but a presumptive identification should be available within 48 hours of culture.

Erythromycin is used for severe campylobacter diarrhea

Erythromycin is the antibiotic of choice for cases of diarrheal disease that are severe enough to warrant treatment. Invasive infections may require treatment with an aminoglycoside.

The preventive measures for salmonella infections described above are equally applicable to the prevention of campylobacter infections, but there are no requirements for the screening of food handlers because contamination of food by this route is very uncommon.

Cholera

Cholera is an acute infection of the gastrointestinal tract caused by the comma-shaped Gram-negative bacterium *V. cholerae (Fig. 20.15)*. The disease has a long history characterized by epidemics and pandemics. The last cases of cholera acquired in the UK were in the last century following the introduction of the bacterium by sailors arriving from Europe, and in 1849 Snow published his historic essay *On the Mode of Communication of Cholera.*

Cholera flourishes in communities with inadequate clean drinking water and sewage disposal

The 1990s have witnessed the seventh pandemic of cholera spreading into Latin America, and the disease remains endemic in South East Asia and parts of Africa and South America. Unlike salmonellae and campylobacter, *V. cholerae* is a free-living inhabitant of fresh water, but causes infection only in humans. Asymptomatic human carriers are believed to be a major reservoir. The disease is spread via contaminated food; shellfish grown in fresh and estuarine waters have also been implicated. Direct person to person spread is thought to be uncommon. Therefore cholera continues to flourish in communities where there is absent or unreliable provision of clean drinking water and sewage disposal. Cases still occur in developed countries, but high standards of hygiene mean that secondary spread should not occur. Over the past 20 years there have been 66 cases reported in the UK and 10 cases in the USA, which amounts to about one case for every 500 000 travellers to areas with endemic cholera.

V. cholerae serotypes are based on somatic (O) antigens

Serotype O1 is the most important and is further divided into two biotypes: classical and El Tor *(Fig. 20.16)*. The El Tor biotype, named after the quarantine camp where it was first isolated from pilgrims returning from Mecca, differs from classical *V. cholerae* in several ways. In particular it causes only a mild diarrhea and has a higher ratio of carriers to cases than classical cholera; carriage is also more prolonged and the organisms survive better in the environment. The El Tor biotype, which was responsible for the seventh pandemic, has now spread throughout the world and has largely displaced the classical biotype.

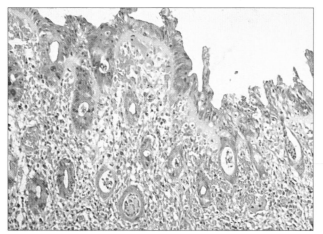

Fig. 20.14 Inflammatory enteritis caused by *Campylobacter jejuni*, involving the entire mucosa, with flattened atrophic villi, necrotic debris in the crypts and thickening of the basement membrane. Cresyl-fast violet stain. (Courtesy of J Newman.)

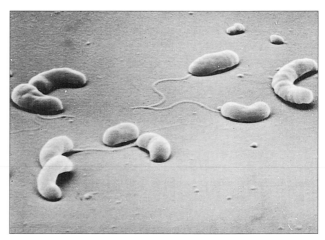

Fig. 20.15 Scanning electron micrograph of *Vibrio cholerae* showing comma-shaped rods with a single polar flagellum. ×13 000. (Courtesy of DK Banerjee.)

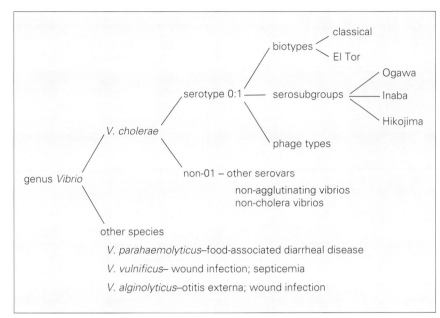

Fig. 20.16 *Vibrio cholerae* serotype O:1, the cause of cholera, can be subdivided into different biotypes with different epidemiologic features, and into serosubgroups and phage types for the purposes of investigating outbreaks of infection. Although *V. cholerae* is the most important pathogen of the genus, other species can also cause infections of both the gastrointestinal tract and other sites.

In 1992 a new non-O1 strain (O139) arose in south India and spread rapidly. It is able to infect O1-immune individuals and cause epidemics, and has been proclaimed as the eighth pandemic strain of cholera. *V. cholerae* O139 appears to have originated from the El Tor O1 biotype when the latter acquired a new O (capsular) antigen by horizontal gene transfer from a non-O1 strain. This provided the recipient strain with a selective advantage in a region where a large part of the population is immune to O1 strains.

Other species of *Vibrio* cause a variety of infections in man *(Fig. 20.16)*. *V. parahaemolyticus* is another cause of diarrheal disease, but this is usually much less severe than cholera (see below).

The symptoms of cholera are caused by an enterotoxin

The symptoms of cholera are entirely due to the production of an enterotoxin in the gastrointestinal tract (see Chapter 12). However, the organism requires additional virulence factors to enable it to survive the host defenses and adhere to the intestinal mucosa. These are illustrated in *Figure 20.17* (see also Chapter 8).

The clinical features of cholera are summarized in *Figure 20.12*. The severe watery non-bloody diarrhea is known as rice water stool because of its appearance *(Fig. 20.18)* and can result in the loss of one liter of fluid every hour. It is this fluid loss and the consequent electrolyte imbalance that results in marked dehydration, metabolic acidosis (loss of bicarbonate), hypokalemia (potassium loss) and hypovolemic shock resulting in cardiac failure. Untreated, the mortality from cholera is 40–60%; rapidly instituted fluid and electrolyte replacement reduces the mortality to less than 1%.

Culture is necessary to diagnose sporadic or imported cases of cholera and carriers

In countries where cholera is prevalent, diagnosis is based on

clinical grounds and laboratory confirmation is rarely sought. It is worth remembering that ETEC infection can resemble cholera in its severity, but for both diseases, fluid and electrolyte replacement are of paramount important. The methods are given in the Appendix.

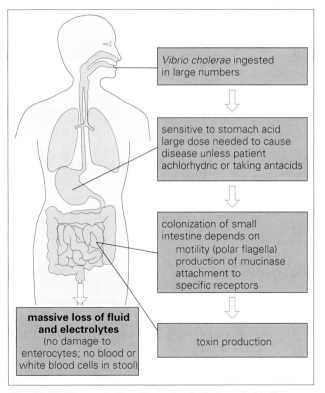

Fig. 20.17 The production of an enterotoxin is central to the pathogenesis of cholera, but the organisms must possess other virulence factors to allow them to reach the small intestine and to adhere to the mucosal cells.

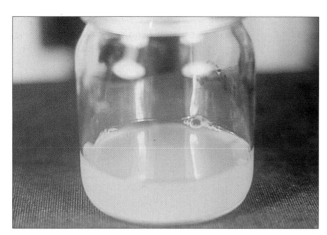

Fig. 20.18 Rice water stool in cholera. (Courtesy of AM Geddes.)

Prompt rehydration with fluids and electrolytes is central to the treatment of cholera

Oral or intravenous rehydration may be used. Antibiotics are not necessary, but tetracycline may be given as some evidence indicates that this reduces the time of excretion of *V. cholerae* thereby reducing the risk of transmission. There have, however, been reports of tetracycline-resistant *V. cholerae* in some areas.

As with other diarrheal disease, a clean drinking water supply and adequate sewage disposal are fundamental to the prevention of cholera. As there is no animal reservoir, it should in theory be possible to eliminate the disease. However, carriage in humans, albeit for only a few weeks, occurs in 1–20% of previously infected patients making eradication difficult to achieve.

Killed whole-cell cholera vaccine is no longer recommended by the WHO

A killed whole-cell vaccine is available and is given parenterally, but is effective in only about 50% of those vaccinated, with protection lasting for only 3–6 months. It is no longer recommended by the World Health Organization (WHO) for travellers to cholera-endemic areas, although it may be required in certain countries. Field trials of various oral vaccines are in progress.

Shigellosis
Symptoms of Shigella infection range from mild to severe depending upon the infecting species

Shigellosis is also known as bacillary dysentery (in contrast to amebic dysentery; see below) because in its more severe form it is characterized by an invasive infection of the mucosa of the large intestine causing inflammation and resulting in the presence of pus and blood in the diarrheal stool. However, symptoms range from mild to severe depending upon the species of *Shigella* involved and on the underlying state of health of the host. There are four species:

- *Shigella sonnei* causes most infections at the mild end of the spectrum.
- *Shigella flexneri* and *S. boydii* usually produce more severe disease.
- *Shigella dysenteriae* is the most serious.

Shigellosis is primarily a pediatric disease. When associated with severe malnutrition it may precipitate complications such as the protein deficiency syndrome 'kwashiorkor'. Like *V. cholerae*, shigellae are human pathogens without an animal reservoir, but unlike the vibrios, they are not found in the environment, being spread from person to person by the fecal–oral route and less frequently by contaminated food and water. Shigellae appear to be able to initiate infection from a small infective dose (10–100 organisms) and therefore spread is easy in situations where sanitation or personal hygiene may be poor (e.g. refugee camps, nurseries, day care centers and institutions for the handicapped).

Shigella diarrhea is usually watery at first, but later contains mucus and blood

Shigellae attach to, and invade, the mucosal epithelium of the distal ileum and colon, causing inflammation and ulceration *(Fig. 20.19)*. However, they rarely invade through the gut wall to the bloodstream. Enterotoxin is produced, but its role in pathogenesis is uncertain since toxin-negative mutants still produce disease.

The main features of shigella infection are summarized in *Figure 20.12*. Diarrhea is usually watery at first, but later contains mucus and blood. Lower abdominal cramps can be severe. The disease is usually self-limiting, but dehydration can occur, especially in the young and elderly. Complications can be associated with malnutrition (see above).

Antibiotics should only be given for severe shigella diarrhea

Rehydration may be indicated. Antibiotics should not be given except in severe cases. Plasmid-mediated resistance is

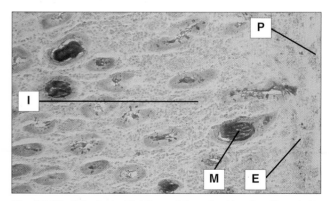

Fig. 20.19 Shigellosis. Histology of the colon showing disrupted epithelium covered by pseudomembrane and interstitial infiltration. Mucin glands have discharged their contents and the goblet cells are empty. Colloidal iron stain. (E, epithelium; I, interstitial infiltration; M, mucin in glands; P, pseudomembrane.) (Courtesy of RH Gilman.)

common and antibiotic susceptibility tests should be performed on shigella isolates if treatment is required.

Education in personal hygiene and proper sewage disposal are important. Cases may continue to excrete shigellae for a few weeks, but longer term carriage is unusual; therefore with adequate public health measures and no animal reservoir, the disease is potentially eradicable.

Other bacterial causes of diarrheal disease

The pathogens described in the previous sections are the major bacterial causes of diarrheal disease. Salmonella and campylobacter infections and some types of *E. coli* infections are most often food-associated, whereas cholera is more often waterborne and shigellosis is usually spread by direct fecal–oral contact. Other bacterial pathogens that cause food-associated infection or food poisoning are described below.

V. parahaemolyticus and Yersinia enterocolitica are foodborne Gram-negative causes of diarrhea

V. parahaemolyticus is a halophilic (salt-loving) vibrio that contaminates seafood and fish. If these foods are consumed uncooked, diarrheal disease can result. The mechanism of pathogenesis is still unclear. Most strains associated with infection are hemolytic due to production of a heat-stable cytotoxin and have been shown to invade intestinal cells (in contrast to *V. cholerae*, which is non-invasive and cholera toxin, which is not cytotoxic).

The clinical features of infection are summarized in *Figure 20.12*. The methods used for the laboratory diagnosis of *V. parahaemolyticus* infection are given in the Appendix. As the special media for cultivating vibrios are not used routinely, the request form accompanying the specimen must provide adequate information about the patient's history and food consumption to indicate to the laboratory that vibrios should be looked for. Prevention of infection depends upon cooking fish and seafood properly.

Yersinia enterocolitica is a member of the Enterobacteriaceae and is a cause of food-associated infection, particularly in colder parts of the world. The reason for this geographic distribution is unknown, but it has been speculated that it is because the organism prefers to grow at temperatures of 22–25°C. *Y. enterocolitica* is found in a variety of animal hosts including rodents, rabbits, pigs, sheep, cattle, horses and domestic pets. Transmission to humans from household dogs has been reported. The organism survives and multiplies, albeit more slowly, at refrigeration temperatures (4°C) and has been implicated in outbreaks of infection associated with contaminated milk as well as other foods.

The mechanism of pathogenesis is unknown, but the clinical features of the disease result from invasion of the terminal ileum, necrosis in Peyer's patches and an associated inflammation of the mesenteric lymph nodes *(Fig. 20.20)*. The presentation, with enterocolitis and often mesenteric adenitis, can easily be confused with acute appendicitis, particularly in children. The clinical features are summarized in *Figure 20.12*. The laboratory diagnosis is

outlined in the Appendix. As with *V. parahaemolyticus*, an indication of a suspicion of yersinia infection is useful so that the laboratory staff can process the specimen appropriately.

Clostridium perfringens and Bacillus cereus are spore-forming Gram-positive causes of diarrhea

The Gram-negative organisms described in the previous sections invade the intestinal mucosa or produce enterotoxins, which cause diarrhea. None of these organisms produce spores. Two Gram-positive species are important causes of diarrheal disease, particularly in association with spore-contaminated food. These are *Clostridium perfringens* and *Bacillus cereus*.

Cl. perfringens is associated with diarrheal diseases in different circumstances and the pathogenesis is summarized in *Figure 20.21*:

- Enterotoxin-producing strains are a common cause of food-associated infection.
- Much more rarely β toxin-producing strains produce an acute necrotizing disease of the small intestine, accompanied by abdominal pain and diarrhea. This form occurs after the consumption of contaminated meat by people who are unaccustomed to a high protein diet and do not have sufficient intestinal trypsin to destroy the toxin. It is traditionally associated with the orgiastic pig feasts enjoyed by the natives of New Guinea, but also occurred in people released from prisoner of war camps.

The clinical features of the common type of infection are shown in *Figure 20.12*. The laboratory investigation of suspected *Cl. perfringens* infection is outlined in the Appendix. The organism is an anaerobe and grows readily on routine laboratory media. Enterotoxin production can be demonstrated by a latex agglutination method.

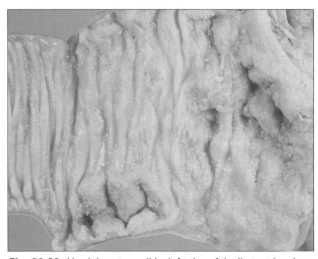

Fig. 20.20 *Yersinia enterocolitica* infection of the ileum, showing superficial necrosis of the mucosa and ulceration. (Courtesy of J Newman.)

Antibacterial treatment of *Cl. perfringens* diarrhea is rarely required. Prevention depends on thorough reheating of food before serving, or preferably avoiding cooking food too long before consumption.

Cl. perfringens is also an important cause of wound and soft tissue infections, as described in Chapter 23.

Bacillus cereus spores and vegetative cells contaminate many foods, and food-associated infection takes one of two forms:
- Diarrhea resulting from the production of enterotoxin in the gut.

- Vomiting due to the ingestion of enterotoxin in food.

Two different toxins are involved, as illustrated in *Figure 20.22*. The clinical features of the infections are summarized in *Figure 20.12*. Laboratory confirmation of the diagnosis requires specific media as described in the Appendix. The emetic type of disease may be difficult to assign to *B. cereus* unless the incriminated food is cultured.

As with *Cl. perfringens*, prevention of *B. cereus* food-associated infection depends upon proper cooking and rapid consumption of food. Specific antibacterial treatment is not indicated.

Antibiotic-associated diarrhea – *Clostridium difficile*
Treatment with broad-spectrum antibiotics can be complicated by *Cl. difficile* diarrhea
All the infections described so far arise from the ingestion of organisms or their toxins. However, diarrhea can also arise

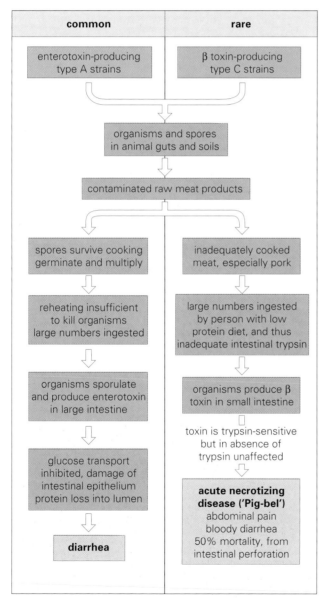

Fig. 20.21 *Clostridium perfringens* is linked with two forms of food-associated infection. The common, enterotoxin-mediated infection (left) is usually acquired by eating meat or poultry that has been cooked enough to kill vegetative cells, but not spores. As the food cools the spores germinate. If reheating before consumption is inadequate (as it often is in mass catering outlets), large numbers of organisms are ingested. The rare form associated with β toxin-producing strains (right) causes a severe necrotizing disease.

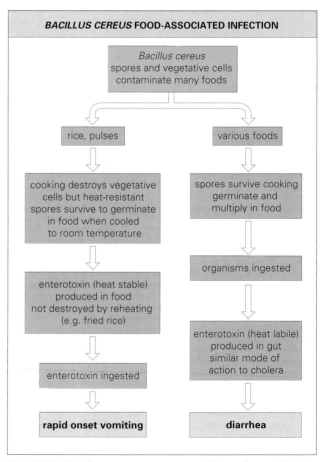

Fig. 20.22 *Bacillus cereus* can cause two different forms of food-associated infection. Both involve toxins.

from disruption of the normal gut flora. Even in the early days of antibiotic use it was recognized that these agents affected the normal flora of the body as well as attacked the pathogens. For example, orally-administered tetracycline disrupts the normal gut flora and patients sometimes become recolonized not with the usual facultative Gram-negative anaerobes, but with *Staphylococcus aureus*, causing enterocolitis, or with yeasts such as *Candida*. Soon after clindamycin was introduced for therapeutic use, it was found to be associated with a severe diarrhea in which the colonic mucosa became covered with a characteristic fibrinous pseudomembrane (pseudomembranous colitis; *Fig. 20.23*). However, clindamycin is not the cause of the condition; it merely inhibits the normal gut flora and allows *Cl. difficile* to multiply. This organism is commonly found in the gut of children and sometimes in adults, but can also be acquired from other patients in hospital by cross-infection. In common with other clostridia, *Cl. difficile* produces exotoxins, two of which have been characterized: one is a cytotoxin and the other an enterotoxin, and both appear to play a role in producing diarrhea.

Although initially associated with clindamycin, *Cl. difficile* diarrhea has since been shown to follow therapy with many other broad-spectrum antibiotics; hence the term antibiotic-associated diarrhea or colitis. The infection is often severe and requires treatment with the anti-anaerobic agent, metronidazole, or with oral vancomycin. However, the recent emergence of vancomycin-resistant enterococci, probably originating in the gut flora, has led to the recommendation that oral vancomycin is avoided wherever possible (see Chapter 30).

Viral diarrhea

Over three million infants die of gastroenteritis each year and viruses are the commonest cause

Non-bacterial gastroenteritis and diarrhea are usually caused by viruses. Infection is seen in all parts of the world, especially in infants and young children *(Fig. 20.24)*. Its impact is staggering – in parts of Asia, Africa and Latin America more than three million infants die of gastroenteritis each year, and children may have a total of 60 days of diarrhea in each year. It has a major effect on nutritional status and growth. In the USA about 200 000 children less than five years of age are hospitalized each year due to infectious gastroenteritis.

Although viruses appear to be the commonest causes of gastroenteritis in infants and young children, viral gastroenteritis is not distinguishable clinically from other types of gastroenteritis. The viruses are specific to humans and infection follows the general rules for fecal–oral transmission. Oral transmission of non-bacterial gastroenteritis was first demonstrated experimentally in 1945, but it was not until 1972 that viral particles were identified in feces by electron microscopy. It has been difficult or impossible to cultivate most of these viruses in cell culture.

Rotaviruses

These are morphologically characteristic viruses *(Fig 20.25)*, with a genome consisting of 11 separate segments of

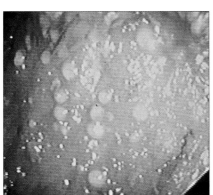

Fig. 20.23
Antibiotic-associated colitis due to *Clostridium difficile*. Sigmoidoscopic view showing multiple pseudomembranous lesions. (Courtesy of J Cunningham.)

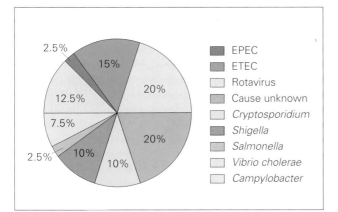

Legend:
- ■ EPEC
- ■ ETEC
- □ Rotavirus
- ■ Cause unknown
- □ *Cryptosporidium*
- ■ *Shigella*
- ▨ *Salmonella*
- □ *Vibrio cholerae*
- □ *Campylobacter*

Fig. 20.24 Diarrheal disease is a major cause of illness and death in children in developing countries. This illustration shows the proportion of infections caused by different pathogens. Note that in as many as 20% of infections a cause is not identified, but many of these are likely to be viral. (Data from the WHO.) (ETEC, enterotoxigenic *Escerichia coli*; ETEC *enterotoxigenic E. coli*.)

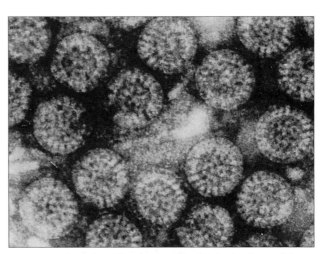

Fig. 20.25 Rotavirus. The virus particles (65 nm in diameter) have a well-defined outer margin and capsules radiating from an inner core to give the particle a wheel-like (hence 'rota') appearance. (Courtesy of JE Banatvala.)

double-stranded RNA. Different rotaviruses infect the young of many mammals, including children, kittens, puppies, calves, foals and piglets, but it is thought that viruses from one host species occasionally cross-infect another. There are at least two human serotypes.

Replicating rotavirus causes diarrhea by damaging transport mechanisms in the gut

The incubation period is 1–4 days. After virus replication in intestinal epithelial cells there is an acute onset of vomiting, which is sometimes projectile, and diarrhea. The replicating virus damages transport mechanisms in the gut and loss of water, salt and glucose causes diarrhea *(Fig. 20.26)*. Infected cells are destroyed, but there is no inflammation or loss of blood. Exceedingly large numbers of virus particles (10^{10}–10^{11}/g) appear in the feces. For unknown reasons, respiratory symptoms (cough, coryza) are quite common. The disease is more severe in infants in developing countries.

Infection is commonest in children under two years of age, and most frequent in the cooler months of the year.

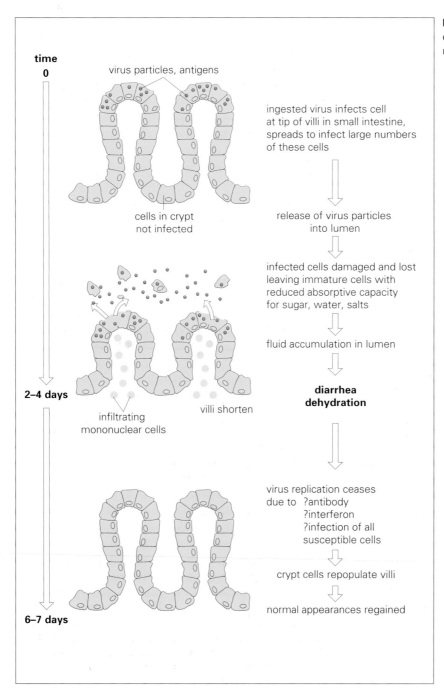

Fig. 20.26 The mechanism of rotavirus diarrhea. Other viruses may have different mechanisms.

time
0

virus particles, antigens

ingested virus infects cell
at tip of villi in small intestine,
spreads to infect large numbers
of these cells

cells in crypt
not infected

release of virus particles
into lumen

infected cells damaged and lost
leaving immature cells with
reduced absorptive capacity
for sugar, water, salts

fluid accumulation in lumen

2–4 days

infiltrating
mononuclear cells

villi shorten

**diarrhea
dehydration**

virus replication ceases
due to ?antibody
?interferon
?infection of all
susceptible cells

crypt cells repopulate villi

normal appearances regained

6–7 days

IgA antibodies in colostrum give protection during the first six months of life. Epidemics are sometimes seen in nurseries. Older children are less susceptible, nearly all of them having developed antibodies, but occasional infections occur in adults.

Rotaviruses are well-adapted intestinal parasites. As few as 10 ingested particles can cause infection, and by generating a diarrhea laden with enormous quantities of infectious particles these organisms have ensured their continued transmission and survival.

Rotavirus particles can be seen in fecal samples by electron microscopy

Laboratory methods are generally not available in developing countries or necessary in developed countries, but during the acute stages the characteristic 65 nm particles can be seen in fecal samples by electron microscopy. They show cubic symmetry and an outer capsid coat arranged like the spokes of a wheel *(Fig. 20.25)*. Viral antigen can be detected in feces by enzyme-linked immunosorbent assay (ELISA) or radioimmunoassay (RIA) methods (see Chapter 14).

Fluid and salt replacement can be life-saving in rotavirus diarrhea

Dehydration occurs readily in infants and fluid and salt replacement orally (or intravenously) can be life-saving. There are no antiviral agents available, but a variety of live attenuated oral vaccines are undergoing trials.

Other viruses
Other viruses causing diarrhea include caliciviruses, astroviruses, adenoviruses, parvoviruses and coronaviruses

Caliciviruses are 27 nm single-stranded RNA viruses that may cause 'winter vomiting disease'. They include the small round-structured viruses. One representative is the Norwalk virus, which has not yet been cultivated *in vitro*, but causes gastroenteritis when fed to adult volunteers. One of the first identified outbreaks was in a school in Norwalk, Ohio in 1969. Infection is common in older children and adults. In 25–50% of cases there may be chills, headache, myalgia or fever as well as nausea, vomiting and diarrhea, but recovery occurs within about 24 hours and laboratory diagnosis is unnecessary. Viruses in this group are often implicated in diarrhea, occurring after eating sewage-contaminated shellfish such as cockles or mussels.

Astroviruses are 28 nm single-stranded RNA viruses of which five serotypes are known. Most infections occur in childhood and are mild. Adenoviruses (especially types 40 and 41) are second to rotaviruses as a cause of acute diarrhea in young children. Most cannot be grown in cell culture. Parvoviruses and coronaviruses have an uncertain role.

Although outbreaks of gastroenteritis often have a viral etiology it may be difficult to be sure about the exact role of a given virus when it is identified in feces.

Food poisoning

In this chapter the term 'food poisoning' is restricted to the diseases caused by toxins elaborated by contaminating bacte-ria in food before it is consumed (see above). The emetic toxin of *B. cereus* fits this definition, as do the diseases associated with the consumption of *Staph. aureus* enterotoxin and *Cl. botulinum* toxin.

Staphylococcus aureus
Five different enterotoxins are produced by different strains of Staph. aureus

Five serologically distinct enterotoxins (A–E) are produced by strains of *Staph. aureus (Fig. 20.27)*. All are heat stable and resistant to destruction by enzymes in the stomach and small intestine. Their mechanism of action is not understood, but they have an effect on the central nervous system that results in severe vomiting within 3–6 hours of consumption. Diarrhea is not a feature and recovery within 24 hours is usual.

Up to 50% of *Staph. aureus* strains produce enterotoxin, and food (especially processed meats) is contaminated by human carriers. The bacteria grow at room temperature and release toxin. Subsequent heating may kill the organisms, but the toxin is stable. Often there are no viable organisms detectable in the food consumed, but enterotoxin can be detected by a latex agglutination test.

Botulism
Exotoxins produced by Cl. botulinum cause botulism

Botulism is a rare but serious disease caused by the exotoxin of *Cl. botulinum*. The organism is widespread in the environment and spores can be isolated readily from soil samples and from various animals including fish. Eight serologically distinct toxins have been identified, but only three – A, B and E – are associated with human disease *(Fig. 20.28)*. The toxins are ingested in food (often canned or reheated) or produced in the gut after ingestion of the organism; they are absorbed from the gut into the bloodstream and then reach their site of action, the peripheral

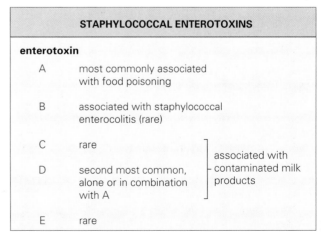

Fig. 20.27 *Staphylococcus aureus* produces five immunologically distinct enterotoxins. Strains may produce one or more of the toxins simultaneously. Enterotoxin A is by far the most common in food-associated disease.

TOXINS OF *CLOSTRIDIUM BOTULINUM*
antigenically distinct polypeptides
types: A ⎫ B ⎬ human disease E ⎭
types: C ⎫ D ⎬ animal botulism
relative heat labile, destroyed at 80°C for 30 minutes
not destroyed by digestive enzymes

Fig. 20.28 Eight different *Clostridium botulinum* toxins have been identified, but of these only three are associated with human disease and two others with botulism in animals. These protein exotoxins are the most potent biologic toxins known to man. They are antigenic and can be inactivated and used to produce antitoxin in animals.

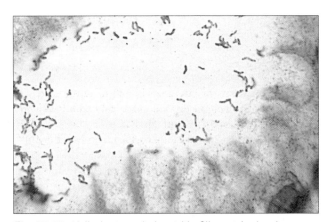

Fig. 20.29 *Helicobacter pylori* gastritis. Silver stain showing numerous spiral-shaped organisms adhering to the mucosal surface. (Courtesy of AM Geddes.)

nerve synapses. The action of the toxin is to block neuro-transmission (see Chapter 12).

Infant botulism is the most common form of botulism

There are three forms of botulism:
- Foodborne botulism.
- Infant botulism.
- Wound botulism.

In foodborne botulism, toxin is elaborated by organisms in food, which is then ingested. In infant and wound botulism, the organisms are respectively ingested or implanted in a wound, and multiply and elaborate toxin *in vivo*. Infant botulism has been associated with feeding babies honey contaminated with *Cl. botulinum* spores.

The clinical disease is the same in all three forms and is characterized by flaccid paralysis leading to progressive muscle weakness and respiratory arrest. Intensive supportive treatment is urgently required and complete recovery may take many months. Improvements in supportive care have reduced the mortality from around 70% to approximately 10%, but the disease, although rare, remains life-threatening.

Laboratory diagnosis of botulism involves injecting fecal and food samples into mice

Laboratory diagnosis depends largely upon demonstrating the presence of toxin by injecting samples of feces and food (if available) into mice that have been protected with botulinum antitoxin or left unprotected. There are no *in vitro* tests routinely available at present. Culture of feces or wound exudate for *Cl. botulinum* should also be performed.

Polyvalent antitoxin is recommended as an adjunct to intensive supportive therapy for botulism

Antibacterial agents are not helpful. It is not practicable to prevent food becoming contaminated with botulinum spores so prevention of disease depends upon preventing the germination of spores in food by:
- Maintaining food at an acid pH.
- Storing food at less than 4°C.
- Destroying toxin in food by heating for 30 minutes at 80°C.

Helicobacter pylori and Gastric Ulcer Disease

Helicobacter pylori is associated with most duodenal and gastric ulcers

It is now well established that the Gram-negative spiral bacterium *H. pylori* is associated with over 90% of duodenal ulcers and 70–80% of gastric ulcers (*Fig. 20.29*). The role of *H. pylori* in functional or non-ulcer dyspepsia, which most commonly presents with persistent or recurrent pain in the upper abdomen in the absence of structural evidence of disease, is less clear. Diagnosis is usually made on the basis of histologic examination of biopsy specimens, although non-invasive tests such as the urea breath test (*H. pylori* produces large amounts of urease) are being increasingly used. *H. pylori* can be cultured in the laboratory, but it is not an easy organism to grow.

The mechanism of pathogenicity has still to be identified, but cytotoxin production has been described. The large amounts of urease produced by the organism may assist its survival in the acid environment of the gastric mucosa.

Eradication of *H. pylori* leads to the remission and healing of ulcers without the need for acid suppression, but successful treatment requires combination therapy. The most promising regimens to date employ the combination of a proton pump inhibitor and two antibiotics (e.g. omeprazole with amoxicillin and metronidazole or clarithromycin (a new macrolide, see Chapter 30).

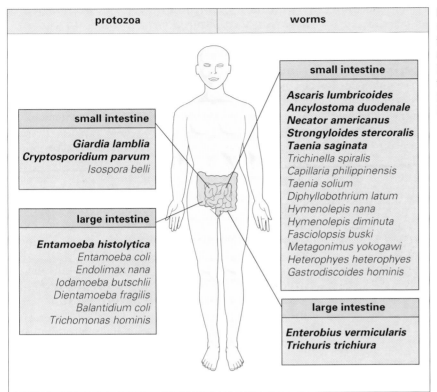

protozoa	worms

small intestine

Giardia lamblia
Cryptosporidium parvum
Isospora belli

large intestine

Entamoeba histolytica
Entamoeba coli
Endolimax nana
Iodamoeba butschlii
Dientamoeba fragilis
Balantidium coli
Trichomonas hominis

small intestine

Ascaris lumbricoides
Ancylostoma duodenale
Necator americanus
Strongyloides stercoralis
Taenia saginata
Trichinella spiralis
Capillaria philippinensis
Taenia solium
Diphyllobothrium latum
Hymenolepis nana
Hymenolepis diminuta
Fasciolopsis buski
Metagonimus yokogawi
Heterophyes heterophyes
Gastrodiscoides hominis

large intestine

Enterobius vermicularis
Trichuris trichiura

Fig. 20.30 Gastrointestinal parasites of man. The majority of these infections are found in developing countries, but all species also occur in the developed world and some have recently come to prominence because of their association with AIDS. The most important parasite species are highlighted in bold type.

Parasites and the Gastrointestinal Tract

Many species of protozoan and worm parasites live in the gastrointestinal tract, but only a few are a frequent cause of serious pathology *(Fig. 20.30)*. These will form the focus of this section.

Transmission of intestinal parasites is maintained by the release of life cycle stages in feces

The different life cycle stages include cysts, eggs and larvae. In most cases new infections depend either directly or indirectly upon contact with fecally-derived material, infection rates therefore reflecting standards of hygiene and levels of sanitation. In general, the stages of protozoan parasites passed in feces are either already infective or become infective within a short time. These parasites are therefore usually acquired by swallowing infective stages in fecally-contaminated food or water. Worm parasites, with two major exceptions (pinworms and tapeworms), produce eggs or larvae that require a period of development outside the host before they become infective. Transmission routes are more complex here:

- Some species are acquired through food or water contaminated with infective eggs or larvae, or are picked up directly via contaminated fingers.
- Some have larvae that can actively penetrate through the skin, migrating eventually to the intestine.
- Others are acquired by eating animals or animal products containing infective stages.

The symptoms of intestinal infection range from very mild, through acute or chronic diarrheal conditions associated with parasite-related inflammation, to life-threatening diseases caused by spread of the parasites into other organs of the body. Most infections fall into the first of these categories; indeed, in many parts of the world, intestinal parasitism is accepted as a normal condition of life.

Protozoan infections

Three species are of particular importance:
- *Entamoeba histolytica*.
- *Giardia lamblia*.
- *Cryptosporidium parvum*.

All three can give rise to diarrheal illnesses, but the organisms have distinctive features that allow a differential diagnosis to be made quite easily *(Fig. 20.31)*.

Entamoeba histolytica
Entamoeba histolytica infection is particularly common in subtropical and tropical countries

Infections with *Entamoeba histolytica* occur worldwide, but are most often found in subtropical and tropical countries where the prevalence may exceed 50%. The trophozoite stages of the amebae live in the large intestine on the mucosal surface, frequently as harmless commensals feeding on bacteria. Reproduction of these stages is by simple binary fission, and there is periodic formation of resistant encysted forms, which pass out of the body. These cysts can survive in the external environment and act as the infective stages; asymptomatic individuals are therefore carriers capable of infecting others. Infection occurs when food or drink is contaminated either by infected food handlers or as a result of inadequate sanitation. Transmission can also take place as a result of anal sexual activity. The cysts pass intact through the stomach when swallowed and excyst in the small intestine, each giving rise to eight progeny. Under certain conditions, still undefined, but including variables of both host and parasite origin, *Entamoeba* can become pathogenic, the amebae invading the mucosa and feeding on host materials including red blood cells, giving rise to amebic colitis.

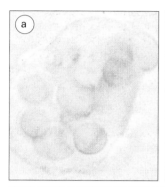

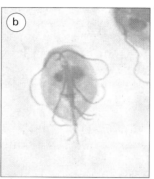

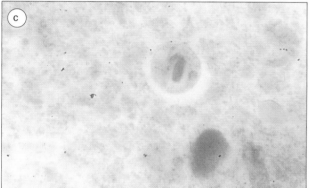

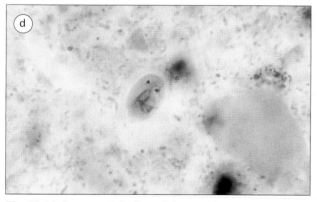

Fig. 20.31 Protozoan infections of the gastrointestinal tract. (a) *Entamoeba histolytica*. Trophozoite found in the acute stage of the disease, which often contains ingested red blood cells. (b) *Giardia lamblia* trophozoite associated with acute infection in man. (Courtesy of DK Banerjee.) (c) Cyst of *E. histolytica*, with only one of the four nuclei visible. The broad chromatid bar is a semicrystalline aggregation of ribosomes. Hematoxylin and eosin stain. (d) Oval cyst of *G. lamblia* showing two of the four nuclei. Iron hematoxylin stain. (Courtesy of R Muller and JR Baker.)

The clinical manifestations of E. histolytica infection vary from asymptomatic to severe dysentery

Infections with commensal forms of the ameba are asymptomatic. Invasion of the mucosa may produce small localized superficial ulcers or involve the entire colonic mucosa with the formation of deep confluent ulcers *(Fig. 20.32)*. The former causes a mild diarrhea, whereas more severe invasion leads to 'amebic dysentery', which is characterized by mucus, pus and blood in the stools. Dysenteries of amebic and bacillary origin can be distinguished by a number of features *(Fig. 20.33)*.

Complications include perforation of the intestine, leading to peritonitis, and extraintestinal invasion. Trophozoites can spread via the blood to the liver, with the formation of an abscess, and may secondarily extend to the lung and other organs. Rarely, abscesses spread directly and involve the overlying skin.

E. histolytica infection can be diagnosed from the presence of characteristic four-nucleate cysts in the stool

These cysts may be infrequent in light infections and repeated stool examination is necessary. Care must be taken

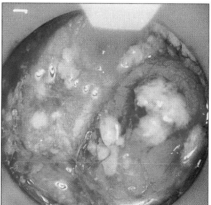

Fig. 20.32 Amebic colitis. Sigmoidoscopic view showing deep ulcers and overlying purulent exudate. (Courtesy of RH Gilman.)

FEATURES OF BACILLARY AND AMEBIC DYSENTERY		
	bacillary	**amebic**
organism	shigella	entameba
polymorphs and macrophages in stool	many	few
eosinophils and Charcot–Leydon crystals in stool	few or absent	often present
organisms in stool	many	few
blood and mucus in stool	yes	yes

Fig. 20.33 Features of bacillary and amebic dysentery.

Entamoeba histolytica	Entamoeba coli	Endolimax nana	Iodamoeba bütschlii	red blood cell

Fig. 20.34 Characterisics of cysts (size and number of nuclei) are used to differentiate pathogenic from non-pathogenic protozoa. A red blood cell is shown for comparison.

to differentiate *E. histolytica* from other non-pathogenic species that might be present *(Fig. 20.34)*. Trophozoites can be found in cases of dysentery (when the stools are loose and wet), but they are fragile and deteriorate rapidly; specimens should therefore be preserved before examination. Several immunologic tests are available, but only indicate whether patients have been exposed to infection at some time in their history, though they can be useful in confirming a preliminary diagnosis.

Acute E. histolytica infection can be treated with metronidazole

Recovery from infection is usual and there is some immunity to reinfection. Treatment may fail to clear the infection completely and the passage of infective cysts can continue. Metronidazole is useful against the extraintestinal sites of infection, but if these become secondarily infected with bacteria, additional antibiotics and drainage are necessary. Prevention of amebiasis in the community requires the same approaches to hygiene and sanitation as those adopted for bacterial infections of the intestine.

Giardia lamblia

Giardia was the first intestinal microorganism to be observed under a microscope. It was discovered by Anton van Leeuwenhoek in 1681, using the microscope he had invented to examine specimens of his own stool. At the present time it is the most commonly diagnosed intestinal parasite in the USA.

Like Entamoeba, Giardia has only two life cycle stages

The two life cycle stages are the flagellate (four pairs of flagella) binucleate trophozoite and the resistant four-nucleate cyst. The trophozoites live in the upper portion of the small intestine, adhering closely to the brush border of the epithelial cells by specialized attachment regions *(Fig. 20.35)*. They divide by binary fission and can occur in such numbers that they cover large areas of the mucosal surface. Cyst formation occurs at regular intervals, each cyst being formed as one trophozoite rounds up and produces a resistant wall. Cysts pass out in the stools and can survive for several weeks under optimum conditions. Infection occurs when the cysts are swallowed, usually as a result of drinking contaminated water. Epidemics of giardiasis have occurred when public drinking supplies have become contaminated, but smaller outbreaks

have been traced to drinking from rivers and streams that have been contaminated by wild animals. The genus *Giardia* is widely distributed in mammals and there is suggestive evidence for cross-infection between certain animal hosts (e.g. beaver) and humans. Much of this is circumstantial, but case reports provide more direct evidence. Recent data suggest that *Giardia* may also be transmitted sexually.

Mild Giardia infections are asymptomatic, more severe infections cause diarrhea

The diarrhea may be:
- Self-limiting, with 7–10 days being the usual course.
- Chronic, and develop into a serious condition, particularly in patients with deficient or compromised immunologic defenses.

It is thought to arise from inflammatory responses triggered by the damaged epithelial cells and from interference with normal absorptive processes. Characteristically the stools are loose, foul-smelling and often fatty.

Diagnosis of Giardia infection is based on identifying cysts or trophozoites in the stool

Repeated examination is necessary in light infections when concentration techniques improve the chances of finding cysts. Duodenal intubation or the use of recoverable swallowed capsules and threads may aid in obtaining trophozoites directly from the intestine.

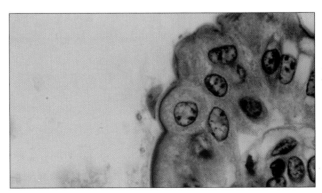

Fig. 20.35 Trophozoite of *Giardia lamblia* attached to the mucosal surface of the small intestine. Iron hematoxylin stain. (Courtesy of R Muller and JR Baker.)

Giardia infection can be treated with a variety of drugs

These include mepacrine hydrochloride, metronidazole and tinidazole, but none is completely successful. Community measures for prevention include the usual concerns with hygiene and sanitation, and improved treatment of drinking water supplies (largely filtration and chlorination) where these are suspected as a source. Care in drinking from potentially-contaminated natural waters is also indicated.

Cryptosporidium parvum
Cryptosporidium parvum is widely distributed in many animals

The implication of *Cryptosporidium parvum* as a cause of diarrhea in humans is comparatively recent (within the last 10–15 years). The parasite is widely distributed in many animals, but is very small and easily overlooked. It has a complex life cycle, going through both asexual and sexual phases of development in the same host. Transmission is by ingestion of about 100 of the resistant oocyst stage (4–5 mm diameter) in fecally-contaminated material *(Fig. 20.36)*. In the small intestine the cyst releases infective sporozoites, which invade the epithelial cells, remaining closely associated with the apical plasma membrane. Here they form schizonts, which divide to release merozoites and these then reinvade further epithelial cells. Eventually a sexual phase occurs and oocysts are released. Transmission probably occurs most often via drinking water contaminated by oocysts, either from other humans or from animals. In 1993, *C. parvum* caused a massive outbreak of watery diarrhea affecting 403 000 people in Milwaukee, USA. It was transmitted through the public water supply and probably originated from cattle.

C. parvum diarrhea ranges from moderate to severe

Symptoms of infection with *C. parvum* range from a moderate diarrhea to a more severe profuse diarrhea that is self-limiting in immunocompetent individuals (lasting up to 20 days), but can become chronic in immunocompromised patients. Cryptosporidiosis is a common infection in people with AIDS. In these individuals diarrhea is prolonged, may become irreversible, and can be life-threatening.

Routine fecal examinations are inadequate for diagnosing C. parvum diarrhea

Concentration techniques and special staining (e.g. modified acid-fast stain) are necessary to recover and identify the oocysts.

Only immunocompromised patients need treatment for C. parvum diarrhea

The macrolide spiramycin has been used for immunocompromised patients with limited success. Public health measures are similar to those outlined for controlling giardiasis, although *Cryptosporidium* is more resistant to chlorination.

Worm infections
The most important intestinal worms clinically are the nematodes known as 'soil-transmitted helminths'

Soil-transmitted helminths fall into two distinct groups:
* *Ascaris lumbricoides* (large roundworm) and *Trichuris trichiura* (whipworm), in which infection occurs by swallowing the infective eggs.
* *Ancylostoma duodenale* and *Necator americanus* (hookworms) and *Strongyloides stercoralis*, which infect by active skin penetration by infective larvae, which then undertake a systemic migration through the lungs to the intestine.

With the exception of *Trichuris* (large intestine), all inhabit the small bowel.

The pinworm or threadworm *Enterobius vermicularis* is perhaps the commonest intestinal nematode in developed countries and is the least pathogenic. The females of this species, which live in the large bowel, release infective eggs onto the perianal skin. This causes itching and transmission usually occurs directly from contaminated fingers, but the eggs are also light enough to be carried in dust.

The soil-transmitted helminths are commonest in the warmer developing countries. About 25% of the world's population carry these worms, children being the most heavily infected section of the population. Transmission is favored where there is inadequate disposal of feces, contamination of water supplies, use of feces (night-soil) as fertilizer, or low standards of hygiene (see below). Vast numbers of eggs are formed by each female (tens of thousands by *Trichuris* and *Ancylostoma* and hundreds of thousands by *Ascaris*).

Life cycle and transmission
Female Ascaris and Trichuris lay thick-shelled eggs in the intestine, which are expelled with feces and hatch after being swallowed by another host

The thick-shelled eggs of *Ascaris* and *Trichuris* are shown in *Figure 20.37*. The eggs require incubation for several days at optimum conditions (warm temperature, high humidity) for the infective larvae to develop. Once this occurs, the eggs remain infective for many weeks or months, depending upon the local microclimate. After being swallowed the eggs hatch in the intestine, releasing the larvae. Those of *Ascaris* penetrate the gut wall and are carried in the blood through the liver to the lungs, climbing up the bronchi and trachea before being swallowed and once again reaching the intestine. The adult worms live freely in the gut lumen, feeding on intestinal

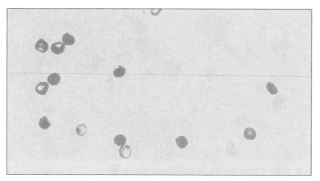

Fig. 20.36 *Cryptosporidium* oocysts in fecal specimen. (Courtesy of S Tzipori.)

contents. In contrast *Trichuris* larvae remain within the large bowel, penetrating into the epithelial cell layer, where they remain as they mature.

Adult female hookworms lay thin-shelled eggs that hatch in the feces shortly after leaving the host

A hookworm egg is shown in *Figure 20.37*. The larvae of these hookworms *(A. duodenale* and *N. americanus)* feed on bacteria until infective, and then migrate away from the fecal mass. Infection takes place when larvae come into contact with unprotected skin (or additionally, in the case of *Ancylostoma,* are swallowed). They penetrate the skin, migrate via the blood to the lungs, climb the trachea and are swallowed. Adult worms attach by their enlarged mouths to the intestinal mucosa, ingest a plug of tissue, rupture capillaries and suck blood.

The adult female Strongyloides lays eggs that hatch in the intestine

The life cycle of *Strongyloides* is similar to that of hookworms, but shows some important differences. The adult worm exists as a parthenogenetic female that lays eggs into the mucosa. These eggs hatch in the intestine and the released larvae usually pass out in the feces *(Fig. 20.37)*. Development outside the host can follow the hookworm pattern, with the direct production of skin-penetrating larvae or may be diverted into the production of a complete free-living generation, which then produces infective larvae. Under certain conditions, and particularly when the host is immunocompromised, *Strongyloides* larvae can reinvade before they are voided in the feces. This process of autoinfection can give rise to the severe clinical condition known as 'disseminated strongyloidiasis'. All soil-transmitted helminths are relatively long-lived (several months to years), but authenticated cases show that strongyloides infections can persist for more than 30 years, presumably through continuous internal autoinfection.

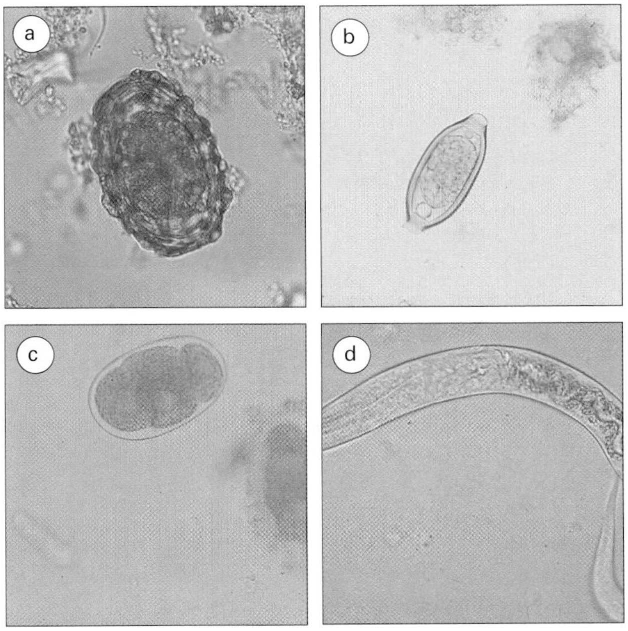

Clinical features

In most individuals, worm infections produce chronic mild intestinal discomfort rather than severe diarrhea or other conditions. Each infection has a number of characteristic pathologic conditions linked with it.

Large numbers of adult Ascaris worms can cause intestinal obstruction

The migration of *Ascaris* larvae through the lungs can cause severe respiratory distress (pneumonitis) and this stage is often associated with pronounced eosinophilia. Intestinal stages of infection can cause abdominal pain, nausea and digestive disturbances. In children with a suboptimal nutritional intake these disturbances can contribute to clinical malnutrition. Large numbers of adult worms can cause a physical blockage in the intestine and this may also occur as worms die following chemotherapy. Intestinal worms tend to migrate out of the intestine, often up the bile duct, causing cholangitis. Perforation of the intestinal wall can also occur. Worms have occasionally been reported in unusual locations, including the orbit of the eye and the (male) urethra. *Ascaris* is highly allergenic and infections often give rise to symptoms of hypersensitivity, which may persist for many years after the infection has been cleared.

Moderate to severe Trichuris infection can cause a chronic diarrhea

As with all intestinal worms, children are the members of the community most heavily infected with *Trichuris*. Although usually regarded as of little clinical significance, recent research has shown that moderate to heavy infections in children can cause a chronic diarrhea *(Fig. 20.38)*, reflected in impaired nutrition and retarded growth. Occasionally heavy infections lead to prolapse of the rectum.

Fig. 20.37 Eggs and larvae of intestinal nematodes passed in feces. (a) Egg of *Ascaris* (fertile). (b) Egg of *Trichuris*. (c) Egg of hookworm. The ovum continues to divide in the fecal sample and may be at the 16- or 32-cell stage by the time the sample is examined. (d) Larva of *Strongyloides stercoralis*. (Courtesy of JH Cross.)

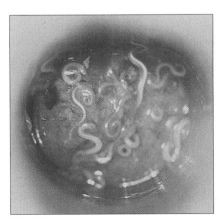

Fig. 20.38 Trichuriasis in a healthy, infected, child. Proctoscopic view showing numerous adult *Trichuris trichiura* attached to the intestinal mucosa. (Courtesy of RH Gilman.)

Hookworm disease can result in an iron-deficiency anemia

Invasion of hookworm larvae through the skin and lungs can cause a dermatitis and pneumonitis, respectively. The blood-feeding activities of the intestinal worms can lead to an iron-deficiency anemia if the diet is inadequate. Heavy infections cause a marked debility and growth retardation.

Strongyloidiasis can be fatal in immunosuppressed people

Heavy intestinal infection with *Strongyloidiasis* causes a persistent and profuse diarrhea with dehydration and electrolyte imbalance. Profound mucosal changes can also lead to a malabsorption syndrome, which is sometimes confused with tropical sprue. People with diseases that suppress immune function such as AIDS and cancer or who are being treated with immunosuppressant drugs are susceptible to the development of disseminated strongyloidiasis. Invasion of the body by many thousands of autoinfective larvae can be fatal.

The commonest sign of pinworm (threadworm) infection is anal pruritus. Occasionally this is accompanied by mild diarrhea. Migrating worms sometimes invade the appendix and have been linked with appendicitis. Invasion of the vagina has been reported in female children.

Laboratory diagnosis

All five of the soil-transmitted species can be diagnosed by finding eggs or larvae in the fresh stool and direct smears or concentration techniques can be used. Immunodiagnosis of intestinal parasites is still at an early stage. Infections with *Ascaris*, hookworms and *Strongyloides* are often accompanied by a marked blood eosinophilia. Although this is not diagnostic, it is a strong indicator of worm infection.

The eggs of Ascaris, Trichuris and hookworms are characteristic

These eggs are shown in *Figure 20.37* and are easily recognizable. Identification of the species of hookworm requires culture of the stool to allow the eggs to hatch and the larvae to mature into the infective third stage. The presence of adult *Ascaris* can sometimes be confirmed directly by radiography *(Fig. 20.39)*.

The presence of larvae in fresh stools is diagnostic of *Strongyloides infection*.

Pinworm infection is diagnosed by finding eggs on perianal skin

Although adult pinworms sometimes appear in the stools, the eggs are seldom seen because they are laid directly onto the perianal skin *(Fig. 20.40)*. They can be found by wiping this area with a piece of clear adhesive tape (the 'Scotch tape' test) and examining the tape under the microscope.

Treatment and prevention

A variety of anthelmintic drugs is available for treating intestinal nematodes. Piperazine has been used with great success against *Ascaris*, hookworms and pinworm, though many more recent drugs (albendazole, mebendazole, levamisole, pyrantel) can also be used and are also effective against trichuriasis and strongyloidiasis (especially albendazole and levamisole). At the community level, prevention can be achieved through improved hygiene and sanitation, making sure that fecal material is disposed of properly.

Other intestinal worms
Many other worm species can infect the intestine, but most are uncommon in developed countries

Of the human tapeworms:

- The beef tapeworm *Taenia saginata*, transmitted through infected beef, is the most widely distributed. However, infection is usually asymptomatic, apart from the nausea felt on passing the large segments! Diagnosis involves finding these segments or the characteristic eggs in the stool *(Fig. 20.41)*.
- *Diphyllobothrium latum*, the broadfish tapeworm, is widely distributed geographically, but infection is restricted to individuals eating raw or undercooked fish carrying the infective larvae. The eggs of this species have a terminal 'lid' and are the diagnostic stage in the stool *(Fig. 20.42)*.
- *Hymenolepis nana*, the dwarf tapeworm, occurs primarily in children, infection occurring directly by swallowing eggs *(Fig. 20.42)*. This worm has the ability to undergo autoinfection within the host's intestine, so that a large number of worms can build up rapidly, leading to diarrhea and some abdominal discomfort.

All these tapeworms can be removed by praziquantel or niclosamide.

Intestinal symptoms (predominantly diarrhea and abdominal pain) are also associated with infections by the nematode *Trichinella spiralis*, which is better known clinically for the pathology caused by the blood-borne muscle phase (see Chapters 23 and 26). Infection with the two species of schistosome associated with mesenteric blood vessels (*Schistosoma*

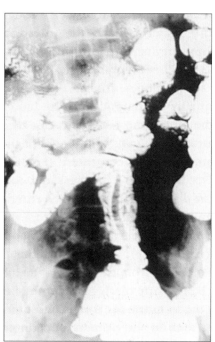

Fig. 20.39 Filling defect in the small intestine due to the presence of *Ascaris* seen on a radiograph after a barium meal. (Courtesy of W Peters.)

japonicum and *S. mansoni*) can also cause symptoms of intestinal disease. As the eggs pass through the intestinal wall they cause marked inflammatory responses, granulomatous lesions form, and diarrhea may occur in the early acute phase. Heavy chronic *S. mansoni* infection is associated with inflammatory polyps in the colon, while severe involvement of the small bowel is more common with *S. japonicum*.

Systemic Infection Initiated in the Gastrointestinal Tract

We opened this chapter by noting that infections acquired by the ingestion of pathogens could remain localized in the gastrointestinal tract or could disseminate to other organs and body systems. Important examples of disseminated infection are the enteric fevers and viral hepatitis type A and E. Listeriosis also appears to be acquired via the gastrointestinal tract. For the sake of clarity and convenience, other types of viral hepatitis will also be discussed in this chapter.

Enteric fevers: typhoid and paratyphoid

The term 'enteric fever' was introduced in the last century in an attempt to clarify the distinction between typhus (see Chapter 30) and typhoid. For many years these two diseases had been confused, as the common root of their names suggests (typhus, a fever with delirium; typhoid, resembling typhus), but even before the causative agents were isolated (typhoid caused by *S. typhi* and typhus caused by *Rickettsia* spp.), it was pointed out that it was 'just as impossible to confuse the intestinal lesions of typhoid with the pathologic findings of typhus as it was to confuse the eruptions of measles with the pustules of smallpox'. In fact, enteric fevers can be caused by *S. paratyphi* as well as *S. typhi*, but the name 'typhoid' has stuck.

S. typhi and *S. paratyphi* types A, B and C cause enteric fevers

These species of *Salmonella* are restricted to humans and do not have a reservoir in animals. Therefore, spread of the infection is from person to person, usually through contaminated food or water. After infection, people can carry the organism for months or years, providing a continuing source from which others may become infected. Typhoid Mary, a cook in New York City in the early 1900s, is one such example. She was a long-term carrier who succeeded in initiating at least 10 outbreaks of the disease.

The salmonellae multiply within, and are transported around, the body in macrophages

After ingestion, the salmonellae that survive the antibacterial defenses of the stomach and small intestine penetrate the gut mucosa through the Peyer's patches, probably in the jejunum or distal ileum *(Fig. 20.43)*. Once through the mucosal barrier, the bacteria reach the intestinal lymph nodes, where they survive and multiply within macrophages (see *Fig. 10.5*). They are transported in the macrophages to the mesenteric lymph nodes and thence to the thoracic duct and are eventually discharged into the bloodstream. Circulating in the blood, the organisms can seed many organs, most importantly in areas where cells of the

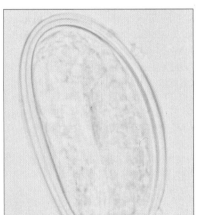

Fig. 20.40 Egg of *Enterobius* on perianal skin. (Courtesy of JH Cross.)

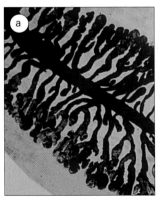
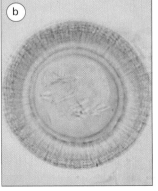

Fig. 20.41 *Taenia saginata.* (a) Gravid proglottids stained with India ink to show numerous side branches. (b) Egg containing six-hooked (hexacanth) larva. (Courtesy of R Muller and JR Baker.)

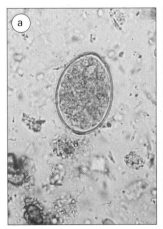
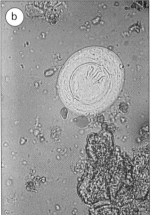

Fig. 20.42 Eggs of (a) *Diphyllobothrium latum* and (b) *Hymenolepis nana*. (Courtesy of R Muller and JR Baker.)

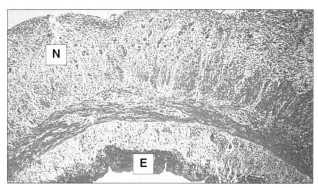

Fig. 20.43 Typhoid. Section of ileum showing a typhoid ulcer with a transmural inflammatory reaction, focal areas of necrosis (N) and a fibrinous exudate (E) on the serosal surface. Hematoxylin and eosin stain. (Courtesy of MSR Hutt.)

Fig. 20.44 Rose spots on the skin in typhoid fever. (Courtesy of WE Farrar.)

reticuloendothelial system are concentrated (i.e. the spleen, bone marrow, liver and Peyer's patches). In the liver they multiply in Kupffer cells. From the reticuloendothelial system the bacteria reinvade the blood to reach other organs (e.g. kidney). The gallbladder is infected either from the blood or from the liver via the biliary tract, the bacterium being particularly resistant to bile. As a result *S. typhi* enters the intestine for a second time in much larger numbers than on the primary encounter and causes a strong inflammatory response in Peyer's patches leading to ulceration, with the danger of intestinal perforation.

Rose spots on the upper abdomen are characteristic, but absent in up to 50% of patients with enteric fever

After an incubation period of 10–14 days (range 7–21 days), the disease has an insidious onset with non-specific symptoms of fever and malaise accompanied by aches and respiratory symptoms, and may resemble a flu-like illness (see Chapter 10). Diarrhea may be present, but constipation is just as likely. At this stage the patient often presents with a pyrexia of unknown origin (PUO; see Chapter 27). In the absence of treatment the fever increases and the patient becomes acutely ill. Rose spots – erythematous maculopapular lesions that blanch on pressure (*Fig. 20.44*) – are characteristic on the upper abdomen, but may be absent in up to 50% of patients. They are transient and disappear within hours to days. Without treatment, an uncomplicated infection lasts 4–6 weeks.

Before antibiotics, 12–16% of patients with enteric fever died, usually of complications

The complications can be classified into:

- Those secondary to the local gastrointestinal lesions (e.g. hemorrhage and perforation; *Fig. 20.45*).
- Those associated with toxemia (e.g. myocarditis, hepatic and bone marrow damage).
- Those secondary to a prolonged serious illness.
- Those resulting from multiplication of the organisms in other sites causing meningitis, osteomyelitis or endocarditis.

Before antibiotics became available, 12–16% of patients died, usually of complications occurring in the third or fourth week of the disease. Relapse after an initial recovery was also common.

1–3% of patients with enteric fever become chronic carriers

Patients usually continue to excrete *S. typhi* in the feces for several weeks after recovery and 1–3% become a chronic carrier, which is defined as *S. typhi* excretion in feces or urine for one year after infection. Chronic carriage is more common in women, in older patients and in those with underlying disease of the gallbladder (e.g. stones) or urinary bladder (e.g. schistosomiasis).

Diagnosis of enteric fever depends upon isolating S. typhi or S. paratyphi using selective media

This cannot be made on clinical grounds alone, although the presence of rose spots in a febrile patient is highly suggestive. Samples of blood, feces and urine should be cultured on selective media. Blood cultures are usually positive during the first two weeks, and feces and urine at 2–4 weeks (see Chapter 14). An antibody response to infection can be detected by an agglutination test (Widal test), but interpretation of the results depends upon a knowledge of the normal antibody titers in the population and whether the patient has been vaccinated. A demonstration of a rising titer between acute and convalescent phase sera is more useful than examination of a single sample. At best the results confirm the microbiologic diagnosis, at worst they are misleading.

Antibiotic treatment should be commenced as soon as enteric fever is diagnosed

Effective antibiotics are chloramphenicol, ampicillin, cotrimoxazole or ciprofloxacin and treatment should continue for at least one week after the temperature has returned to normal. Isolates of *S. typhi* resistant to one or more of the above agents have been reported. Many other agents are active *in vitro*, but do not achieve a clinical cure, presumably because they do not reach the bacteria in their intracellular location.

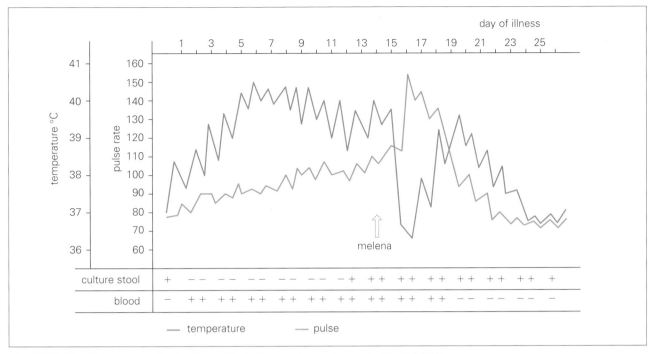

Fig. 20.45 The clinical course of typhoid fever. Chart of temperature, pulse rate and bacteriologic findings in a patient whose illness was complicated by massive hemorrhage. (Courtesy of HL DuPont.)

Prevention of enteric fever involves public health measures, treating carriers and vaccination

Breaking the chain of spread of infection from person to person depends upon good personal hygiene, adequate sewage disposal and a clean water supply. These conditions exist in the developed world where outbreaks of enteric fever are rare, but still occur.

Typhoid carriers are a public health concern and should be excluded from employment involving food handling. Every effort should be made to eradicate carriage by antibiotic treatment and if this is unsuccessful, removal of the gallbladder (the most common site of carriage) should be considered.

A killed vaccine against *S. typhi* and one which includes *S. paratyphi* are available and are recommended for travellers to developing countries; protection, however, is incomplete. Side effects of vaccination include pain at the site of injection, fever and headache. A live oral vaccine (strain Ty 21a) is now available, but protection appears to be short-lived.

Listeriosis
Listeria infection is associated with pregnancy and reduced immunity

Listeria monocytogenes is a Gram-positive coccobacillus that is widespread among animals and in the environment. It is becoming increasingly recognized as a foodborne pathogen, associated particularly with uncooked foods such as paté, contaminated milk, soft cheeses and coleslaw. It is likely that a large number of organisms must be ingested to cause disease, but the ability of the organism to multiply, albeit slowly,

at refrigeration temperatures allows an infective dose to accumulate in goods stored in this way. Even then, the population at risk appears to be limited to:
- Pregnant women, with the possibility of infection of the baby in the uterus or during birth.
- Immunocompromised people.

The disease usually presents as meningitis (see Chapters 22 and 38).

Hepatitis
There are at least six different hepatitis viruses

Hepatitis means inflammation and damage to the liver, and can be caused by viruses and less commonly bacteria (e.g. *Leptospira* spp.) or other microorganisms. The disease picture varies from malaise, anorexia and nausea to acute life-threatening liver failure, which is rare. More than 50% of the liver must be damaged or destroyed before liver function fails. Regeneration of liver cells is rapid, but fibrous repair, especially when infection persists, can lead to cirrhosis.

At least six different viruses are referred to as hepatitis viruses *(Fig. 20.46)* and generally they cannot be distinguished clinically. Other viruses cause hepatitis as part of a disease syndrome and are dealt with elsewhere. Dramatic elevations of serum aminotransferase concentration (alanine aminotransferase, ALT; aspartate aminotransferase, AST) are characteristic of acute viral hepatitis. Specific laboratory tests for hepatitis A and B viruses have been available for some years, and tests for others, originally referred to as 'nonA-nonB' viruses are now becoming available. Except in the cases of hepatitis A and B, there are no licensed vaccines, and

VIRAL HEPATITIS								
virus	virus group	type of virus	mode of infection	incubation period	frequency of infection in UK/USA	severity of hepatitis	persistent carriage of virus	other comments
hepatitis A (HAV)	enterovirus 72	ssRNA	fecal–oral	2–4 weeks	+ +	±	−	common in UK and USA
hepatitis B (HBV)	hepadnavirus	dsDNA	from blood (also sexual)	1–3 months	±	+ +	+	carriage associated with liver cancer
hepatitis C (HCV)	togavirus	ssRNA	from blood (?also sexual)	2 months	±	+	±	uncommon in UK, USA
hepatitis D (HDV)	very small	ssRNA	from blood	2–12 weeks	±	+	+	needs concurrent hepatitis B virus infection
hepatitis E* (HEV)	calicivirus	ssRNA	fecal–oral	6–8 weeks	−	±	−	common in Far East
yellow fever	togavirus	ssRNA	mosquito	3–6 days	−	+ +	−	no person-to-person spread

Fig. 20.46 The main viruses causing hepatitis in humans. Other viruses causing hepatitis include Epstein–Barr virus (mild hepatitis in 15% of infected adults and adolescents) and rarely herpes simplex virus, while intrauterine infection with rubella or cytomegalovirus causes hepatitis in the newborn.) *Hepatitis F (HFV) is of uncertain status; hepatitis G (HGV), a flavivirus, is spread via the blood. (ds, double-stranded; ss, single-stranded.)

except for interferons (IFNS; hepatitis B and C) there are no specific treatments.

Hepatitis A

This disease is caused by a typical enterovirus (single-stranded RNA) referred to as hepatitis A virus (HAV) or enterovirus 72. There is only one serotype.

HAV is transmitted by the fecal–oral route

Virus is excreted in large amounts in feces (10^8 infectious doses=g) and spreads from person to person by contact (hands) or by contamination of food or water. The incubation period between infection and illness is 2–4 weeks; virus is present in feces 1–2 weeks before symptoms appear and during the first week (sometimes also the second and third week) of the illness. Person to person transmission can lead to outbreaks in places such as schools and camps and viral contamination of water or food is a common source of infection *(Fig. 20.47)*. In developed countries, 20–50% of adults have been infected and have antibody, whereas in developing countries infection is more common and over 90% of adults have been infected.

Clinically, hepatitis A is milder in young children than in older children and adults

After infection, the virus enters the blood from unknown sites in the gastrointestinal tract, where it may replicate. It then infects liver cells, passing into the biliary tract to reach the intestine and appear in feces *(Fig. 20.48)*. Relatively small amounts of virus enter the blood at this stage. Events during

Hepatitis A

In August 1988 the Florida Department of Health and Rehabilitation Services traced 61 people who had suffered serologically-confirmed infection with HAV. These individuals resided in five different states, but 59 of them had eaten raw oysters from the same growing areas in Bay County coastal waters. The oysters had been gathered illegally from outside the approved harvesting areas and were contaminated with HAV. The mean incubation period of the disease was 29 days (range 16–48 days). Probable sources of fecal contamination near the oyster beds included boats with inappropriate sewage disposal systems and discharge from a local sewage treatment plant that contained a high concentration of fecal coliforms.

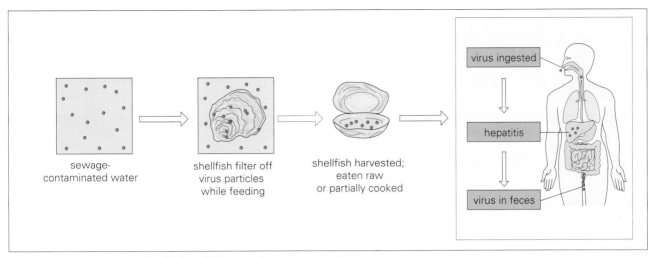

Fig. 20.47 Contamination of shellfish by HAV can lead to human infection.

the rather lengthy incubation period are poorly understood, but liver cells are damaged, possibly by a direct viral action. Common clinical manifestations are fever, anorexia, nausea, vomiting; jaundice is more common in adults. The illness generally has a more sudden onset than hepatitis B.

The best laboratory method for diagnosis is to detect hepatitis A-specific IgM antibody in serum or to demonstrate the antigen in the feces using an ELISA method (see Chapter 14).

Pooled normal immunoglobulin contains antibody to HAV, and gives approximately 1–2 months of protection when injected into travellers to developing countries. There is no antiviral therapy, but an effective formaldehyde-inactivated vaccine is now available.

Hepatitis B

This disease is caused by hepatitis B virus (HBV), a hepadna (hepatitis DNA) virus (see Appendix, and below) containing a partially double-stranded circular DNA genome and

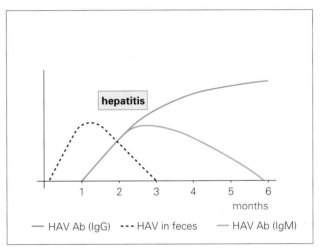

Fig. 20.48 The clinical and virologic course of hepatitis A virus (HAV). (Ab, antibody.)

— HAV Ab (IgG)   --- HAV in feces   — HAV Ab (IgM)

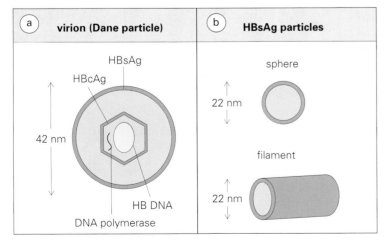

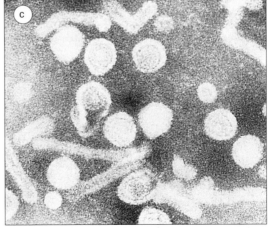

Fig. 20.49 During acute infection and in some carriers there are 10^6–10^7 infectious (Dane) particles/µl of serum (a), and as many as 10^{12} HBsAg particles/µl (b). (c) Electron micrograph showing Dane particles and HbsAg particles. (Courtesy of JD Almeida.)

three important antigens – HBsAg, HBcAg, and HBeAg *(Figs 20.49, 20.50)*. There is only one serotype in the sense that infection with a given strain of HBV confers resistance to all strains, but antigenic variation in HBsAg gives four sub-types (adw, adr, ayn and ayr). These do not differ in virulence or chronicity, but are useful in epidemiologic studies.

HBV is transmitted in blood

HBV is present in blood and can spread:

- Between intravenous drug misusers or male homosexuals.
- Between mother and child (intrauterine, peri- and post-natal infection; see Chapter 22).
- In association with tattooing, earpiercing and acupuncture.
- Probably heterosexually when there are genital ulcers.

Bloodsucking arthropods do not appear to be important. As blood contains up to one million infectious doses/μl , invisible amounts of blood can transmit the infection. Virus carriers, of which there are about 350 million worldwide, play a major role in transmission.

HBV is not directly cytopathic for liver cells and the pathology is largely immune-mediated

After entering the body there is probably a preliminary period of virus replication in lymphoid tissue, following which the virus reaches the blood, and then the liver. This results in inflammation and necrosis. Much of the pathology is immune mediated, for instance attack on infected liver cells by virus-specific Tcs. It is not known why the incubation period is so long (1–3 months). As the first virus-specific antibodies are formed there may be a brief prodromal illness with a rash and arthralgia. This is seen in 10–20% of icteric (jaundiced) patients and is due to the formation of immune complexes between HBs and anti-HBs antibody in the circulation in antigen excess (free antibody then being undetectable). These are deposited in the skin and joints for example. (see Chapter 12).

As liver damage increases, clinical signs of hepatitis appear *(Fig. 20.51)*; the disease is generally more severe than hepatitis A. The immune response slowly becomes effective, virus replication is curtailed, and eventually, although sometimes not for many months, the blood becomes non-infectious. The host's

HEPATITIS B ANTIGENS AND ANTIBODIES	
HBsAg	envelope (surface) antigen of HBV particle also occurs as free particle (spheres and filaments) in blood; indicates infectivity of blood
HBsAb	antibody to HBsAg; provides immunity; appears late (not in carriers)
HBcAg	antigen in core of HBV
HBcAb	antibody to HBcAg; appears early
HBeAg	antigen derived from core; indicates transmissibility
HBeAb	antibody to HBcAg; indicates low transmissibility

Fig. 20.50 Characteristics of hepatitis B virus (HBV) antigens (Ag) and antibodies (Ab).

α and β IFN responses to the infection are specifically suppressed by the gene products of this resourceful viral parasite.

Certain groups of people are more likely to become carriers of hepatitis B

About 10% of infected individuals fail to eliminate the virus from the body and become virus carriers. The blood remains infectious, often for life, and although continuing liver damage can cause chronic hepatitis, the damage is often so mild that the carrier remains in good health. Certain groups of people are more or less likely to become carriers as follows:

- People with a more vigorous immune response to the infection clear the virus more rapidly, but tend to suffer a more severe illness.
- Immunodeficient patients develop a milder disease, but are more likely to become carriers.
- There is a marked age-related effect. In Taiwan, for instance, 90–95% of perinatally infected infants became carriers compared with 23% of those infected at 1–3 years of age and only 3% of those infected as university students.
- Sex is another factor, with males being more likely to become carriers than females.

In countries where infection in infancy and childhood is

Hepadnaviruses

Hepadnaviruses are also found in woodchucks, ground squirrels and Pekin ducks. In each case the infection persists in the body, with HBs-like particles in the blood and chronic hepatitis and liver cancer as sequelae. These viruses often infect non-hepatic cells. In northeast USA for instance, 30% of woodchucks carry their own type of hepadnavirus and most develop liver cancer by later life. The virus replicates not only in liver cells, but also in lymphoid cells in the spleen, peripheral blood and thymus and in pancreatic acinar cells and bile duct epithelium.

common (possibly because there is a high carrier rate in mothers), overall carrier rates are higher. Therefore in West Africa where more than 70% of the population have antibodies, 12–20% of the population are carriers, whereas in western Europe and North America up to 5% of the population have antibodies and 0.9% are carriers.

Complications of hepatitis B are cirrhosis and hepatocellular carcinoma

Complications of hepatitis B include:
- Cirrhosis, as a result of chronic active hepatitis.
- Hepatocellular carcinoma. Hepatitis B carriers are 200-times more likely to develop liver cancer than non-carriers. This is not seen until 20–30 years after the infection. The cancer cells contain multple integrated copies of HBV DNA (integration takes place in infected liver cells after about two years of carriage) and this could be the carcinogenic factor. Alternatives would be the constant regenerative mitosis of liver cells in response to chronic infection or the presence of an unknown co-carcinogen.

Detection of HBeAg means that there are large amounts of virus in the blood

HBsAg appears in the serum during the incubation period and as the amount increases it signifies that infectious ('Dane') particles are also present (Fig. 20.51). The HBsAg concentration generally falls and finally disappears during recovery and convalescence, but remains in carriers. As HBsAg disappears, anti-HBs antibody becomes detectable and can be used for diagnosis. Before it becomes detectable, anti-HBC IgM may only be a matter of injection. Anti-HBs is demonstrable in previously infected non-carriers. If HBeAg is detected there are large amounts of virus in the blood and after HBeAg disappears anti-HBe antibody becomes detectable.

Genetically engineered hepatitis B vaccine is safe and effective

There is no standard antiviral therapy. However, large doses of α/β IFN have been used to clear the virus, sometimes permanently, from carriers.

A vaccine is available. Originally it consisted of purified HBsAg prepared from the serum of carriers and wash chemically-treated to kill any contaminating viruses, but the current vaccine is genetically engineered HBsAg produced in yeasts. Two to three injections of vaccine generally give good protection, and vaccination is recommended, especially for those frequently exposed to blood or blood products such as surgeons and other health care workers, dentists, multiply-transfused or dialysed patients, sexual contacts of acute hepatitis B cases, morticians, and intravenous drug misusers. One problem is that up to 10% of normal individuals fail to produce the protective anti-HBs antibody, even when revaccinated. This could be due to genetically determined defects in the

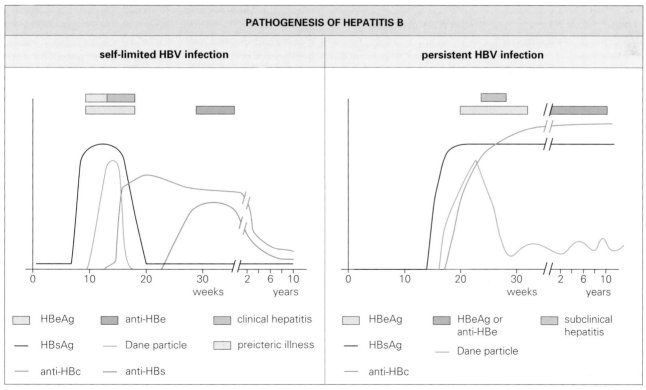

Fig. 20.51 Hepatitis B virus (HBV). (a) Clinical and virologic course of hepatitis B, with recovery.
(b) Clinical and virologic course in a carrier of hepatitis B. Results for HBV DNA polymerase and DNA are not routinely available, but parallel those for HBeAg. (Redrawn from WE Farrar, MJ Wood, JA Innes et al. Infectious Diseases, 2nd edition. Mosby International, 1992.)

immune repertoire or because of the induction of immune suppressor cells.

After accidental exposure to infection, hepatitis B immunoglobulin (HBIg) can be used to provide immediate passive protection. This is prepared from the serum of hemophiliacs or others with high titers of antibody to HBs.

In areas of high hepatitis B endemicity such as parts of West Africa, HBIg administered within 24 hours of birth followed by vaccination prevents children of infected mothers becoming carriers.

Hepatitis C
Hepatitis C virus is the commonest cause of transfusion-associated hepatitis

Hepatitis C virus (HCV) was discovered in 1989 as the cause of 90–95% of cases of transfusion-associated nonA-nonB hepatitis. It is a single-stranded RNA virus related to the flaviviruses and pestiviruses. The viral RNA was extracted from blood, a complementary DNA (cDNA) clone was made, and viral protein produced. Antibody to viral protein could then be tested for in sera. The discovery of HCV was a *tour de force* in molecular virology; although it has been cloned it has still not been visualized or grown in the laboratory.

HCV spreads in the same way as hepatitis B

HCV is present in blood (about 10^4–10^5 infectious doses/ml), and spreads in the same way as hepatitis B, by blood transfusion, intravenous drug misuse and from mother to infant; sexual transmission is uncommon. There may be other methods of transfer.

About 50% of patients with HCV develop chronic active hepatitis

The incubation period is 2–4 months, at which stage mild disease occurs in about one in 10 individuals. Nothing is known of its pathogenesis. Virus is often detectable in the blood after recovery from the illness, and carriers are a source of infection. In Europe and the USA up to 1% of apparently healthy individuals have antibody and may be infectious. About 50% of patients develop chronic active hepatitis and 20% progress to cirrhosis. Infection is also associated with liver cancer.

If antibody is present it is possible that the virus is also present and the patient is infectious, but this is not necessarily the case. Virus-specific cDNA can be tested for by the polymerase chain reaction.

Results of treatment with IFN$_\alpha$ and ribavirin have been encouraging

There is no vaccine. As HCV is now the commonest cause of transfusion-associated hepatitis, blood donors are routinely tested for antibody to hepatitis C.

Hepatitis D
Hepatitus D virus can only multiply in a cell infected with HBV

This is caused by hepatitis D virus (HDV or delta virus), which has a very small circular single-stranded RNA genome and is a defective virus, so-named because it can successfully multiply in a cell only when the cell is infected with HBV at the same time (see Appendix). When HDV buds from the surface of a liver cell it acquires an envelope consisting of HBs *(Fig. 20.52)*. The HBs envelope makes the 35–37 nm virus particle infectious by attaching it to hepatic cells.

Spread of HDV is similar to that of HBV and HBC

Infected blood contains very large amounts of virus (up to 10^{10} infectious doses/ml in experimentally-infected chimpanzees) and transmission includes heterosexual transmission.

When HDV infection accompanies, or is added to, HBV infection the resulting disease is more severe than with HBV alone. Infection is uncommon in the UK and USA, but common in parts of South America and Africa. Worldwide it is occurs in approximately 5% of HBV carriers.

The laboratory test is for HDAg ('delta' antigen) or antibody to HDAg. HBsAg will be present, although not necessarily at a detectable concentration.

There is no vaccine, but vaccination against hepatitis B prevents infection with hepatitis D.

Hepatitis E
Hepatitis E virus spreads by the fecal–oral route

This disease, also known as enteric nonA-nonB hepatitis, is caused by a small single-stranded RNA virus, probably a calicivirus. The virus is excreted in feces and spreads by the fecal–oral route. Although uncommon in developed countries, it occurs as a waterborne infection in India and may be responsible for 50% of cases of sporadic hepatitis in developing countries. The incubation period is 6–8 weeks. The disease is generally mild, but is severe in pregnant women with a high mortality (up to 20%) involving disseminated intravascular coagulation during the third trimester. The virus is eliminated from the body on recovery and there are no carriers. The possible protective value of passively-administered normal immunoglobulin is being investigated. Serologic tests are also being developed.

Hepatitis F, hepatitis G

Approximately 5–10% of hepatitis cases known to be transmitted by blood transfusion cannot be attributed to a known virus. Perhaps there are even more human hepatitis viruses

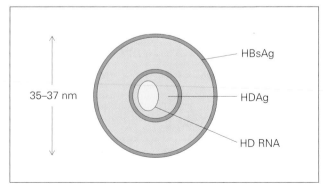

Fig. 20.52 Structure of hepatitis D virus in serum. (Ag, antigen.)

waiting to be discovered. Hepatitis F virus (a virus of uncertain status) and hepatitis G virus (a flavivirus) have been described and cause persistent infection and viremia.

Parasitic infections affecting the liver
An inflammatory response to the eggs of Schistosoma mansoni results in severe liver damage

Liver pathology in parasitic infections is most severe in *S. mansoni*. infection. Although the worms of *S. mansoni* spend only a relatively short time in the liver before moving to the mesenteric vessels, eggs released by the females can be swept by the bloodstream into the hepatic circulation and be filtered out in the sinusoids. The inflammatory response to these trapped eggs is the primary cause of the complex changes that result in hepatomegaly, fibrosis and the formation of varices *(Fig. 20.53)*.

Whereas schistosomiasis is widespread in tropical and subtropical regions, other parasitic infections affecting the liver are much more restricted in their distribution (e.g. clonorchiasis, fasciolasis, hydatid disease).

In Asia, infections with the human liver fluke *Clonorchis sinensis* are acquired by eating fish infected with the metacercarial stage. Juvenile flukes released in the intestine move up the bile duct and attach to the duct epithelium, feeding on the cells and blood and tissue fluids. In heavy infections there is a pronounced inflammatory response, and proliferation and hyperplasia of the biliary epithelium, cholangitis, jaundice and liver enlargement are possible consequences. There may be an association with cholangiocarcinoma, but there is little evidence for this in humans.

A number of animal liver flukes can also establish themselves in humans. These include species of *Opisthorchis* (in Asia and Eastern Europe) and the common liver fluke *Fasciola hepatica*. In general the symptoms associated with these infections are similar to those described for *C. sinensis*. Other parasitic infections associated with liver pathology are malaria, leishmaniasis, extraintestinal amebiasis, hydatid disease and ascariasis.

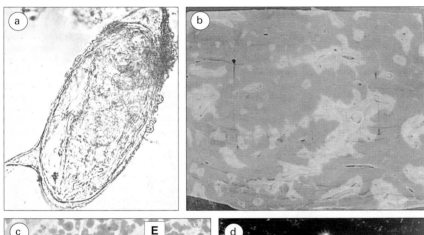

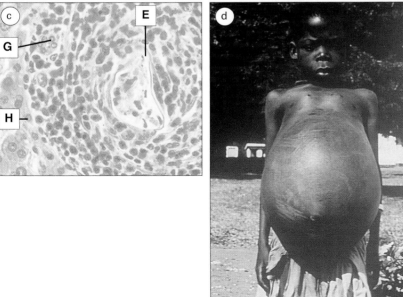

Fig. 20.53 The portal cirrhosis of *Schistosoma mansoni* is the end result of huge numbers of granulomas formed around worm eggs deposited in the liver. In the related *Schistosoma haematobium* infection, a similar process occurs in the wall of the bladder. (a) Egg of *S. mansoni*. ×400. (Courtesy of R Muller.) (b) Pipe-stem cirrhosis in the liver as a result of coalescent calcified granulomas. (Courtesy of R Muller.) (c) Cellular reaction around an egg in the liver. E, egg containing miracidium; G, giant cell; H, hepatic cell. (Courtesy of R Muller.) (d) Clinical schistosomiasis with massive hepatosplenomegaly and ascites due to portal obstruction. (Courtesy of G Webbe.)

Liver abscesses
Despite its name an amebic liver abscess does not consist of pus

E. histolytica can escape from the gastrointestinal tract and cause disease in other sites, including the liver (see above). However, the term 'amebic liver abscess' is not strictly accurate because the lesion formed in the liver consists of necrotic liver tissue rather than pus. True liver abscesses – walled-off lesions containing organisms and dead or dying polymorphs (pus) – are frequently polymicrobial, containing a mixed flora of aerobic and anaerobic bacteria *(Fig. 20.54)*. Lesions caused by *Echinococcus granulosus* in hydatid disease can become secondarily infected with bacteria. The source of infection may be local to the lesion or another body site, but is usually undiagnosed. Broad spectrum antimicrobial therapy is required to cover both aerobes and anaerobes.

Biliary tract infections
Infection is a common complication of biliary tract disease

Although infection is not often the primary cause of disease in the biliary tract, it is a common complication. Many patients with gallstones obstructing the biliary system develop infective complications caused by organisms from the normal gastrointestinal flora such as enterobacteria and anaerobes. Local infection can result in cholangitis and subsequent liver abscesses or invade the bloodstream to cause septicemia and generalized infection. Removing the underlying obstruction in the biliary tree is a prerequisite to successful therapy. Antibacterial therapy is usually broad-spectrum, covering both aerobes and anaerobes.

Peritonitis and intra-abdominal sepsis

The peritoneal cavity is normally sterile, but is in constant danger of becoming contaminated by bacteria discharged through perforations in the gut wall arising from trauma (accidental or surgical) or infection. The outcome of peritoneal contamination depends upon the volume of the inoculum (1 ml of gut contents contains many millions of microorganisms), and the ability of the local defenses to wall off and destroy the microorganisms.

Peritonitis is usually caused by Bacteroides fragilis mixed with facultative anaerobes

Although the gut contains an enormous range of different bacterial species, peritonitis and intra-abdominal abscesses are usually caused by only a few, primarily strict, anaerobes of the *Bacteroides fragilis* group mixed with facultative anaerobes such as *E. coli*. It is unusual to find a single species causing the infection. *Mycobacterium tuberculosis* and *Actinomyces* can also cause intraperitoneal infection *(Fig. 20.55)*.

Peritonitis usually begins as an acute inflammation in the abdomen and progresses to the formation of localized intra-abdominal abscesses. In the absence of appropriate antibiotic therapy the infection is frequently fatal and even with appropriate treatment, the mortality remains at 1–5%. Antibiotic therapy must be chosen to cover both aerobic and anaerobic pathogens. Suitable regimens include a combination of gentamicin (for the aerobic Gram-negative rods), ampicillin (for

enterococci) and metronidazole (to cover the anaerobes). Mycobacterial infection requires specific antituberculous therapy (see Chapter 30), while actinomycosis responds well to prolonged treatment with penicillin.

Summary

The length and complexity of the gastrointestinal tract is matched by the variety of microorganisms that can be acquired by this route, causing damage locally or invading to cause disseminated disease. Diarrheal disease is a major cause of morbidity and mortality in malnourished populations in the developing world and will only be combatted successfully when there are adequate public health measures. Meanwhile in the developed world, diarrheal disease is still common and causes severe illness in the very young and the very old. Certain infections such as typhoid are initiated in the gastrointestinal tract, but cause systemic disease, while hepatitis A is acquired and excreted by the intestinal route. The remaining members of the hepatitis 'alphabet' are also dealt with in this chapter. Infections result not only from the ingestion of pathogens from an external source, but also from the normal flora of the gastrointestinal tract if there are accidental or manmade breaches of the mucosa as microorganisms can then 'escape' and cause intra-abdominal sepsis.

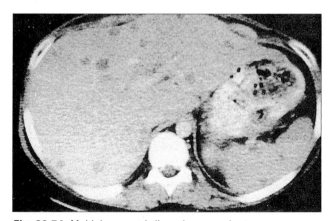

Fig. 20.54 Multiple pyogenic liver abscesses due to *Pseudomonas aeruginosa*. (Courtesy of N Holland.)

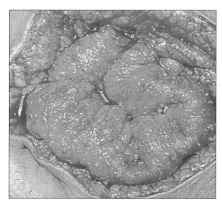

Fig. 20.55 Tuberculous peritonitis. Edematous bowel with multiple lesions on the peritoneal surface. (Courtesy of M Goldman.)

- Diarrheal disease is a major cause of morbidity and mortality in the developing world. A wide range of diverse microbes cause infections of the gastrointestinal tract. Diarrhea, the most common symptom, ranges from mild and self-limiting to severe with consequent dehydration and death.
- Gastrointestinal pathogens are transmitted by the fecal–oral route. They may invade the gut, causing systemic disease (e.g. typhoid), or multiply and produce locally acting toxins and damage only the gastrointestinal tract (e.g. cholera). The number of organisms ingested and their virulence attributes are critical factors determining whether infection becomes established.
- Microbiologic diagnosis is usually impossible without laboratory investigations, but the patient's history, including food and travel history, provides useful pointers.
- The major bacterial causes of diarrhea are E. coli, salmonellae, Campylobacter, V. cholerae and shigellae. Other less common causes include Cl. perfringens, B. cereus, V. parahaemolyticus and Y. enterocolitica. Food poisoning (i.e. the ingestion of bacterial toxins in food) is caused by Staph. aureus and Cl. botulinum.
- E. coli is the major bacterial cause of diarrhea in developing countries and of traveller's diarrhea. Distinct groups within the species (ETEC, EHEC, EPEC and EIEC) have different pathogenic mechanisms – some are invasive, others toxigenic.
- Salmonellae and Campylobacter are common in the developed world, have large animal reservoirs and spread via the food chain. Both cause disease by multiplication in the gut and the production of locally acting toxins.
- V. cholerae and shigellae have no animal reservoirs and the diseases are potentially eradicable. Transmission is prevented by good hygiene, clean drinking water and hygienic disposal of feces. The pathogenesis of cholera depends upon production of cholera enterotoxin, which acts on the gastrointestinal mucosal cells. In contrast, Shigella invades the mucosa, causing ulceration and bloody diarrhea, symptoms similar to those of amebic dysentery.
- H. pylori is associated with gastritis and duodenal ulcers. Removal of the bacterium by combination treatment with antibiotics and proton pump inhibitors reduces symptoms and encourages healing.
- Disruption of the normal bacterial flora of the gut (usually due to antibiotic treatment) allows organisms normally absent or present in small numbers (e.g. Cl. difficile) to multiply and cause antibiotic-associated diarrhea.
- Viral gastroenteritis causes appalling morbidity and mortality, especially in young children in the developing world. The chief culprits are the rotaviruses, which are specific to humans, spread by the fecal–oral route and restrict their multiplication to the gastrointestinal epithelial cells, which they destroy. Very small numbers can initiate infection and multiply in the gut to produce enormous numbers for excretion and transmission to new hosts.
- Ingestion of food or water contaminated with S. typhi or S. paratyphi can result in the systemic infection enteric (typhoid) fever. These pathogens invade the gut mucosa and are ingested by, and survive in, macrophages. They are transported via the lymphatics to the bloodstream from whence they seed many organs and give the characteristic multisystem disease. Positive diagnosis depends upon culture of the organism. Specific antibiotic therapy is required and specific prevention is achievable through immunization.
- Hepatitis is usually caused by viruses and there are at least six different types (hepatitis A–G), from different virus groups. Hepatitis A and E are transmitted by the fecal–oral route and the rest by contaminated blood or the sexual route. Infection with HBV and HBC often leads to chronic hepatitis or liver cancer.
- Many protozoa and worms live in the intestine, but relatively few cause severe diarrhea. Important protozoa are E. histolytica, G. lamblia and Cryptosporidium, which are acquired by ingestion of infective stages in fecally contaminated food or water. Important worms are Ascaris, Trichuris and the hookworms. They have more complex routes of transmission with the eggs or larvae requiring a development period outside the human host.
- Parasitic infections involving the liver include infections by S. mansoni in the tropics and subtropics, and C. sinensis, the human liver fluke, in Asia. Other parasitic infections with important liver pathology include malaria, leishmaniasis, extraintestinal amebiasis, hydatid disease and ascariasis.
- Infection of the biliary tree is usually secondary to obstruction. The normal intestinal flora cause mixed infections, which may extend to produce liver abscesses and septicemia.
- Peritonitis and intra-abdominal sepsis follow contamination of the normally sterile abdominal cavity with intestinal microbes. The presentation is acute and infection can be fatal. Antibiotic therapy against both aerobic and anaerobic bacteria is essential.

A 24-year-old astrologer with a history of intravenous drug abuse sees his doctor because he has felt tired and unwell for the past few weeks. He has noticed that his urine is very dark, he feels nauseated, and does not feel like eating, and he has developed right-sided abdominal discomfort. A friend thinks that he looks 'yellow'. On examination he is tattooed, has yellow sclerae, and is tender in the right upper quadrant of his abdomen. His liver is enlarged, firm and smooth.

The results of investigations including the liver function tests are: AST, 1200 IU/l; ALT, 1000 IU/l; ALP, 100 IU/l; bilirubin, 60 μmol/l.)
1. What is the most likely diagnosis and what is the differential diagnosis of a viral hepatitis in this setting?
2. What investigations would you perform?
3. How would you manage this man?
4. What other factors are important regarding the control of infection?

In September 1994, 80 cases of F. S. enteritidis gastroenteritis were reported from Minnesota, USA, plus 14 cases from South Dakota and 48 from Wisconsin. All had eaten a certain brand of nation-wide distributed ice-cream. The outbreak caused an estimated total of 2000 cases of illness in 41 different states (MMWR 1994; 43:740–741.)

1. Why was ice-cream involved and where did the bacteria come from?
2. What treatment would you have recommended for the patients?
3. What actions would you have recommended in the ice-cream plant?

An 11-month-old baby girl is admitted to the pediatric unit with a two-day history of fever, vomiting, and copious watery diarrhea. She was a full-term normal delivery and has two siblings, one of whom had a mild diarrheal illness that cleared up four days earlier.

On examination she is unwell, mildly dehydrated, and febrile with a temperature of 38°C. Her abdomen is soft and there are no other findings of note.

1. What would be your immediate management of this baby?
2. What viral causes of diarrhoea are most likely?
3. How would a viral infection be diagnosed?
4. What is the natural course of the infection?

Further Reading

Blacklow NR, Greenberg HB. Viral gastroenteritis. *New Engl J Med* 1991;**325**:252–264.

Farrar WE, Wood MJ, Innes JA *et al*. Infectious Diseases, 2nd edition. London: Mosby International, 1992.

Field M, Rao MC, Chang FB. Intestinal electrolyte transport and diarrheal disease. *N Engl J Med* 1989;**321**:800–806.

Gross RJ. The pathogenesis of *Escherichia coli* diarrhoea. *Rev Med Microbiol* 1991;**2**:37–44.

Lemon SM. Type A viral hepatitis: new developments in an old disease. *N Engl J Med* 1985;**313**:1059–1067.

McMahon BL, Alward WLM, Hall DB *et al*. Acute hepatitis B infection: relation of age to the clinical expression of disease and subsequent development of the carrier state. *J Infect Dis* 1985;**151**: 599–603.

Moayyedi P, Anthony TR. *Helicobacter pylori*: the research explosion. *Curr Opin Infect Dis* 1995;**8**:374–379.

Nair GB, Albert MJ, Shimada T *et al*. *Vibrio cholerae* O139 Bengal: the new serogroup causing cholera. *Rev Med Microbiol* 1996;**7**:43–51.

World Health Organization. *Readings on Diarrhoea. Student Manual.* (WHO/CDD/SER/90,13) Geneva: World Health Organization, 1990.

Introduction

During pregnancy certain infections in the mother can be more severe than usual or reactivate
During pregnancy a novel set of potentially susceptible tissues appear, including the fetus, the placenta and the lactating mammary glands. The placenta acts as an effective barrier, protecting the fetus from most circulating microorganisms, and the fetal membranes shield the fetus from microorganisms in the genital tract. Perforation of the amniotic sac, for instance, at a late stage of pregnancy, often results in fetal infection.

A few particular infections of the infant occur at or around the time of birth

The infant may be directly exposed during passage down a birth canal that is infected with gonococci, chlamydia or herpes simplex virus, or is contaminated with fecal bacteria from the mother. In the immediate postnatal period, the mother's blood (hepatitis B virus) or milk (human T cell lymphotropic virus type 1, HTLV1) can also be a source of infection. Here we describe infections that occur during pregnancy and around the time of birth, and discuss their effects on the mother, the fetus and the neonate.

Infections Occurring in Pregnancy

Immune and hormonal changes during pregnancy worsen or reactivate certain infections

The fetus may be considered as an immunologically incompatible transplant that must not be rejected by the mother. Reasons for the failure to reject the fetus include:
- The absence or low density of major histocompatibility complex (MHC) antigens on placental cells.
- A covering of antigens with blocking antibody.
- Subtle defects in the maternal immune responses.

A severe or generalized immunosuppression in the mother would be undesirable because it would mean potentially disastrous susceptibility to infectious disease. Certain infections, however, are known to be more severe *(Fig. 21.1)* and certain persistent infections reactivate *(Fig. 21.2)* during pregnancy. The hormonal changes that accompany pregnancy can also increase susceptibility. The picture is further complicated when there is malnutrition, which in itself impairs host defenses by weakening immune responses, decreasing metabolic reserves and interfering with the integrity of epithelial surfaces.

The fetus has poor immune defenses

Once the fetus is infected it is exquisitely susceptible because:
- IgM and IgA antibodies are not produced in significant amounts until the second half of pregnancy.
- There is no IgG antibody synthesis.
- Cell-mediated immune responses are poorly developed or absent, with inadequate production of the necessary cytokines.

Indeed if the fetus were able to generate a vigorous response to maternal antigens, a troublesome graft-versus-host reaction could be unleashed.

INFECTIONS THAT ARE MORE SEVERE DURING PREGNANCY	
infection	**comments**
malaria	?depressed cell-mediated immunity
viral hepatitis	?additional metabolic burden of pregnancy
influenza	higher mortality during pandemics
poliomyelitis	paralysis more common
urinary tract infections	cystitis; pyelonephritis more common; atony of bladder and ureter leads to less effective flushing, emptying
candidiasis	vulvovaginitis
listeriosis	influenza-like illness
coccidioidomycosis	leading cause of maternal mortality in endemic areas in SW USA and Latin America

Fig. 21.1 The effect of pregnancy on the severity of infectious disease.

INFECTIONS THAT CAN REACTIVATE DURING PREGNANCY	
infection	**phenomenon**
polyomavirus (JC, BK)	viruses appear in urine
cytomegalovirus	increased shedding from cervix virus in milk of nursing mother
herpes simplex virus	increased replication in cervical region
Epstein–Barr virus	increased antibody titers increased shedding of virus in oropharynx

Fig. 21.2 Reactivation of persistent infections during pregnancy.

Most microorganisms have sufficient destructive activity to kill the fetus once it is infected, leading to spontaneous abortion, or stillbirth. Here, our interests focus on the few microorganisms that are capable of more subtle, non-lethal effects. They overcome the placental barrier by infecting it so that the infection then spreads to the fetus. They can then interfere with fetal development or cause lesions so that a live but damaged baby is born.

Congenital Infections

Intrauterine infection may result in death of the fetus or congenital malformations

After primary infection during pregnancy, certain microorganisms enter the blood, establish infection in the placenta, and then invade the fetus. The fetus sometimes dies, leading to abortion, but when the infection is less severe, as in the case of a relatively non-cytopathic virus, or when it is partially controlled by the maternal IgG response, the fetus survives. It may then be born with a congenital infection, often showing malformations or other pathologic changes. The infant is generally small and fails to thrive. It produces specific antibodies, but often, for instance with cytomegalovins (CMV), fails to generate an adequate virus-specific cell-mediated immune response, remaining infected for a long period. Hence, the lesions may progress after birth. It is a striking feature of these infections that they are generally mild or unnoticed by the mother.

Important causes of congenital infections are shown in *Figure 21.3*. Viruses that induce fetal malformations (i.e. act as teratogens) share certain characteristics with other teratogens such as drugs or radiation *(Fig. 21.4)*. The fetus tends to show similar responses (e.g. hepatosplenomegaly, encephalitis, eye lesions, low birth weight) to different infectious agents and the diagnosis is difficult on purely clinical grounds. Most of these infections (rubella, CMV, syphilis) can also, at times, kill the fetus. They generally follow primary infection of the mother during pregnancy, so their incidence depends upon the proportion of non-immune females of childbearing age. Routine antenatal screening for antibodies to rubella, syphilis and HIV identifies susceptible (rubella) and infected (syphilis, HIV) mothers. In the case of CMV, an earlier infection can reactivate during pregnancy and lead to fetal infection. Partial control of the infection by maternal antibody under these circumstances means that the baby is generally born normal. Congenital syphilis can also result from earlier untreated infection of the mother.

There is no good evidence to suggest that maternal mumps, influenza or poliovirus infection during pregnancy leads to harmful effects in the fetus, but the human parvovirus (see Chapter 23) occasionally causes fetal damage or death (in about 10% of cases) following maternal infection in early pregnancy. The infected fetus develops severe anemia with pallor, ascites and hepatosplenomegaly (hydrops fetalis) following extensive growth of the virus in the liver and elsewhere.

Congenital rubella
The fetus is particularly susceptible to rubella infection when maternal infection occurs during the first three months of pregnancy

At this time the heart, brain, eyes and ears are being formed and the infecting virus interferes with their development. If the fetus survives it may show certain abnormalities *(Fig. 21.5)*. About 25% of congenitally infected children eventually develop insulin-dependent diabetes mellitus, but rubella is a very uncommon cause of this disease. The virus replicates in the pancreas.

The classic features of congenital rubella infection were first described by Gregg in Australia in 1941, long before the virus had been isolated and characterized. Not all fetuses are

CONGENITAL *(IN UTERO)* INFECTIONS	
microorganism	**effects**
rubella virus	congenital rubella
cytomegalovirus (CMV)	congenital CMV – deafness, mental retardation
human immuno-deficiency virus (HIV)	congenital infection – childhood AIDS; about 1 in 5 infants born to infected mothers are infected *in utero*
varicella–zoster virus (VZV)	skin lesions; musculoskeletal, CNS abnormalities severe disease in newborn if mother infected too late in pregnancy to have provided transplacental IgG for fetus*
herpes simplex virus (HSV)	neonatal HSV infection, often disseminated – infection *in utero* is rare
hepatitis B virus	congenital hepatitis B – persistent infection*†
Treponema pallidum	congenital syphilis – classical syndrome
Toxoplasma gondii	congenital toxoplasmosis
Listeria monocytogenes	congenital listeriosis – pneumonia septicemia, meningitis*
Mycobacterium leprae	congenital infection common in mothers with lepromatous leprosy

* infection also occurs during and immediately after birth
† protection of newborn by hepatitis B vaccine plus specific immunoglobulin is probably less effective after *in utero* infection

Fig. 21.3 Maternal infections that are transmitted to the fetus. Congenitally infected babies may be symptomless, especially in cytomegalovirus infection. They are often small, fail to thrive or show detectable abnormalities later in childhood. In all cases the baby remains infected, often for long periods, and may infect others.

affected; in one study detectable congenital defects were seen in 15.3% of cases when maternal rubella occurred in the first month of pregnancy, 24.6% in the second month, 17.5% in the third month and 6.5% in the fourth month. The figure for the first month is relatively low because fetal death is a common sequel at this stage.

Congenital rubella causes malformations as a result of:
- A primary effect on blood vessels in the developing organs.
- A virus-mediated inhibition of mitosis which contributes to the reduced number of cells and the small size of rubella babies.

Congenital rubella can affect the eye, heart, brain and ear

Clinical manifestations of congenital rubella include low birth weight and eye *(Fig. 21.6)* and heart lesions. Effects on the brain and ears may not become detectable until later in childhood in the form of mental retardation and deafness. There is a 15% mortality in infants showing signs of infection at birth, often associated with hypogammaglobulinemia.

Fetal rubella IgM is found in cord blood

Infected fetuses produce their own IgM molecules to rubella virus, which can be detected in cord blood. Maternal IgG antibodies are also present and together with interferons help control the spread of infection in the fetus. Virus can be isolated from the infant's throat or urine. The infant sheds virus into the throat and urine for several months and can infect susceptible individuals.

Congenital rubella is completely preventable by vaccination

Vaccination with live attenuated virus vaccine is given during childhood, usually with the combined MMR (mumps, measles and rubella) vaccine (see Chapter 31). Pregnancy is a contraindication to vaccination and the only safe time during

COMPARISON BETWEEN TERATOGENIC VIRUSES AND OTHER TERATOGENS		
	viral teratogens (e.g. rubella)	other teratogens (e.g. drugs, radiation)
critical stages of susceptibility during pregnancy (organogenesis)	+	+
fetal death a possible outcome	+	+
maternal effects minimal or absent	+	+
cause retarded fetal growth	+	+
increase in frequency of naturally occurring abnormalities	–	+
influence of genetic factors in mother/fetus	–	+

Fig. 21.4 Teratogenic viruses show many similarities to other types of teratogen.

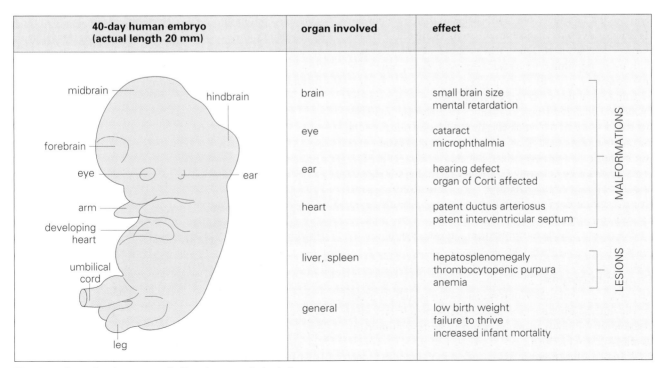

40-day human embryo (actual length 20 mm)	organ involved	effect	
	brain	small brain size mental retardation	MALFORMATIONS
	eye	cataract microphthalmia	
	ear	hearing defect organ of Corti affected	
	heart	patent ductus arteriosus patent interventricular septum	
	liver, spleen	hepatosplenomegaly thrombocytopenic purpura anemia	LESIONS
	general	low birth weight failure to thrive increased infant mortality	

Fig. 21.5 Organ involvement and effects in congenital rubella.

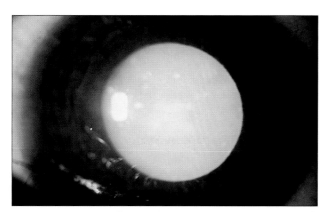

Fig. 21.6 Cataract in congenital rubella. (Courtesy of RJ Marsh and S Ford.)

reproductive life is the immediate postpartum period. This is an interesting example of a vaccine that is given to protect an as yet non-existent individual (the future fetus), the infection being only subclinical or mild in the mother. Until effective vaccines became available in the late 1960s, rubella was an important cause of congenital heart disease, deafness, blindness and mental retardation. The virus continues to circulate in the community and damage fetuses in countries with less extensive rubella vaccination.

Congenital CMV infection
Mothers with a poor T cell proliferative response to CMV antigens are more likely to infect their fetus

After primary maternal infection during pregnancy, about 40% of fetuses are infected and 5% of these show signs at birth. It is not known whether the fetus is especially vulnerable at certain stages of pregnancy. The fetus is also infected following pregnancy reactivation of CMV in immune (seropositive) mothers, but fetal damage is then uncommon. As many as 1–2% of infants born in the USA are infected (less in the UK) and up to about 10% of these are symptomatic, with up to one million infectious doses of virus present per ml of urine.

Clinical features of congenital CMV (see also Chapter 24) include mental retardation, spasticity, eye abnormalities, hearing defects, hepatosplenomegaly, thrombocytopenic purpura and anemia *(Fig. 21.7)*. Deafness and mental retardation may not be detectable until later in childhood.

Diagnosis is by detecting CMV-specific IgM antibodies in cord blood, and more reliably by virus isolation from the throat or urine. Live attenuated vaccines are presently being developed (AD169 and Towne strains) and in preliminary studies no one who became pregnant after vaccination transmitted the virus to the infant.

Congenital syphilis
As a result of routine serologic screening for syphilis in antenatal clinics and treatment with penicillin (see Chapter 19), congenital syphilis is now rare, but is more common in developing countries.

Clinical features in the infant include rhinitis (snuffles), skin and mucosal lesions, hepatosplenomegaly, lymphadenopathy,

and abnormalities of bones, teeth and cartilage (saddle-shaped nose). Pregnancy often masks the early signs of syphilis, but antibodies will be present in the mother and *Treponema pallidum*-specific IgM antibodies in the fetus.

Treatment of the mother before the fourth month of pregnancy prevents fetal infection.

Congenital toxoplasmosis
Acute asymptomatic infection by Toxoplasma gondii during pregnancy can cause fetal malformation

Approximately 35% of healthy adults are seropositive for *Toxoplasma gondii*. Clinical features of congenital toxoplasmosis in the infant include convulsions, microcephaly, chorioretinitis, hepatosplenomegaly and jaundice, with later hydrocephaly, mental retardation and defective vision (see Chapter 16). There are often no detectable abnormalities at birth, but signs (e.g. chorioretinitis, see *Fig 16.7*) generally appear within a few years. The incidence of fetal infection and damage (leading to abortion, stillbirth or disease in the newborn) increases from 14% when maternal infection is in the first trimester to 59% when in the third trimester.

Toxoplasma-specific IgM antibodies may be detected in cord blood. Treatment of a pregnant woman or an infected infant is with spiramycin or (with care to avoid toxicity) sulphonamide or pyrimethamine.

There is no vaccine. Prevention is by avoidance of primary infection via cysts from cat feces or lightly cooked meat during pregnancy.

Congenital HIV infection
Approximately 20% of infants born to mothers with HIV are infected in utero

Clinically congenital HIV infection manifests as poor weight gain, susceptibility to sepsis, developmental delays, lymphocytic pneumonitis, oral thrush, enlarged lymph nodes, hepatosplenomegaly, diarrhea and pneumonia, and some infants develop encephalopathy and AIDS by one year of age. Infection may also take place during or shortly after birth.

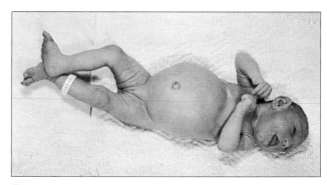

Fig. 21.7 Microcephaly with associated severe psychomotor retardation and hepatosplenomegaly in congenital cytomegalovirus infection. (Courtesy of WE Farrar.)

Laboratory diagnosis is at present difficult (see Chapter 19). If IgG antibodies are present they are of maternal origin and can persist for at least one year. There is no satisfactory test for HIV-specific IgM antibodies, which would signify *in utero* infection. Reliable blood tests for viral antigens or nucleic acid sequences would solve this problem.

Congenital and neonatal listeriosis
Maternal exposure to animals or foods infected with Listeria can lead to fetal death or malformations

Listeria monocytogenes is a small Gram-positive rod, which is motile and β-hemolytic. It is distributed worldwide in a great variety of animals including cattle, pigs, rodents and birds and the bacteria occur in plants and in soil. *Listeria* can grow at regular refrigeration temperatures (e.g. 3–4°C). Transmission to man is by:

- Contact with infected animals and their feces.
- Consumption of unpasteurized milk or soft cheeses or contaminated vegetables.

Up to 70% of people may carry *Listeria* in the gut for short periods without disease. In the UK in 1988 there were 291 reported cases of Listeriosis, 115 of them pregnancy-associated, and this declined to 59 cases in 1990, 11 of them pregnancy-associated.

L. monocytogenes in the pregnant woman causes a mild influenza-like illness or is asymptomatic, but there is a bacteremia, which leads to infection of the placenta and then the fetus. This may cause abortion, premature delivery, neonatal septicemia or pneumonia with abscesses or granulomas. The infant can also be infected shortly after birth, for instance from other babies or from hospital staff and this may lead to a meningitic illness.

L. monocytogenes is isolated from blood cultures, cerebrospinal fluid (CSF) or skin lesions.

Treatment is with penicillin or ampicillin, which may need to be combined with gentamicin to achieve a bactericidal effect. There are no vaccines.

Pregnant women should avoid exposure to infected material, but the exact source of infection is generally unknown.

Infections Occurring Around the Time of Birth

Effects on the fetus and neonate

The routes of infection in the fetus and neonate are shown in *Figure 21.8*.

Viral infections (e.g. rubella, CMV) are generally less damaging to the fetus when the maternal infection occurs late in pregnancy, but primary infection with varicella-zoster virus (VZV) at this time can lead to limb deformities and other severe lesions in the newborn.

Bacterial infections originating from the vagina and perineum are more important than viral infections late in pregnancy, especially occurring when the fetal membranes have been ruptured for more than 1–2 days, and result in chorioamnionitis, maternal fever, premature delivery and stillbirth. Infants of low birth weight (less than 1500 g) tend to be more

severely affected. Bacteria involved include:

- Group B hemolytic streptococci.
- *Escherichia coli.*
- *Klebsiella.*
- *Proteus.*
- *Bacteroides.*
- Staphylococci.
- *Mycoplasma hominis.*

These infections may also be acquired after delivery to give later onset disease.

Neonatal septicemia often progresses to meningitis

Meningitis (see Chapter 22, *Fig. 22.10*) is frequently fatal unless treated. Clinical diagnosis is difficult because the infant shows generalized signs such as respiratory distress, poor feeding, diarrhea and vomiting, but early diagnosis is essential

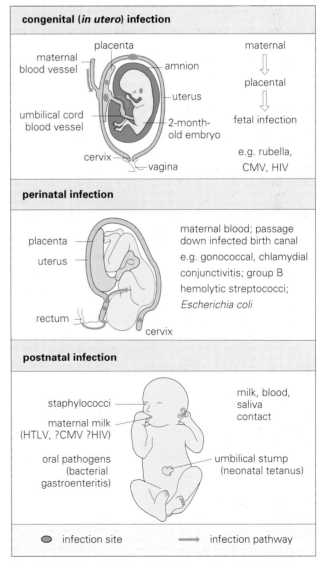

Fig. 21.8 Routes of infection in the fetus and neonate. (CMV, cytomegalovirus; HIV, human immunodeficiency virus; HTLV, human T cell lymphotropic virus.)

and emergency treatment is required. 'Blind' antibiotic treatment should be started as soon as CSF (Gram stain and culture) and blood samples have been taken.

Fetal infection can occur during labor or breast feeding

Fetal infection during labor results from direct contact with the infecting microorganism as the fetus passes down an infected birth canal *(Fig. 21.9)*. For instance, cutaneous lesions of herpes simplex may develop one week after delivery with generalized infection and severe central nervous system (CNS) involvement, and gonococci *(Fig. 21.10)*, chlamydia or staphylococci (see Chapter 16) can infect the eye to cause ophthalmia neonatorum.

Maternal blood can be a source of hepatitis B virus infection during or shortly after birth and 80–90% of infants from hepatitis B virus carrier mothers become infected and then carry the virus. This is preventable by giving the vaccine plus specific immunoglobulin to the newborn.

Human milk may contain rubella virus, CMV, HTLV1, and (probably) HIV. Virus titers are generally low and, except in the case of HTLV1, milk is not thought to be an important source of infection. However, it makes sense to pasteurize milk in human milk banks, just as we pasteurize cows' milk.

Effects on the mother
Puerpural sepsis is prevented by aseptic techniques

After delivery (or abortion) a large area of damaged vulnerable uterine tissue is exposed to infection. Puerpural sepsis (childbed fever) was a major cause of maternal death in Europe in the nineteenth century. In 1843 Oliver Wendell Holmes made the unpopular suggestion that it was carried on the hands of doctors, and four years later Ignaz Semmelweiss in Vienna showed how it could be prevented if doctors and midwives washed their hands before attending a woman in labor and practiced aseptic techniques. This is because:

- Group A β-hemolytic streptococci are the major culprits and come from the nose, throat or skin of hospital attendants.
- Other possible organisms include anaerobes such as *Clostridium perfringens* or *Bacteroides* and *E. coli* and are derived from the mother's own fecal flora.

Puerpural sepsis carried a mortality rate of up to 10% until the 1930s, but now, like septic abortion, is uncommon in developed countries. Predisposing factors include premature rupture of the membranes, instrumentation and retained fragments of membrane or placenta. High vaginal swabs and blood cultures should be taken if there is postnatal pyrexia or an offensive discharge.

Other neonatal infections

Infection may be transmitted to the newborn infant during the first week or two after birth rather than during delivery as follows:

- Group B β-hemolytic streptococci and Gram-negative bacilli (see above) acquired by cross-infection in the nursery, can still cause serious infection at this time, often with meningitis (see Chapter 22).
- Herpes simplex virus may come from cold sores or herpetic whitlows of attending adults.

Fig. 21.9 Neonatal infections acquired during passage down an infected birth canal.

NEONATAL INFECTIONS ACQUIRED DURING PASSAGE DOWN INFECTED BIRTH CANAL		
infectious agent	site of infection	phenomenon
Neisseria gonorrhoeae	conjunctiva	neonatal conjunctivitis (ophthalmia neonatorum)
Chlamydia trachomatis	conjunctiva, respiratory tract	neonatal conjunctivitis (ophthalmia neonatorum) neonatal pneumonia
herpes simplex virus	?	neonatal herpetic infection*
genital papillomavirus	respiratory tract	laryngeal warts in young children
group B streptococci** gram-negative bacilli (*E. coli* etc.)	respiratory tract	septicemia; death if not treated
Candida albicans	?	neonatal oral thrush

* although preventable by cesarean section, it is often difficult to detect maternal genital infection; infants can be treated prophylactically with acyclovir

** up to 30% of women carry these bacteria in the vagina or rectum

- Staphylococci from the noses and fingers of adult carriers may cause staphylococcal conjunctivitis or 'sticky eye' (see Chapter 16), skin sepsis in the neonate, and sometimes the staphylococcal 'scalded skin' syndrome *(Fig. 21.11)* due to a specific 'epidermolytic' staphylococcal toxin.

During the first week or two of life the nose of the neonate becomes colonized with *Staphylococcus aureus*, which can enter the nipple during feeding to cause a breast abscess. These infections are preventable if hospital staff pay vigorous attention to handwashing and aseptic techniques.

If hygienic practices are poor the umbilical stump, especially in developing countries, may by infected with *Clostridium tetani*, usually because instruments used to cut the cord are contaminated with bacterial spores, resulting in neonatal tetanus *(Fig. 21.12)*. It can be prevented by immunizing mothers with tetanus toxoid.

In developing countries, gastroenteritis is an important problem during the neonatal period as well as during infancy

Diarrhea leading to water and electrolyte depletion is particularly serious in low birth weight infants. Causative agents include strains of *E. coli* and salmonellae rather than rotaviruses. Breast feeding gives some protection by supplying specific antibodies and other less well characterized protective factors.

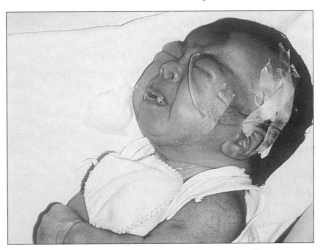

Fig. 21.12 Tetanus. Risus sardonicus in a newborn infant. (Courtesy of WE Farrar.)

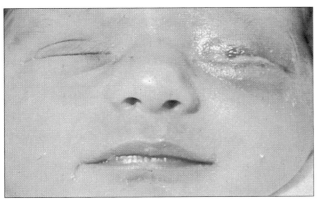

Fig. 21.10 Gonococcal ophthalmia neonatorum. Signs appear 2–5 days after birth. The inflammation and edema are more severe than with chlamydia infection. (Courtesy of JS Bingham.)

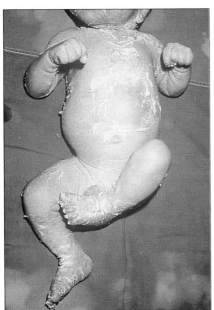

Fig. 21.11 Staphylococcal scalded skin syndrome. There are large areas of epidermal loss where bullae have burst. (Courtesy of L Brown.)

- During pregnancy certain infections (coccidioidomycosis, influenza) can be more severe than usual and there can be reactivation of certain persistent infections (polyomaviruses, CMV).
- A few infections are able to pass to the fetus via the placenta and cause damage.
- These infections are generally mild or subclinical in the mother (rubella, CMV, toxoplasmosis), but this is not always the case (syphilis).
- Once infected the fetus may die, but more importantly may survive and be born with the infection (HIV, toxoplasmosis), often showing characteristic malformations (rubella, syphilis).
- Rubella is the only congenital infection that can at present be prevented by vaccination.
- Infection during birth or shortly afterwards can cause local disease (conjunctivitis due to gonococci or chlamydia) or occasionally severe life-threatening illness (*E. coli* meningitis, herpes simplex virus infection).

A pediatrician is called to the postnatal ward by a midwife. She is anxious about a baby born 12 hours ago. The child is the mother's first baby. The labor was long and the delivery difficult and eventually forceps had to be used. The mother's membranes ruptured 12 hours before the baby was born. The mother had a fever of 38.5 °C during the last stages of labor, which has persisted since her arrival on the postnatal ward.

The baby had Apgar scores of 1 at 1 minute and 9 at 5 minutes. On examination, the baby is lethargic and pale. He has a faint systolic murmur, crepitations in both lung fields, and his liver is palpable below the costal margin. He is transferred to the Special Care Unit.

1. What is the likely diagnosis?
2. How would you investigate this baby?
3. What are the risk factors in his mother's history?

Further reading

Kovar IZ. Neonatal and pediatric infections. *Curr Opin Infect Dis* 1990;**3**:479–500.

Preece P, Pearl K, Peckham C. Congenital cytomegalovirus. *Arch Dis Child* 1984;**59**:1120–1126.

Scott GB, Hutto C, Makuch RW *et al*. Survival in children with perinatally acquired human immunodeficiency virus type I infection. *N Engl J Med* 1989;**311**:1791–1796.

Wilfert CM, Wilson W, Luzuriaga K. Pathogenesis of pediatric human immunodeficiency virus type 1 infection. *J Inf Dis* 1994;**170**:286.

Introduction

Central nervous system infections are usually bloodborne or invade via peripheral nerves
The brain and spinal cord are protected from mechanical pressure or deformation by enclosure in rigid containers (skull and vertebral column), which also act as barriers to the spread of infection. The blood vessels and nerves that traverse the walls of the skull and vertebral column are the main routes of invasion. Bloodborne invasion is the commonest (e.g. poliovirus or meningococcus). Invasion via peripheral nerves is less common – for example by herpes simplex virus, varicella-zoster virus and rabies virus. Local invasion from infected ears or sinuses, local injury or congenital defects such as spina bifida, also occurs, while invasion from the olfactory tract (e.g. amebic meningitis) is rare.

Here we discuss the main routes of central nervous system invasion by microorganisms (see also Chapter 7) and the body's response, followed by a more detailed discussion of the diseases that result.

Invasion of the Central Nervous System

Natural barriers act to prevent bloodborne invasion

Bloodborne invasion takes place across:

- The blood–brain barrier to cause encephalitis.
- The blood–cerebrospinal fluid (CSF) barrier to cause meningitis (*Fig. 22.1*).

The blood–brain barrier consists of tightly joined endothelial cells surrounded by glial processes, while the brain–CSF barrier at the choroid plexus consists of endothelium with fenestrations, and tightly joined choroid plexus epithelial cells. Microbes can traverse these barriers by:

- Growing across, infecting the cells that comprise the barrier.
- Being passively transported across in intracellular vacuoles.
- Being carried across by infected white blood cells.

In the case of viruses, examples of each mechanism are known. Poliovirus, for instance, invades the central nervous system (CNS) across the blood–brain barrier. After oral ingestion of virus, a complex stepwise series of events provides the mechanism for CNS invasion (Fig. 22.2). Poliovirus also invades the meninges after localizing in vascular endothelial cells, and can cross the blood–CSF barrier. Mumps virus behaves in the same way, as do circulating Haemophilus influenzae, meningococci or pneumococci. Once infection has reached the meninges and CSF, the brain substance can in turn be invaded if the infection crosses the pia. In poliomyelitis, for instance, a meningitic phase often precedes encephalitis and paralysis.

CNS invasion, however, is a rare event because most microorganisms fail to pass from blood to the CNS across the natural barriers. A large variety of viruses can grow and cause disease if introduced directly into the brain, but circulating viruses generally fail to invade, and CNS involvement by polio, mumps, rubella or measles viruses is seen in only a very small proportion of infected individuals. The factors that determine such CNS invasion are unknown.

Invasion of the CNS via peripheral nerves is a feature of herpes simplex virus, varicella-zoster virus and rabies infections

Herpes simplex virus (HSV) and varicella-zoster virus (VZV) present in skin or mucosal lesions (see Chapter 23), travel up axons using the normal retrograde transport mechanisms that can move virus particles (as well as foreign molecules such as tetanus toxin) at the rate of about 200 mm/day, to reach dorsal root ganglia. Rabies virus, introduced into muscle or subcutaneous tissues by the bite of a rabid animal, infects muscle fibers and muscle spindles after binding of the virus to

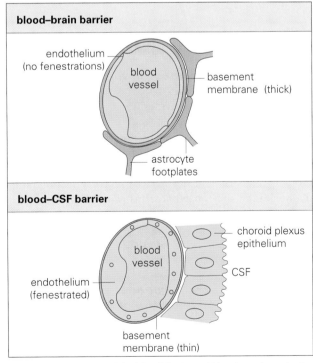

Fig. 22.1 Structures of the blood–brain and blood–cerebrospinal fluid (CSF) barriers.

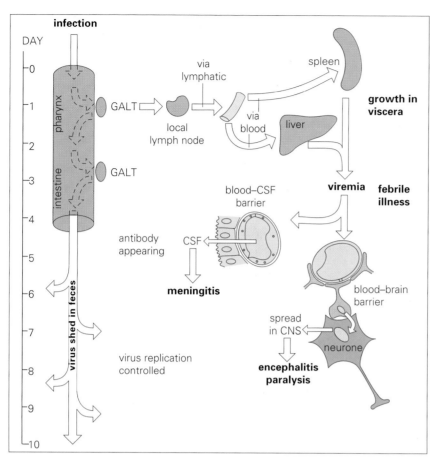

Fig. 22.2 The mechanism of central nervous system (CNS) invasion by poliovirus. (CSF, cerebrospinal fluid; GALT, gut-associated lymphoid tissue).

the nicotinic acetylcholine receptor. It then enters peripheral nerves and travels to the CNS, to reach glial cells and neurones, where it multiplies.

The Body's Response to Invasion

CSF cell counts increase in response to infection

The response to invading viruses is reflected by an increase in lymphocytes (mostly T cells) and monocytes in the CSF *(Fig. 22.3)*. A slight increase in protein also occurs, the CSF remaining clear. This condition is termed 'aseptic' meningitis. The response to pyogenic bacteria shows a more spectacular and more rapid increase in polymorphonuclear leukocytes and proteins *(Fig. 22.4)*, so that the CSF becomes visibly turbid. This condition is termed 'septic' meningitis. Certain slower growing or less pyogenic microorganisms induce less dramatic changes, such as in tuberculous or listerial meningitis.

The pathologic consequences of CNS infection depend upon the microorganism

In the CNS itself viruses can infect neural cells, sometimes showing a marked preference. Polio and rabies viruses, for instance, invade neurones whereas JC virus invades oligodendrocytes. Because there is very little extracellular space, spread is mostly direct from cell to cell along established nervous pathways. Invading bacteria and protozoa generally induce more dramatic inflammatory events, which limit local spread so that infection is soon localized to form abscesses.

Viruses induce perivascular infiltration of lymphocytes and monocytes, sometimes, as in the case of polio, with direct damage to infected cells. The pathogenesis of viral encephalomyelitis is illustrated on p. 305. Associated immune responses not only to viral, but also often to host CNS components play a part (see 'postvaccinial encephalitis' on p. 309). Infiltrating B cells produce antibody to the invading microorganism and T cells react with microbial antigens to release cytokines that attract and activate other T cells and macrophages. The pathologic condition evolves over the course of several days and, occasionally, when partly controlled by host defenses, over the course of years – for example subacute sclerosing panencephalitis (SSPE). Bacteria cause more rapidly evolving pathologic changes, with local responses to bacterial antigens and toxins playing an important part.

In all cases, a degree of inflammation and edema that would be trivial in striated muscle, skin or liver may be life-threatening when it occurs in the vulnerable 'closed box' containing the leptomeninges, brain and spinal cord. It may be several weeks after clinical recovery before cellular infiltrations are removed and histologic appearances are restored to normal.

CNS invasion only rarely assists in the transmission of infection

From the point of view of a parasitic microorganism that needs to be transmitted to a fresh host, invasion of the CNS is generally foolish because it damages the host, or at least

CSF CHANGES DURING CENTRAL NERVOUS SYSTEM INFECTION

	cells/μl	protein mg/dl	glucose mg/dl	causes
normal	0–5	15–45	45–85	—
septic (purulent) meningitis	200–20 000 (mainly neutrophils)	high (>100)	<45	bacteria amebae brain abscess
aseptic* meningitis or meningo-encephalitis	100–1000 (mainly mononuclear)	moderately high (50–100)	normal**	viruses tuberculosis leptospira fungi brain abscess partly treated bacterial meningitis

* aseptic because the CSF is sterile on regular bacteriologic culture

** low (<45) in the case of tuberculosis, fungi, leptospira

Fig. 22.3 Changes in cerebrospinal fluid (CSF) in response to invading microbes.

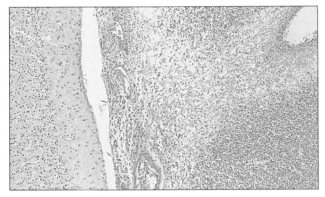

Fig. 22.4 Bacterial meningitis. Exudate of acute inflammatory cells in the subarachnoid space. Hematoxylin and eosin stain. (Courtesy of P Garen.)

unnecessary. The only occasions on which it makes sense are:

• When dorsal root ganglion neurones are invaded as an essential step in establishing latency (HSV and VZV). This gives a mechanism for reactivation and further episodes of shedding from mucosal or skin lesions.

• In the case of rabies (see below), where CNS invasion in the animal host is necessary for two reasons. First, it enables the virus to spread from the CNS down peripheral nerves to the salivary glands, from which transmission takes place. Second, invasion of the limbic system of the brain causes a change in behavior of the infected animal so that it becomes less retiring, more aggressive and more likely to bite, thus transmitting the infection. Invasion of the limbic system can be regarded as a fiendish strategy on the part of rabies virus to promote its own transmission and survival.

Bacterial Meningitis

Acute bacterial meningitis is a life-threatening infection, needing urgent specific treatment

It is more severe, but less common, than viral meningitis (see p. 302). The important causative agents (shown in *Figure 22.5.*) *Neisseria meningitidis*, *Haemophilus influenzae* and *Streptococcus pneumoniae* invade the meninges in healthy individuals and account for more than 75% of cases of bacterial meningitis. These three pathogens have several virulence factors in common *(Fig. 22.6)*, including possession of a polysaccharide capsule *(Fig. 22.7)*.

Meningococcal meningitis
Neisseria meningitidis is carried by 20% of the population but in epidemics higher rates are seen

Neisseria meningitidis is a Gram-negative diplococcus, which closely resembles *N. gonorrhoeae* in structure (see Chapter 19), but with an additional polysaccharide capsule that is antigenic and by which the serotype of *N. meningitidis* can be recognized. The bacteria are carried asymptomatically in up to 20% of the population, attached by their pili to the epithelial cells in the nasopharynx. Invasion of the blood and meninges is a rare and poorly understood event. The known virulence factors are summarized in *Figure 22.6*. People possessing specific complement-dependent bacterial antibodies to capsular antigens are protected against invasion. Those with C5–C9 complement deficiencies show increased susceptibility to bacteremia (as they do to *N. gonorrhoeae* bacteremia; see Chapter 19). Young children who have lost the antibodies acquired from their mother, and adolescents who have not previously encountered the infecting serotype, and

NON-VIRAL MENINGITIS – CAUSES, TREATMENT AND PREVENTION		
pathogen	**treatment***	**prevention**
Neisseria meningitidis	penicillin (or chloramphenicol)	rifampin prophylaxis for close contacts polysaccharide vaccine (poor protection against group B)
Haemophilus influenzae	ampicillin** ceftriaxone or cefotaxime (or chloramphenicol)	polysaccharide vaccine against type B (Hib)
Streptococcus pneumoniae	penicillin*** (or ceftriaxone or chloramphenicol)	prompt treatment of otitis media and respiratory infections polyvalent (23 serotypes) polysaccharide vaccine
Escherichia coli (and other coliforms) group B streptococci	gentamicin + cefotaxime or ceftriaxone (or chloramphenicol)**	no vaccines available
Listeria monocytogenes	penicillin or ampicillin + gentamicin	
Mycobacterium tuberculosis	isoniazid and rifampin and pyrazinamide ± streptomycin	BCG vaccination isoniazid prophylaxis for contacts recommended in USA
Cryptococcus neoformans	amphotericin B and flucytosine	no vaccines available

* treatment should be initiated immediately and the susceptibilty of the infecting isolate confirmed in the laboratory

** if isolate is shown to be susceptible (10–20% of isolates are resistant because they produce a plasmid coded beta-lactamase)

*** in areas of high prevalence of penicillin resistant pneumococci initial treatment with ceftriaxone may be advised until susceptibility of isolate is known

Fig. 22.5 The important causative agents of non-viral meningitis, their treatment and prevention. (BCG, bacille Calmette–Guérin.)

therefore have no type-specific immunity, are those most often infected. Person to person spread takes place by droplet infection, and is facilitated by other (viral) respiratory infec-

BACTERIAL MENINGITIS – VIRULENCE FACTORS FOR MAJOR PATHOGENS			
virulence factor	**bacterial pathogen**		
	Neisseria meningitidis	*Haemophilus influenzae*	*Streptococcus pneumoniae*
capsule	+	+	+
IgA protease	+	+	+
pili	+	+	–
endotoxin	+	+	–
outer membrane proteins	?	+	–

Fig. 22.6 Virulence factors in bacterial meningitis.

tions that cause increased respiratory secretions, and by overcrowding. During outbreaks of meningococcal meningitis the carrier rate may reach 70%. In the UK and USA serotype B infections are the commonest, but in Africa, China and South America there have been repeated epidemics due to serotypes A and C.

Clinical features of meningococcal meningitis include a hemorrhagic skin rash

After an incubation period of 1–3 days, the onset of meningococcal meningitis is sudden with a sore throat, headache, drowsiness and signs of meningitis (fever, irritability, neck stiffness). There is often a hemorrhagic skin rash with petechiae, reflecting the associated septicemia (*Fig. 22.8*). In about 35% of patients this septicemia is fulminating, with complications due to disseminated intravascular coagulation, endotoxemia and shock, and renal failure. In the most severe cases there is an acute Addisonian crisis, with bleeding into the brain and adrenal glands (Waterhouse–Friderichsen syndrome). Mortality from meningococcal meningitis reaches 100% if untreated, but

CAPSULES – IMPORTANT VIRULENCE FACTORS

pathogen	capsule	important type	vaccine
Neisseria meningitidis	polysaccharide	A, B, C, Y, W-135	good for A and C; poor for B
Haemophilus influenzae	polysaccharide	b	Hib vaccine for <1-year-olds
Streptococcus pneumoniae	polysaccharide	many	pneumovax:23-valent most common types
group B streptococcus	polysaccharide rich in sialic acid	(Ia, Ib, II) III in neonatal meningitis	– ? future
Escherichia coli		KI in meningitis	– ? future

Fig. 22.7 Polysaccharide capsules are important virulence factors in the pathogenesis of bacterial meningitis.

remains around 10% even if treated. However, serious sequelae are uncommon in survivors compared with the outcome of *H. influenzae* or *Strep. pneumoniae* meningitis *(Fig. 22.9)*.

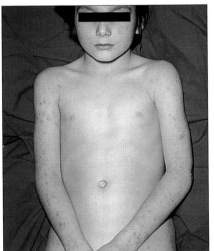

Fig. 22.8 Meningococcal septicemia showing a mixed petechial and maculopapular rash on the extremities and exterior surfaces. (Courtesy of WE Farrar.)

A diagnosis of acute meningitis is usually suspected on clinical examination

Laboratory identification of the bacterial cause of acute meningitis is essential so that appropriate antibiotic therapy can be given and prophylaxis of contacts initiated. Preliminary results should be available within an hour of receipt of the CSF sample in the laboratory. Results of culture of CSF and blood should follow after 24 hours (see Chapter 14). Serology is not helpful in the diagnosis because the infection is too acute for an antibody response to be detectable.

Bacterial meningitis is a medical emergency

Antibiotic therapy (usually penicillin or ampicillin) should be instigated if the diagnosis is suspected *(Fig. 22.5)*. Early treatment saves lives, although it may make recovery of viable organisms from specimens more difficult.

Close contacts in the family ('kissing contacts') should be given rifampin chemoprophylaxis for 2–3 days. Note that penicillin is not used for prophylaxis because it does not eliminate nasopharyngeal carriage of meningococci. Patients should be given a course of rifampin to clear carriage after the acute phase of the infection has passed. Sulfonamides can

BACTERIAL MENINGITIS – CLINICAL FEATURES

pathogen	host (patient)	important clinical features	mortality (as % of treated cases)	sequelae (as % of treated cases)*
Neisseria meningitidis	children and adolescents	acute onset (6–24 hours) skin rash	7–10	< 1
Haemophilus influenzae	children <5 years of age	onset often less acute (1–2 days)	5	9
Streptococcus pneumoniae	all ages, but especially children <2 years of age and elderly	acute onset may follow pneumonia and/or septicemia in elderly	20–30	15–20

* major central nervous system deficit; in addition, up to 10% of patients develop deafness

Fig. 22.9 Clinical features of bacterial meningitis.

no longer be relied upon for prophylaxis because resistance in meningococci is common.

Haemophilus meningitis
Type b H. influenzae causes meningitis in infants and young children

H. influenzae is a Gram-negative coccobacillus. 'Haemophilus' means 'blood-loving', and the name 'influenzae' was given because it was originally thought to be the cause of influenza, but is now known to be a common secondary invader in the lower respiratory tract. There are six types (a–f) of *H. influenzae*, distinguishable serologically by their capsular polysaccharides:

- Unencapsulated strains are common and are present in the throat of most healthy people.
- The capsulated type b, a common inhabitant of the respiratory tract of infants and young children (where it may cause infection: see Chapter 21), very occasionally invades the blood and reaches the meninges.

Maternal antibody protects the infant up to 3–4 months of age, but as it wanes there is a 'window of susceptibility' until the child produces his/her own antibody. Anticapsular antibodies are good opsonins (see Chapter 10), which allow the bacteria to be phagocytosed and killed, but children do not generally produce them until 2–3 years of age, possibly because these antibodies are T independent. In addition to the capsule, *H. influenzae* has several other virulence factors, as shown in *Figure 22.6*.

Acute H. influenzae meningitis is commonly complicated by severe neurologic sequelae

The incubation period of *H. influenzae* meningitis is 5–6 days and the onset is often more insidious than that of meningococcal or pneumococcal meningitis *(Fig. 22.9)*. The condition is less frequently fatal, but there is a 10% higher incidence of serious sequelae (hearing loss, delayed language development, mental retardation and seizures) than with meningococcal infection *(Fig. 22.9)*.

General diagnostic features are the same as for meningococcal meningitis, as explained above. For laboratory diagnosis see Chapter 14. It is important to note than the organisms may be difficult to see in Gram-stained smears of CSF, particularly if they are present in small numbers.

Hib vaccine is effective for children from six months of age

General features of treatment are referred to above under meningococcal meningitis; details are summarized in *Figure 22.5*. An effective *H. influenzae* vaccine (Hib), suitable for children of six months of age and upwards, is now available. Close contacts of patients are sometimes given rifampin prophylaxis.

Pneumococcal meningitis
Streptococcus pneumoniae is a common cause of bacterial meningitis, particularly in children and the elderly

Strep. pneumoniae was first isolated more than 100 years ago and has since received intensive study both as a pathogen and as the subject of early work on bacterial transformation. Despite this, relatively little is known about its virulence attributes apart from its polysaccharide capsule *(Figs 22.6* and

22.7), and the pneumococcus remains a major cause of morbidity and mortality. (Pneumococcal respiratory tract infections are reviewed in Chapter 16.)

Strep. pneumoniae is a capsulate Gram-positive coccus carried in the throats of many healthy individuals. Invasion of the blood and meninges is a rare event, but is more common in the very young (less than two years of age), in the elderly, in those with sickle cell disease, in debilitated or splenectomized patients and following head trauma. Susceptibility to infection is associated with low levels of antibodies to capsular polysaccharide antigens: antibody opsonizes the organism and promotes phagocytosis, thereby protecting the host from invasion. However, this protection is type-specific and there are more than 85 different capsular types of *Strep. pneumoniae*.

The clinical features of pneumococcal meningitis are summarized in *Figure 22.9*, and the general diagnostic features are the same as for meningococcal meningitis described above. Details are referred to in Chapter 14.

Treatment and prevention of pneumococcal meningitis are summarized in *Figure 22.5*. In countries where penicillin-resistant pneumococci are prevalent, attention should be paid to the antibiotic susceptibility of the infecting strain. The role of the 23-valent polysaccharide vaccine in the prevention of meningitis is uncertain. It is not very effective on children under two.

Listeria monocytogenes meningitis
Listeria monocytogenes causes meningitis in immunocompromised adults

Listeria monocytogenes is a Gram-positive coccobacillus and is an important cause of meningitis in immunocompromised adults, especially in renal transplant and cancer patients. It also causes intrauterine infections and infections of the newborn, as summarized in Chapter 21. *L. monocytogenes* is less susceptible than *Strep. pneumoniae* to penicillin and the recommended treatment is a combination of penicillin or ampicillin with gentamicin.

Neonatal meningitis

This can be caused by a wide range of bacteria but the most frequent are *Escherichia coli* and group B hemolytic streptococci *(Fig. 22.10*; see also Chapter 20).

Neonatal meningitis is fatal in about 35% of cases

It also often leads to permanent neurologic sequelae such as cerebral or cranial nerve palsy, epilepsy, mental retardation or hydrocephalus. This is partly because the clinical diagnosis of meningitis in the neonate is difficult, perhaps with no more specific signs than fever, poor feeding, vomiting, respiratory distress or diarrhea. In addition the possible range of organisms is wide, 'blind' antibiotic therapy in the absence of susceptibility tests may not be optimal, and many antibiotics inadequately penetrate the CSF. Host defenses are poor, especially in low birth weight (less than 1000 g) babies.

Tuberculous meningitis

Patients with tuberculous meningitis always have a focus of infection elsewhere, but 25% have no clinical or historic evidence of such an infection. In more than 50% of cases, meningitis is associated with acute miliary tuberculosis *(Fig. 22.11)*.

NEONATAL MENINGITIS		
group B streptococci and neonatal meningitis		
group B streptococci *(Streptococcus agalactiae)* are normal inhabitants of the female genital tract and may be acquired by the neonate		
	at or soon after birth	in the nursery
	early onset disease	**late onset disease**
age	<7 days	1 week–3 months
risk factors	heavily colonized mother lacking specific antibody premature rupture of membranes pre-term delivery prolonged labor, obstetric complications	lack of maternal antibody exposure to cross-infection from heavily colonized babies poor hygiene in nursery
type of disease	generalized infection including bacteremia, pneumonia and meningitis	predominantly meningitis
type of group B streptococcus	all serotypes but meningitis mostly due to type III	90% type III
outcome	approximately 60% fatal; serious sequelae in many survivors	approximately 20% fatal
treatment	take blood and CSF for culture treat on suspicion gentamicin and ampicillin or cefotaxime/ceftriaxone	treat on suspicion take blood and CSF for culture gentamicin and ampicillin or cefotaxime/ceftriaxone
prevention	antibiotic treatment does not reliably abolish carriage in mother; not recommended 'blind' treatment of sick baby who has risk factors future: ?? immunize antibody-negative females of child-bearing age	good hygienic practices in nursery do not allow mothers to handle other babies

Fig. 22.10 Group B streptococci are a major cause of neonatal meningitis. (CSF, cerebrospinal fluid.)

Tuberculous meningitis usually presents with a gradual onset over a few weeks

There is a gradual onset of generalized illness beginning with malaise, apathy and anorexia and proceeding within a few weeks to photophobia, neck stiffness and impairment of consciousness. Occasionally the onset is much more rapid and may be mistaken for a subarachnoid hemorrhage. The variability of presentation means that the clinician needs to maintain an awareness of possible tuberculous meningitis to make the diagnosis. A delay in making the diagnosis and in starting appropriate antimicrobial therapy *(Fig. 22.5)* results in serious complications and sequelae.

Spinal tuberculosis is uncommon now except in developing countries; bacteria in the vertebrae destroy the intervertebral discs to form epidural abscesses. These compress the spinal cord and lead to paraplegia.

Fungal Meningitis

Cryptococcus neoformans and *Coccidioides immitis* can invade the blood from a primary site of infection in the lungs and thence to the brain to cause meningitis.

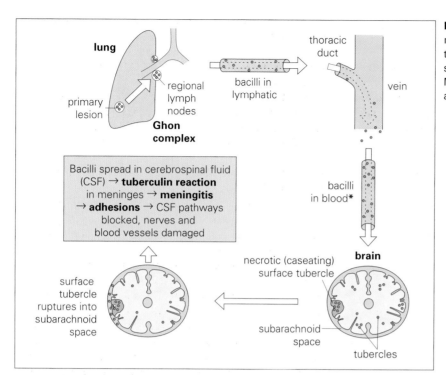

Fig. 22.11 The association between acute miliary tuberculosis and meningitis. (*Leads to miliary tuberculosis – Latin: milium, millet seed – each tubercle resembles a millet seed. Miliary tuberculosis also occurs in the lungs and elsewhere.)

Cryptococcus neoformans meningitis is seen in patients with depressed cell-mediated immunity

It therefore occurs in AIDS patients. The onset is usually slow, over days or weeks. The capsulate yeasts can be seen in India ink-stained preparations of CSF *(Fig. 22.12)* and can be cultured (see Chapter 14). Antigen detection is also a useful diagnostic tool and evidence of a decline in antigen and an increase in antibody levels in the CSF can be used as a measure of successful therapy. Treatment with the antifungal drugs amphotericin B and flucytosine in combination is recommended.

Coccidioides immitis infection is common in particular geographic locations

These locations are notably Southwest USA, Mexico and South America. CNS infection occurs in fewer than 1% of infected individuals, but is fatal unless treated. It may be part of the generalized disease or may represent the only extrapulmonary site. The organisms are rarely visible in the CSF and cultures are positive in less than 50% of cases, but the diagnosis can be made by demonstrating complement-fixing antibodies in the serum. Treatment with amphotericin B or miconazole is recommended.

Protozoal Meningitis

Free-living amebae (*Naegleria* or *Hartmanella* spp.) can multiply in stagnant fresh water in warm countries, especially in the sludge at the bottom of lakes and swimming pools. They reach the meninges via the olfactory tract and cribriform plate, and cause an acute or subacute meningitis. These slowly motile amebae can be seen on careful examination of a fresh wet sample of CSF. The mortality rate from such infection is high.

Viral Meningitis

Viral meningitis is the commonest type of meningitis

It is a milder disease than bacterial meningitis, with headache, fever and general illness, but less neck stiffness. The CSF is clear and bacteria free, and the cells are mainly lymphocytes, although polymorphonuclear leukocytes may be present in the early stages *(Fig. 22.3)*. The causes of viral meningitis are listed in *Figure 22.13*, but viruses are isolated from the CSF in less than 50% of cases. As there are many types of enteroviruses (32 echoviruses, 29 coxsackieviruses, three polioviruses) and infection is commonly asymptomatic, a virus isolated from the throat or stool of a child with mild meningitis may be of no etiologic significance. In contrast to bacterial meningitis, and in spite of the fact that there are no antiviral drugs (except for HSV), complete recovery is the rule.

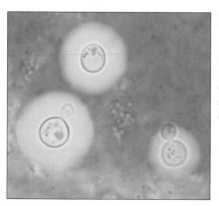

Fig. 22.12 *Cryptococcus neoformans* in India ink-stained preparation of cerebrospinal fluid sediment. (Courtesy of AE Prevost.)

Encephalitis

Encephalitis is usually caused by viruses
The causes and pathogenesis of viral encephalitis are shown in *Figure 22.14* and *Figure 22.15*. Characteristically, there are signs of cerebral dysfunction such as abnormal behavior, seizures and altered consciousness, often with nausea, vomiting and fever.

Toxoplasma gondii and *C. neoformans* can also cause life-threatening encephalitis or meningoencephalitis. This is particularly likely in those with defective cell-mediated immunity, and cerebral malaria as a complication of *Plasmodium falciparum* infection is frequently fatal. Encephalitis may occur in Lyme disease *(Borrelia burgdorferi)* and Legionnaires' disease *(Legionella pneumophila)*, but the relative importance of bacterial invasion, bacterial toxins and immunopatholog is unknown.

HSV encephalitis is the commonest severe sporadic encephalitis
There are two forms of HSV encephalitis:
- One form occurs following primary and generalized infection in infancy.
- Another form, seen in adults, is probably due to virus reactivation in the trigeminal ganglia (see Chapter 15), the infection then passing back to the temporal lobe of the brain.

Herpetic skin or mucosal lesions may be present. The diagnosis is indicated by clinical signs of a space-occupying lesion in the temporal lobe and a computerized tomographic (CT) or radioactive (technetium-99) brain scan *(Fig. 22.16)*. Brain biopsy is sometimes justified. The 70% mortality rate

VIRAL MENINGITIS		
virus	**virus group**	**comments**
herpes simplex virus	alpha herpesvirus	uncommon; may follow genital infection with HSV2
mumps	paramyxovirus	a quite common complication
lymphocytic choriomeningitis	arenavirus	uncommon infection from urine etc. of mice, hamsters carrying the virus
poliovirus, coxsackievirus, echovirus etc.	picornaviruses (enterovirus group)	commonly seen (especially due to echoviruses) although an uncommon complication of infection
Japanese encephalitis	togavirus	India, South East Asia, Japan
Eastern and Western equine encephalitis	togavirus	East and West USA
louping ill	togavirus	Scotland
HIV	retrovirus	may occur early after infection

Fig. 22.13 Causes of viral meningitis.

in untreated patients is greatly reduced by early treatment with acyclovir.

Other herpesviruses less commonly cause encephalitis
With VZV, encephalitis generally occurs as a sequel to reactivation, and with cytomegalovirus (CMV) either during primary infection *in utero* (see Chapter 21) or reactivation as a complication of immunodeficiency (e.g. in AIDS).

Poliovirus used to be a common cause of encephalitis
In the great 1916 polio epidemic in New York City, 9000 cases of paralysis, nearly all in children less than five years of age, were reported. CNS disease occurs in less than 1% of those infected. After an initial 1–4 days of fever, sore throat, malaise, meningeal signs and symptoms appear, followed by involvement of motor neurones and paralysis *(Fig. 22.2)*. In spite of the fact that there are successful vaccines and we now have sophisticated information about the structure *(Fig. 22.17)* and replication of the virus, the disease poliomyelitis is still common in developing countries (there were 200 000 cases in India in 1989). The disease is completely preventable by vaccination (see Chapter 29) and has been disappearing in developed countries since vaccination programs were first carried out in the 1950s *(Fig. 22.18)*. There are three serologic (antigenic) types of poliovirus, with little cross-reaction between them, so that antibody to each type is necessary for protection. At least 75% of paralytic cases are due to type 1 polioviruses.

Other enteroviruses (coxsackieviruses, echoviruses) also occasionally cause encephalitis.

Mumps virus is a common cause of mild encephalitis
Asymptomatic CNS invasion may be common because there are increased numbers of cells in the CSF in about 50% of patients with parotitis; on the other hand, meningitis and encephalitis are often seen without parotitis.

Rabies encephalitis
There are 35 000 cases of human rabies worldwide each year
The causative agent of rabies is a rhabdovirus, a bullet-shaped single-stranded RNA virus. The virus is excreted in the saliva of infected dogs, foxes, jackals, wolves, skunks, raccoons and vampire bats, and transmission to man follows a bite or salivary contamination of other types of skin abrasions or wounds. Some species of animal (e.g. foxes) are more infectious than others because larger amounts of virus (up to 10^6 infectious doses/ml) are present in their saliva. The infection is eventually fatal, although the course of the disease varies considerably between species. If an apparently healthy dog is still healthy 10 days after biting a human, rabies is extremely unlikely. However, the virus may be excreted in the dog's saliva before the animal shows any clinical signs of disease.

The virus can infect all warm-blooded animals. Rabies from vampire bats causes more than one million deaths/year in cattle in Central and South America. Dogs transmit most of the 35 000 cases of human rabies that occur in the world each year. In all the mainland masses, the infection maintains itself in non-human mammalian hosts; islands such as Australia, Great Britain, Japan, Hawaii, most of the Caribbean islands, and also Scandinavia, are free of rabies because of strict controls over the importation of animals such as dogs and cats. In the USA, the incidence of human

CAUSES OF ENCEPHALITIS		
cause	**infectious agent**	**comment**
viruses (sporadic occurrence)	herpes simplex virus	infant and adult forms distinguished
	mumps	much less common than meningitis
	varicella-zoster virus	a rare complication of ophthalmic zoster
	cytomegalovirus	*in utero* and in immunosuppressed (e.g. AIDS)
	rabies	in India 15–20 000 deaths/year, in USA less than 10
	louping ill	one of tick-borne encephalitis virus complex (others cause Russian spring–summer encephalitis etc.)
	retroviruses HTLV1	tropical spastic paraparesis in small proportion of those infected
	HIV	subacute encephalitis (often together with other central nervous system infections)
viruses (may be outbreaks)	polio and other enteroviruses	uncommon; may be spastic paralysis
	eastern and western equine encephalitis	mosquito-borne togaviruses
	St Louis encephalitis virus	
	Japanese encephalitis virus	
	Californian encephalitis virus	mosquito-borne bunyavirus
slow viruses	rubella	infection *in utero* (microcephaly etc.) or subacute sclerosing panencephalitis (SSPE)-type disease
	measles	SSPE following uncomplicated measles after interval of up to 10 years
	JC virus (progressive multifocal leukoencephalopathy)	usually in immunocompromised
atypical agents of scrapie group (non-viral)	? prions	Creutzfeldt–Jakob disease (CJD) and kuru in humans incubation period up to 20 years 'spongiform' encephalopathy
post-vaccinial or post-infectious	?	occurs as a rare complication 2–3 weeks after exposure to certain viruses (e.g. measles) or vaccines; strong autoimmune component
protozoa and fungi	*Toxoplasma gondii*	encephalitis a rare complication
	Cryptococcus neoformans	meningoencephalitis
	Plasmodium falciparum	cerebral malaria
	Trypanosoma spp.	sleeping sickness in Africa
bacteria	*Treponema pallidum*	rare
	Mycoplasma pneumoniae	rare
	Borrelia borgdorferi	uncommon

Fig. 22.14 Infectious causes of encephalitis. (HTLV, human T cell lymphotropic virus.)

rabies has been falling since the 1940s and 1950s, when most cases followed exposure to infected dogs. Since then the source has more often been non-domesticated animals such as skunks, raccoons and bats, or exposure to dogs in other countries.

Raccoon rabies spread slowly northwards from Florida in the 1950s, and in the 1980s caused an explosive epidemic in Virginia, Maryland and the District of Colombia. This outbreak was due to the importation of raccoons from infected areas for sporting purposes.

The incubation period in humans is generally 4–13 weeks, although it may occasionally be as long as six months, possibly due to a delay in virus entry into peripheral nerves. The virus travels up peripheral nerves (see above) and, in general, the further the bite is from the CNS, the longer the incubation period. For instance, a bite on the foot gives a longer incubation period than a bite on the face.

While the virus is travelling up the axons of motor or sensory neurones, there is no detectable antibody or

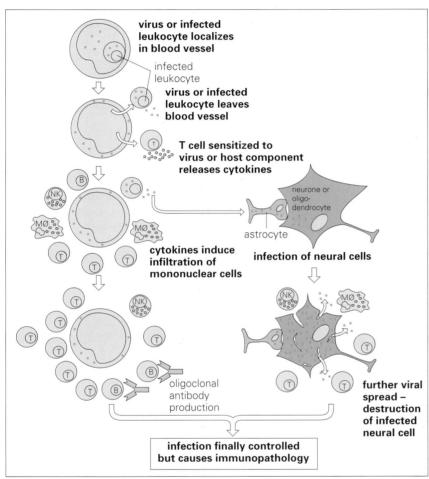

Fig. 22.15 The pathogenesis of viral encephalomyelitis. (MØ, macrophage; NK, natural killer cell.)

virus or infected leukocyte localizes in blood vessel

infected leukocyte

virus or infected leukocyte leaves blood vessel

T cell sensitized to virus or host component releases cytokines

neurone or oligo-dendrocyte

astrocyte

cytokines induce infiltration of mononuclear cells

infection of neural cells

oligoclonal antibody production

further viral spread – destruction of infected neural cell

infection finally controlled but causes immunopathology

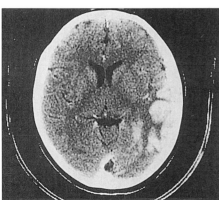

Fig. 22.16 Herpes simplex encephalitis. Computerized tomographic scan showing enhancement of gyral structures in the left temporal lobe and associated cerebral edema. (Courtesy of Dr J Curé.)

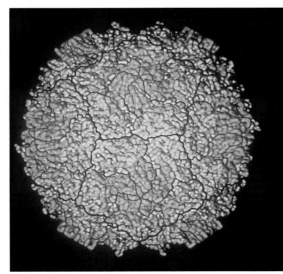

Fig. 22.17 Computer graphic model of the surface of a poliovirus based on X-ray diffraction studies. The capsid protein subunits visible on the surface of the virus particle are viral protein 1 (VP1) in blue, VP2 in green and VP3 in gray. (Courtesy of AJ Olson, Research Institute of Scripps Clinic, La Jolla, California.)

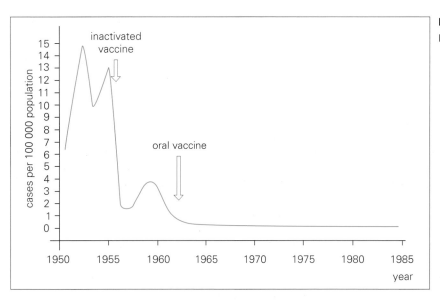

Fig. 22.18 The incidence of paralytic poliomyelitis in the USA from 1951–85.

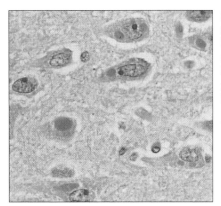

Fig. 22.19 Multiple cytoplasmic Negri bodies in pyramidal neurones of the hippocampus in rabies. (Courtesy of P Garen.)

cell-mediated immune response, possibly because antigen remains sequestered in infected muscle cells. Hence, passively administered immunoglobulin may be given during the incubation period.

Once in the brain, the virus spreads from cell to cell until a large proportion of neurones is infected, but there is little cytopathic effect, even when viewed by electron microscopy, and almost no cellular infiltration. The striking symptoms of this disease are largely due to dysfunction rather than visible damage to infected cells. The change in behavior of infected animals results from virus invasion of the limbic system.

Clinical features of rabies include muscle spasms, convulsions and hydrophobia

After developing a sore throat, headache, fever and discomfort at the site of the bite, the patient becomes excited, with muscle spasms and convulsions. Involvement of the muscles of swallowing when attempting to drink water gave the old name for rabies – hydrophobia – as the symptoms are sometimes precipitated by the mere sight of water.

Once rabies has developed it is fatal, death occurring following cardiac or respiratory arrest. Paralysis is often a major feature of the disease. One or two patients treated in intensive care units have recovered, but with serious neurologic sequelae.

Rabies can be diagnosed by detecting viral antigen

Laboratory diagnosis can be made by the detection of viral antigen by immunofluorescence observations on skin biopsies, corneal impression smears or brain biopsy. Characteristic intracytoplasmic inclusions (Negri bodies) are seen in neurones (*Fig. 22.19*).

There is no treatment except supportive nursing.

Many countries have developed vaccination programs for domestic dogs (e.g. France) and in Canada and elsewhere wild foxes have been vaccinated by dropping food baited with live virus vaccine from the air. For the rabies-free countries, constant vigilance at borders and strict quarantine regulations are necessary to prevent the introduction of infected animals. In 1886 there were 36 human rabies deaths in England, 11 of them in London. As recently as 1906, rabies was still endemic in England, and there were deaths due to rabies in the deer in Hampton Court Park, London.

After exposure to a possibly infected animal immediate preventive action should be taken

This action includes:

- Prompt cleaning of the wound (alcoholic iodine, debridement).
- Confirmation of whether or not the animal is rabid (clinical observation of suspected dogs, histologic observation of the brain of other suspected species).
- Administration of human rabies immunoglobulin, to ensure prompt passive immunization – 50% of the dose is given into the wound and 50% intramuscularly.
- If the risk is definite, active immunization with killed diploid cell-derived rabies virus (see Chapter 31). The

chances of preventing the disease are greater when vaccination is begun as early as possible after infection.

Togavirus meningitis and encephalitis
Numerous arthropod-borne togaviruses can cause meningitis or encephalitis

These togaviruses are listed in *Figures 22.13* and *22.14*, and sometimes cause outbreaks of infection. In different parts of the world different mammals, birds or even reptiles act as reservoirs and there are a variety of arthropod (mosquito and tick) vectors. Usually less than 1% of humans infected develop neurologic disease (see Chapter 25). There may be a febrile illness, but asymptomatic infection is common. In California, for instance, western equine encephalomyelitis (WEE) virus and St Louis encephalitis (SLE) virus are prevalent and transmitted by the mosquito *Culex tarsalis*; a WEE vaccine is available, but only for horses.

Japanese encephalitis virus infection is common in India and can result in a mortality of more than 50% in older age groups; a vaccine for humans has been developed.

Retrovirus meningitis and encephalitis
HIV can cause subacute encephalitis, often with dementia

HIV (see Chapter 19) often invades the CNS shortly after initial infection, resulting in an increase in cells in the CSF and a mild meningitic illness. At a later stage, and quite independently of the disease picture that results from immune deficiency – AIDS-related complex (ARC), a subacute encephalitis may develop, often with dementia (AIDS dementia complex). This is sometimes difficult to distinguish from the neurologic disease caused by microorganisms such as *T. gondii, C. neoformans,* cytomegalovirus and JC virus. The brain is shrunken with enlarged ventricles and vacuolation of myelin tracts. HIV mainly infects macrophages and microglia in the CNS and because the clinical disease is more severe than might be expected from the pathologic changes, additional pathogenic mechanisms have been proposed. For instance, there are amino acid sequence similarities between the HIV envelope protein gp120 and certain transmitter molecules, so that HIV-derived molecules could block the action of natural neurotransmitters.

Some of those infected with human T cell lymphotropic virus type 1 (HTLV1) develop the disease 'tropical spastic paraparesis'. The spinal cord is involved, but little is known of the pathogenesis.

Neurologic Diseases of Possible Viral Etiology

It has often been suggested that certain neurologic diseases of unknown origin, including multiple sclerosis, amyotrophic lateral sclerosis, Parkinson's disease, schizophrenia and senile dementia, have a viral origin. Although so far there is no acceptable evidence for this, it is possible that viruses may, at times, trigger dangerous autoimmune-type responses in the CNS.

Slow Virus Infection

In these rare infections a virus (rubella, measles or JC virus) invades the CNS, but virus growth is slow, often incomplete, and partially controlled by host defenses (see Chapter 11); clinical disease appears after an incubation period of up to 10 years. For instance:

* In otherwise uncomplicated measles, CNS invasion can take place and eventually result in SSPE.
* Rubella very occasionally causes a similar disease to SSPE but, more commonly, like CMV, it invades the brain of the fetus, interfering with development to cause mental retardation.
* JC virus (a polyomavirus) occasionally invades oligodendrocytes in immunodeficient people and eventually gives rise to progressive multifocal leukoencephalopathy (PML).

Brain Abscesses

Brain abscesses are usually associated with predisposing factors

Since the development of antibiotics, brain abscesses have become rare and usually follow surgery or trauma, chronic osteomyelitis of neighboring bone, septic embolism or chronic cerebral anoxia. They are also seen in children with congenital cyanotic heart disease in whom the lungs fail to filter off circulating bacteria. Acute abscesses are caused by various bacteria, generally of oropharyngeal origin, including anaerobes. There is usually a mixed bacterial flora. Chronic abscesses are often due to *Mycobacterium tuberculosis* or *C. neoformans.*

Brain abscesses are diagnosed clinically and by scans. If an abscess is suspected, lumbar puncture is contraindicated, but if performed generally shows raised CSF cells and proteins *(Fig. 22.3).* Treatment is by surgical drainage if the abscess is well encapsulated, and antibiotics should be given for at least one month.

Other infections that may manifest as chronic meningitis or brain abscess are summarized in *Figure 22.20.*

Encephalopathy Due to Scrapie-Type Agents

Scrapie-type agents are closely associated with host-coded prion protein

Scrapie-type agents form a closely related group, infect a variety of mammals, including humans, and are all transmissible to laboratory rodents or primates. They show a number of remarkable features, and nearly all our knowledge comes from experiments in laboratory mice and from molecular biology. These features of scrapie-type agents include the following:

* They replicate extremely slowly, taking more than one week to double in number. Hence the incubation period is long, usually a large fraction of the life span.
* They are of virus size, but are not true viruses, since they

appear to contain neither DNA nor RNA. A prion protein, closely associated with the infectious agent, is host-coded but slightly altered in the infected brain; the abnormal form accumulates in nerve cells. Replication occurs by conversion of host prion protein into the abnormal form. Is the prion protein the actual infectious agent? Although mice with

INFECTIOUS DISEASES THAT MAY BE MANIFEST AS CHRONIC MENINGITIS OR BRAIN ABSCESS	
bacterial	
tuberculosis	*Mycobacterium tuberculosis*
syphilis	*Treponema pallidum*
brucellosis	*Brucella abortus*
Lyme disease	*Borrelia burgdorferi*
nocardiosis*	*Nocardia asteroides*
actinomycosis*	*Actinomyces fumigatus*
fungal	
cryptococcosis	*Cryptococcus neoformans*
coccidioidomycosis	*Coccidioides immitis*
histoplasmosis	*Histoplasma capsulatum*
candidiasis	*Candida albicans*
blastomycosis*	*Blastomyces dermatitidis*
parasitic	
toxoplasmosis*	*Toxoplasma gondii*
cysticercosis*	*Taenia solium*
* disease manifest as brain abscess	

Fig. 22.20 Infections causing chronic meningitis or brain abscess.

inactivated prion protein genes are insusceptible to infection, no one has yet shown that the abnormal form of the protein, when manufactured in the laboraory, is infectious.
- They show amazing resistance to heat, chemical agents and irradiation, and are not completely killed by boiling or immersion for years in formalin.
- They cannot be cultivated in test tubes, and since there is no antibody or other immune response to infection, diagnosis is by clinical appearances and characteristic pathologic changes in the brain. Microscopic vacuoles are seen, giving a spongiform appearance, with little or no inflammatory response. The infectious agent is restricted to the CNS and lymphoid tissues.
- There is no treatment and no vaccine, and the disease is lethal.

In animals, infection seems to have originated from sheep and goats with scrapie *(Fig. 22.21)*, which has been present in Europe for 200–300 years. Affected animals itch and scrape themselves against posts for relief.

Creutzfeldt–Jakob Disease
Creutzfeldt–Jakob disease is a rare chronic encephalopathy of humans with associated dementia

The natural mode of transmission of Creutzfeldt–Jakob disease (CJD) is unknown, and it does not appear to be acquired from sheep. A few cases have resulted from eating bovine spongiform encephalopathy (BSE)-contaminated food and it has been occasionally transmitted from person to person by:
- Neurosurgical stereotactic electrodes that have been incompletely sterilized between patients.
- Corneal grafts.
- Injections of growth hormone preparations extracted from pooled 'normal' human pituitary glands before genetically engineered growth hormone became available. A total of 15–20 cases have been reported, with incubation periods of up to 19 years.

About 10% of CJD occurs in families where affected individuals have mutations in the gene coding for the prion protein. The abnormal prion protein is more easily converted into the pathogenic form, and this can occur spontaneously.

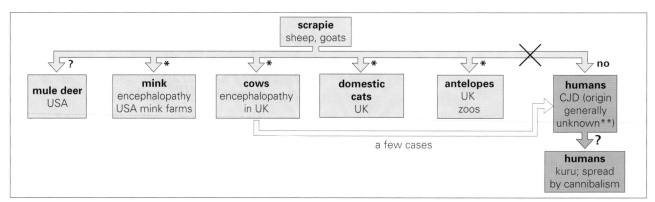

Fig. 22.21 The spread of scrapie agents between species. Nearly all have been transmitted to laboratory rodents and primates. (* Infections transferred by scrapie-infected sheep material present in foodstuff; **10% of cases are familial. Most of these have mutations at amino acid residue 129 of the prion protein, which are thought to cause spontaneous conversion of the protein into the pathogenic form.)

In this case CJD is transmitted vertically rather than horizontally (see Chapter 8) and the borderline between infection and heredity becomes indistinct. It is possible that most CJD is due to somatic mutations in the prion gene.

Kuru was a fatal neurologic disease with cerebellar signs exclusive to the Fore tribes in Papua New Guinea

A total of 3700 cases occurred in a population of 35 000, and transmission from human to human was associated with ritual cannibalism involving the consumption of the body of a dead member of the family. The disease was most common in adult females, so that in some villages the men outnumbered the women by three to one. Adult males rarely participated in the ritual and were less commonly affected. Although transmission was clearly associated with cannibalism, infection may have taken place via abrasions on the fingers and mouth rather than in the gastrointestinal tract. There was a remarkable absence of communicability from person to person, and none of the hundreds of children born and suckled by mothers with kuru developed the disease.

The incubation period of kuru was 4–20 years. No cases have been seen in those born since 1957, when cannibalism ceased. In some villages it was the commonest cause of death, and because deaths were attributed to sorcery, the second commonest cause of death was reprisal murder! A suggested origin of kuru was from the cannibalistic consumption of a missionary who was dying from CJD.

Two other rare neurologic diseases of humans are due to prion-type agents

These are:
- Gerstmann–Sträussler–Scheinker syndrome (GSS).
- Fatal familial insomnia.

In fatal familial insomnia there is loss of ability to sleep and death within 1–2 years.

Postvaccinial and Postinfectious Encephalitis

Encephalitis following viral infection or vaccination possibly has an autoimmune basis

Encephalitis very occasionally occurs 1–2 weeks after apparently normal measles, and even less commonly after varicella. It is also seen after *Mycoplasma* infection and various influenza-like illnesses. Virus is generally not recoverable from the CNS and the perivascular infiltration, sometimes with demyelination, suggests an autoimmune pathogenesis. A similar condition occurs after administration of brain-derived inactivated rabies vaccines (now obsolete), and after other immunizations with non-infectious materials. The clinical picture resembles experimental allergic encephalitis, and is probably due to autoimmune responses triggered by the infection or by the injected material.

An analogous inflammatory demyelinating condition of the peripheral nervous system (the Guillain–Barré syndrome)

has been associated with a variety of viral infections, as well as with immunization with non-infectious material. In 1976, most adults in the USA were given inactivated influenza virus vaccine, which resulted in a small but highly significant number of cases of Guillain–Barré syndrome.

CNS Disease Due to Helminth Parasites

Toxocara infection can result in granuloma formation in the brain and retina

The cat and dog roundworms *Toxocara cati* and *Toxocara canis* infect humans, usually children, when *Toxocara* eggs derived from kitten or puppy feces are ingested (see Chapter 3). Although transmission can be direct in cats and dogs, it is thought that these parasites originally required rodents as intermediate hosts, the life cycle being completed when these animals were eaten by cats or dogs. After ingestion by humans, the eggs hatch and the larvae migrate from the gut to the liver, lung, eye (see Chapter 16), brain, kidney, and muscles as in the rodent. Granulomas form around the larvae, which in the brain may cause epilepsy, and in the retina a tumor-like mass can cause detachment and eventually blindness. There is usually a marked eosinophilia. However, infection is often asymptomatic.

Serum can be tested for fluorescent antibody to *Toxocara* antigen. The disease is prevented by de-worming puppies and kittens, and by reducing the pollution of children's play areas by dog excreta.

Hydatid disease is characterized by cyst formation in the liver, lungs, brain and kidney

Hydatid disease is caused by the tapeworm *Echinococcus granulosus* (see Chapter 3) which has a worldwide distribution, especially in sheep-rearing areas. When humans ingest eggs from infected dogs, the embryos emerge, migrate through the gut to the portal blood vessels, and subsequently develop into hydatid cysts, especially in the liver, but also in the lungs, brain and kidney. Disease is caused by local pressure from the cyst, and sometimes hypersensitivity reactions to hydatid antigens. Neurologic symptoms include nausea and vomiting, seizures and altered mental status.

Hydatid disease is diagnosed by detecting antibody to hydatid antigens, and by CT scanning, radiography or ultrasound examination to demonstrate cysts (*Fig. 22.22*). The disease is prevented by interrupting the natural dog–sheep, dog–goat, or other carnivore–herbivore transmission cycle.

Cysticercosis is characterized by cyst formation in the brain and eye

Cysticercosis results from infection with *Taenia solium*, a human tapeworm. The eggs present in human feces infect pigs, which develop cysts in muscle tissue ('measly pork') and are a source of further human infection. Occasionally the eggs produced in the human intestine re-infect the same individual, perhaps as a result of ingesting fecal material. After passing through the gut wall, the parasite develops into cysts,

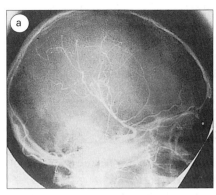

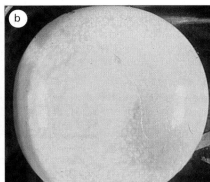

Fig. 22.22 Echinococcosis. (a) Cerebral angiography showing displacement of vessels by a large frontal mass. (b) Cyst removed from patient in (a). (Courtesy of H Whitwell.)

most commonly in the brain *(Fig. 22.23)*, or eye causing epilepsy or encephalopathy. Diagnosis is by detecting specific antibody in serum or CSF, and visualizing cysts by CT scans, magnetic resonance imaging or radiography.

Tetanus and Botulism

Several bacteria release toxins that act on the nervous system (see Chapter 12), but do not themselves invade the CNS. In the case of *Clostridium tetani* and *Clostridium botulinum*, the major clinical impact is neurologic.

Tetanus
C. tetani toxin is carried to the CNS in peripheral nerve axons
Tetanus spores are widespread in soil and originate from the feces of domestic animals. The spores enter a wound and if necrotic tissue or the presence of a foreign body permits local and anaerobic growth of bacteria, the toxin tetanospasmin (see Chapter 12) is produced. All strains of *Cl. tetani* produce the same toxin. The wound can be anything from a small gardener's scratch or cut to a large automobile or battlefield injury. However, in as many as 20% of cases there is no history of injury. Infection of the umbilical stump can cause neonatal tetanus, which in 1993 killed 560 000 infants in developing countries (see Chapter 21).

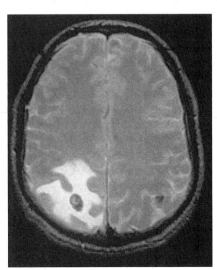

Fig. 22.23 Cerebral cysticercosis. Magnetic resonance imaging scan showing a cyst containing a developing larva. (Courtesy of J Curé.)

The toxin is carried in peripheral nerve axons and probably in the blood to the CNS, where it binds to neurones and blocks the release of inhibitory mediators in spinal synapses, causing overactivity of motor neurones. It can also pass up sympathetic nerve axons and lead to overactivity of the sympathetic nervous system.

Clinical features of tetanus include muscle rigidity and spasms
After a period of 3–21 days, but sometimes longer, there are exaggerated reflexes, muscle rigidity and uncontrolled muscle spasms. Lockjaw (trismus) is due to contraction of jaw muscles. Dysphagia, 'risus sardonicus' (a sneering appearance), neck stiffness and opisthotonos (especially in neonatal tetanus; see Chapter 21) are also seen. Muscle spasms may lead to injury and eventually there is respiratory failure. Tachycardia and sweating can result from effects on the sympathetic nervous system. Mortality is up to 50%, depending upon the severity and quality of treatment.

The diagnosis is clinical. Organisms are rarely isolated from the wound, and only a small number of bacteria are needed to form enough toxin to cause disease.

Human antitetanus immunoglobulin should be given as soon as tetanus is suspected clinically
The wound should be excised if necessary and penicillin given to inhibit bacterial replication. Muscle relaxants are used and, if necessary, respiratory support in an intensive care unit.

Immunization with toxoid prevents tetanus, the effects of the vaccine lasting for 10 years after the last dose. Wounds should be cleansed, necrotic tissue and foreign bodies removed, and a tetanus toxoid booster given. Those with badly contaminated wounds should also be given tetanus immunoglobulin and penicillin.

In developing countries, routine immunization of women with tetanus toxoid and improved hygienic birth practices are having a significant impact in reducing the rates of neonatal tetanus.

Botulism
Spores of *Cl. botulinum* are widespread in soil and contaminate vegetables, meat, and fish. When foods are canned or preserved without adequate sterilization (often at home),

contaminating spores survive and can germinate in the anaerobic environment, leading to the formation of toxin.

Cl. botulinum toxin blocks acetylcholine release from peripheral nerves

Pre-formed botulinus toxin is ingested, then absorbed from the gut into the blood (see Chapter 20). It acts on peripheral nerve synapses by blocking the release of acetylcholine (see Chapter 11). It is therefore a type of food poisoning that affects the motor and autonomic nervous systems. Sometimes spores contaminate a wound and the toxin is then absorbed from this site. If the organism is ingested by infants, in the honey smeared on pacifiers for instance, it can multiply in the gut and produce the toxin, causing infant botulism.

Clinical features of botulism include weakness and paralysis

After an incubation period of 2–72 hours, there is descending weakness and paralysis, with dysphagia, diplopia, vomiting, vertigo and respiratory muscle failure. There is no abdominal pain, diarrhea or fever. Infants develop generalized weakness ('floppy babies'), but usually recover.

Botulism is treated with antibodies and respiratory support

A diagnosis of botulism is mainly clinical. The toxin can be demonstrated in contaminated food and occasionally in the patient's serum.

Antibodies (preferably human) specific for types A, B and E toxins are given (types C and D cause botulism in birds) plus respiratory support. The mortality is less than 20%, depending upon the success of the respiratory support.

Prevention is by avoidance of imperfectly sterilized canned or preserved food. Contaminated cans are often swollen due to the release of gas by clostridial enzymes. Home preserved foods are often incriminated, but fruit, with its acidic pH, usually prevents the development of the spores. The toxin is heat labile and is destroyed by adequate cooking (80°C for four minutes). The spores can, however, survive for up to two hours at boiling point (100°C).

- Microbial invasion of the CNS is uncommon, due to the presence of the blood–brain or blood–CSF barriers, which limit the spread of infection.
- Once infectious agents have traversed these barriers they generally cause neurological disease by involving the meninges (meningitis) or the brain substance (encephalitis).
- Viral meningitis is the commonest condition, bacterial meningitis the next commonest, with cerebral abscesses and viral encephalitis as rarities. The spinal cord (in myelitis) or peripheral nerves (in neuritis) are occasionally affected.
- Disease results from interference with the function of infected nerve cells (e.g. rabies), from direct damage to infected nerve cells (e.g. poliomyelitis), or from the inflammatory sequel to CNS invasion (e.g. bacterial meningitis, viral encephalitis).
- Because the anatomically defined compartments of the nervous system are adjacent or interconnected, more than one of them can be involved in a given infectious disease.
- CNS disease is sometimes seen in the helminth infections toxocariasis, hydatid disease and cysticercosis.
- CNS disease can also result when bacterial neurotoxins reach the CNS either from extraneural sites of growth (tetanus) or from contaminated food (botulism).

A 45-year-old bank manageress is brought to hospital by ambulance having collapsed in the street. She is unable to give a history, but a passerby had said that she suddenly collapsed having left a shop and then had a seizure. The police contact her husband who tells them that she has been complaining of a headache for the past few days and has been acting in a slightly strange way. She has no relevant past medical history, has not had a seizure before, and is on no medication. On examination she is drowsy, confused and has a temperature of 38°C. She has no focal neurologic signs, although her reflexes are brisk. The rest of her examination is normal. Fundoscopy reveals no papilloedema and examination of her oropharynx and ears is normal. Investigations include a full blood count, which is normal, and urea and electrolytes, including a blood glucose level, which are also normal.

1. What urgent investigations would you perform?
2. A CT scan shows an area of low density attenuation in the left temporal lobe and no evidence of cerebral edema or midline shift. Results of a lumbar puncture are: CSF appearance clear, white cell count 50/mm3 (all lymphocytes), zero red cells, protein 0.9 g/dl; CSF glucose 3.3 mmol/l; blood glucose 5 mmol/l; no organisms seen on Gram stain. What diagnoses would you consider in the light of these results and the clinical history?
3. How would you manage and treat her?

Further Reading

Fishbein DB, Robinson LE. Rabies. *N Engl J Med* 1993;**329**:1632.

Johnson RT. The pathogenesis of acute viral encephalitis and post infectious encephalomyelitis. *J Inf Dis* 1987;**155**:359.

Mestel R. Putting prions to the test. *Science* 1996;**273**:184–189.

Prusiner SB. Molecular biology of prion diseases. *Science* 1991;**252**: 1515–1522.

Quagliarello V, Schell WM. Bacterial meningitis: pathogenesis, pathophysiology, and progress. *N Engl J Med* 1992;**327**:864–872.

Weinstein L. Tetanus. *N Engl J Med* 1973;**289**:1293.

Infections of the Skin, Muscle, Joints, Bone and Hemopoietic System

Introduction

Healthy intact skin protects underlying tissues and provides excellent defense against invading microbes

The microbial load of normal skin is kept in check by various factors, as shown in *Figure 23.1*. Alterations in these factors (e.g. prolonged exposure to moisture) upsets the ecologic balance of the commensal flora, and predisposes to infection.

A small number of microbes cause diseases of muscle, joints or the hemopoietic system. Invasion of these sites is generally from the blood, but the reason for localization to particular tissues is often obscure. Circulating microbes tend to localize in growing or damaged bones (acute osteomyelitis) and in damaged joints, but we do not know why coxsackieviruses or *Trichinella spiralis* invade muscle. On the other hand some viruses infect a given target cell and plasmodia invade erythrocytes because they have specific attachment sites for these cells.

Infections of the Skin

In addition to being a structural barrier, the skin is colonized by an array of organisms which forms its normal flora. The relatively arid areas of the forearm and back are colonized with fewer organisms, predominantly Gram-positive bacteria and yeasts. In the moister areas, such as the groin and the armpit, the organisms are more numerous and more varied and include Gram-negative bacteria. The normal flora of the skin plays an important role, as does the normal flora in other body sites, in defending the surface from 'foreign invaders'.

An appreciation of the structure of the skin helps in understanding the different sorts of infection to which the skin and its underlying tissues are prone *(Fig. 23.2)*. If organisms breach the stratum corneum the host defenses are mobilized, the epidermal Langerhans' cells elaborate cytokines, neutrophils are attracted to the site of invasion and complement is activated via the alternative pathway.

Microbial disease of the skin may result from any of three lines of attack

These lines of attack are:
- Breach of intact skin, allowing infection from the outside.
- Skin manifestations of systemic infections, which may arise as a result of bloodborne spread from the infected focus to the skin or by direct extension (e.g. draining sinuses from actinomycotic lesions or necrotizing anaerobic infection from intra-abdominal sepsis).
- Toxin-mediated skin damage due to production of a microbial toxin at another site in the body (e.g. scarlet fever, toxic shock syndrome).

The sequence of events in the pathogenesis of mucocutaneous lesions caused by bacterial, fungal and viral infections is outlined in *Figure 23.3*. Breaches in the skin range from microscopic to major trauma, which may be accidental (e.g. lacerations or burns) or intentional (e.g. surgery). Hospitalized patients are liable to other skin breaches (e.g. pressure sores and intravenous catheter insertions), which

may become infected (see Chapter 34). Infections in compromised individuals such as burn patients will be discussed in Chapter 28. Here we will consider primary infections of the skin and underlying soft tissues, together with mucocutaneous lesions resulting from certain systemic viral infections. Systemic bacterial and fungal infections that cause mucocutaneous lesions are summarized in *Figure 23.4*.

Bacterial Infections of Skin, Soft Tissue and Muscle

These can be classified on an anatomic basis

The classification depends upon the layers of skin and soft tissue involved, although some infections may involve several components of the soft tissues:

FACTORS CONTROLLING THE SKIN'S MICROBIAL LOAD
the limited amount of moisture present
acid pH of normal skin
surface temperature < optimum for many pathogens
salty sweat
excreted chemicals such as sebum, fatty acids and urea
competition between different species of the normal flora

Fig. 23.1 The number of bacteria on the skin vary from a few hundred per cm^2 on the arid surfaces of the forearm and back, to tens of thousands per cm^2 on the moist areas such as the axilla and groin. This normal flora plays an important role in preventing 'foreign' organisms from colonizing the skin, but it too needs to be kept in check.

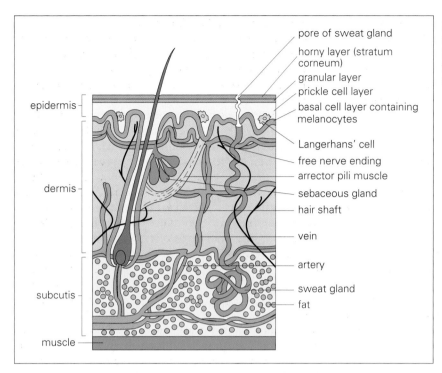

Fig. 23.2 Infection of the skin and soft tissue can be related to the anatomy of the skin. Pathogens usually enter the lower layers of the epidermis and dermis only after the skin surface has been damaged.

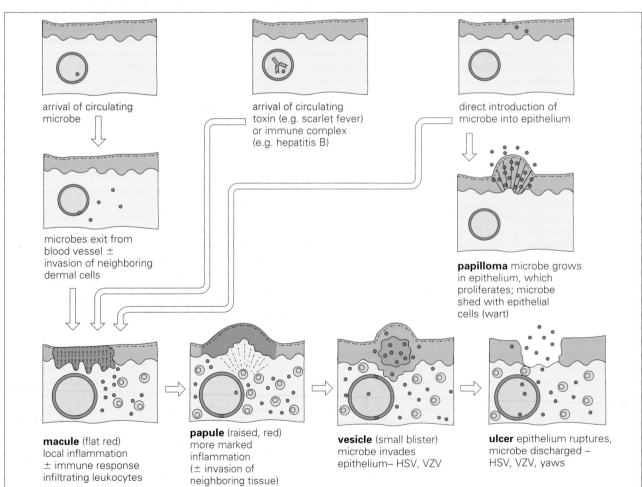

Fig. 23.3 The pathogenesis of mucocutaneous lesions. In different infections the starting point (arrival of microbe or toxin or immune complex) and the final picture (e.g. maculopapular rash, vesicle) will be different. (HSV, herpes simplex virus; VZV, varicella-zoster virus.)

- Abscess formation. Boils and carbuncles are the result of infection and inflammation of the hair follicles in the skin (folliculitis).
- Spreading infections. Impetigo is limited to the epidermis and presents as a bullous, crusted or pustular erupt`n of the skin. Erysipelas involves the blocking of dermal lymphatics and presents as a well-defined, spreading erythematous inflammation, generally on the face, legs or feet, and often accompanied by pain and fever. If the focus of infection is in the subcutaneous fat, cellulitis, a diffuse form of acute inflammation, is the usual presentation.
- Necrotizing infections. Fasciitis describes the inflammatory response to infection of the soft tissue below the dermis. Infection spreads, often with alarming rapidity, along the fascial planes causing disruption of the blood supply. Gangrene or myonecrosis may follow infection associated with ischemia of the muscle layer. Gas resulting from the fermentative metabolism of anaerobic organisms may be palpable in the tissues (gas gangrene).

The common causative organisms are shown in *Figure 23.5*. Note that the same pathogen (e.g. *Streptococcus pyogenes*) can cause different infections in different layers of the skin and soft tissue.

Staphylococcal skin infections
Staphylococcus aureus is the most common cause of skin infections and provokes an intense inflammatory response

Staphylococcus aureus causes minor skin infections such as boils or abscesses as well as more serious postoperative wound infection. Infection may be acquired by 'self-inoculation' from a carrier site (e.g. the nose) or acquired by contact with an exogenous source, usually another person. People who are nasal carriers of virulent *Staph. aureus* may suffer from recurrent boils, but an inoculum of about 100 000 organisms is thought to be required in the absence of a wound or foreign body. *Staph. aureus* can also cause serious skin disease due to toxin production (scalded skin syndrome, toxic shock syndrome; see below).

A boil begins, within 2–4 days of inoculation, as a superficial infection in and around a hair follicle (folliculitis; *Fig. 23.6*). In this site the organisms are relatively protected from the host defenses, multiply rapidly and spread locally. This provokes an intense inflammatory response with an influx of neutrophils. Fibrin is deposited, and the site is walled off. Abscesses typically contain abundant yellow creamy pus formed by the massive number of organisms and necrotic white cells. They continue to expand slowly, eventually erode

SKIN MANIFESTATIONS OF SYSTEMIC INFECTIONS CAUSED BY BACTERIA AND FUNGI		
organism	**disease**	**skin manifestation**
Salmonella typhi *Salmonella paratyphi* B	enteric fever	'rose spots' containing bacteria
Neisseria meningitidis	septicemia, meningitis	petechial or maculopapular lesions containing bacteria
Pseudomonas aeruginosa	septicemia	ecthyma gangrenosum, skin lesion pathonomomic if infected with this organism
Treponema pallidum *Treponema pertenue*	syphilis yaws	disseminated infectious rash seen in secondary stage of disease, 2–3 months after infection
Rickettsia prowazeki *Rickettsia rickettsiae* *Rickettsia conori*	typhus spotted fevers	macular or hemorrhagic rash
Streptococcus pyogenes	scarlet fever	erythematous rash caused by erythrogenic toxin
Staphylococcus aureus	toxic shock syndrome	rash and desquamation due to toxin
Blastomyces dermatitidis	blastomycosis	papule or pustule develops into granuloma lesions containing organisms
Cryptococcus neoformans	cryptococcosis	papule or pustule, usually on face or neck

Fig. 23.4 Skin lesions are often associated with systemic infection with particular bacteria and fungi. The lesions may provide useful diagnostic aids. Sometimes they are a site from which organisms are shed.

DIRECT ENTRY INTO SKIN OF BACTERIA AND FUNGI		
structure involved	**infection**	**common cause**
keratinized epithelium	ringworm	dermatophyte fungi (*Trichophyton, Epidermophyton* and *Microsporum*)
epidermis	impetigo	*Streptococcus pygenes* and/or *Staphylococcus aureus*
dermis	erysipelas	*Strep. pyogenes*
hair follicles	folliculitis boils (furuncles) carbuncles	*Staph. aureus*
subcutaneous fat	cellulitis	*Strep. pyogenes*
fascia	necrotizing fasciitis	anaerobes and microaerophiles, usually mixed infections
muscle	myonecrosis gangrene	*Clostridium perfringens* (and other clostridia)

Fig. 23.5 Direct introduction of bacteria or fungi into the skin is the most common route of skin infection. Infections range from mild, often chronic, conditions such as ringworm to acute and life-threatening fasciitis and gangrene. Relatively few species are involved in the common infections.

the overlying skin, 'come to a head' and drain. Drainage inwards can result in seeding of the staphylococci to underlying body sites to cause serious infections such as peritonitis, empyema or meningitis.

Staph. aureus infections are often diagnosed clinically and treatment includes drainage and antibiotics

Staph. aureus is the most common cause of boils, and diagnosis is made on clinical grounds. Isolation and further identification of the infecting staphylococcus in hospital patients and staff is important in the investigation of hospital infections (see Chapter 34).

Treatment involves drainage and this is usually sufficient for minor lesions but antibiotics may be given in addition when the infection is severe and the patient has a fever. Most *Staph. aureus* are beta-lactamase producers and therefore enzyme-stable penicillins such as cloxacillin or flucloxacillin are indicated. Treatment with these agents does not necessarily eradicate carriage of the staphylococci.

Recurrent infections may be prevented by treating nasal carriers of *Staph. aureus* with nasal creams containing antibiotics such as bacitracin or neomycin; mupirocin has been used successfully for carriers of methicillin-resistant staphylococci (see Chapter 34). Good skin care and personal hygiene should be encouraged.

Staphylococcal scalded skin syndrome is caused by toxin-producing Staph. aureus

This condition, also known as 'Ritter's disease' in infants and 'Lyell's disease' or 'toxic epidermal necrolysis' in older children, occurs sporadically and in outbreaks. It is caused by strains of *Staph. aureus* producing a toxin known as 'exfoliatin' or 'scalded skin syndrome toxin'. The initial skin lesion may be minor, but the toxin causes destruction of the inter-

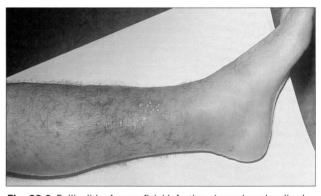

Fig. 23.6 Folliculitis. A superficial infection shown here localized in the hair follicles on the leg. The boils contain creamy-yellow pus and masses of bacteria. *Staphylococcus aureus* is the most common cause. (Courtesy of A du Vivier.)

cellular connections and separation of the top layer of the epidermis. Large blisters are formed, containing clear fluid, and within one or two days the overlying areas of skin are lost *(Fig. 23.7)* leaving normal skin underneath. The baby is irritable and uncomfortable, but rarely severely ill. However, treatment should take into account the risk of increased loss of fluid from the damaged surface and fluid replacement may be needed. A beta-lactamase stable penicillin (e.g. cloxacillin) should be administered parenterally.

Toxic shock syndrome is caused by toxic shock syndrome toxin-producing Staph. aureus

This systemic infection came to prominence through its association with tampon use by healthy women, but it is not confined to women and can occur as a result of *Staph. aureus* infection at non-genital sites. There is septicemia and toxemia,

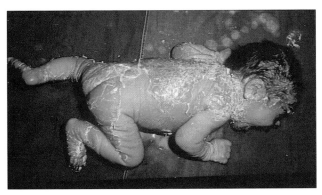

Fig. 23.7 Scalded skin syndrome results from infection of the skin with strains of *Staphylococcus aureus* producing a specific toxin, which destroys the intercellular connections in the skin resulting in large areas of desquamation. The appearance may be confused with a burn. (Courtesy of A du Vivier.)

and skin manifestations include a rash followed by desquamation of the skin, particularly on the soles and palms *(Fig. 23.8)*.

Streptococcal skin infections
Streptococcal skin infections are caused by Strep. pyogenes (group A streptococci)

Streptococcal impetigo develops independently of streptococcal upper respiratory tract infection, and although up to 35% of patients carry the same strain in their nose or throat, colonization may well occur after the skin has become infected. The organisms are acquired through contact with other people with infected skin lesions and may first colonize and multiply on normal skin before invasion through minor breaks in the epithelium and the development of lesions. The various risk factors involved in the development of streptococcal impetigo are shown in *Figure 23.9*. *Strep. pyogenes* may also infect deeper in the dermis causing erysipelas.

Strep. pyogenes possesses certain surface proteins (M and T), which are antigenic. The species can be subdivided (typed) on the basis of these antigens, and it has been recognized that certain M and T types are associated with skin infection (and these differ from the types associated with sore throats). T proteins play no known role in virulence and their function is unknown. M proteins are important virulence factors because they inhibit opsonization and confer on the bacterium resistance to phagocytosis.

Clinical features of streptococcal skin infections are typically acute

They develop within 24–48 hours of skin invasion and trigger a marked inflammatory response as the host attempts to localize the infection *(Figs 23.10, 23.11)*. *Strep. pyogenes* elaborates a number of toxic products and enzymes, such as hyaluronidase, which help the organism to spread in tissue. Lymphatic involvement is common, resulting in lymphadenitis and lymphangitis.

Lysogenic strains of *Strep. pyogenes* produce erythrogenic toxin. This has potent effects on the immune system, and also acts on skin blood vessels to cause the diffuse erythematous rash of scarlet fever, which may occur with streptococcal pharyngitis.

About 5% of patients with erysipelas go on to develop bacteremia and this infection carries a high mortality if untreated.

Certain M types (e.g. M49) of Strep. pyogenes are associated with acute glomerulonephritis

Acute glomerulonephritis (AGN) occurs more often after skin infections than after infections of the throat (see Chapter 15). It is characterized by the deposition of immune complexes on the basement membrane of the glomerulus, but the precise role of the streptococcus in the causation is still

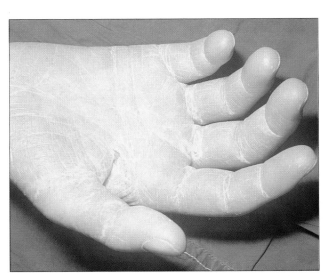

Fig. 23.8 Toxic shock syndrome results from systemic infection with *Staphylococcus aureus*, but has skin manifestations in the form of desquamation, particularly of the palm and soles. (Courtesy of MJ Wood.)

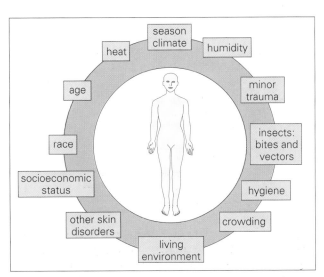

Fig. 23.9 Various factors are involved in the development of streptococcal skin infections. Particular M types of *Streptococcus pyogenes* have a predilection for skin, but various factors predispose the host (usually a child) to infection. Mixed infections with *Staphylococcus aureus* are also common.

unclear (see Chapter 12); 10–15% of individuals infected with a nephritogenic strain will develop AGN about 2–3 weeks after the primary infection. Most people recover completely and recurrence after a subsequent streptococcal infection is rare. Rheumatic fever (see p. 000) very rarely follows skin infections with *Strep. pyogenes*.

Streptococcal skin infections are usually diagnosed clinically and treated with penicillin

Gram stains of pus from vesicles in impetigo show Gram-positive cocci and culture reveals *Strep. pyogenes* sometimes mixed with *Staph. aureus (Fig. 23.12)*. In erysipelas, skin cultures are often negative, although culture of fluid from the advancing edge of the lesion may be successful.

Penicillin is the drug of choice, administered orally or intramuscularly in the long-acting benzathine formulation. Erythromycin should be used for penicillin-allergic patients (although the prevalence of resistance in streptococci is increasing). Severe infections may require hospitalization.

Impetigo is prevented by improving the host factors associated with acquisition of the disease, as illustrated in *Figure 23.9*. Since AGN rarely recurs on subsequent streptococcal infection, long-term prophylaxis with penicillin is not indicated (in contrast to the long-term prophylaxis following rheumatic fever, see Chapter 15).

Cellulitis and gangrene
Cellulitis is an acute spreading infection of the skin that involves subcutaneous tissues

Cellulitis extends deeper than erysipelas and usually originates either from superficial skin lesions such as boils or ulcers or following trauma. It is rarely bloodborne, but conversely it may lead to bacterial invasion of the bloodstream. Infection develops within a few hours or days of trauma and quickly produces a hot red swollen lesion *(Fig. 23.13)*. Regional lymph nodes are enlarged and the patient suffers malaise, chills and fever.

The great majority of cases of cellulitis are caused by *Strep. pyogenes* and *Staph. aureus*. Occasionally, in patients who have had particular environmental exposure, other organisms may be implicated. For example, *Erysipelothrix rhusiopathiae* is associated with cellulitis in butchers and fishmongers, while *Vibrio vulnificus* and *Vibrio alginolyticus* may complicate traumatic wounds acquired in salt water environments (see Chapter 20).

The pathogen causing cellulitis is isolated in only 25–35% of cases and initial therapy should cover streptococci and staphylococci

Attempts can be made to confirm the clinical diagnosis by culture of:
- Aspirates from the advancing edge of the cellulitis.
- The site of trauma (if present).
- Skin biopsies.
- Blood.

Treatment should be initiated on the basis of the clinical diagnosis because of the rapid progression of the disease, particularly when caused by *Strep. pyogenes*. Initial therapy should cover both streptococci and staphylococci, and a combination of benzylpenicillin and a beta-lactamase stable penicillin such as cloxacillin should be given.

Anaerobic cellulitis may develop in areas of traumatized or devitalized tissue

Such damaged tissue is associated with surgical or traumatic wounds or is found in ischemic extremities. Diabetic patients are particularly prone to anaerobic cellulitis of their feet *(Fig. 23.14)*. The causative organisms depend upon the circumstances of the trauma: infections in the lower parts of the body are most often caused by organisms from the fecal flora whereas wounds from human bites are infected with oral organisms. Foul-smelling discharge, marked swelling and gas in the tissues are characteristic of anaerobic cellulitis and a mixture of organisms is usually cultured from the wound. Treatment needs to be aggressive to halt the spread of infec-

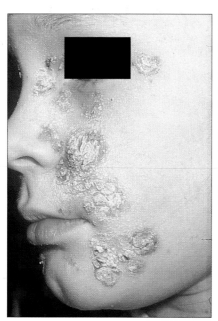

Fig. 23.10 Impetigo is a condition limited to the epidermis, with typically yellow, crusted lesions. It is commonly caused by *Streptococcus pyogenes* either alone or together with *Staphylococcus aureus*. (Courtesy of MJ Wood.)

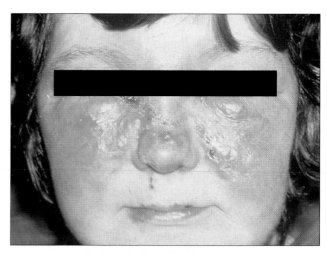

Fig. 23.11 Erysipelas. Infection with *Streptococcus pyogenes* involving the dermal lymphatics and giving rise to a clearly demarcated area of erythema and induration. When the face is involved there is often a typical 'butterfly-wing' rash, as shown here. (Courtesy of MJ Wood.)

tion and both antibiotics and surgical debridement are required. Osteomyelitis (see below) is a common sequela.

Synergistic bacterial gangrene is a relentlessly destructive infection

This rare infection is caused by a mixture of organisms, typically microaerophilic streptococci and *Staph. aureus*. The gangrene most commonly follows surgery in the groin or genital area, starting at the site of a drain or suture. Cellulitis develops in the surrounding skin and extends rapidly (within hours), leaving a black necrotic center. The condition is often fatal, and treatment requires radical excision of the necrotic area and systemic antibiotic therapy.

Necrotizing fasciitis, myonecrosis and gangrene
Necrotizing fasciitis is a frequently fatal mixed infection caused by anaerobes and facultative anaerobes

Although apparently resembling synergistic bacterial gangrene, necrotizing fasciitis is a much more acute and highly toxic infection, causing widespread necrosis and undermining of the surrounding tissues, such that the underlying destruction is more widespread than the skin lesion *(Fig. 23.15)*. Patients deteriorate rapidly and frequently die. Radical excision of all necrotic fascia is an essential part of therapy, along with antibiotics given both locally to the wound and systemically.

Traumatic or surgical wounds can become infected with *Clostridium* species

Clostridium tetani gains access to the tissues through trauma to the skin, but the disease it produces is entirely due to the production of a powerful exotoxin (see Chapter 12).

Gas gangrene or clostridial myonecrosis can be caused by several species of clostridia, but *Clostridium perfringens* is the most common. The organism and its spores are found in the soil and in human and animal feces, and can therefore gain access to traumatized tissues by contamination from these sources. Infection develops in areas of the body with poor blood supply (anaerobic), and the buttocks and perineum are common sites, particularly in patients with ischemic vascular disease or peripheral arteriosclerosis. The organisms multiply in the subcutaneous tissues producing gas and an anaerobic cellulitis, but a characteristic feature of clostridial infection is that the organisms invade deeper into the muscle, where they cause necrosis and produce bubbles of gas, which can be felt in the tissue and sometimes seen in the wound *(Fig. 23.16)*. The infection proceeds very rapidly and causes acute pain. Much of the damage is due to the production by *Cl. perfringens* of a lecithinase (also known as alpha toxin), which hydrolyzes the lipids in cell membranes resulting in cell lysis and death *(Fig. 23.17)*. The presence of dead and dying tissue further compromises the blood supply and the organisms multiply and produce more toxin and more damage. Other extracellular enzymes may also play a role in helping the clostridia to spread.

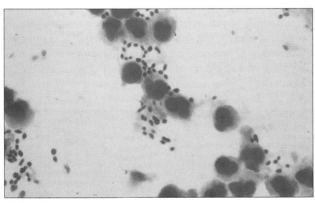

Fig. 23.12 Gram-positive cocci in pus.

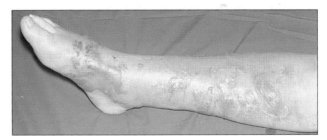

Fig. 23.13 When the focus of infection is in the subdermal fat, cellulitis – a severe and rapidly progressive infection – is the typical presentation. Large blisters and scabs may also be present on the skin surface. (Courtesy of MJ Wood.)

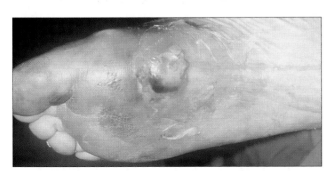

Fig. 23.14 Severe progressive cellulitis of the foot. Such cellulitis is usually caused by anaerobic bacteria or a mixture of aerobes and anaerobes and is a particular problem in diabetic patients with peripheral vascular and neuropathic damage. (Courtesy of JD Ward.)

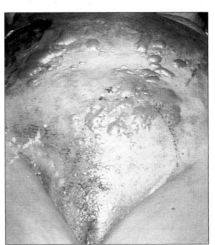

Fig. 23.15 Necrotizing fasciitis of the abdominal wall. In patients such as this, infection can be seen rapidly spreading from its origin and causing deep and widespread necrosis. Complete debridement and intensive antimicrobial therapy is required, but the condition is often fatal. (Courtesy of WM Rambo.)

If the toxin escapes from the affected area and enters the blood-stream, there is massive hemolysis, renal failure and death.

Amputation may be necessary to prevent further spread of clostridial infection

Because of the rapid progression and fatal outcome of this type of clostridial infection, gangrenous areas require immediate surgery to excise all the affected tissue and amputation may be necessary. Anti-alpha toxin may help if given early enough and treatment in a hyperbaric oxygen chamber has also been recommended to improve the oxygenation of the tissue and amputation may be necessary. Antibiotics (penicillin or metronidazole) should be considered only as adjuncts to, not in place of, surgical debridement.

Prevention of infection is of foremost importance. Wounds should be cleaned and debrided early to remove dead and poorly perfused tissue, which the anaerobes favor. Prophylactic antibiotics (penicillin or metronidazole) should be given preoperatively to patients having elective surgery of body sites liable to contamination with fecal flora (see Chapters 30 and 34).

Propionibacterium acnes and acne
P. acnes goes hand in hand with the hormonal changes of puberty which result in acne

An increased responsiveness to androgenic hormones leads to increased sebum production plus increased keratinization and desquamation in pilosebaceous ducts. Blockage of ducts turns them into sacs in which *P. acnes* and other members of the normal flora (e.g. micrococci, yeasts, staphylococci) multiply. *P. acnes* acts on sebum to form fatty acids and peptides, which together with enzymes and other substances released from bacteria and polymorphs, cause the inflammation *(Fig. 23.18)*. Comedones are greasy plugs composed of a mixture of keratin, sebum and bacteria and capped by a layer of melanin (blackheads in popular terminology) *(Fig. 23.19)*.

Treatment of acne includes long-term administration of oral antibiotics

The antibiotics used to treat acne are usually one of the tetracyclines, or erythromycin. Other treatments include skin care, keratolytics and, in severe cases, synthetic vitamin A derivatives such as isoretinoin. Orally administered antibiotics reduce the surface numbers of *P. acnes* only 10-fold, but are also thought to influence metabolic activity. Acne can be a problem for teenagers, but often disappears in older age groups as the sebaceous follicles become less active.

Other Gram-positive rods related to *P. acnes* such as corynebacteria and brevibacteria, can cause skin infections.

Mycobacterial Diseases of the Skin

Leprosy
Leprosy affects 12–15 million people worldwide

Leprosy has been recognized since biblical times, but in the past the word was a generic term applied to several different diseases and also implying 'moral uncleanliness'. Leprosy is thought to have spread to Europe in the sixth century, and by the thirteenth century there were some 200 leper hospitals in England. Over the centuries that followed leprosy declined in incidence and by the fifteenth century was no longer endemic in England; in contrast tuberculosis was on the increase. Now leprosy is rare in the UK and USA.

Leprosy is caused by Mycobacterium leprae

Mycobacterium leprae appears to be confined to humans and no animal reservoir has been defined, although it is possible that one exists unrecognized. Transmission of infection is directly related to overcrowding and poor hygiene. Relatively

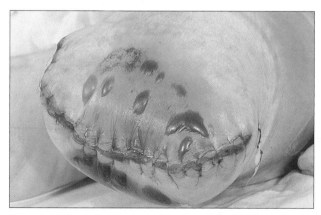

Fig. 23.16 Gas gangrene caused by *Clostridium perfringens*. Organisms from the fecal flora may contaminate a wound and grow and multiply in poorly perfused (anaerobic) tissue. Infection spreads rapidly and gas can be felt in the tissue and seen on radiographs. (Courtesy of J Newman.)

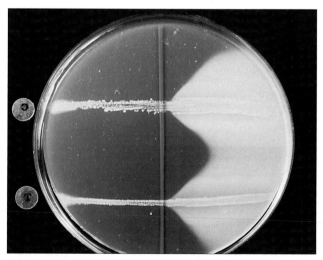

Fig. 23.17 The Nagler reaction. *Clostridium perfringens* produces alpha toxin, which is a lecithinase. If the organism is grown on a medium containing egg yolk (lecithin) enzyme activity can be detected as opacity around the line of growth (right). If anti-alpha toxin is applied to the surface of the plate before inoculation of the organism, the action of the toxin is inhibited (left). This test can be used to confirm the identity of a clostridial isolate.

few organisms are shed from skin lesions, but nasal secretions of patients with lepromatous leprosy are laden with *M. leprae*. Arthropod vectors may play a role in transmission. Leprosy is

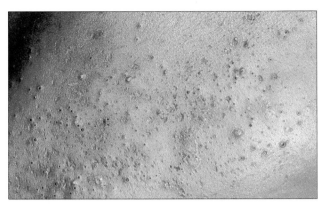

Fig. 23.18 Typical lesions of acne. 'Blackheads' are seen when plugs of keratin block the pilosebaceous duct. (Courtesy of A du Vivier.)

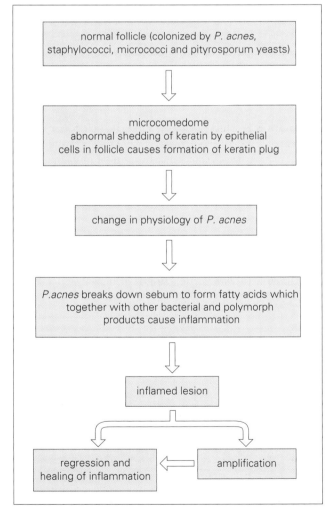

Fig. 23.19 The proposed mechanism of the pathogenesis of acne. Hormonal changes in the host initiate the formation of comedones from normal follicles and thereby change the environment of *Propionibacterium acnes* and its physiologic properties. *P. acnes* is also known to be an immunostimulator.

not highly contagious and prolonged exposure to an infected source is necessary; it seems that children living under the same roof as an open case of leprosy are most at risk. Ironically, because the lesions of leprosy are more obvious, patients were in the past excluded from the community and gathered in leper colonies, whereas tuberculosis is much more contagious, but people with tuberculosis were not shunned.

The clinical features of leprosy depend upon the cell-mediated immune response to M. leprae

M. leprae cannot be grown in artificial culture media and little is known about its mechanism of pathogenicity. Two animal models have been used: infection in the armadillo and in the footpads of mice. The organism grows better at temperatures below 37°C, hence its concentration in the skin and superficial nerves, and it grows extremely slowly; in the mouse footpad the generation time is 11–13 days. Likewise in man the incubation period may be many years.

M. leprae grows intracellularly, typically within skin histiocytes and endothelial cells and the Schwann cells of peripheral nerves. The immune response is all important in deciding the type of disease.

M. leprae shares many pathobiologic features with *M. tuberculosis*, but the clinical manifestations of the diseases are quite different. After an incubation period of several years, the onset of leprosy is gradual and the spectrum of disease activity is very broad depending upon the presence or absence of a cell-mediated immune (CMI) response to *M. leprae* (Fig. 23.20). At one end of the spectrum is tuberculoid leprosy (TT), characterized by blotchy red lesions with anesthetic areas on the face, trunk and extremities *(Fig. 23.21)*. There is palpable thickening of the peripheral nerves because the organisms multiply in the nerve sheaths. The local anesthesia renders the patient prone to repeated trauma and secondary bacterial infection. This disease state is equivalent to secondary tuberculosis (see Chapter 17), with a vigorous CMI response leading to phagocytic destruction of bacteria, and exaggerated allergic responses. TT carries a better prognosis than lepromatous leprosy (LL) and in some patients is self-limiting, but in others may progress across the spectrum towards LL.

In LL there is extensive skin involvement with large numbers of bacteria in affected areas. As the disease progresses there is loss of eyebrows, thickening and enlargement of the nostrils, ears and cheeks, resulting in the typical leonine (lion-like) facial appearance *(Fig. 23.22)*. There is progressive destruction of the nasal septum and the nasal mucosa is loaded with organisms *(Fig. 23.23)*. This form of the disease is equivalent to miliary tuberculosis (see Chapter 17) with a weak CMI response and many extracellular organisms visible in the lesions. The gross deformities characteristic of late disease result primarily from infectious destruction of the naso-maxillary facial structures, and secondarily from pathologic changes in the peripheral nerves predisposing to repeated trauma of the hands and feet and subsequent superinfection with other organisms.

Whether a patient develops TT or LL may in part be genetically determined. Patients with intermediate forms of the disease may progress to either extreme.

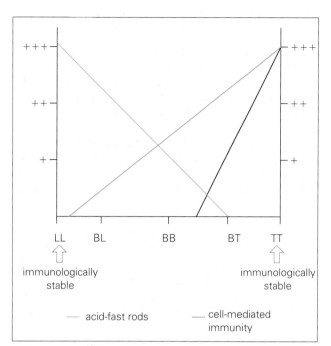

Fig. 23.20 Immunologic responses in leprosy. In tuberculoid leprosy (TT) the patient is capable of mounting an effective cell-mediated immune (CMI) response, which makes it possible for macrophages to destroy the organisms and contain the infection. At the other extreme, in lepromatous leprosy (LL) the patient is incapable of producing a CMI response and the organisms multiply unhindered. These patients have many acid-fast rods in their skin and nasal secretions, and are much more infectious than TT patients.

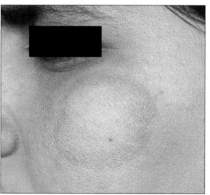

Fig. 23.21 Tuberculoid leprosy – a characteristic dry blotchy lesion on the face, but the diagnosis needs to be confirmed by microscopic examination of skin biopsy *(Fig. 23.24)*. (Courtesy of the Institute of Dermatology.)

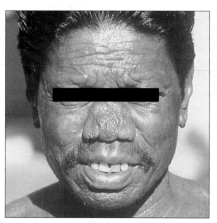

Fig. 23.22 Extensive skin involvement in lepromatous leprosy results in a characteristic leonine appearance. (Courtesy of DA Lewis.)

M. leprae are seen as acid-fast rods in nasal scrapings and lesion biopsies

An alertness to the possibility of leprosy when confronted with a patient with dermatologic, neurologic or multisystem complaints is of fundamental importance. Although the majority of cases are in people who are not native to Europe or the USA, the diagnosis should also be considered in those who have worked in endemic areas.

Nasal scrapings and biopsies of skin lesions should be stained by Ziehl–Neelsen or auramine stain (see Appendix) to demonstrate acid-fast rods. In LL these are numerous, but in TT few if any organisms are seen, but the appearance of granulomas is sufficiently typical to allow the diagnosis to be made *(Fig. 23.24)*. Remember that, in contrast to *M. tuberculosis*, the organism cannot be grown *in vitro*.

Treatment
Leprosy is treated with dapsone given as part of a multidrug regimen to avoid resistance

If the disease is diagnosed early and treatment initiated promptly the patient has a much better prognosis. Dapsone (see Chapter 30) had long been the mainstay of therapy, but multidrug therapy is now used because of dapsone resistance:

- For LL, triple therapy with dapsone, rifampin and clofazimine (or ethionamide) is given for a minimum of two years and may be life-long or until all skin scrapings and biopsies are negative for acid-fast rods.
- For TT, a combination of dapsone and rifampin for six months is recommended, the rationale being that in this form of disease there are many fewer organisms and therefore less chance of emergence of resistant mutants.

As a result of multidrug therapy, which is reasonably cheap, well tolerated and effects a complete cure, steady progress is being made towards the elimination of leprosy as a public health problem.

Destruction of the organisms by effective antimicrobial therapy may result in an inflammatory response, erythema nodosum leprosum, which may be severe and, occasionally, fatal. Treatment with corticosteroids or thalidomide may be indicated.

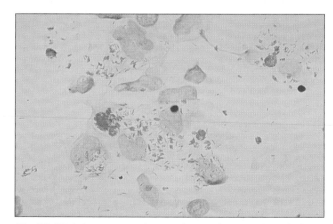

Fig. 23.23 In lepromatous leprosy the nasal mucosa is packed with *Mycobacterium leprae*, seen here in an acid-fast stain (Ziehl–Neelsen) of nasal scrapings. (Courtesy of I Farrell.)

Dapsone prophylaxis is advised for household contacts of LL cases

Although leprosy is not highly contagious, prophylaxis for household contacts (particularly children) of LL cases is advisable.

Trials aimed to determine the role of bacille Calmette-Guérin (BCG) immunization for the prevention of leprosy have shown conflicting results. A vaccine of heat-killed *M. leprae* is being tested, but it will be some time before the long-term follow-up necessary for such a slowly developing disease will be complete.

Other mycobacterial skin infections
Mycobacterium marinum, Mycobacterium ulcerans and *M. tuberculosis* also cause skin lesions

Mycobacterium marinum and *Mycobacterium ulcerans* are two slow-growing mycobacterial species that prefer cooler temperatures and cause skin lesions. As its name suggests, *M. marinum* is associated with water and marine organisms. Human infections follow trauma, often minor such as a graze acquired while climbing out of a swimming pool or while cleaning out an aquarium, which becomes contaminated with mycobacteria from the wet environment. After an incubation period of 2–8 weeks, initial lesions appear as small papules, which enlarge and suppurate and may ulcerate. Histologically, the lesions are granulomas and hence the name 'swimming pool granuloma' or 'fish-tank granuloma' *(Fig. 23.25)*. Sometimes the nodules follow the course of the draining lymphatic and produce an appearance that may be mistaken for sporotrichosis (see below).

M. ulcerans causes chronic, relatively painless cutaneous ulcers known as 'Buruli ulcers'. This disease is prevalent in Africa and Australia, but is rarely seen elsewhere.

Tuberculosis of the skin is exceedingly uncommon. Infection can occur by direct implantation of *M. tuberculosis* during trauma to the skin (lupus vulgaris) or may extend to the skin from an infected lymph node (scrofuloderma).

Fungal Infections of the Skin

Fungal infections of the skin may be confined to the very outermost layer (superficial mycoses) or penetrate into the epidermal or dermal layers (subcutaneous mycoses). In addition, some systemic fungal infections acquired by the airborne route have skin manifestations *(Fig. 23.4)*.

Superficial mycoses – the dermatophytes

Superficial fungal infections are among the most common infections in humans. The important causative agents are the dermatophyte fungi of the genera *Epidermophyton*, *Trichophyton* and *Microsporum*, and the yeast *Malassezia furfur*.

Dermatophyte infections are spread by arthrospores shed from the primary host

The dermatophytes are known as zoophilic, anthropophilic or geophilic depending upon their primary source (animal, human or soil). Their geographic distribution and routes of transmission to man therefore depend upon their normal habitat *(Fig. 23.26)*. In temperate countries, *Trichophyton verrucosum*, the cause of cattle ringworm, and *Microsporum canis*, which causes infections in cats and dogs, are the most common zoophilic causes of human infection. Geophilic species such as *Microsporum gypseum* are uncommon causes of human disease, but are seen in people who have appropriate exposure, such as gardeners and agricultural workers. The anthropophilic dermatophytes are the most common causes of dermatophyte infections. The species differ in their geographic distribution and in their predilection for different body sites (see below).

Infections are spread by contact with arthrospores, the thick-walled vegetative cells formed by dermatophyte hyphae *(Fig. 23.27)*, which are shed from the primary host probably in skin scales and hair and can survive for months.

Dermatophytes invade skin, hair and nails

The dermatophytes are keratin-loving organisms and invade the keratinized structures of the body (i.e. skin, hair and nails).

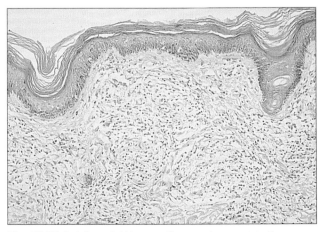

Fig. 23.24 In tuberculoid leprosy the organisms are much more sparse but characteristic granulomas form in the dermis, as shown in this histologic preparation. (Courtesy of CJ Edwards.)

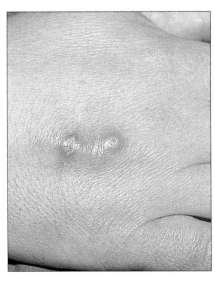

Fig. 23.25 Fish tank granuloma caused by *Mycobacterium marinum* infection of a lesion acquired while cleaning out a fish tank. (Courtesy of MJ Wood.)

The arthrospores adhere to keratinocytes, germinate and invade. The latin word 'tinea' (meaning a maggot or grub) or ringworm is used for dermatophyte infections because they were originally thought to be caused by a worm-like parasite. Thus tinea capitis affects the hair and skin of the scalp, tinea corporis the body, and tinea pedis the feet *(Fig. 23.28)*.

The typical lesion of dermatophyte infection is an annular scaling patch with a raised margin. The main symptom is itching, but this is variable in degree. The skin is often dry and scaly and sometimes cracks (e.g. between the toes in tinea pedis), while infections of hair cause hair loss *(Fig. 23.29)*. The degree of associated inflammation varies with the infecting species, usually being greater with zoophilic than with anthropophilic species. Individuals also differ in their susceptibility to

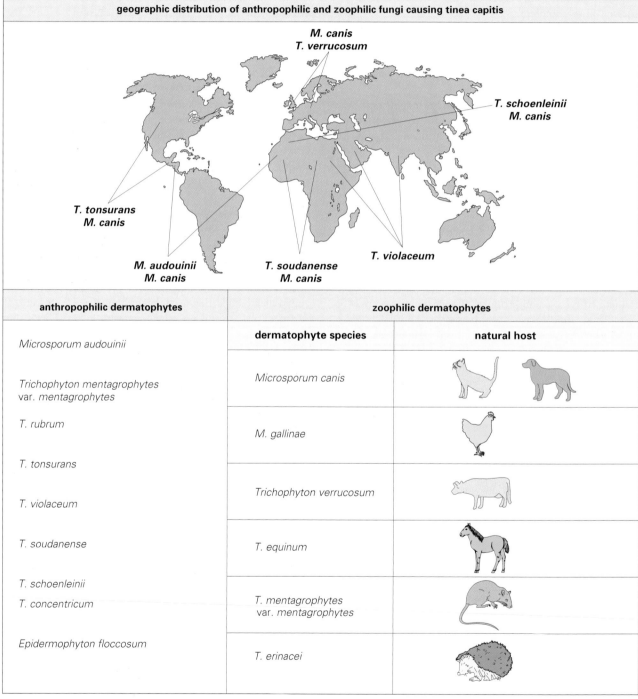

Fig. 23.26 Three genera of dermatophytes are important causes of disease: *Microsporum*, *Trichophyton* and *Epidermophyton*. Within each genus there are anthropophilic, zoophilic and geophilic species. The natural host and therefore distribution of anthropophilic species varies. *Microsporum gypseum* is the geophilic species of importance.

infection, but the factors determining these differences are not clearly understood. Likewise dermatophyte species differ in their ability to elicit an immune response; some, such as *Trichophyton rubrum*, cause chronic or relapsing conditions, whereas other species induce long-term resistance to reinfection. In some patients circulating fungal antigens give rise to immunologically-mediated hypersensitivity phenomena in the skin (e.g. erythema or vesicles) known as dermatophytid reactions. When the skin becomes cracked and macerated as a result of infection, it is liable to superinfection with other organisms such as Gram-negative bacteria in moist sites.

Very rarely, dermatophytes invade the subcutaneous tissues via the lymphatics causing granulomas, lymphedema and draining sinuses. Further extension to sites such as the liver and brain may be fatal.

Most dermatophyte species fluoresce under ultraviolet light

This feature can be used as a diagnostic aid, particularly for tinea capitis, in the clinic. Laboratory diagnosis depends upon microscopic examination for fungal hyphae and culture on Sabouraud agar of scrapings or clippings from lesions (*Fig. 23.30*, see Chapter 18 and Appendix). Dermatophytes infecting hair show a characteristic distribution, which may be helpful for identification:

- Some, such as most *Microsporum* species, form arthrospores on the outside of the hair shaft (ectothrix infections).
- The majority of *Trichophyton* infections form arthrospores within the hair shaft (endothrix infection, *Fig. 23.31*).

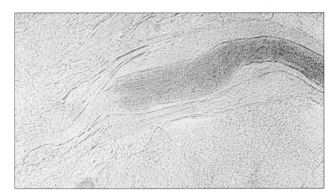

Fig. 23.27 Arthrospores of *Trichophyton tonsurans* in an infected hair shaft. These thick-walled spores are the form in which infection is spread. They can survive in the environment for weeks or months before infecting a new host. (Courtesy of AE Prevost.)

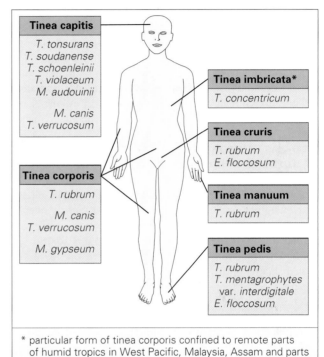

Fig. 23.28 Tinea (or ringworm) is the disease of skin, hair and nails caused by dermatophyte fungi. Different species have predilections for different body sites. (E., Epidermophyton; M., Microsporum; T., Trichophyton.)

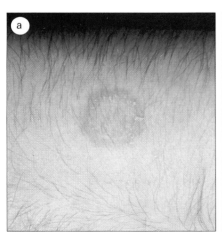
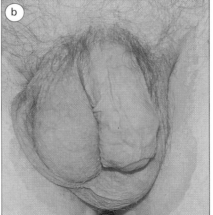
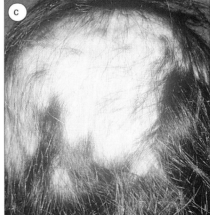

Fig. 23.29 (a) Classic annular lesion of tinea corporis, caused here by infection with a *Microsporum* species. (Courtesy of AE Prevost.) (b) Tinea cruris or 'jock itch' is a scaly rash on the thighs; the scrotum is usually spared. (Courtesy of MJ Wood.) (c) Tinea capitis is characterized by scaling on the scalp and hair loss. Some dermatophytes fluoresce under ultraviolet light and this can be an aid to diagnosis. (Courtesy of MH Winterborn.)

Confirmation of identity depends upon the colonial and microscopic characteristics of the fungi cultured on Sabouraud agar *(Fig. 23.32)*. Growth may take up to two weeks, but identification is not difficult and is useful for determining the source of infection.

Dermatophyte infections are treated topically if possible

However, infections of nails and hair are better treated by oral antifungal drugs. A range of agents is available for topical treatment (see Chapter 30), both antifungals (e.g. miconazole) and keratolytic agents such as Whitfield's ointment (a mixture of salicylic and benzoic acids). The orally administered agent most commonly used is griseofulvin. Scalp infections take 6–12 weeks to respond, fingernail infections up to six months and toenail infections one year or longer. The relapse rate of treated nail infections is high and many physicians advise against treatment unless there is pain or more widespread skin involvement.

Pityriasis versicolor
M. furfur is the cause of pityriasis or tinea versicolor

The yeast *M. (Pityrosporum) furfur* is a common skin inhabitant. The change from commensalism to pathogenicity appears to be associated with the phase change from yeast to hyphal forms of the fungus, but the stimulus for this is unknown. Infections are usually confined to the trunk or proximal parts of the limbs and are associated with hypo- or hyperpigmented macules that coalesce to form scaling plaques. The lesions are not usually itchy and in some patients they resolve spontaneously.

Pityrosporum yeasts are also thought to be involved in the pathogenesis of seborrheic dermatitis.

Diagnosis of pityriasis versicolor can be confirmed by direct microscopy of scrapings

Direct microscopy of scrapings shows characteristic round yeast forms *(Fig. 23.33)* and treatment with a topical azole antifungal (see above) or with selenium sulphide (2%) lotion is appropriate.

Candida and the skin
Candida requires moisture for growth

The relative dryness of most areas of skin limits the growth of fungi such as *Candida* that require moisture. *Candida* is found in low numbers on healthy intact skin, but rapidly colonizes damaged skin and intertriginous sites (apposed skin sites which are often moist and become chafed, *Fig. 23.34*). *Candida* also colonizes the oral and vaginal mucosa and overgrowth may result in disease in these sites (thrush, see Chapter 19). However, a substantial lowering of host resistance (e.g. neutropenia) is necessary for *Candida* to invade deeper subcutaneous tissue, and disseminated candidiasis does not often originate from skin infection unless there is instrumentation through infected areas (see Chapter 28). Chronic mucocutaneous candidiasis is associated with a specific immune defect and is discussed in Chapter 28.

Subcutaneous mycoses
Subcutaneous fungal infections can be caused by a number of different species

Lesions usually develop at sites of trauma (a thorn, a bite) where the fungus becomes implanted. With the exception of sporotrichosis, subcutaneous fungal infections are rare but similar diseases can be caused by certain bacteria such as *Actinomyces* and atypical mycobacteria, and therefore it is important to establish the etiology in order to select optimal

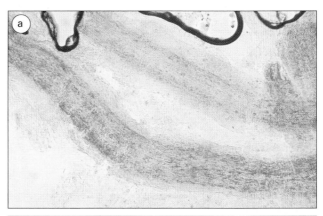

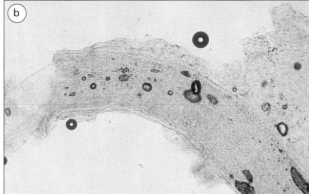

Fig. 23.31 Dermatophytes may form arthrospores within the hair shafts (endothrix infection) as shown in (a) and less commonly outside the shaft (ectothrix infection) as shown in (b). (Courtesy of Y Clayton and G Midgley.)

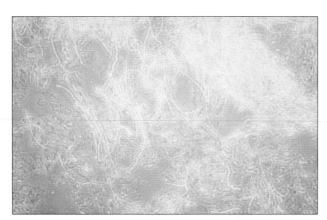

Fig. 23.30 Dermatophyte infection. Samples of skin, hair and nails need to be be 'cleared' by treatment with potassium hydroxide before examining under the microscope for the presence of fungal hyphae. (Courtesy of RY Cartwright.)

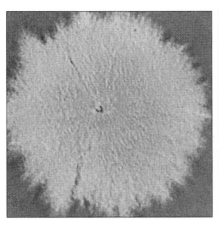
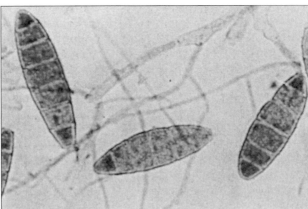

Fig. 23.32
Macroscopic growth (colony) and microscopic preparation showing the macroconidia of *Microsporum gypseum*.

therapy. The fungi involved are difficult to eradicate with antifungal agents, and surgical intervention, in the form of excision or amputation, is often required.

Sporotrichosis is a nodular condition caused by Sporothrix schenckii

Sporothrix schenckii is a saprophytic fungus that is widespread in nature in soil, on rose and *Berberis* bushes, tree bark and sphagnum moss. Infection is acquired through trauma (e.g. a thorn) and is an occupational hazard for people such as farmers, gardeners and florists. A small papule or subcutaneous nodule develops at the site of trauma one week to six months after inoculation and infection spreads, producing a series of secondary nodules along the lymphatics that drain the site (*Fig. 23.35*). Diagnosis is made by culture of draining or aspirated material onto Sabouraud agar. Treatment with oral potassium iodide is effective for cutaneous lymphatic disease.

Disseminated disease can occur following cutaneous or pulmonary infection with *S. schenckii*. It is more common in compromised patients such as those with carcinoma or sarcoidosis, but many cases occur in people in whom no underlying disease is recognized. Treatment with amphotericin B is indicated and the prognosis is often poor.

Systemic fungal infections with skin manifestations include blastomycosis and cryptococcosis

Skin lesions are the most common presenting symptom of blastomycosis. This disease, caused by *Blastomyces dermatitidis*, is acquired by aspiration of the fungal spores and invasion and bloodborne spread of infection from the primary site in the lung. Blastomycosis is one of the endemic fungal diseases of Central and North America and Africa and can be a systemic disease in apparently immunologically normal hosts (*Fig. 23.36*). It also causes disease in horses and dogs.

Cryptococcus neoformans is a yeast that causes infection of the lungs. Bloodborne dissemination occurs and the organism has a particular predilection for the central nervous system (CNS), but skin and bones are also common sites of infection. Many patients with disseminated infection have no demonstrable underlying disease, but immunocompromised patients are more prone to rapidly progressive disease (see Chapter 33).

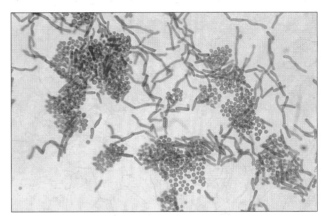

Fig. 23.33 Infected skin scales stained to show the thick-walled yeast forms of *Malassezia furfur* and the short angular hyphae. (Courtesy of Y Clayton and G Midgley.)

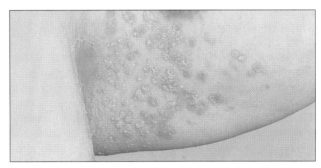

Fig. 23.34 *Candida* infection of the skin. Here, infection has occurred between two apposing skin surfaces, which provide a suitably moist environment for this yeast to multiply. (Courtesy of A du Vivier and St Mary's Hospital.)

Parasitic Infections of the Skin

The skin is a major route of entry for parasites, which may:
- Penetrate directly (e.g. schistosomes, nematodes).
- Be injected by blood-feeding vectors.

Many of these parasites leave the skin almost immediately, but some remain there and others may become trapped. A few parasites actually exit from the body through the skin.

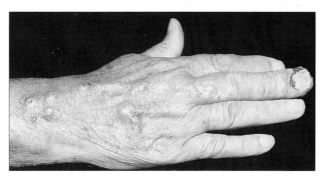

Fig. 23.35 Sporotrichosis spreading up the draining lymphatics of the hand following a primary infection in the nailbed of the third finger. (Courtesy of TF Sellers, Jr.)

Pathologic responses to parasites associated with the skin range from mild to disablingly severe. Some species causing severe conditions are described briefly below.

Leishmaniasis may be cutaneous and mucocutaneous

Two major disease complexes caused by the protozoans *Leishmania* affect the skin and both are transmitted by the bite of sandfly vectors:

- The cutaneous leishmaniases, which occur in both the Old World (Asia, Africa, S. Europe) and New World (Central and South America), include conditions ranging from localized self-healing ulcers to non-curing, disseminated lesions akin to leprosy in appearance.
- In the New World, mucocutaneous leishmaniases are conditions where the parasite is localized in the skin or invades skin–mucous surfaces (nose, mouth) giving rise to chronic disfiguring conditions. Leishmaniasis is discussed in detail in Chapter 25.

Schistosome infection can cause a dermatitis

Transmission of schistosomes from the snail vector is achieved by active skin penetration by the larvae (see Chapter 25). With those species adapted to man, this stage of infection can give rise to a dermatitis. A similar, though more pronounced, skin reaction is seen when bird schistosomes invade. This condition, known as 'swimmer's itch', is relatively common where natural water used for recreation is populated with aquatic birds. Topical anti-inflammatory treatments are effective therapy.

Cutaneous larval migrans is characterized by itchy inflammatory hookworm trails

Human hookworms (the nematodes *Ancylostoma* and *Necator*) invade the body through the skin, the infective larvae burrowing into the dermis and then migrating via the blood to eventually reach the intestine. Invasion may cause dermatitis, and this becomes more severe upon repeated infection. Humans, however, can also be invaded by the larvae of the cat and dog species of hookworm. Infection is acquired when exposed skin comes into contact with soil that has been contaminated by animals carrying the adult worms in their

intestines. Eggs in the feces hatch to produce the infective larvae, which remain viable for prolonged periods. As the human host is foreign for these species the larvae fail to escape from the dermis after invasion, and may live for some time, migrating parallel to the skin and leaving intensely itchy sinuous inflammatory trails, which are easily visible at the surface *(Fig. 23.37)*. Topical treatment can be used to control inflammation, together with an anthelmintic such as thiabendazole.

Onchocerciasis is characterized by hypersensitivity responses to larval antigens

Onchocerciasis is also known as river blindness. The adult stages of *Onchocerca volvulus* live for many years in subcutaneous nodules. Female worms release live microfilarae, which migrate away from the nodules, remaining largely in the dermal layers. They can invade the eye causing river blindness (see Chapter 16). The slow build-up of parasite numbers, and the development of a hypersensitivity response to the antigens released by living and dying larvae, give rise to inflammatory skin conditions. In the early stages these appear as erythematous papular rashes accompanied by intense itching. Later on there is skin thickening, elasticity is lost and excessive wrinkling occurs; depigmentation is also common. The microfilarae can be killed by ivermectin treatment, but the skin conditions, once advanced, are irreversible. Dermal inflammatory conditions are not uncommon during infections with other filarial nematodes.

Arthropod infections
Some flies, mainly in the tropics and subtropics, lay their eggs on the skin

Myiasis is a condition associated with invasion of the body by the larvae (maggots) of dipterous flies. Many species of fly have a cycle in which the larvae feed and grow just below the skin of a mammal, escaping before or after pupation to release the aerial adult forms. Female flies lay eggs or larvae directly onto the skin, and larvae may then invade wounds or natural orifices. The activities and feeding of the larvae cause intense painful reactions, and large lesions may develop. A number of species have been found in humans, and infections have been recorded in many countries, although primarily in tropical and subtropical regions. Treatment involves removal of the larvae, alleviation of symptoms and prevention of secondary infection.

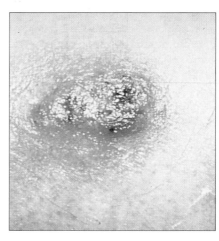

Fig. 23.36 Typical skin lesion of blastomycosis. Infection is acquired by the respiratory route and the primary site of infection is the lung. However, in chronic blastomycosis the skin is the most common extrapulmonary site of infection. (Courtesy of KA Riley.)

Maggots were once used medically to eat away necrotic tissue from wounds, and maggots ('worms') of some species feed on corpses.

Certain ticks, lice and mites live on blood or tissue fluids from humans

Some feed non-selectively on humans and other species are host specific. The feeding processes, and the inevitable release of saliva, give rise to skin irritation, which becomes more intense as the body responds immunologically to the proteins present in the saliva. Prolonged feeding, as practiced by ticks, may leave painful lesions in the skin, which can became secondarily infected. Species such as lice and scabies mites, which spend the greater part or the whole of their lives on the human body, can cause severe skin conditions when populations accumulate. These conditions arise from:

- The activity of the insects themselves.
- Their production of excreta.
- The oozing of blood and tissue fluids from the feeding sites.
- The host's inflammatory reaction.

Pediculosis— infection with head and body lice of the genus *Pediculus*— can, when severe, give rise to encrusting inflammatory masses in which fungal infections may establish. Good personal hygiene prevents infestation; use of insecticidal creams, lotions, shampoos and powders containing malathion or carbaryl helps to clear the insects directly.

The scabies mite has a more intimate contact with the human host than lice, living its whole life in burrows within the skin. The female lays eggs into these burrows, and so the area of infection can spread to cover large areas of the body from the original site, which is usually on the hands or wrists (*Fig. 23.38*, see Chapter 19). Infection causes a characteristic rash with itching, and secondary infections may follow scratching. Very heavy infections may develop in immunocompromised individuals or in people who are unable to care adequately for themselves. Under these conditions there is extensive thickening and crusting of the skin (Norwegian scabies). Treatment with malathion, gamma benzene hexachloride or lindane is recommended; benzyl benzoate can also be used on unbroken skin.

Mucocutaneous Lesions Caused by Viruses

Mucocutaneous lesions caused by viruses can be divided into:
- Those in which the virus remains restricted to the body surface at the site of initial infection.
- Those in which the virus causes mucocutaneous lesions after spreading systemically through the body (*Fig. 23.39*).

The infections that spread systemically can in turn be divided into:
- Those in which the skin lesions (vesicular) are sites of virus growth and are infectious.
- Those in which the skin lesions (maculopapular) are non-infectious and immunologically mediated.

The skin rash has a characteristic distribution in many infectious diseases, but with the exception of zoster the reason for this is unknown.

Rashes are particular features of human infection and are rare in animals. This is because human skin is naked and is a turbulent highly reactive tissue in which immune and inflammatory events are clearly visible. Rashes are not often in themselves a source of suffering but they may be very helpful for the clinician who needs to make a diagnosis. The veterinarian is less privileged because the skin of most other mammals is largely covered with fur and skin lesions generally involve hairless areas such as udders, scrotums, ears, prepuces, teats, noses or paws, which have the human properties of thickness, sensitivity and vascular reactivity.

Papillomavirus infection
About 70 different types of papillomavirus can infect humans

Papillomaviruses are small (55 nm) icosahedral double-stranded DNA viruses and cause skin papillomas (warts). The 70 different types that can infect humans show less than 50% cross-hybridization of DNA, although not all types are common. Human papillomaviruses (HPV) are species-specific and distinct from animal papillomaviruses. They are highly adapted to human skin and mucosa and are ancient associates of our species, and therefore for most of the time

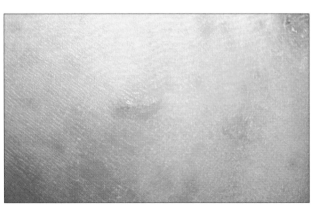

Fig. 23.37 Cutaneous larval migrans (creeping eruption), showing the raised inflammatory track left by the invading hookworm larvae. (Courtesy of A du Vivier.)

Fig. 23.38 A characteristic cutaneous burrow in scabies. (Courtesy of MJ Wood.)

MUCOCUTANEOUS LESIONS CAUSED BY VIRUSES			
	virus	**lesion**	**virus shedding from lesion**
no systemic spread	papilloma (wart)	common wart plantar wart genital wart	+
	molluscum contagiosum (poxvirus)	fleshy papule	+
	orf (poxvirus from sheep, goats)	papulovesicular	+
systemic spread	herpes simplex varicella-zoster	vesicular (neural spread and latency)	+
	coxsackievirus A (9, 16, 23)	vesicular, in mouth (herpangina)	+
	coxsackievirus A16	vesicular (hand, foot and mouth disease)	+
	human parvovirus (B19)	facial maculopapular (erythema infectiosum)	–
	human herpesvirus 6	exanthem subitum (roseola infantum)	–
	measles	maculopapular skin rash	–
	rubella echoviruses (4, 6, 9,16)	maculopapular not distinguishable clinically	–
	dengue and other arthropod transmitted viruses	maculopapular	–

Fig. 23.39 Mucocutaneous lesions caused by viruses. The pathogenesis of these diseases is illustrated in *Figure 23.3*. Papillomas and vesicular lesions are generally sites of virus shedding. The distribution as well as the nature of the lesion can be important in diagnosis (e.g. varicella), but many maculopapular rashes are clinically indistinguishable.

they cause little or no disease. They show some adaptation to definite sites on the body:

- At least five types (HPV 6, 11, 16, 18, 32) regularly infect the genital areas and are sexually transmitted.
- HPV 1 and 4 tend to cause plantar warts.
- HPV 2, 3 and 10 cause warts on the knees and fingers.

Papillomaviruses are generally transmitted by direct contact, but they are stable and can also be spread indirectly. For instance, plantar warts can be acquired from contaminated floors or from the non-slip surfaces at the edges of swimming pools, and in a given individual warts can be spread from one site to another by shaving.

Papillomavirus infects cells in the basal layers of skin or mucosa

After entering the body via surface abrasions the virus infects cells in the basal layers of the skin or mucosa *(Fig. 23.3)*. There is no spread to deeper tissues. Virus replication is slow and is critically dependent upon the differentiation of host cells. Viral DNA is present in basal cells, but viral antigen and infectious virus are produced only when the cells begin to become squamified and keratinized as they approach the surface (see Chapter 14). The infected cells are stimulated to divide and finally, 1–6 months after initial infection, the mass of infected cells protrudes from the body surface to form a visible papilloma or wart *(Fig. 23.40)*. There is marked proliferation of prickle cells and vacuolated cells are present in the more superficial layers. Warts can be:

- Filiform with finger-like projections.
- Flat topped.
- Flat because they grow inwards due to external pressure (plantar warts).
- A cauliflower-like protuberance (e.g. genital warts).
- A flat area of dysplasia on the cervix.

Immune responses eventually bring virus replication under control and, several months after infection, the wart regresses. Antibodies are demonstrable, but CMI responses are more important in recovery. It seems likely that viral DNA remains in a latent state in the basal cell layer, infecting an occasional stem cell, and is therefore retained within the layer as epidermal cells differentiate and are shed from the surface. Hence, when patients are subsequently immunocompromised (e.g. post-transplant) crops of warts may result from reactivation of latent virus in the skin.

Papillomavirus infections are associated with cancer of the cervix, vulva, penis and rectum

The association between genital warts and cancer of the cervix, vulva, penis and rectum is referred to in Chapter 12. It is not clear whether this association is causal or merely casual. There is no evidence that regular skin warts are involved in the development of skin cancer. There is, however, a rare autosomal recessive disease, epidermodysplasia verruciformis, characterized by multiple warts containing many different types of wart virus and poorly understood immunologic defects. Warts may undergo malignant change in these patients.

A diagnosis of papillomovirus infection is clinical and there are many treatments

Wart viruses cannot be cultivated in the laboratory, and at present serologic tests are neither useful nor available.

An astounding variety of treatments have been used for warts, some of them doubtless seeming effective because warts eventually disappear without treatment. Post-hypnotic suggestion has at times been successful. Current treatments include the application of karyolytic agents such as salicylic acid and destruction of wart tissue by freezing with dry ice (solid carbon dioxide) or with liquid nitrogen. The latter is the most commonly used and most effective treatment.

Molluscum contagiosum is an umbilicated lesion caused by a poxvirus

The poxvirus infects epidermal cells to form a fleshy lesion, often with an umbilicated center *(Fig. 23.41)*. It only infects humans and is spread by contact, or in the case of genital lesions, by sexual intercourse. There are two antigenically distinct types. Poxvirus particles can be seen by electron microscopy (see Chapter 3).

Orf is a papulovesicular lesion caused by a poxvirus

Orf (contagious pustular dermatitis) is an uncommon infection of the epidermis and is acquired by direct contact with infected sheep or goats. There is a papulovesicular lesion, generally on the hands, which may ulcerate.

Herpes simplex virus infection

Herpes simplex virus infection is universal and occurs in early childhood

Herpes simplex virus (HSV) is a medium-sized (120 nm) double-stranded DNA virus of the herpesvirus group. Two types, HSV1 and HSV2, are distinguishable antigenically. They cause a wide variety of clinical syndromes, the basic lesion being an intraepithelial vesicle, from which the virus is shed. Infection is usually transmitted from the saliva or cold sores of other individuals and frequently by kissing.

Clinical features of HSV infection are vesicles and latency

After infection the virus replicates in cells in the oral mucosa and forms virus-rich vesicles. The patient suffers at most a mild febrile illness. The vesicles ulcerate and become coated with a whitish-grey slough *(Fig. 23.42)*.

During the primary infection, virus particles enter sensory nerve endings in the lesion and are transported to the dorsal root (trigeminal) ganglion, where they initiate latent infection in sensory neurones (see Chapter 11). The lesion resolves as antibody and CMI responses develop. The latent virus remains in the sensory ganglion for life, and under certain circumstances can reactivate and spread down sensory nerves to cause cold sores at the site of the original infection *(Fig. 23.43)*.

Primary infection can also occur in:

- The eye, to cause conjunctivitis and keratitis, often with vesicles on the eyelids (see Chapter 16).
- The finger, to cause herpetic whitlow.
- Other skin sites following direct contact with infected individuals where there is rubbing or trauma. This is seen for instance in rugby football ('scrum pox') or in wrestlers ('herpes gladiatorum').
- The genital tract (see Chapter 19). Although HSV2 arose as a sexually transmitted variant of HSV1, the sites infected by the two types are now less clearly distinct.

Serious complications associated with HSV infection include:

- Herpetic infection of eczematous skin areas leading to severe disease in young children *(Fig. 23.44)*.

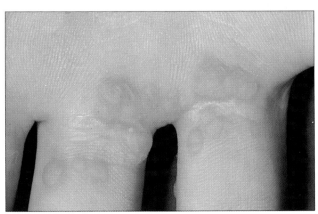

Fig. 23.40 Common warts (papillomas) on the hand. (Courtesy of MJ Wood.)

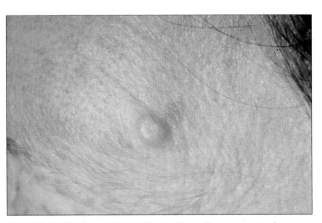

Fig. 23.41 Single umbilicated lesion in molluscum contagiosum. (Courtesy of MJ Wood.)

- Acute necrotizing encephalitis following either primary infection or reactivation (see Chapter 22).
- Neonatal infection acquired from the genital tract of the mother (see Chapter 21).
- Primary or reactivating HSV infection in immunocompromised individuals, causing very severe disease (see Chapter 28).

HSV reactivation is provoked by a variety of factors

In healthy individuals HSV reactivation is provoked by:
- Certain febrile illnesses (e.g. common cold, pneumonia).
- Direct sunlight.
- Stress.
- Menstruation (see Chapter 14).
- Immunocompromise.

Reactivation is more severe in immunocompromised patients (see Chapter 28).

A sensory prodrome (pain, burning, itching) precedes the appearance of the lesion and is due to virus activity in sensory neurones. The lesion, a so-called 'cold sore', generally occurs around the mucocutaneous junctions in the nose or mouth *(Fig. 23.45)*. Less commonly, when the ophthalmic branch of the trigeminal ganglion is involved, the lesion is a dendritic ulcer of the cornea. Large amounts of

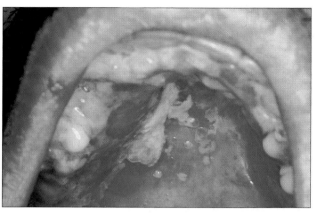

Fig. 23.42 Primary herpes simplex virus infection. There are shallow ulcers with white exudate on the palate and gums. (Courtesy of JA Innes.)

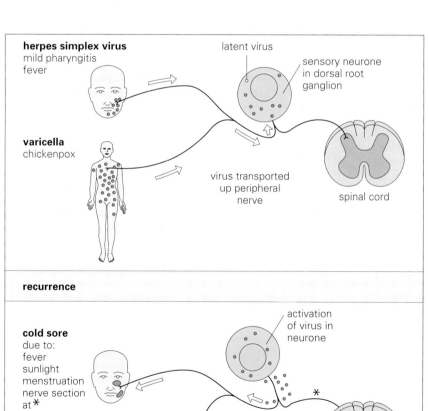

Fig. 23.43 Pathogenesis of cold sores and zoster. In both herpes simplex virus and varicella-zoster virus infections the virus in mucocutaneous nerve endings travels up the axon to reach the sensory neurones, where it becomes latent. Recurrences are due to reactivation of the virus within the neurone to become infectious followed by passage of virus down the axon to mucocutaneous site(s) and local spread and replication to form clinical lesion(s).

virus are shed in the cold sore, which scabs over and heals over the course of about one week. Occasionally the sensory prodrome occurs without proceeding to a cold sore (see also varicella-zoster virus [VZV] recurrence below).

HSV is readily isolated from vesicle fluid and infection is treated with acyclovir

HSV is also readily isolated from saliva or conjunctival fluid, and causes a distinct cytopathic effect in human embryo lung and other cells. Significant rises in complement fixing antibodies may be useful in diagnosing primary infection, but recurrent infection rarely leads to a rise in titer.

Acyclovir has revolutionized the treatment of HSV infection (see Chapter 30), and can be used either topically or systemically. It is relatively non-toxic and acts specifically in virus-infected cells. Recurrent herpetic eruptions have been successfully treated with low doses of acyclovir twice daily for up to three years.

Other topical treatments include 0.1% idoxuridine for herpes keratitis or 5–40% idoxuridine in dimethylsulfoxide for herpetic skin lesions.

VZV infection
VZV causes chickenpox (varicella) and zoster (shingles) and is highly contagious

VZV is a medium-sized (100–200 nm diameter) double-stranded DNA virus of the herpesvirus group and is morphologically indistinguishable from HSV. There is only one serologic type. The virus grows more slowly than HSV and is not released from the infected cell. Infection is by inhalation of droplets from respiratory secretions and saliva, or by direct contact from skin lesions. Primary infection with VZV causes varicella (chickenpox). Immunity develops and prevents reinfection (a second attack of varicella), but the virus persists in the body and later in life, after reactivation, causes zoster (shingles). Nearly all humans worldwide are infected during childhood. The vesicles of zoster are slightly less infectious, but are an important source of varicella in the community (see Chapter 11).

Varicella is characterized by crops of vesicles that develop into pustules and then scab

After primary infection, the virus passes across surface epithelium in the respiratory tract to infect mononuclear cells, and is then carried to lymphoid tissues. There are no symptoms and no detectable lesions at the site of entry into the body. The virus slowly replicates in lymphoreticular tissues for about a week, and then enters the blood in association with mononuclear cells and is seeded out to epithelial sites. These are mainly the respiratory tract and the skin, but also include the mouth, often the conjunctiva, and probably also the alimentary and urinogenital tracts. In the skin, for unknown reasons, the trunk, face and scalp are especially involved. At these epithelial sites the virus exits from small blood vessels, infecting subepithelial and finally epithelial cells. Multinucleated giant cells with intranuclear inclusions are present in the lesions. In the oropharynx and respiratory tract the virus reaches the surface and is shed to the exterior to infect other individuals about two weeks after initial infection. In the skin it takes a day or two longer, and it is at this stage, when the characteristic varicella vesicles appear, that a clinical diagnosis can be made *(Fig. 23.46)* The mean incubation period is 14 days (range 10–23 days).

The patient remains well until a day or two before the rash, when there may be slight fever and malaise, but the illness is usually mild and often unnoticed. The vesicles appear first on the trunk, then on the face and scalp, and less commonly on arms and legs. They often come in 'crops' over the course of several days, then develop into pustules, break down, and scab over. The lesions are deeper than with HSV and scarring is more common. Lesions in the mouth may be painful.

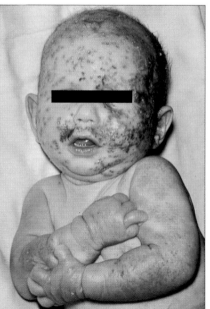

Fig. 23.44 Eczema herpeticum due to herpes simplex virus infection in an infant. (Courtesy of MJ Wood.)

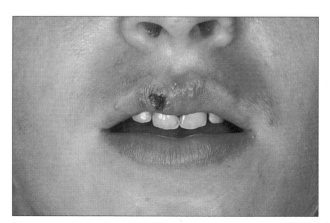

Fig. 23.45 Recurrent herpes simplex virus vesicles on the mucocutaneous margin of the lip. (Courtesy of A du Vivier.)

Varicella is usually more severe and more likely to cause complications in adults

The skin lesions of varicella can become infected with staphylococci or streptococci to produce secondary impetigo, but varicella in a child is characteristically a very mild illness. The main complications are:

- Interstitial pneumonia, which can be detected radiologically, although it is often subclinical, in up to 20% of adults with varicella. Secondary bacterial pneumonia can also occur.
- CNS involvement, which may consist of a lymphocytic meningitis or an encephalomyelitis (see Chapter 22).

Thrombocytopenia can occur, but it is usually symptomless. In immunocompromised patients, particularly children with leukemia, varicella can be a life-threatening disease.

After primary infection during pregnancy the virus may infect the fetus (see Chapter 21), but maternal antibody is present by then and the infection is generally without serious consequences. However, when the mother is infected a few days after delivery the infant is exposed without the protection of maternal antibody and can suffer a serious disease.

Zoster results from reactivation of latent VZV

During primary infection, VZV in mucocutaneous lesions enters sensory nerve endings and establishes latent infection in sensory neurones in dorsal root ganglia (*Fig. 23.43*). Later in life reactivation can occur to cause zoster in the dermatome at the site of the reactivation. Thoracic dermatomes are most commonly involved because the original varicella lesions are commonest here. Zoster is unilateral because the reactivation is a localized event in a single dorsal root ganglion. Zoster therefore originates from inside the body and is not directly acquired from either varicella or zoster in other individuals. During reactivation in sensory neurones (*Fig. 23.43*), there is paraesthesia and pain. Pain may be severe and precedes the development of the erythematous rash in which virus-rich vesicles appear (*Fig. 23.47*) by several days. It takes a few days for the virus to travel down peripheral nerves and multiply in the skin. Fever and malaise may accompany the rash. Sometimes the immune response controls the reactivating virus before skin lesions have had time to form, and in this case the sensory phenomena occur without the skin eruption.

Conditions that predispose to zoster include:

- Increasing age. Although zoster is very occasionally seen in childhood, its incidence increases with increasing age, rising from 3/1000/year in 50–59 year olds to 10/1000/year in 80–89 year olds.
- Immunocompromise due to leukemia, lymphoma, AIDS, renal transplant or other drug-induced immunosuppression. For instance, zoster occurs in about 20% of patients with Hodgkin's disease.
- Fractures or tumors affecting the brain or spinal cord.

The skin areas affected by zoster reflect the distribution of the original varicella rash, as might be expected from its pathogenesis (*Fig. 23.43*). Hence the trunk is most commonly involved. Ophthalmic zoster involving the upper eyelid, forehead and scalp is a particularly unpleasant manifestation.

Postherpetic neuralgia is a common complication of zoster

In the healthy host postherpetic (postzoster) neuralgia is common, especially in the elderly. The pain, which can be severe early in the illness, continues for up to several months after the lesions have resolved. It is difficult to treat.

In immunocompromised patients zoster may be severe. A few days after the localized eruption, the virus, with inadequate control by cell-mediated immunity, spreads via the blood to produce skin and visceral lesions throughout the body. Hemorrhagic complications and pneumonia may occur.

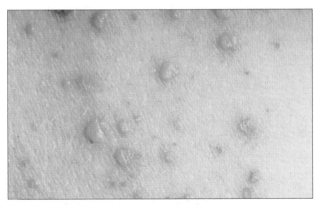

Fig. 23.46 Early rash in varicella (chickenpox), with macules, papules and vesicles. (Courtesy of MJ Wood.)

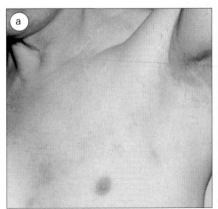
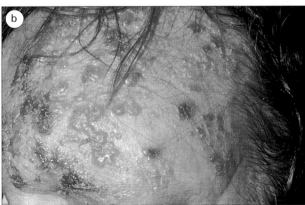

Fig. 23.47 Zoster rash. (a) A band of faint erythema, an early sign of shingles, along an intercostal nerve. (b) Rash affecting the ophthalmic division of the trigeminal nerve. (Courtesy of MJ Wood.)

VZV is difficult to isolate

Isolation of VZV is difficult and is not routinely attempted in laboratories. Herpesvirus particles can be seen by electron microscopy in vesicle fluid, but are indistinguishable from HSV particles. In varicella, and usually in zoster, a rise in complement fixing antibody titer between acute and convalescent sera is detectable. Past immunity is determined from the presence of antibodies by enzyme-linked immunosorbent assay (ELISA) or other tests.

Treatment of varicella is often symptomatic, but famciclovir can be used for zoster

Varicella skin lesions are treated with baths and soothing applications to relieve itching and to prevent scratching and secondary infection. VZV is much less sensitive than HSV to acyclovir, but this drug, or the more readily absorbed derivative famciclovir, is used orally to treat zoster. Severe infections can be treated with intravenous acyclovir. VZV immune globulin contains a high titer of human antibody to the virus, and is used to prevent varicella in vulnerable individuals after exposure.

A live attenuated vaccine is available to protect immunocompromised children, but is not yet approved for general use.

Rashes caused by coxsackieviruses and echoviruses
Coxsackieviruses and echoviruses cause a variety of exanthems (skin rashes)

Sometimes such infections are accompanied by an enanthem (lesions on internal epithelial surfaces such as the oral cavity). These infections are generally seen in young children, are not usually distinguishable on clinical examination, and are not severe. These viruses are also responsible for illnesses affecting the CNS (see Chapter 22), the upper respiratory tract (see Chapter 15), and striated and heart muscle (see below).

Coxsackievirus A lesions are usually vesicular and occur mostly on the buccal mucosa and the tongue. Most children complain of a sore mouth or tongue and there is slight fever. When vesicular lesions are also seen on the skin, principally on the hands, feet and buttocks, the condition is called 'hand, foot and mouth disease' (Fig. 23.48). The virus is present in the lesions and coxsackievirus A16 is the commonest cause.

Maculopapular rashes resembling rubella are common manifestations of echovirus infection; a number of different serotypes may be involved.

Rashes caused by human parvovirus
Parvovirus B19 causes slapped cheek syndrome

Parvoviruses are very small (22 nm diameter) single-stranded DNA viruses. The defective parvoviruses (see Appendix, p. 000) require a helper (adeno-) virus to replicate, and are called 'adeno-associated viruses'; there are four serotypes and infection is common, but they have not been implicated in any human disease. There is a non-defective parvovirus (B19) that grows in mitotically active cells. It causes a febrile illness in children with a characteristic maculopapular rash on the face ('slapped cheek syndrome'). The condition is referred to as 'erythema infectiosum' and sometimes 'fifth disease', it being the fifth of the six common exanthematous infections recognized by nineteenth century physicians.

Symptomless parvovirus infection is common and spreads by respiratory droplets

Nearly 50% of the population has parvovirus antibodies. The virus grows in hemopoietic cells in the bone marrow and although this normally causes no more than a temporary and barely detectable fall in hemoglobin levels, it can lead to serious consequences in those with chronic anemia. In children with sickle cell anemia for instance, the effect on erythropoiesis may cause an aplastic crisis. The virus can also cause arthralgia when it infects adults. Parvovirus B19 was first discovered by electron microscopy and cannot be isolated in cell culture. Virus-specific IgM antibody tests are available.

Other Infectious Causes of Maculopapular Rashes

Maculopapular rashes are seen in many other virus infections. These appear to be immune-mediated, there being little or no viral invasion of the skin and no shedding of virus from the skin.

Human herpesvirus 6 (HHV6) infects nearly all humans during the first five years of life (see Chapter 24). Although it grows in T and B cells, its main clinical manifestation is a maculopapular rash known as exanthem subitum or roseola infantum. After an incubation period of about two weeks there is fever for a few days with cervical lymphadenopathy, the rash appearing 1–2 days after disappearance of the fever.

The maculopapular rashes caused by measles and rubella viruses, and the maculopapular rashes seen in certain arthropod-borne virus infections (e.g. dengue) and in zoonotic virus infections (e.g. Marburg disease) are referred to in Chapters 24, 25 and 26. A maculopapular rash is often seen in the prodromal stage of hepatitis B virus infection (see Chapter 19), and is immune complex-mediated.

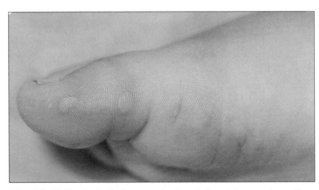

Fig. 23.48 Vesicular lesions on the foot in hand, foot and mouth disease. (Courtesy of MJ Wood.)

Other bacterial, fungal and rickettsial infections produce a variety of rashes or other skin lesions

Most of these are referred to elsewhere in this book, and they are listed in *Figure 23.4*. Rashes in rickettsial infections are often striking, as in the case of Rocky Mountain spotted fever or typhus (see Chapter 25). Most rickettsia invade vascular endothelial cells, from whence they are shed into the blood to infect blood-sucking arthropod vectors. Invasion of vascular endothelial cells in the skin provides the basis for the skin rash but is not a source of direct shedding to the exterior.

Kawasaki Syndrome

Kawasaki syndrome is an acute vasculitis and is probably caused by superantigen toxins

The Kawasaki syndrome is a childhood illness of uncertain etiology. Patients, who are generally less than four years of age, develop fever, conjunctivitis and a rash. There is dryness and redness of the lips and red palms and soles with some edema, desquamation of fingertips, often arthralgia and myocarditis, which gives a case mortality of about 2%. The basic pathology is an acute vasculitis, and 20% of untreated patients develop coronary artery aneurysms. The disease is commoner in those of Asian ancestry, but occurs worldwide. There is no clear evidence for person to person transmission, but it is thought to be of infectious origin, and is probably due to the superantigen toxins (see Chapter 11) of *Staph. aureus* or *Strep. pyogenes*.

Treatment, which prevents the aneurysms if given early enough, is high-dose intravenous immunoglobulin.

Viral Infections of Muscle

Viral myositis, myocarditis and pericarditis
Some viruses, particularly coxsackievirus B, cause myocarditis and myalgia

Group B, and to a lesser extent group A, coxsackieviruses and certain enteroviruses, are the main viral causes of myocarditis and pericarditis. Both conditions are seen principally in adult males and are important because they can be mistaken for myocardial infarction, yet the prognosis is good and complete recovery is the rule. These infections are transmitted by the fecal–oral route and occasionally from pharyngeal secretions. Ingested coxsackieviruses spread from the pharynx or gut wall to the lymphatics and then to the blood. Invasion of striated muscles, heart or pericardium takes place across small blood vessels and results in acute inflammation. In the heart and pericardium this gives rise to dyspnea, pain in the chest, and sometimes mimics a myocardial infarction. Mumps and influenza are less common causes of myocarditis or pericarditis. Rubella (see Chapter 21) can cause myocarditis and associated congenital lesions in the fetus.   .

Group B coxsackieviruses also cause pleurodynia or epidemic myalgia. This condition is sometimes called 'Bornholm disease', after the Danish island where there was an extensive outbreak in 1930. There is pain and inflammation involving intercostal or abdominal muscles.

Influenza (especially influenza B in children) can cause pain and tenderness in muscles, but it is not known whether this is associated with viral invasion of muscle. Myalgias are also seen in dengue and in rickettsial and other febrile infections and are probably caused by circulating cytokines.

Coxsackievirus may be isolated from throat swabs, fecal specimens or occasionally pericardial fluid. Rising titers of neutralizing antibody or the presence of IgM antibodies in ELISA may be demonstrable.

There are no specific treatments and no vaccines for coxsackievirus infections.

Postviral fatigue syndrome
It has been difficult to establish postviral fatigue syndrome as a clinical entity

The postviral fatigue syndrome or chronic fatigue syndrome is sometimes referred to as myalgic encephalomyelitis, but this is inappropriate because there is no evidence for CNS pathology. It consists of:

* Chronic and severe muscle weakness, lasting at least six months, often as a sequel to an acute febrile illness.
* Severe tiredness.
* Less regularly associated symptoms such as depression, headache and anxiety.

It is more reliably identified when the first two symptoms appear in a previously healthy individual with no history of psychosomatic illness. Several viruses have been suggested as causes. A small proportion of cases appear to be due to chronic infection with Epstein–Barr virus (EBV). There have been repeated claims for the role of coxsackie B viruses, based on antibody tests and on the detection of a virus-specific protein in the serum of patients, but these results have not been widely confirmed and the picture remains unclear. Occasional reports have associated the condition with HHV6 and with other viruses. It has also been suggested that it is due to 'allergic reactions' triggered by virus infection.

Parasitic Infections of Muscle

Relatively few parasites commonly invade muscle tissues or cause serious disease. Three are described here to illustrate the variety of organisms and the range of pathology.

Trypanosoma cruzi infection
Trypanosoma cruzi is a protozoan and causes Chagas' disease

Chagas' disease is also known as American trypanosomiasis (see Chapter 25). The disease is restricted to Central and South America, where it affects an estimated 10–12 million people. It is a zoonosis, and *Trypanosoma cruzi* has been isolated from more than 150 species of mammal. The parasite is carried by blood-sucking bugs, which deposit infective trypomastigote stages on to the skin as they defecate while feeding. If these are rubbed into mucous membranes or wounds, the parasites penetrate cells, transform into amastigotes and proliferate. The infected cells then burst, liberating trypomastigotes, and a local lesion is formed. The parasite is dispersed around the body to reinvade other cells. Major sites of infection include the CNS, intestinal myenteric plexus, reticuloendothelial system and cardiac muscle.

Chagas' disease is complicated by heart failure many years later

Disease occurs as an acute febrile phase, with intense inflammatory changes, and as a chronic phase that becomes apparent years later. In the chronic phase there is gradual tissue destruction with autoimmune damage playing an important role. The parasite invades the myofibrils of the heart (see *Fig. 25.19*), and muscle fibrils and Purkinje fibers may be replaced by fibrous tissue. As a result of the conduction defects this causes, the heart enlarges, there are cardiac arrhythmias and heart failure can occur. Enlargement of the esophagus and colon is sometimes seen, due to destruction of nerve cells in the myenteric plexus.

Nifurtimox is used to treat the acute phase, but the chronic disease is irreversible. At present no vaccine is available, and prevention of infection is the most important measure.

Taenia solium infection
The larval stages of Taemia solium may invade body tissues

Tapeworms are intestinal parasites, but the larval stages of a number of species may invade deeper tissues. The most important of these are the larvae of:
- *Echinococcus granulosus* (which causes hydatid disease, see Chapter 31).
- The pork tapeworm *Taemia solium*.

Humans acquire *T. solium* infection by eating undercooked infected pig meat in which the cysticercus larvae are found as small, bladder-like structures in the muscle tissue. These larvae are digested out from surrounding muscle in the intestine and mature into the adult tapeworm, which may reach a length of several metres. *T. solium* is unusual in that its eggs can hatch directly in the human intestine. This may result from accidental swallowing of water contaminated with eggs, but can occur directly from the eggs released by adult worms. If hatching occurs, the larvae cross the intestinal wall and are carried via the blood to internal organs. Sites of development include the CNS and body muscles. In the latter, the cysts eventually become calcified and can be seen on radiography (*Fig. 23.49*). Muscle infection is not serious, being largely asymptomatic. Infections are common in many parts of the world, particularly South and Central America and Asia. Avoidance of undercooked pork products is the safest precaution and infections can be treated with praziquantel.

Trichinella spiralis infection
The larvae of Trichinella spiralis invade striated muscle

The life cycle of this nematode has many unique features. The parasite is able to infect almost any warm-blooded animal, and has a life cycle in which a complete generation (infective stage to infective stage) develops within the body of a single host. Transmission depends upon the ingestion of muscle tissue containing viable infective larvae. As far as humans are concerned, the commonest route of transmission is through infected pig meat, but many other meat sources have been known to transmit infection (e.g. bear, boar, horse). Infections occur worldwide. When infected undercooked meat is eaten, the larvae are digested out from surrounding muscle in the small intestine and develop rapidly into the adult worms. These live in the mucosa, the females releasing newborn larvae directly into the intestinal tissues, from where the larvae are carried in blood or lymph around the body. Eventually the larvae penetrate striated muscles where they mature into the infective stage, transforming muscle cells into a parasite-sustaining nurse cell (see *Fig. 26.14*).

Light infections are asymptomatic, but the migration and penetration of the larvae is associated with inflammatory reactions, which can be severe and life-threatening when a person is heavily infected. A variety of symptoms are associated with this phase, of which fever, muscle pains, weakness and eosinophilia are characteristic. Myocarditis may also occur, although the parasite does not develop in the heart.

The muscle stage of infection can be treated with mebendazole; corticosteroids may also be required.

Joint and Bone Infections

Joints and bones will be considered separately for convenience, but joint lesions often spread to involve neighboring bone, and vice versa (e.g. in tuberculosis).

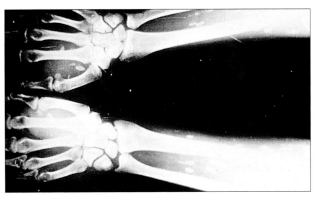

Fig. 23.49 Radiograph showing numerous calcified cysts of *Taenia solium* in the forearms. (Courtesy of R Muller and JR Baker.)

Reactive arthritis, arthralgia and septic arthritis

Arthralgia and arthritis occur in a variety of infections and are often immunologically mediated

Examples of such infections are outlined in *Figure 23.50*. Joints can become infected by the hematogenous route or directly following trauma or surgery, but in many cases the condition is immunologically mediated rather than due to microbial invasion of the joint. The microbe responsible is at a distant site in the body and causes a 'reactive arthritis'. Reactive arthritis and arthralgia occur after certain enteric bacterial infections, and the arthralgia in rubella and hepatitis B infections is of similar origin. In this type of arthritis more than one joint is usually affected.

Ankylosing spondylitis is associated with *Klebsiella* infection and it has been suggested that the antigenic similarity between *Klebsiella* and HLA B27 antigens provokes a cross-reactive immune response that causes the disease. So far there is no evidence that rheumatoid arthritis is caused by either viruses or other microbes.

Circulating bacteria sometimes localize in joints, especially following trauma

Such bacterial localization can then cause a suppurative (septic) arthritis. Generally a single joint is involved. Joints are very susceptible, particularly if they are already damaged for instance by rheumatoid arthritis, or if a prosthesis has been inserted. Knees are most commonly affected, followed by hips, ankles (see *Fig. 19.12b*) and elbows. Signs include a fever, joint pain, limitation of movement and swelling, and usually a joint effusion. Bacteria can be isolated from the joint fluid or seen in the centrifuged deposit, and the commonest organism is *Staph. aureus*. Sometimes the source of the circulating bacteria is obvious (e.g. a septic skin lesion), but often no source is apparent.

ARTHRALGIA AND ARTHRITIS IN INFECTIOUS DISEASES		
	infectious agent	**comments**
viral arthritis	hepatitis B	occurs in prodromal period; due to circulating immune complexes
	rubella	especially in young women, often follows live virus vaccine
	mumps	unusual, mostly in men
	Ross River and other togaviruses	mosquito-transmitted infections in Australia (Ross River) and Africa
	parvovirus	may follow adult infection
reactive arthritis	*Campylobacter, Yersinia,* salmonellae, shigellae, *Chlamydia trachomatis* (Reiter's syndrome*)	'post-infectious' arthritis, HLA B27-associated, no bacterial invasion of joint, immune mediated
septic arthritis	*Staphylococcus aureus*	commonest cause of suppurative arthritis
	salmonellae	occurs in children
	Haemophilus influenzae	occurs in children
	Neisseria gonorrhoeae	may affect multiple joints
	Mycobacterium tuberculosis	often with bone lesions, especially weight bearing joints and bones
	Borrelia burgdorferi	arthritis a late feature of Lyme disease
	streptococci, *Pseudomonas aeruginosa*	uncommon
	Mycoplasma hominis	bacteria can enter maternal blood during delivery and invade joints; uncommon
	Sporothrix schenckii	fungal infection of joints
* urethritis, arthritis, uveitis ± mucocutaneous lesions; complicates 1–2% of cases of chlamydial urethritis		

Fig. 23.50 Arthralgia and arthritis in infectious diseases.

Osteomyelitis
Bone can become infected by adjacent infection or hematogenously

As with joints, infection can be by the direct route (e.g. from a nearby focus of infection, after fractures, after orthopedic surgery) or from circulating microbes. The commonest cause of hematogenous osteomyelitis is *Staph. aureus*, but when infection is from a neighboring site it is generally mixed, with Gram-negative rods and occasionally anaerobes also present. There seems to be no equivalent to reactive arthritis, in which inflammation is due to infection at a distant site.

Acute osteomyelitis typically involves the growing end of a long bone, where sprouting capillary loops adjacent to epi-physeal growth plates promote the localization of circulating bacteria. It therefore tends to be a disease of children and ado-lescents, and may follow non-penetrating injury to the bone.

Osteomyelitis results in a painful tender bone lesion and a general febrile illness.

Osteomyelitis is treated with antibiotics and sometimes surgery

The infection is diagnosed from blood cultures taken before the start of antimicrobial therapy or if there is an open lesion, from a bone biopsy. Periosteal reaction and bone loss may be visible radiologically *(Fig. 23.51)*. Treatment is begun on a 'most likely' basis (cloxacillin for penicillinase-producing *Staph. aureus*) as soon as microbio-logic samples have been taken.

Osteomyelitis can become chronic, especially when there are necrotic bone fragments to act as a continued source of

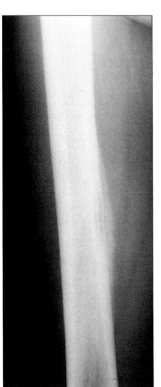

Fig. 23.51 Acute staphylococcal osteomyelitis in the femur of a 24-year-old woman. There is a well-defined periosteal reaction in relation to the midshaft of the femur and an underlying lucency. (Courtesy of AM Davies.)

infection. Surgical intervention for debridement and drainage, as well as prolonged courses of antibiotics, may be necessary.

Tuberculosis may affect the spine, the hip, the knee and the bones of the hands and feet, and in developed countries is particularly seen in immigrants from the Indian subconti-nent. Constitutional disturbances are often absent, but the site is generally painful and pressure from a tuberculous abscess in the spine can cause paraplegia.

Infections of the Hemopoietic System

Many infectious agents cause changes in circulating blood cells
Examples of such agents include:
* *Bordetella pertussis*, which causes lymphocytosis.
* EBV and cytomegaloviruses, which cause mononucleosis.
* Plasmodia, which cause anemia and thrombocytopenia.

A smaller number of infectious agents act directly on cells in the bone marrow (human parvovirus) or cause malignant transformation of lymphocytes – for example human T cell lymphotropic virus (HTLV) type 1 and HTLV2. The range of possibilities is summarized in *Figure 23.52*. HTLV1 and 2 are mentioned in Chapters 19 and 22, but are described more fully below.

HTLV1 infection
HTLV1 is mainly transmitted by maternal milk
HTLV1 was first isolated in 1980 from a patient with adult T cell leukemia. Infection is widespread, especially in certain islands in the West Indies and Japan where 5–15% of the population are seropositive, and also in South America and parts of Africa. Transmission is primarily via maternal milk, less effectively via homosexual and heterosexual routes, and by blood in intravenous drug misusers.

HTLV1 infects T cells and up to 5% of those infected develop T cell leukemia
As HTLV1 infects T cells blood is infectious. In addition, the infection is persistent. The tax (transcriptional activator) protein (coded by the pxV region of the viral genome) stim-ulates transcription of host genes controlling production of interleukin-2 (IL-2), IL-2 receptor and other molecules. Infected T cells proliferate, and if in addition there are certain chromosomal abnormalities, malignant transformation takes place.

Clinically, the patient develops a mild febrile disease with lymphadenopathy. The skin is often involved (nodules, plaques) and pleural effusion or aseptic meningitis can occur. There is also increased susceptibility to opportunist infections (*Pneumocystis carinii*, cytomegalovirus) associ-ated with depressed delayed hypersensitivity responses to tuberculin. Polymyositis has been described. Up to 5% of infected individuals eventually develop T cell leukemia, and others (about the same proportion) progress to 'tropical' spastic paraparesis, a myelopathy in which there is primary demyelination (see Chapter 22). Neural cells do not appear to be infected and it is not known how the virus causes a neurologic disease.

HTLV1-specific antibodies are demonstrable, but false positive results can occur. Retrovir inhibits viral replication, but is not known to influence the leukemia or the myelopathy once they have appeared. Seropositive individuals are assumed to be infectious and should not donate blood or organs.

HTLV2 infection

HTLV2 was first isolated in 1982 from a patient with T cell hairy leukemia, although it is not the usual cause of this condition. HTLV2 is closely related to HTLV1, and is not distinguishable by routine laboratory tests. Almost nothing is known of its distribution, transmission or natural history.

MICROBES AFFECTING BLOOD CELLS OR HEMOPOIESIS			
microbe	**disease**	**effect**	**mechanism**
Plasmodium spp.	malaria	anemia	replication in erythrocytes
Babesia spp.	babesiosis (uncommon, tick-borne)	anemia	replication in erythrocytes
Bartonella brucelliformis	oroya fever* (rare, sandfly-transmitted, occurs in Peru)	anemia	replication in erythrocytes
Ehrlichia sp. (Rickettsiae)	human Ehrlichiosis (tick transmitted in Southern USA and Japan)	leucopenia thrombocytopenia	replication in leukocytes
human parvovirus	erythema infectiosum	temporary fall in hemoglobin levels (adult) aplastic crisis (child with chronic anemia)	replication in erythropoietic cells
Colorado tick fever virus	Colorado tick fever	no effect on survival of infected erythrocytes	replication in erythropoietic cells
human T cell lymphotropic virus (HTLV)1, HTLV2	T cell leukemia, lymphoma	malignant transformation of infected T cells	replication in T cells
HIV **	AIDS	immunosuppression	infection of CD4-positive T cells
Epstein-Barr virus (EBV)	infectious mononucleosis	thrombocytopenia (common) anemia (complication)	autoantibody to platelets, erythrocytes
cytomegalovirus (CMV)	congenital CMV complication of adult infection	anemia, thrombocytopenia	infection of, or autoantibody to, erythrocytes, platelets

*a cutaneous form (Verrugas) also occurs; in 1885 a Peruvian medical student, Daniel Carrion, demonstrated the common bacterial origin by inoculating himself with infected blood from the cutaneous form of the disease and developing oroya fever

** many other viruses infect immune cells and depress immune responses less dramatically (e.g. CMV, measles)

Fig. 23.52 Microbes affecting blood cells or hemopoiesis.

- The intact skin is an invaluable barrier that defends the body against invasion.
- A wide range of organisms is associated with skin infection and disease.
- Bacteria, fungi and viruses usually gain access through breaches of the barrier caused by trauma.
- Some parasites initiate their own penetration into the skin (leptospirosis, schistosomiasis).
- Other microbes are introduced into the skin by arthropod vectors.
- Once in the skin, microbes cause local infections or disseminate through the body to distant sites.
- Pathogens may be acquired by other routes, disseminate in the body and then localize in the skin or cause toxic or immunopathologic manifestations in the skin.

- Superficial infections of the skin are among the commonest human infections (boils, impetigo, warts, acne, ringworm).
- Invasion of pathogens deeper into dermal and subdermal tissues may produce severe infections that can be rapidly fatal, as in gangrene, or slow but progressive deformation and destruction, as in leprosy.
- Infections of muscle usually arise from invasion from the outside whereas infections of joints are more often bloodborne.
- Bone infections may arise either by local spread from an infected joint or as a result of hematogenous seeding.
- Bone marrow cells or leukocytes may be invaded by viruses that interfere with hemopoiesis (parvovirus), cause malignant transformation (HTLV1 and 2), or interfere with the immune system (EBV, HIV).

A four-year-old boy has been referred to the clinic with a history of a painful arm. He fell while on a climbing frame five days ago and lacerated his right forearm. He has become more unwell in the last 24 hours with a fever, vomiting and abdominal pain. On examination he is miserable, dehydrated and feverish. His right forearm is exquisitely tender over the area of the wound. His abdomen is tender, but there is no rebound tenderness or guarding. His chest is clear.

1. What is the likely diagnosis?
2. What investigations would you perform?
3. The results of investigations are hemoglobin 15 g/dl and white cell count 24×10^9/l with 90% neutrophils, and blood cultures grow *Staph. aureus* sensitive to flucloxacillin. A radiograph of the forearm shows soft tissue swelling over the affected area of the forearm.

A two-year-old girl develops a fine erythematous rash together with the sudden onset of a high fever. She is up to date with her immunisation schedule and her doctor sees her at home.

On examination she is unwell with a fever and rash. There are no other findings of note.

1. What is the differential diagnosis?
2. The diagnosis is invariably a clinical diagnosis, but if this child is admitted to hospital she may be further investigated. What investigations would you perform if she is admitted?

A 35-year-old man sees his doctor with a two-day history of a painful swollen left knee joint. He is a regular rugby player and thinks that he may have twisted his leg while playing the previous weekend. He also reported a slight feeling of 'flu' with some generalized aching and fever. He is normally healthy.

On examination he is flushed and his temperature is 37.8°C. His left knee is red and tender to touch. There is some swelling in the soft tissues. Movements in all directions are limited by pain. There are no palpable lymph nodes. The rest of the examination is normal.

1. What are the most common infectious causes of acute monoarthritis.
2. What other points may be helpful in the history?
3. How is the diagnosis made?
4. What would you advise on treatment?

Further Reading

Bisno AL, Stevens DL. Streptococcal infections of skin and soft tissues. *N Engl J Med* 1996;**334**:240.

Demeter LM, Reichman RC. Human papillomavirus. *Curr Opin Infect Dis* 1990;**3**:796–804.

Jones HE, Reinhardt JH, Renaldi MG. Acquired immunity to dermatophytes. *Arch Dermatol* 1974;**109**:840.

Miller AE. Selective decline in cellular immune response to varicella–zoster in the elderly. *Neurology* 1980;**30**:582–587.

Roth RR, James WD. Microbial ecology of the skin. *Ann Rev Microbiol* 1988;**42**:411–464.

Rous BT. Herpes simplex virus; pathogenesis, immunobiology, and control. *Curr Topics Microbiol Immunol* 1992;**179**:1–179.

Straus SE, Ostrove JM, Inchauspé G. Varicella–zoster virus infections: Biology, natural history, treatment and prevention. *Ann Int Med* 1988;**108**:221–237.

Swartz MN. The chronic fatigue syndrome – one entity or many? *N Engl J Med* 1988;**319**:1726–1727.

Introduction

The infectious agents described in the previous chapters characteristically cause diseases in which damage and symptoms predominate in a particular part of the body, even though spread to other systems may occur. Thus, tuberculosis, typhoid and syphilis are considered in chapters on the respiratory tract, intestine and urinogenital tract, respectively, these being the main sites involved in infection and/or transmission. Many other microbes cannot be so easily pigeon-holed.

Some important and common virus infections cause diseases that are not localized to any one body system

These multisystem infections are discussed in this chapter. The viruses described occur in all parts of the world, and are exclusively human infections. Some of them, like the viruses included in Chapter 23 such as herpes simplex virus (HSV), varicella-zoster virus (VZV) and human papillomavirus (HPV), cause skin rashes (exanthems), but the ones described in this chapter differ because they are not primarily dermatotropic. Most of them involve young children, but some such as mumps and Epstein–Barr virus (EBV) cause more severe illness when primary infection takes place during adolescence or adult life. This is more common in developed countries, especially with EBV, where individuals often escape infection during childhood. Some (measles, mumps, rubella) are readily controllable by vaccines, but so far this has been achieved only in developed countries.

Measles

Measles has several special features. These are as follows:

- Nearly all infected individuals become unwell and develop disease. This is in contrast to most other viral infections, in which a significant proportion of individuals undergo an asymptomatic or subclinical infection.
- The disease is so characteristic that a clinical diagnosis can nearly always be made without the need for laboratory help. We can recognize measles as described one thousand years ago by the Arabian physician Rhazes.
- There is only one antigenic type of measles virus.
- After infection there is complete resistance to reinfection, which is probably life-long. Second attacks are almost unknown.
- Measles is highly infectious, and nearly all susceptible children contract the disease on exposure. Until recently measles was regarded as a routine inescapable part of childhood, and more than 99% of individuals were infected.
- There is a striking contrast between measles in well-nourished children with good access to medical care (i.e. in developed countries) and measles under conditions of malnutrition or starvation or with poor medical services (i.e. developing countries, *Fig. 24.1*).

Etiology and transmission
Measles outbreaks occur every few years in unvaccinated populations

The basic virology of this paramyxovirus is described in Chapter 3 and in the Appendix (see p. 000). Transmission takes place readily via respiratory droplets. Although the virus is soon inactivated as it dries on surfaces, it is more stable in droplets suspended in the air. In unvaccinated populations, outbreaks tend to occur every few years when the number of susceptible children reaches a high enough level.

Clinical features of measles include respiratory symptoms, Koplik's spots and a rash

The pathogenesis of measles is illustrated in Chapter 13. The inhaled virus enters the body at unknown sites in the upper or lower respiratory tract and spreads to subepithelial and local lymphatic tissues, without causing detectable lesions or symptoms. During the next few days the virus slowly spreads and multiplies in lymphoid tissues elsewhere in the body, including the spleen. The virus then enters the blood in larger amounts and about one week after infection is seeded out to a variety of epithelial sites. Clinical signs soon appear in the respiratory tract where there are only one or two layers of epithelial cells to traverse. The patient is well until 9–10 days after infection and then develops an acute respiratory illness with a runny nose, fever and cough. Conjunctivitis is also a feature and as a result of the large amounts of virus being shed in respiratory secretions, the patient is highly infectious. The diagnosis may be suspected during this prodromal illness, especially after known exposure to measles. It takes a day or two longer for the foci of infection at mucosal and skin surfaces to cause lesions. Koplik's spots appear inside the cheek *(Fig. 24.2)*, and shortly afterwards the unmistakable maculopapular rash *(Fig. 24.3)* is seen, first on the face, then spreading down the body to the extremities. The diagnosis is now clear.

Measles rash results from a cell-mediated immune response

Antibodies are formed, but a cell-mediated immune (CMI) response is needed to control the growth of virus in the lungs and elsewhere. Without it the virus continues to grow and gives rise to giant cell pneumonia (see Chapter 16). The CMI response is also responsible for the skin lesions, which

CLINICAL IMPACT OF MEASLES

site of virus growth	well-nourished child good medical care	malnourished child poor medical care
lung	temporary respiratory illness	life-threatening pneumonia
ear	otitis media quite common	otitis media more common more severe
oral mucosa	Koplik's spots	severe ulcerating lesions
conjunctiva	conjunctivitis	severe corneal lesions secondary bacterial infection blindness may result
skin	maculopapular rash	hemorrhagic rashes may occur ('black measles')
intestinal tract	no lesions	diarrhea – exacerbates malnutrition, halts growth, impairs recovery
urinary tract	virus detectable in urine	no known complications
overall impact	**serious disease in a small proportion of those infected**	**major cause of death in childhood (estimated one million deaths/year worldwide)**

Fig. 24.1 The clinical impact of measles depends upon the host. Measles is a much more serious disease in malnourished children with poor access to medical care. The same epithelial surfaces are infected, but more extensively and with more serious sequelae.

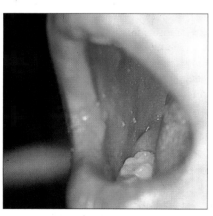

Fig. 24.2 Koplik's spots seen as minute white dots on the inflamed buccal mucosa of a patient with measles. (Courtesy of MJ Wood.)

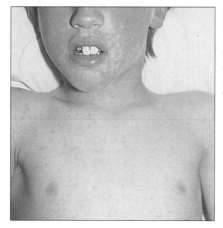

Fig. 24.3 Maculopapular rash on the face and trunk of a patient with measles. (Courtesy of MJ Wood.)

are not seen in patients with serious defects in this type of immunity. Children with agammaglobulinemia, on the other hand, have a normal course of disease, develop normal immunity, and can be protected by vaccination. In uncomplicated cases recovery is rapid.

During measles, as in a variety of other acute infections, there are temporary defects in immune responses to unrelated antigens. For instance, at about the time the rash appears, individuals who are known to be tuberculin-positive give negative skin test responses to tuberculin. This returns to normal in about a month. During the 'virgin-soil' epidemic, when measles reappeared after a long absence in Southern Greenland, in 1953, and adults as well as children were infected, there was increased mortality in those previously infected with tuberculosis.

Complications of measles are particularly likely among children in developing countries

Complications of measles include:

- Opportunistic bacterial superinfections, which are quite common, especially otitis media and pneumonia, as a result of virus damage to respiratory surfaces.
- A primary measles virus pneumonia (giant cell pneumonia), which is seen in patients with serious CMI response defects.
- Encephalitis, which occurs in about 1 in 1000 cases (see Chapter 27);
- Very rarely, subacute sclerosing panencephalitis (SSPE). This develops 1–10 years after apparent recovery from acute infection.

Children in countries where there is poor medical care and malnutrition develop a more serious disease *(Fig. 24.1)*, especially during famine. This is attributable to:

- Poor local mucosal defenses, which can be improved by vitamin A administration.
- Impaired immune defenses due to protein–calorie malnutrition, with the added impact of measles virus-induced immunosuppression.
- Poor medical services, with less ready availability of antibiotics to control secondary infection.
- High levels of bacterial contamination of the environment.
- Exposure to a larger virus dose – a possible factor if others with severe measles shed larger amounts of virus from the respiratory tract.

Diagnosis, treatment and prevention

Measles is usually diagnosed clinically, there is no antiviral treatment but there is a vaccine

Greater than fourfold rises in antibody titer can be detected in difficult cases. Virus isolation in cell culture is rarely necessary.

A live attenuated vaccine has been available since 1963. It is effective, safe and long-lasting, and is combined with mumps and rubella vaccines (MMR vaccine; see Chapter 31). Before a vaccine became available, measles killed 7–8 million children each year worldwide. This has now (1996) been reduced to one million, and if the mass immunization programs used in the Americas and Europe are applied to developing countries, the World Health Organization (WHO) suggests that measles could be eliminated from the world by the year 2010.

Mumps

Mumps virus is spread by intimate contact and infects the salivary glands

There is only one serotype of this single-stranded RNA paramyxovirus. It spreads by airborne droplets, salivary secretions and possibly urine. Intimate contact is necessary, either at school (peak incidence is at 5–14 years of age) or in crowded adult communities (e.g. prisons, garrisons, ships).

After entry into the body at unknown sites, probably in the upper respiratory tract, the virus spreads systemically, undergoing a lengthy period of growth in lymphoid tissues (lymphocytes and monocytes) and reticuloendothelial cells. After approximately 7–10 days the virus re-enters the blood and localizes in salivary and other glands (Fig. 24.4). Infected cells lining the ducts degenerate and finally, after an incubation period of 18–21 days, the inflammation, with lymphocyte infiltration and often edema, results in disease. After a prodromal period of malaise and anorexia lasting 1–2 days, the parotid gland becomes painful, tender and swollen, and is sometimes accompanied by submandibular gland involvement (Fig. 24.5). This is the classic sign of mumps although it is present only in 30–40% of infections. CMI as well as antibody responses appear, and the patient usually recovers within one week. There is life-long resistance to reinfection. However, other tissues in the body may be invaded, with clinical consequences as outlined in Figure 24.6.

Mumps is diagnosed on the basis of parotitis—there is no specific treatment, but there is a vaccine

Laboratory diagnosis is made:
- By isolating virus in cell culture from saliva, cerebrospinal fluid (CSF) or urine.
- By detecting a greater than fourfold rise in antibody, mumps-specific IgM antibody and complement fixing (CF) antibody to the soluble, nucleocapsid (S) mumps antigen. These antibodies disappear within months and suggest recent infection. CF antibody to the viral envelope (V) antigen persists for years.

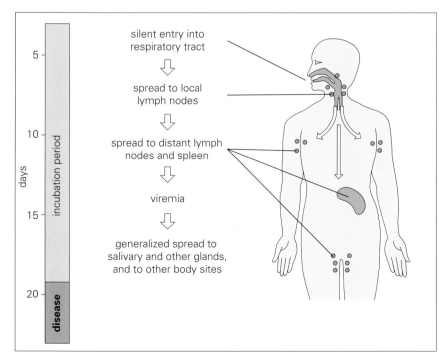

Fig. 24.4 The pathogenesis of mumps. Understanding the pathogenesis of this infection helps to explain the disease picture, sites of shedding and the complications that can arise, but little is known about the events that occur during the first week of infection.

Treatment and prevention

There is no specific treatment, but mumps is prevented by a single injection of attenuated live virus vaccine, which is safe and effective. This is usually given in combination with measles and rubella vaccines (MMR vaccine).

Rubella

Rubella virus infection causes a multisystem infection, but its main impact is on the fetus

There is only one serotype of this single-stranded RNA togavirus and its principal impact is on the fetus (see Chapter 21). It is transmitted by droplet infection, and is less contagious than measles, but more so than mumps.

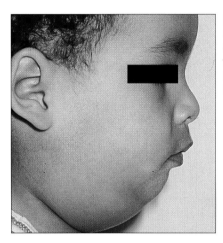

Fig. 24.5 Enlarged submandibular glands in a child with mumps. (Courtesy of JA Innes.)

After entering the body silently at unknown sites in the respiratory tract, the virus grows for a period in local lymphoid tissues, followed by spread to the spleen and to lymph nodes elsewhere in the body. One week after infection further multiplication in these tissues leads to viremia and localization of virus in the respiratory tract and skin, and sometimes the placenta, joints, and kidney. The pathogenesis of rubella is outlined in *Figure 24.7* and the clinical consequences of infection in various tissues of the body are shown in *Figure 24.8*. After an incubation period of 14–21 days there is a mild disease, with fever, malaise and an irregular maculopapular rash lasting three days. Enlarged lymph nodes are often evident behind the ear, but the infection is commonly subclinical.

Rubella is diagnosed serologically—there is no treatment, but there is a vaccine

Clinical diagnosis of rubella is sometimes possible. Laboratory diagnosis is made by demonstrating rubella-specific IgM antibodies or a fourfold or greater rise in radioimmunoassay (RIA) or enzyme-linked immunosorbent assay (ELISA) antibodies (see Chapter 14). Virus isolation from the throat is rarely indicated – the virus fails to damage cells in culture and indirect methods are needed to demonstrate its growth.

There is no antiviral treatment. A live attenuated rubella vaccine that is safe and effective is given by injection, generally in combination with measles and mumps vaccines (MMR vaccine). Prevention of congenital rubella is referred to in Chapter 21.

PATHOGENESIS OF MUMPS		
site of growth	**result**	**comment**
salivary glands	inflammation, parotitis virus shed in saliva (from three days before to six days after symptoms)	often absent; can be unilateral
meninges brain	meningitis ⎤ ⎬ up to seven days after parotitis encephalitis ⎦	common (in about 10% cases) less common; complete recovery is the rule; deafness is a rare complication
kidney	virus present in urine	no clinical consequences
testis, ovary	epididymo-orchitis; rigid tunica albuginea around testis makes orchitis more painful and more damaging in male	common in adults (20% in adult males); often unilateral; not a significant cause of sterility
pancreas	pancreatitis	rare complication (possible role in juvenile diabetes mellitus)
mammary gland	virus detectable in milk; mastitis in 10% post-pubertal females	–
thyroid	thyroiditis	rare
myocardium	myocarditis	rare
joints	arthritis	rare

Fig. 24.6 Clinical consequences of mumps virus invasion of different body tissues.

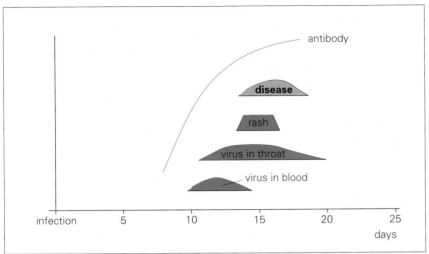

Fig. 24.7 The pathogenesis of rubella. Rubella is generally a very mild, often subclinical infection, but it can cause arthritis and has a major impact when it infects the fetus.

PATHOGENESIS OF RUBELLA		
site of virus growth	**result**	**comment**
respiratory tract	virus shedding but symptoms minimal (mild sore throat, coryza, cough)	patient infectious five days before to three days after symptoms
skin	rash	often fleeting, atypical; immunopathology involved (Ag–Ab complexes)
lymph nodes	lymphadenopathy	more common in posterior triangle of neck or behind ear
joints	mild arthralgia, arthritis	immunopathology involved (circulating immune complexes)
placenta/fetus	placentitis fetal damage	congenital rubella

Fig. 24.8 Clinical consequences of rubella virus invasion of different body tissues.

Cytomegalovirus Infection

Cytomegalovirus can be transmitted by saliva, urine, blood, semen and cervical secretions

Cytomegalovirus (CMV) is the largest human herpesvirus (HHV) *(Fig. 24.9)*, and there is only one serotype. As with animal CMVs it is species specific; humans are the natural hosts and animal CMVs do not infect humans. The name refers to the multinucleated cells, which together with the intranuclear inclusions, are characteristic responses to infection with this virus. Transmission is via saliva, and CMVs were originally called 'salivary gland' viruses.

Urine is an additional source of infection in children, and in infected pregnant women the virus can spread via the blood to the placenta and fetus. Semen and cervical secretions may also contain virus and it can therefore be spread by sexual contact. It is often present in milk in small quantities, but this is of doubtful significance in transmission. In hospitals it can be transmitted by blood transfusions and organ transplants.

CMV infection is often asymptomatic, but can reactivate and cause disease when CMI defenses are impaired

After clinically silent infection of unknown cells in the upper respiratory tract, CMV spreads locally to lymphoid tissues

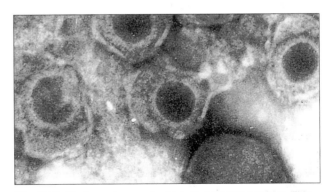

Fig. 24.9 Electron micrograph of cytomegalovirus particles. This is the largest human herpesvirus, with a diameter of 150–200nm, and a dense DNA core. (Courtesy of DK Banerjee.)

and then systemically in circulating lymphocytes and mono-cytes to involve lymph nodes and the spleen. The infection then localizes in epithelial cells in salivary glands and kidney tubules, and in cervix, testes and epididymis, from where the virus is shed to the outside world *(Fig. 24.10).*

Infected cells may be multinucleated or bear intranuclear inclusions, but pathologic changes are minor and infection is generally asymptomatic. In young adults, a glandular fever type illness can occur, but without heterophil anti-bodies (see below). There is fever and lethargy, and abnor-mal lymphocytes and mononucleosis in blood smears. The virus inhibits T cell responses and there is a temporary reduction in their immune reactivity to other antigens.

Although specific antibodies and CMI responses are gen-erated, these fail to clear the virus (see Chapter 11), which often continues to be shed in saliva and urine for many months. The infection is, however, eventually controlled by CMI mechanisms, although infected cells remain in the body throughout life and can be a source of reactivation and disease when CMI defenses are impaired.

CMV owes its success in our species to its ability to evade immune defenses. For instance, it presents a poor target for Tc by interfering with the transprt of major histocompati-bility complex (MHC) class 1 molecules to the cell surface (see Chapter 9), and it induces Fc receptors on infected cells (see Chapter 11).

CMV infection can cause fetal malformations and pneumonia in immunodeficient patients

In the natural host, the human infant or child, CMV causes no illness and at most a mild illness in adults. Two circum-stances, however, interfere with this harmonious host–para-site balance:

- Primary infection during pregnancy allows spread of virus from the blood to the placenta and then to the fetus resulting in congenital abnormalities as described in Chapter 21. Reactivation of infection during pregnancy also occurs and leads to fetal infection, but rarely to con-genital abnormalities.
- In immunodeficient patients such as bone marrow or kid-ney transplant recipients and AIDS patients (see Chapter 28), CMV infection causes an interstitial pneumonia with infiltrating infected mononuclear cells. Focal cerebral 'micronodular' lesions, again with infected mononuclear cells, also occur, together with a variety of other compli-cations, including retinitis.

Clinical diagnosis of primary infection is rarely possible, because it is so commonly asymptomatic. The virus can be isolated in cell culture from the throat or urine. This gener-ally takes a few days, the viral antigens being identified in cells by fluorescent antibody staining. In lung biopsies mult-inucleated cells or cells with prominent intranuclear inclu-sions may be seen. Antibody tests (fourfold or greater rise) can also be used.

Ganciclovir is often effective treatment of CMV retinitis and pneumonia

While ganciclovir or dihydroxypropoxymethylguanine (DHPG, ganciclovir) is often an effective treatment, acyclovir is ineffective.

There is no vaccine, but trials of live and inactivated vac-cines have been carried out. Contact between congenitally-infected children and susceptible pregnant women should be avoided. Blood for transfusion of newborns, and kidneys and bone marrow for transplantation, should preferably come from CMV antibody-negative donors.

CYTOMEGALOVIRUS (CMV) INFECTION		
site of infection	**result**	**comment**
salivary glands	salivary transmission	importance of kissing and contaminated hands
tubular epithelium of kidney	virus in urine	probable role in transmission
cervix testis/epididymis	sexual transmission	up to 10^7 infectious doses/ml of semen in an acutely infected male
lymphocytes macrophages	virus spread through body via infected cells mononucleosis may occur immunosuppressive effect	probable site of persistent infection
placenta fetus	congenital abnormalities	greatest damage in fetus after primary maternal infection rather than reactivation

Fig. 24.10 The effects of cytomegalovirus (CMV) infection. CMV is a 'well-behaved' parasite, causing little or no damage to the host unless it infects the fetus or placenta to cause congenital abnormalities or it reactivates following depressed cell-mediated immunity (post-transplant, AIDS) to cause viremia, fever, hepatitis or pneumonia.

EBV Infection

EBV is transmitted in saliva

EBV, like CMV, is species specific. EBV is structurally and morphologically identical to other herpesviruses (see Chapter 3), but is antigenically distinct. A major antigen is the viral capsid antigen (VCA) used in diagnostic tests. Other useful antigens diagnostically are the early antigens (EA) which are produced before viral DNA synthesis, and the EBV-associated nuclear antigens (EBNA), which are located in the nucleus of the infected cells. Humans are the natural hosts.

EBV is transmitted by the exchange of saliva, for instance during kissing. It is a worldwide infection. In developing countries infection takes place, probably via fingers and close contact in early childhood and is subclinical. In developed countries infection is generally delayed until adolescence or early adult life (peak incidence 15–25 years), and in most cases causes illness.

The clinical features of EBV infection are immunologically mediated

Clinical and immunologic events in EBV infection are illustrated in *Figure 24.11*. EBV replicates in B lymphocytes, after making a specific attachment to the C3d receptor (CD21) on these cells, and also in certain epithelial cells. The pathogenesis of the disease and the clinical features can be accounted for on this basis. Virus is shed in saliva from infected epithelial cells and possibly lymphocytes in salivary glands, and from the oropharynx, with clinically silent spread to B lymphocytes in local lymphoid tissues and elsewhere in the body (lymph nodes, spleen).

T lymphocytes respond immunologically to the infected B cells (outnumbering the latter by about 50 to 1) and appear in peripheral blood as 'atypical lymphocytes' *(Fig. 24.12)*. Much of the disease is attributable to an immunologic civil war, as specifically activated T cells respond to the infected B cells. In the naturally-infected infant or small child these immune responses are weak and there is generally no clinical disease. Older children, however, become unwell, and young adults especially develop infectious mononucleosis or glandular fever 4–7 weeks after initial infection. This is characterized by fever, sore throat (see Chapter 15), often with petechiae on the hard palate, lymphadenopathy and splenomegaly, with anorexia and lethargy as prominent features. Hepatitis may occur, with mild elevations of hepatocellular enzymes in 90% of cases and jaundice in 9%. Rarely there is encephalitis.

The symptoms are presumably due to the action of cytokines released during the intense immunologic activity. The infected B cells are stimulated to differentiate and produce antibodies; this polyclonal activation of B cells is responsible for the production of heterophil antibodies (reacting with erythrocytes of sheep or horses) and a variety

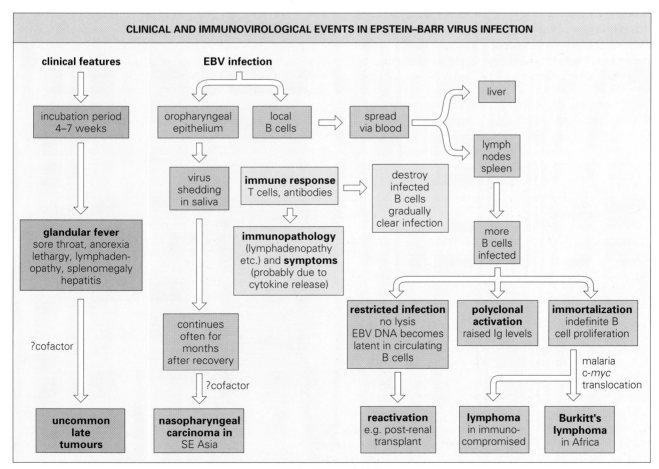

Fig. 24.11 Clinical and immunovirologic events in Epstein–Barr virus (EBV) infection in adolescents or adults. A milder, often subclinical infection occurs in children.

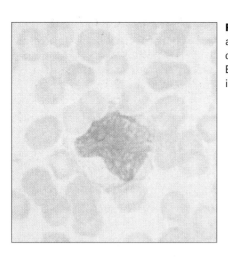

Fig. 24.12 An atypical lymphocyte characteristic of Epstein–Barr virus infection.

of autoantibodies. Spontaneous recovery usually occurs in 2–3 weeks, but the symptoms may persist for a few months. The virus stays in the body in spite of antibody and CMI responses, and saliva often remains infectious for months after clinical recovery.

The autoantibodies produced in response to EBV infection include IgM antibodies to erythrocytes (cold agglutinins), which are present in most cases. About 1% of cases develop an autoimmune hemolytic anemia, which subsides within 1–2 months.

Less than 1% of cases develop neurologic complications (aseptic meningitis, encephalitis) nearly always with complete recovery. A 'hairy tongue' condition caused by EBV replication in squamous epithelial cells in the tongue occurs in immunodeficient patients.

EBV remains latent in a small proportion of B lymphocytes

EBV is well equipped to evade immune defenses (see Chapter 11). It acts against complement and interferon, and produces a fake Il-10 molecule that interferes with the action of the hosts own Il-10 (an important immunoregulatory cytokine). EBV also prevents apoptosis (lysis) of infected cells, and the boldness of its strategy has enabled it to take up permanent residence within the immune system.

EBV DNA is present in episomal form in a small proportion of B lymphocytes and a few copies are integrated into the cell genome. Later in life, immunodeficiency can lead to reactivation of infection so that EBV reappears in the saliva, usually with no clinical symptoms; this occurs in more than 50% of renal transplant patients.

There is a variety of laboratory tests for diagnosing infectious mononucleosis

Infectious mononucleosis is diagnosed clinically by the characteristic syndrome and the appearance of the throat. Laboratory diagnosis is by:

- Demonstrating atypical lymphocytes, comprising up to 30% of nucleated cells, in a blood smear.
- Demonstrating heterophil antibodies to horse (or sheep) erythrocytes in the 'monospot' test. These are present in 90% of cases, but less commonly in infected children.

Titers fall during recovery and disappear by six months, so previous infection is not detected.
- Demonstrating EBV-specific antibody. IgM antibody to the VCA indicates current infection, and IgG antibody past infection. Antibody to the various forms of EBNA persist for life.
- Demonstrating EBV itself by cultivation of cells from clinical samples with cord blood lymphocytes and testing for transformation of the lymphocytes. This is difficult and rarely undertaken.
- Demonstrating EBV DNA by DNA hybridization or the polymerase chain reaction.

These methods are being developed and refined.

Treatment of EBV infection is limited

At present there is no reliable antiviral agent, although high doses of acyclovir are sometimes useful. There is no vaccine, but trials are in progress using various viral envelope glycoproteins.

Burkitt's lymphoma
EBV is closely associated with Burkitt's lymphoma in African children

Burkitt's lymphoma (*Fig. 24.13*) is virtually restricted to parts of Africa and Papua New Guinea, so it is clear that EBV alone is not enough to cause the lymphoma. The most likely co-carcinogen is malaria, which acts by weakening T cell control of EBV infection and perhaps by causing polyclonal activation of B cells, the increased turnover rendering them more susceptible to neoplastic transformation.

EBV is closely associated with other B cell lymphomas in immunodeficient patients

For example, B cell lymphomas occur in 1–10% of renal and heart transplant patients surviving up to 15 years, especially when primary EBV infection occurs during immunosuppression. EBV DNA and EBNA is found in the tumor

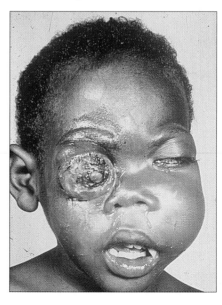

Fig. 24.13 Burkitt's lymphoma affecting the maxilla and eye in an African child. (Courtesy of DH Wright.)

cells, which also show a translocation of the *c-myc* onco-gene on chromosome 8 to the immunoglobulin heavy chain locus on chromosome 14 (see Chapter 12).

EBV infection is also closely associated with nasopharyngeal carcinoma

Nasopharyngeal carcinoma (NPC) is a very common cancer in China and Southeast Asia. EBV DNA (100 episomal copies/cell) and EBNA are detectable in the tumor cells and a co-carcinogen (possibly ingested nitrosamines from pre-served fish) is likely. Host genetic factors controlling human leukocyte antigens (HLA) and immune responses may confer susceptibility to NPC.

Other Human Herpesvirus (HHV) Infections

HHV6 is present in the saliva of over 85% of adults and causes roseola infantum

HHV6 was discovered in 1988 – the preceding 5 HHV being HSV1, HSV2, VZV, CMV and EBV – and its behavior and natural history are still being studied. Infection, which occurs in the first three years of life, is worldwide. The virus replicates in T and B cells and also in the oropharynx, from where it is shed into saliva. The virus persists in the body after initial infection.

HHV6 is the cause of exanthem subitum (or roseola infantum), a very common acute febrile illness in infants and young children. After an incubation period of about two weeks there is onset of fever which lasts for several days. The disease is mild and within two days of the fever subsiding a maculopapular rash is seen (*Fig. 24.14*).

HHV7 is present in the saliva of over 75% of adults

HHV7 has been isolated from CD4-positive T cells. Infection, as determined by seroconversion, was reported in most children but later than in the case of HHV6. The virus persists in the saliva, but it is not yet known whether it is a significant cause of disease.

HHV8 is associated with all forms of Kaposi's sarcoma

HHV8 is yet another recently discovered human herpesvirus, being detectable in the epithelial cells of Kaposi's sarcoma. It is also present in semen, especially in HIV-infected individuals, but its occurrence in the general population is unclear.

Smallpox

Smallpox (variola) was a major scourge of humankind for at least 3000 years. It was caused by a poxvirus and spread from person to person by contact with skin lesions and via the respiratory tract. The disease was severe, with a generalized rash (*Fig. 24.15*), and was fatal in up to 40% of cases, depending upon the strain of virus.

Global smallpox eradication was officially certified in December 1979

During the first part of the twentieth century smallpox was largely eradicated from Oceania, North America and Europe by widespread vaccination, as originally developed by Edward Jenner (see Chapter 31), using a live attenuated strain of

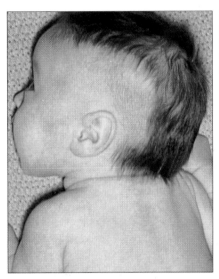

Fig. 24.14
Maculopapular rash in roseola infantum. (Courtesy of MJ Wood.)

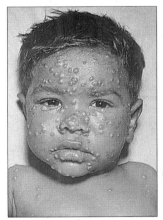
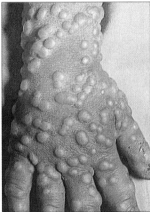
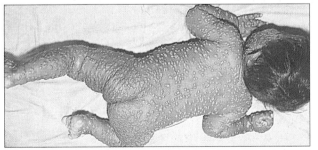

Fig. 24.15 Smallpox. These pictures were used as smallpox recognition cards by the World Health Organization during its smallpox eradication campaign. After upper respiratory tract infection, the virus reached the skin where it replicated to cause a widespread vesiculopustular rash, with later scarring, especially on the face. The fatality rate was up to 40%, depending upon the age of the host and the strain of the virus. (Courtesy of the World Health Organization.)

virus (vaccinia virus), together with strict controls at frontiers. In 1967, the WHO started a campaign to eradicate smallpox from the world, focusing on South America, Africa, India and Indonesia, making use of vaccination, surveillance and containment of cases. Despite such daunting difficulties as cultural barriers, warfare and transport to remote areas, the campaign was successful. Occasional cases had continued to occur in the USA until the 1940s, and in 1974 there were 218 000 cases worldwide, mostly in Asia, but the last case was recorded in Somalia in October 1977. The total cost to the WHO was about $US 150 million.

Global eradication of smallpox was possible for a variety of reasons

These reasons are as follows:

- There were no subclinical infections, so cases could be readily identified.
- The virus was eliminated from the body on recovery, with no carriers.
- Humans were the only host (no animal reservoir).
- An effective vaccine was available.

For a few years there were concerns about monkeypox, a simian disease caused by a similar virus and acquired by contact with infected monkeys in Africa. It is, however, poorly transmitted from human to human. It has at last been agreed that stocks of smallpox virus held in laboratories in Atlanta, USA and Moscow, Russia will be destroyed in 1997, giving sufficient time for the complete sequencing of the viral DNA.

- Measles, mumps, rubella, CMV, EBV, HHV6 and HHV7 are multisystem worldwide infections. These are essentially childhood infections and they generally have more serious consequences if infection is delayed until adolescence or adult life.
- Measles always gives rise to a detectable clinically characteristic illness, whereas mumps may be subclinical, and laboratory tests are often needed for the diagnosis of rubella, CMV and EBV infections.
- Complications in the adolescent or adult involve the central nervous system or testis (mumps), the conceptus (CMV, rubella) and the liver (EBV), and in certain parts of the world EBV infection can result in the development of lymphoma or NPC.
- Safe and effective vaccines are banishing measles, mumps, rubella, polio and many other infections from developed countries, but as long as a reservoir of these diseases remains elsewhere in the world they could reappear in force if barriers break down or immunity in the population is allowed to wane.
- Smallpox, once a major worldwide virus infection, often with fatal consequences, was eradicated from the world in 1980.

A 19-year-old philosophy student sees the college doctor because she has been feeling tired since starting her third term three weeks previously. She has been feverish and sweaty, and has had a sore throat and some abdominal discomfort. On examination she has a temperature of 38.5°C, cervical lymphadenopathy, a few palatal petechiae, an inflamed pharynx, and tender smooth splenomegaly. The results of investigations are: hemoglobin 14 g/dl; white cell count 4×10^9/l with atypical lymphocytes; alanine transaminase 300 IU/l; aspartate transaminase 350 IU/l.

1. What is the differential diagnosis?
2. How would you investigate this woman for EBV infection?
3. The results of the monospot test are as follows: agglutination with unadsorbed serum to which the indicator horse red blood cells are added; agglutination with guinea pig (antigen) cells to which horse red blood cells are added; no agglutination with OCS cells to which horse red blood cells are added; VCA IgM and EA IgM positive; EA IgG positive with a titer of 640. How would you interpret these results?
4. What are the more common complications of EBV infection?
5. What would be your advice to this patient?

Further Reading

Behbehani AM. The smallpox story: life and death of an old disease. *Microbiol Rev* 1983;**47**:455–509.

Koster FT, Curlin GC, Aziz KMA, *et al*. Synergistic impact of measles and diarrhoea on nutrition and mortality in Bangladesh. *Bull WHO* 1981;**59**:901–908.

Mach M, Stamminger T, Jahn G. Human cytomegalovirus: recent aspects from molecular biology. *J Gen Virol* 1989;**70**:3117–3146.

Masucci MG, Ernberg I. Epstein–Barr virus: adaptation to a life within the immune system. *Trends Microbiol* 1994;**2**:125–130.

Neiderman JC, Miller G, Pearson HA, *et al*. Infectious mononucleosis: EB virus shedding in saliva and oropharynx. *N Engl J Med* 1976;**294**:1355–1359.

Smith GL. Virus strategies for evasion of the host response to infection. *Trends Microbiol* 1994;**2**:81–88.

Introduction

Certain insects and arachnids inject parasites into human blood

At least 85% of all known animal species are arthropods, and among them two classes make a major contribution to disease by transmitting parasites from one individual to another. These are the six-legged 'insects' and the eight-legged 'acarine arachnids'. Their habit of feeding on human blood allows them to both ingest parasites from and inject them into the bloodstream. The most important diseases transmitted in this way are discussed in this chapter.

In sparsely populated areas transmission by insects is an effective means of spread

Disease transmission by insects has major implications for the host, the vector and the parasite. To consider the parasite first, it requires the organism to be present in the right place (in the blood) and at the right time (some insects, for example, bite only at night). Blood is an inhospitable environment and this may require quite subtle evasion mechanisms for parasite survival. In addition, the conditions found in the vector are likely to be extremely different from those in the human host, and the parasite may have to make a remarkably complex transition in a short time. With the larger protozoal and helminth parasites this transition often involves clearly visible changes in appearance and is responsible for much of the complicated nomenclature of parasite 'life cycles'. Since some insect vectors have lifespans hardly longer than those of their parasites, there is considerable wastage due to death of the vector before the parasite has matured to the infective stage for man. A difference of a few days in a mosquito's lifespan can make an enormous difference in the effectiveness of malaria transmission, and indeed this simple factor is believed to underlie much of the difference between the African pattern of endemic infection and the Indian pattern of sporadic epidemics. However, what may be lost from wastage is more than compensated for by the enormously increased distance over which dissemination of the parasite can occur.

Vector transmission of disease means that the disease may be controlled by controlling the vector

This is, however, much easier said than done, as was discovered during the attempts to eradicate malaria by dichlorodiphenyltrichloroethane (DDT) spraying of the mosquito breeding areas. In the event the mosquitoes developed resistance and more damage was done to the environment than to the insects. Nevertheless, vector control remains a highly desirable goal in relation to the diseases discussed in this chapter and is, for instance, the only reason malaria is not endemic in northern Europe.

Another potential advantage for the host is that it is sometimes possible to immunize specifically against the transmission stage of the parasite. Again malaria can serve as an example – vaccines against the gametocytes and gametes having been clearly shown to completely block transmission in animal models. Once transmission is blocked there is a mathematically calculable possibility that the disease will die out.

Arbovirus Infections

Arboviruses are arthropod-borne viruses

A wide range of about 500 different viruses is transmitted by arthropods such as ticks, mosquitoes and sandflies. These arboviruses multiply in the arthropod vector, and for each virus there is a natural cycle involving vertebrates (various birds or mammals) and arthropods. The virus enters the arthropod when it takes a blood meal from the infected vertebrate, and passes through the gut wall to reach the salivary gland where replication takes place. Once this has occurred, 1–2 weeks after ingesting the virus, the arthropod becomes infectious, and can transmit virus to another vertebrate during a blood meal. Certain arboviruses that infect ticks are also transmitted directly from adult tick to egg (vertical transmission), so that future generations of ticks are infected without the need for a vertebrate host.

Only a small number of arboviruses are important causes of human disease

Arboviruses tend to replicate in vascular endothelium, the central nervous system (CNS), skin and muscle, and are therefore multisystem infections. They are generally named after the clinical disease (yellow fever) or the place where they were first discovered (Rift Valley fever, Japanese encephalitis). A few (e.g. Ross River virus in Australia and the Pacific) cause arthritis.

The human stage of the virus cycle may be essential (urban yellow fever, dengue), there being no other vertebrate host, or it may be 'accidental' from the virus's point of view, with humans acting as 'dead end' hosts who do not form a necessary part of the natural cycle (e.g. equine encephalitides).

Yellow fever

Yellow fever virus is transmitted by mosquitoes and is restricted to Africa, Central and South America and the Caribbean

Yellow fever virus is a flavivirus and there is only one antigenic type. It was taken to the Americas by the early slave traders and the first recorded case was in Yucatan in 1640. Yellow fever virus is transmitted by two different cycles:

- From human to human by the mosquito *Aedes aegypti*. The infection can be maintained in this way as 'urban' yellow fever.
- From infected monkeys to humans by mosquitoes such as *Haemagogus*. This is 'jungle' yellow fever and is seen in Africa and South America.

Yellow fever is not transmitted directly from human to human.

Clinical features of yellow fever may be mild, but liver damage can prove fatal

The virus enters dermal tissues or blood vessels at the site of a mosquito bite and spreads through the body, infecting vascular endothelium and liver. After an incubation period of 3–6 days there is a sudden onset of fever, headache and muscular aches. Although mild cases occur, prostration and shock are not uncommon, and severe liver damage may result in death. Coagulation defects (largely due to prothrombin deficiency) cause hemorrhage into the gastrointestinal tract (hematemesis) and elsewhere. Renal damage is also seen, with proteinuria and occasionally tubular necrosis.

The diagnosis is usually clinical, there is no specific treatment, but there is a vaccine

Virus can be isolated from blood during the acute stage and a postmortem diagnosis can be made from the severe midzonal changes and acidophilic inclusion bodies seen in the liver.

The best prevention is to give the live attenuated '17D' yellow fever vaccine to those who may be exposed. Protection lasts at least 10 years and vaccination is necessary for entry into and travel through endemic areas. Vaccination is also a legal requirement for travellers from endemic areas to other countries where the disease does not occur (e.g. from tropical Africa to India). As with all arthropod-borne infections, control of arthropod vectors (insecticides, attention to breeding sites) and reduced exposure (insect repellents, mosquito nets) are also important.

Dengue fever
Dengue virus is transmitted by mosquitoes and occurs in South East Asia, the Pacific area, India and the Caribbean

Dengue virus is a flavivirus with four antigenic subtypes. The mosquito *A. aegypti* is the principal human vector. The virus also circulates in monkeys and can be transmitted by mosquitoes to cause 'jungle' dengue in humans, a disease analogous to jungle yellow fever.

Dengue fever may be complicated by dengue hemorrhagic fever shock syndrome

Dengue virus replicates in monocytes and possibly in vascular endothelium. After an incubation period of 4–8 days there is malaise, fever, headache, arthralgia, nausea and vomiting, and sometimes a maculopapular rash. On recovery, prostration and depression are quite common.

Dengue hemorrhagic fever shock syndrome is a particularly severe form of disease and occurs in children in endemic areas, with a mortality of up to 10%. The pathogenesis of this syndrome is shown in *Figure 25.1*. After an earlier attack of dengue, antibodies are formed that are specific for that serotype. On subsequent infection with a different serotype the antibodies bind to the virus and not only fail to neutralize it (as might be expected for a different subtype), but actually enhance its ability to infect monocytes. The Fc portion of the virus-bound immunoglobulin molecule attaches to Fc receptors on monocytes and entry into the cell by this route increases the efficiency of infection. Infection of increased numbers of monocytes results in an increased release of cytokines into the circulation (see Chapter 12) and this leads to vascular damage, shock and hemorrhage, especially into the gastrointestinal tract and skin. Similar 'enhancing' antibodies are formed in many other virus infections, but it is only in dengue hemorrhagic fever that they are known to play a pathogenic role.

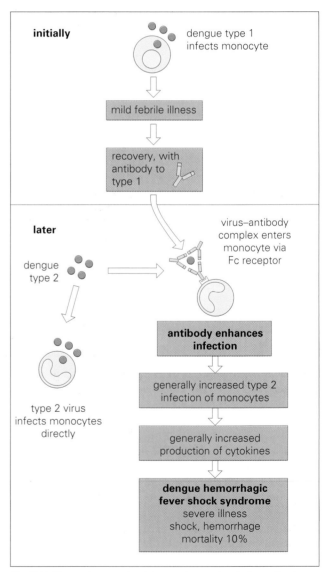

Fig. 25.1 The pathogenesis of dengue hemorrhagic fever shock syndrome. There are four serotypes of dengue virus. Types 1 and 2 are illustrated as an example. Antibody to type 1 binds to type 2 without preventing infection with type 2.

There is no antiviral therapy or vaccine for dengue fever

There is the obvious danger that a vaccine could induce a dangerous type of antibody.

Arbovirus encephalitis
The encephalitic arboviruses only occasionally cause encephalitis

Five of the nine encephalitic arboviruses listed in *Figure 25.2* cause disease in the USA, and although most infections are subclinical or mild, encephalitis can occur. The virus replicates in the CNS, but a cell-mediated immune response to infection makes a major contribution to the encephalitis. Vaccines against Western equine encephalitis (WEE), Eastern equine encephalitis (EEE) and Venezuelan equnine encephalitis (VEE), each of which may cause disease in horses, have been used for laboratory workers, and a Japanese encephalitis vaccine is available in Japan and India. Laboratory diagnosis is carried out in special centers, occasionally by virus isolation, but more commonly by demonstrating a rise in specific antibody.

Arboviruses and Hemorrhagic Fevers

Arboviruses are major causes of fever in endemic areas of the world

Arbovirus infections are often subclinical or mild, but occasionally there is a severe hemorrhagic illness. Some of the best known of these infections are listed in *Figure 25.3*. Laboratory diagnosis by isolation of virus or by demonstration of a rise in antibody is possible in special centers.

Rickettsial Infections

Rickettsiae are small bacteria and infections tend to be persistent or become latent

Rickettsiae are small bacteria (see Chapter 3 and Appendix) that multiply by binary fission, and with the exception of *Rochalimaea quintana*, the causative agent of 'trench fever', are obligate intracellular parasites. Howard T Ricketts identified 'Rocky Mountain spotted fever' in 1906 and showed that it was transmitted transovarially in ticks. All rickettsiae

ARBOVIRUSES THAT CAN CAUSE ENCEPHALITIS				
virus and disease	**geographic distribution**	**vector for human infection**	**vertebrate reservoir**	**severity of infection**
Eastern equine encephalitis (alphavirus)	USA (Atlantic Gulf states)	*Aedes* spp. mosquitoes	wild birds, horses (dead-end hosts)	50% case fatality
Western equine encephalitis (alphavirus)	USA (west of Mississippi)	*Culex* spp. mosquitoes	wild birds, horses (dead-end hosts)	up to 2% case fatality
St Louis encephalitis (flavivirus)	USA (southern, Central and western States)	*Culex* spp. mosquitoes	wild birds	10% case fatality
California encephalitis (bunyavirus)	USA (northern and Central States)	*Aedes* spp. mosquitoes	small mammals	fatalities rare
Japanese encephalitis (flavivirus)	Far East, South East Asia	*Culex* spp. mosquitoes	birds, pigs	8% case fatality
Murray valley encephalitis (flavivirus)	Australia	*Culex* spp. mosquitoes	birds	up to 70% case fatality (variable)
tick-borne encephalitis (flavivirus)	Eastern Europe	tick	mammals, birds	up to 10% case fatality (variable)
Venezuelan encephalitis (alphavirus)	Southern USA Central and South America	mosquito	rodents	70% case fatality (cases rare)
Powassan (flavivirus)	USA, Canada	tick	rodents	cases rare

Fig. 25.2 Arboviruses causing encephalitis. The great majority of infections are either subclinical or are associated with non-specific febrile illness (e.g. 70% case fatality in encephalitis due to Venezuelan encephalitis virus, but only 3% develop encephalitis).

ARBOVIRUSES THAT CAN CAUSE FEVERS AND HEMORRHAGIC DISEASES				
viruses	**disease**	**geographic distribution**	**vector**	**animal reservoir**
yellow fever (alphavirus)	fever, hepatitis	Africa, Central and South America	mosquito *Aedes* spp.	nil (monkeys for jungle type)
dengue (4 serotypes) (flavivirus)	fever, rash (hemorrhagic shock syndrome)	India, South East Asia, Pacific, South America, Caribbean	mosquito	nil
Kyasanur forest (flavivirus)	hemorrhagic fever	India	tick	monkeys, rodents
Ross river (alphavirus)	fever, arthralgia arthritis	Australia, Pacific Islands	mosquito	birds
Rift valley fever (bunyavirus)	fever sometimes hemorrhage	Africa	mosquito	sheep, cattle camels
sandfly fever (bunyavirus)	fever (mild disease)	Asia, South America, Mediterranean	sandflies	gerbils
Congo-Crimean hemorrhagic fever (bunyavirus)	fever, hemorrhage	Asia, Africa	tick	rodents
Colorado tick fever (reovirus)	fever, myalgia	USA (Rocky Mountains)	tick	rodents
La Crosse (bunyavirus)	fever	USA	mosquito	rodents, etc.

Fig. 25.3 Arboviruses causing fevers and hemorrhagic diseases. There are many other less important arboviruses. For example, there are almost 200 in the bunyavirus family, most of which are anthropod-borne, with about 40 occasionally causing human disease.

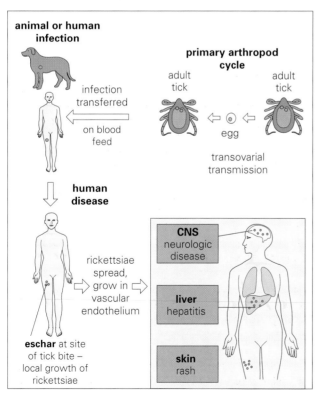

Fig. 25.4 Typical events in rickettsial infection. There is no direct person to person spread. Q fever is atypical (see text). Typhus is unusual because the infected arthropod transmits from person to person, eventually dies and there is no eschar. (CNS, central nervous system.)

except *Coxiella burnetii* (which causes Q fever; see Chapter 26) are transmitted to humans by arthropods *(Fig. 25.4)* and all except epidemic typhus have a vertebrate reservoir. Rickettsiae probably arose as parasites of blood-sucking or other arthropods in which they were maintained by vertical transmission, transfer to the arthropod's vertebrate host being initially 'accidental' and not necessary for rickettsial survival. The infected arthropod does not appear to be adversely affected. *Rickettsia prowazekii* is perhaps a more recent parasite of the human body louse, because the louse dies 1–3 weeks after infection. As with most arthropod-borne infections, transmission from person to person does not occur.

Typical clinical symptoms of rickettsial infection are fever, headache and rash

Rickettsiae multiply in vascular endothelium to cause pathology (vasculitis) in skin, CNS and liver, and hence are multisystem infections *(Fig. 25.5)*. In spite of immune responses there is a tendency for rickettsial infections to persist in the body for long periods or become latent.

Except for Q fever, the typical clinical features are fever, headache and rash. A history suggesting contact with rickettsial vectors or reservoir animals may suggest a diagnosis (e.g. camping, working, engaging in military activities in endemic areas).

Laboratory diagnosis is based on serologic tests

Complement fixation tests are specific for different rickettsiae, and a 4-fold or greater rise in titer can be demonstrated.

PRINCIPAL RICKETTSIAL DISEASES OF HUMANS

	organism	disease	arthropod vector	vertebrate resevoir	clinical severity	geographic distribution
spotted fevers***	R. rickettsii	Rocky Mountain spotted fever	tick*	dogs, rodents	+	Rocky Mountain states, eastern USA
	R. akari	rickettsial pox	mite*	mice	–	Asia, Far East, Africa, USA
	R. conorii	Mediterranean spotted fever	tick	dogs	+	Mediterranean
typhus	R. prowazekii	epidemic typhus	louse	human**	++	Africa, South America
	R. typhi	endemic typhus	flea	rodents	–	worldwide
	R. tsutsugamushi	scrub typhus	mite*	rodents	++	Far East
others	Coxiella burnetii	Q fever	none	sheep, goats, cattle	+	worldwide
	Rochalimaea quintana	trench fever	louse	human	+	Asia, Africa Central and South America [†]
	Ehrlichia chaffeensis [††]	fever (ehrlichiosis)	tick	?	+	USA Japan (E. sennetsu)

*   vertically transmitted in arthropod
**   non-human vertebrates are possibly also involved
*** other rickettsiae cause similar tick-borne fevers in Africa, India, Australia
[†] multiply extracellularly; 1 million soldiers infected in the First World War
[††] isolated at Fort Chaffe Arkansas; Parasitizes lymphocytes, monocytes, neutrophils

Fig. 25.5 The principal rickettsial diseases in humans.

Microimmunofluorescence tests (IgG and IgM) are also used and are more sensitive. Infected patients also make antibody to the rickettsiae that cross-react with the O antigen polysaccharide of various strains of *Proteus vulgaris*, as detected by agglutination in the Weil–Felix test. The agglutination pattern with three strains of *Proteus* can be used to identify the rickettsiae. Although the phenomenon is of interest, the test is not of great value because of false positive and false negative results. Earlier diagnosis can often be made by fluorescent antibody staining of skin biopsy material. Isolation of rickettsiae is difficult and dangerous and laboratory infections have occurred.

All rickettsiae are susceptible to tetracyclines

Chloramphenicol is an alternative treatment.

Prevention is based on reducing exposure to ticks. A killed *R. prowazekii* vaccine is available for the military, and a killed *C. burnetii* vaccine for those at risk (e.g. veterinarians, shepherds).

Rocky Mountain spotted fever
Rocky Mountain spotted fever is transmitted by dog ticks and has a mortality of up to 10%

The rickettsiae causing this disease are carried by the dog tick (*Dermacentor variabilis*) or by wood ticks (*Dermacentor andersoni*) and are transmitted vertically from adult tick to egg. Human infection occurs in the warm months of the year

as ticks become active. Children are most commonly infected, but their disease is milder.

The rickettsiae multiply in the skin at the site of the tick bite, then spread to blood and infect vascular endothelium in the lung, spleen, brain and skin. After an incubation period of about one week there is onset of fever, severe headache and myalgia, and often respiratory symptoms. A generalized maculopapular rash appears a few days later, often becoming petechial or purpuric (*Fig. 25.6*). There is splenomegaly, and neurologic involvement is frequent, with later onset of clotting defects (disseminated intravascular coagulation), shock and death. Fatal cases are usually those with a delayed diagnosis. Peak mortality (10%) is seen in 40–60 year olds.

Mediterranean spotted fever
Mediterranean spotted fever is transmitted by dog ticks and has a mortality of up to 10%

Mediterranean spotted fever is caused by *Rickettsia conorii*, carried by the dog tick *Rhipicephalus sanguineus*. Human infection, which occurs mainly in October, is known in all Mediterranean countries and can occur in urban as well as rural areas. After an incubation period of about one week, 50% of cases develop fever, headache and myalgia, and 2–4 days later a rash, especially on the palms and soles. The bite usually goes unnoticed as it is caused by immature ticks and is painless; a

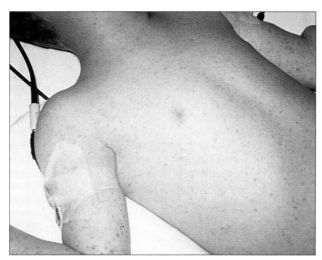

Fig. 25.6 Generalized maculopapular rash with petechiae in Rocky Mountain spotted fever. (Courtesy of TF Sellers, Jr.)

local lesion is not usually seen. Mortality in hospitalized cases is similar to that of Rocky Mountain spotted fever (up to 10%).

Rickettsialpox
Rickettsialpox is a mild infection
About five days after the bite of an infected mite a local eschar develops, followed one week later by fever and headache. After a few days a generalized papulovesicular rash then appears. The disease is, however, mild.

Epidemic typhus
Epidemic typhus is transmitted by the human body louse
Epidemic typhus is transmitted from person to person by *Pediculus corporis*. The rickettsiae (*R. prowazekii*) multiply in the gut epithelium of the louse and are excreted in feces during the act of biting. The rickettsiae enter the skin when the bite is scratched. The disease cannot maintain itself unless enough people are infested with lice. Epidemic typhus is therefore classically associated with poverty and war, when clothes and bodies are washed less frequently. There were 30 million cases in Eastern Europe and the Soviet Union from 1918–1922. The disease is seen in Africa and South America, but the last case in the USA was in 1922. As there is no direct person to person spread, outbreaks can be terminated by delousing campaigns.

Untreated epidemic typhus has a mortality as high as 40%
Rickettsiae proliferate at the site of the bite and then spread in the blood to infect vascular endothelium in skin, heart, CNS, muscle and kidney. About one week after the louse bite (there is no eschar) the infected person develops fever, headache and flu-like symptoms. The generalized maculopapular rash appears 5–9 days later and sometimes there is severe meningoencephalitis with delirium and coma. In untreated cases mortality can be as high as 40%, due to peripheral vascular collapse or secondary bacterial pneumonia.

Convalescence may take months. In some individuals the rickettsiae are not eliminated from the body on clinical recovery and remain in the lymph nodes. As much as 50 years later, the infection can reactivate to cause Brill–Zinsser disease, and the patient once again acts as a source of infection for any lice that may be present.

Endemic typhus
Endemic typhus is caused by *Rickettsia typhi* and is transmitted to humans by the rat flea. The disease is similar to epidemic typhus, but is less severe.

Scrub typhus
Scrub typhus is caused by *Rickettsia tsutsugamushi* and is transmitted to humans by trombiculid mites (chiggers). It occurs only in the Far East; cases were seen in American soldiers in Vietnam. The rickettsiae are maintained in the mites by transovarial transfer and are transmitted to humans or rodents during feeding. There is an eschar, and a macular rash appears after about five days of illness.

Borrelia Infections

Relapsing fever
The epidemic form of relapsing fever is caused by Borrelia recurrentis, which is transmitted by human body lice
Borrelia recurrentis is a spirochete consisting of an irregular spiral, 10–30 μm long, and is highly flexible, moving by rotation and twisting.

Epidemics of relapsing fever *(Fig. 25.7)* are due to transmission of infection by the human body louse. Bacteria multiply in the louse, and when louse bites are rubbed the lice are crushed

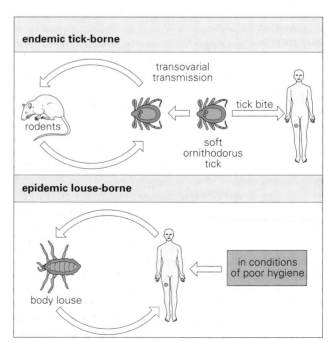

Fig. 25.7 Transmission in relapsing fever.

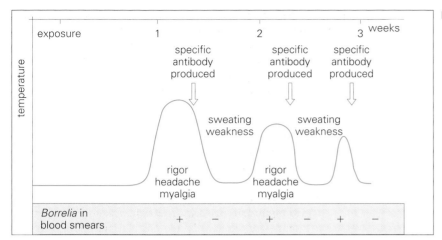

Fig. 25.8 Course of events in relapsing fever.

and the bacteria are introduced into the bite wound. Lice are essential for person to person transmission of louse-borne relapsing fever. As with other louse-borne infections (e.g. typhus), spread of the disease in humans is favored when people rarely wash and when clothes are not changed (e.g. in wars, natural disasters). The last great epidemic in North Africa and Europe during the Second World War, caused 50 000 deaths.

The endemic form of relapsing fever in humans is transmitted by tick bites

Infection with other species of *Borrelia* is endemic in rodents in many parts of the world, including western USA, and *Borrelia* is transmitted by soft ticks of the genus *Ornithodoros*. In the tick, the bacteria are transmitted transovarially from generation to generation. Also, ticks survive for up to 15 years between feeds, which helps maintain the endemic cycle of tick-borne relapsing fever.

Relapsing fever is characterized by repeated febrile episodes due to antigenic variation in the spirochetes

The bacteria multiply locally and enter the blood. After an incubation period of 3–10 days there is a sudden onset of illness with chills and fever, lasting for 3–5 days (*Fig. 25.8*). The afebrile period lasts about a week before there is a second attack of fever, which is followed by another afebrile period. Generally there are 3–10 such episodes, of diminishing severity. More serious illness can occur if there is extensive growth of bacteria in the spleen, liver and kidneys.

Agglutinating and lytic antibodies are formed against the infecting bacteria, which are cleared from the blood. Under the 'pressure' of this immune response a new antigenic type emerges and is free to multiply and cause a fresh febrile episode. Antigenic variation involves switching of the variable major protein (VMP) on the bacterial surface. The *Borrelia* have arrays of VMP genes that are activated by gene conversion. A single cloned bacterium can give rise spontaneously to more than 20 serotypes and switching occurs at a rate of 1:1000–1:10 000 per cell generation. Similar phenomena are seen in trypanosomes. Direct person to person transmission does not occur. Mortality with endemic (tick-borne) relapsing fever is less than 5%, but may be up to 40% in epidemic (louse-borne) relapsing fever.

Relapsing fever is diagnosed in the laboratory and treated with tetracycline

The bacteria can be cultivated in the laboratory and can be seen in Giemsa-stained smears of blood taken during the febrile period (*Fig. 25.9*). Complement fixation antibody tests are available, but are rarely useful because of the problem of antigenic variation.

Tetracycline is used in treatment and to prevent relapses. The best preventative measure is avoidance of arthropod vectors.

Lyme disease
Lyme disease is caused by Borrelia spp. and is transmitted by Ixodes ticks

Lyme disease occurs in Europe, the USA and most continents of the world, and is named after the town in Connecticut, USA where the first cases were recognized in 1975. It is caused by *Borrelia burgdorferi* (USA) or other species of *Borrelia*. The natural cycle of infection takes place in mice and deer in whom it is transmitted by hard ticks of the genus *Ixodes* (*Fig. 25.10*). Human infection follows the bite of an infected tick (larval, nymph or adult form). In Europe and the USA, infection is more common in summer months when recreational exposure to infected ticks is more likely. Person to person transmission does not occur.

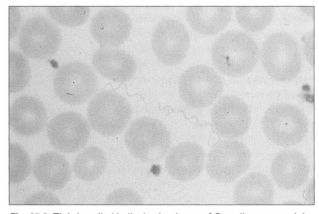

Fig. 25.9 Tightly coiled helical spirochetes of *Borrelia recurrentis* in the blood of a patient with relapsing fever. (Courtesy of TF Sellers.)

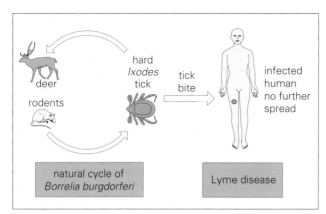

Fig. 25.10 Transmission of Lyme disease.

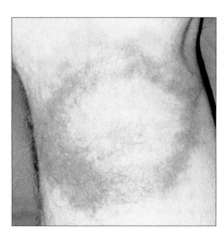

Fig. 25.11 Rash of erythema chronicum migrans on the leg in Lyme disease. (Courtesy of E Sahn.)

Erythema chronicum migrans is a characteristic feature of Lyme disease

The bacteria multiply locally, and after an incubation period of about one week fever, headache, myalgia, lymphadenopathy, and a characteristic lesion at the site of the tick bite develop. The skin lesion is called 'erythema chronicum migrans' *(Fig. 25.11)*, its name describing its main features. It begins as a macule and enlarges over the next few weeks, remaining red and flat, but with the center clearing, until it is several inches in diameter. In 50% of patients fresh transient lesions appear on the skin elsewhere in the body. Immunologic findings include circulating immune complexes and sometimes elevated serum IgM levels and cryoglobulins that contain IgM.

Lyme disease commonly causes additional disease one week to two years after the initial illness

In 75% of untreated patients, in spite of antibody and T cell responses to the *Borrelia*, there are additional later manifestations of disease. These are seen from one week to more than two years after the onset of illness. The first of these manifestations to appear are neurologic (meningitis, encephalitis, peripheral neuropathy) and cardiologic (heart block, myopericarditis). The second of these manifestations to appear are arthralgia and arthritis, which may persist for months or years. Immune complexes are found in affected joints. These late manifestations are immunologic in origin, and are probably due to antigenic cross-reactivity between *Borrelia* and host tissues. The *Borrelia* themselves are rarely detectable at this stage.

Lyme disease is diagnosed serologically and treated with antibiotic

The *Borrelia* are rarely seen in skin biopsies but can some-

HUMAN MALARIA PARASITES				
species	***Plasmodium falciparum***	***P. vivax***	***P. malariae***	***P. ovale***
major distribution	West, East and Central Africa, Middle East Far East, South America	India, North and East Africa, South America, Far East	tropical Africa, India, Far East	tropical Africa
common name	malignant tertian	benign tertian	quartan	ovale tertian
duration of liver stage (incubation period)	6–14 days	12–17 days (with relapses up to 3 years)	13–40 days (with relapses up to 20 years)	9–18 days (with rare relapses)
duration of asexual blood cycle (fever cycle)	48 hours	48 hours	72 hours	50 hours
major complications	cerebral malaria anemia hypoglycemia jaundice pulmonary edema shock	–	nephrotic syndrome	–

Fig. 25.12 Human malaria parasites. The most important and life-threatening complications occur with *Plasmodium falciparum*, hence its old name 'malignant tertian malaria'.

times be isolated from biopsies obtained at an early stage, although this may take weeks. Serologic tests such as enzyme-linked immunosorbent assay (ELISA) are more useful. Specific IgM antibodies are detected 3–6 weeks after infection and IgG antibodies at a later stage. Antigenic cross-reactivity may result in false positive results.

Penicillin or tetracycline are effective and penicillin can be used to treat the late arthritis.

Prevention of Lyme disease is by avoidance of tick bites.

Protozoal Infections

Malaria

Egyptian papyruses from the sixteenth century BC chronicle the association between fever, shivering, and enlargement of the spleen. Since the Middle Ages, Europe knew this condition as malaria, although the causative organism was not identified until 1880. Four species of *Plasmodium* cause malaria in man, of which *P. falciparum* is the most virulent *(Fig. 25.12)*. In addition, occasional infections may occur with the simian parasites *P. knowlesi*, *P. cynomolgi* and *P. simium*.

Malaria is initiated by the bite of an infected female anopheline mosquito

Malaria is therefore restricted to areas where these mosquitoes can breed. At present this includes most of the tropics between 60°N and 40°S (except areas more than about 2000 m above sea level), with a major impact in Africa, India, the Far East and South America. Early hopes of eradication via mosquito control and chemotherapy have been dashed by the emergence of drug resistance and, globally, malaria is now on the increase. About 35% of the world's population is estimated to be infected, with some 10 million new cases annually and perhaps two million deaths. As a result of increased air travel, new cases are regularly seen in the developed world, and unless the diagnosis is constantly borne in mind, vital treatment may be withheld, with fatal results. Malaria can also be transmitted by blood transfusion or needle accidents, and, very rarely, from mother to fetus.

The life cycle of the malaria parasite comprises three stages

The malaria parasite has the most complex life cycle of any human infection, comprising three quite distinct stages and characterized by alternating extracellular and intracellular forms, as described in detail in *Figures 25.13* and *25.14*.

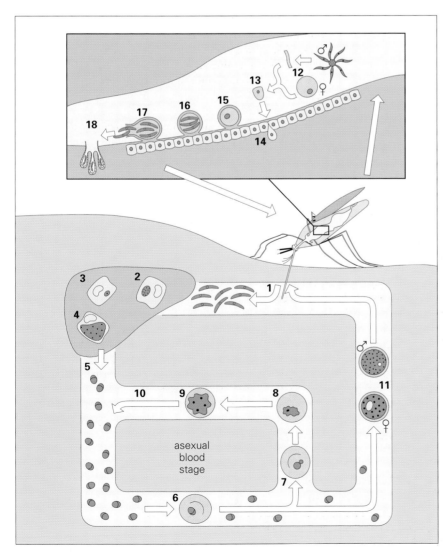

Fig. 25.13 The life cycle of malaria in man and mosquito. In the symptomless pre-erythrocytic stage, sporozoites from the saliva of an infected *Anopheles* mosquito are injected into the human bloodstream when the mosquito bites (1). They then enter the parenchymal cells of the liver (2), where they mature in approximately two weeks into tissue schizonts (4), finally rupturing to produce 10 000–40 000 merozoites (5). These circulate in the blood for a few minutes before entering the red blood cells (6) to initiate the asexual blood stage. Some parasites, however, remain within the liver to lie dormant as hypnozoites (3), which are the cause of relapses. Once in the red blood cells, the merozoites mature into the ring form (7), trophozoite (8) and schizont (9), which complete the cycle by maturing to release merozoites back into the circulation (10). This cycle may last for months or even years. Some merozoites, however, go on to initiate the sexual stage, maturing within the red blood cells to form male and female gametocytes (11), which can be taken up by the *Anopheles* mosquito on feeding. On entering the gut of the insect, the male gametocyte exflagellates (12) to form male microgametes, which fertilize the female gamete to form the zygote (13). This then invades the gut mucosa (14), where it develops into an oocyst (15). This develops to produce thousands of sporozoites (16), which are released into the gut (17), finally migrating to the salivary glands of the insect (18), whence the cycle begins again.

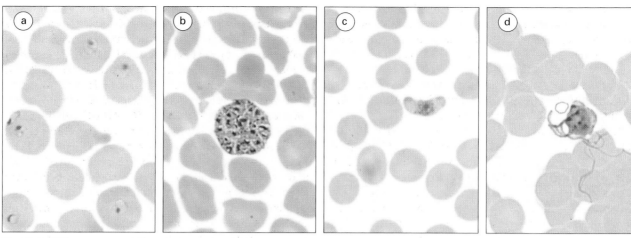

Fig. 25.14 Different stages of the malaria parasites.(a) *Plasmodium falciparum* ring forms in red blood cells. (b) *Plasmodium vivax* erythrocytic schizont. (c) *P. falciparum* female gametocyte. (d) *P. vivax* male gametocytes exflagellating to form microgametes 20–25 µm long.

The genetic recombination allowed by the sexual stage of the process is one element in the remarkable antigenic diversity seen within malaria parasite populations. It is interesting to note that successful transmission of malaria depends crucially upon the mosquito surviving long enough for sporozoites to develop, and that quite small species differences in mosquito lifespan can drastically affect transmission; this may be an important cause of regional differences in malaria incidence.

The symptoms of malaria, which range from fever to fatal cerebral or renal disease, are associated exclusively with the asexual blood stage *(Fig. 25.13)*. Invasion of red cells requires at least two separate receptor–receptor interactions, and the lack of one red cell surface molecule, the 'Duffy' antigen, explains the resistance to *P. vivax* of most West Africans. Other genetic traits that appear to have been selected because they contribute to resistance to malaria include hemoglobin S (sickle cell), β-thalassemia, and glucose-6-phosphate dehydrogenase deficiency.

Clinical features of malaria include a fluctuating fever and drenching sweats

The clinical picture of malaria depends upon the age and immune status of the patient, as well as the species of parasite. The most characteristic feature is fever, which closely follows rupture of erythrocytic schizonts and is thought to be mainly due to the induction of cytokines such as interleukin-1 (IL-1) and tumor necrosis factor (TNF). Because of their regular and synchronous cycle times, the different species of malaria give characteristic patterns of fever, with either a 48-hour (tertian, i.e. days 1 and 3) or 72-hour (quartan, i.e. days 1 and 4) periodicity *(Fig. 25.15)*. A typical paroxysm of fever starts with a feeling of intense cold with shivering followed by a hot dry stage and finally a period of drenching sweats. Headache, muscle pains and vomiting are common. *P. falciparum* infections do not always display the typical periodicity, causing a daily evening fever due to superimposed nonsynchronous

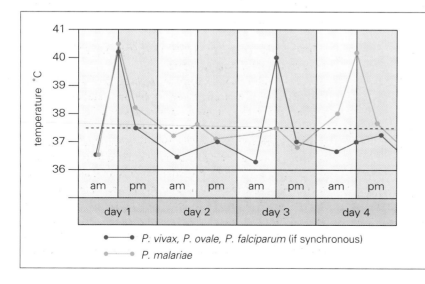

Fig. 25.15 Malaria fever charts showing cyclical fluctuations in temperature. The peaks coincide with the maturation and rupture of the intraerythrocytic schizonts, occurring every 48 hours (*Plasmodium falciparum, Plasmodium vivax* and *Plasmodium ovale*) or every 72 hours (*Plasmodium malariae*), when the cycles are synchronized.

parasite cycles. It is in such cases that the diagnosis is likely to be missed and the symptoms attributed to influenza or some other pyrexial disease. Enlargement of the spleen and liver is common and anemia almost invariable.

Complications of malaria include cerebral malaria, severe anemia, hypoglycemia, lactic acidosis and glomerulonephritis

In the absence of treatment or reinfection, P. vivax, P. ovale and P. malariae malaria are normally self-limiting, but relapses may occur. P. falciparum malaria, however, is frequently fatal during the first 2–3 weeks due to the development of a variety of complications (Fig. 25.12). Relapses may occur after months or even years, especially in P. vivax malaria due to parasites that lie dormant in the liver ('hypnozoites').

In areas where malaria is endemic, complicated P. falciparum malaria is most common in children aged between six months and five years, and in pregnant, particularly primagravid, women. However, it can occur at any age in the non-immune (e.g. tourists). The most dangerous complication is

stage	mechanism
sporozoites	antibody
liver stage	cytotoxic T cells TNF IFN-α IL-1
merozoites	antibody
asexual erythrocyte stage	antibody ROI RNI ECP TNF
gametocytes	antibody ?cytokines
gametes	antibody

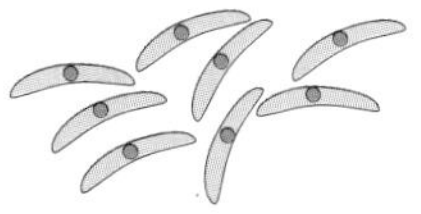

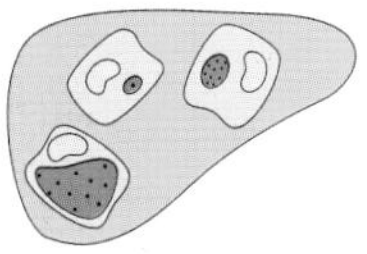

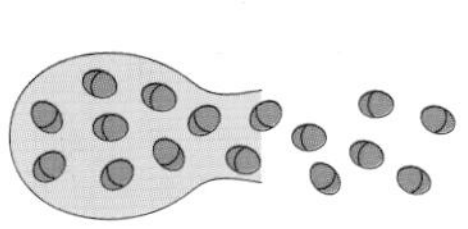

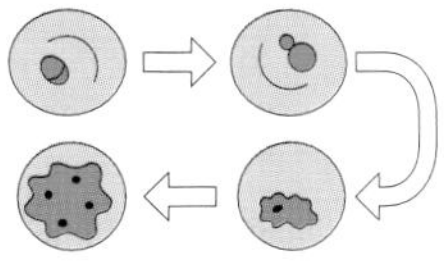

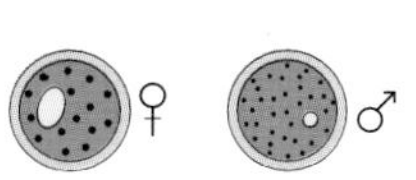

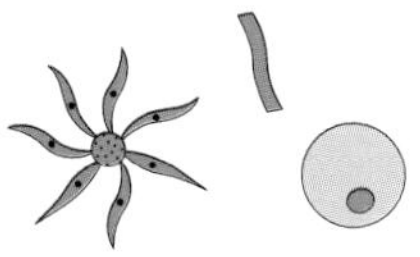

Fig. 25.16 Immunity to malaria. The principal mechanisms thought to be responsible for immunity at each stage of the cycle. (IFN, interferon; IL, interleukin; TNF, tumor necrosis factor; ROI, reactive oxygen intermediates; RNI, reactive nitrogen intermediates; ECP, eosinophil cationic proteins.)

'cerebral malaria', with progressive headache, neck stiffness, convulsions and coma. There is much debate as to whether this is caused by sludging or binding of parasitized red cells in cerebral capillaries, by increased permeability of the blood–brain barrier, or by excessive induction of cytokines such as TNF. If successfully treated, however, it usually leaves little or no impairment of cerebral function, although neurologic and psychiatric sequelae may occur in 5–10% of childhood cases.

Severe anemia is also common, due partly to red cell destruction and partly to dyserythropoiesis in the bone marrow; the spleen appears to be the major site of red cell removal. Of the other complications, hypoglycemia and lactic acidosis are thought to be important contributors to mortality. Reduced food intake, impaired liver gluconeogenesis and possible glucose consumption by the large number of parasites may all be involved, and a role for TNF has been proposed, as it has for many of the complications. Immune complex glomerulonephritis is common, and there is a particular tendency to develop progressive nephrotic disease in P. malariae (quartan) malaria.

Malaria has an immunosuppressive effect
The strong epidemiologic correlation between malaria and endemic Burkitt's lymphoma is generally attributed to a weakening of T cell cytotoxicity against Epstein–Barr virus (EBV)-infected cells. The immunosuppressive effect of malaria may also interfere with the efficacy of vaccines against, for example, common virus or bacterial infections.

Immunity to malaria develops gradually and seems to need repeated boosting
Immunity to malaria develops in stages and in endemic areas children who survive early attacks become resistant to severe disease by about the age of five years. Parasite levels fall progressively until adulthood when they are low or absent most of the time. A period of one year spent away from exposure is sufficient for most of this immunity to wane, suggesting that repeated boosting is needed to maintain it. The actual mechanisms are controversial and seem to involve both antibody and cell-mediated immunity (Fig. 25.16). At least 20 proteins from the various stages of the life cycle have been characterized and investigated as possibly relevant immunogens and/or vaccine candidates.

Malaria is diagnosed by finding parasitized red cells in a blood film
The blood film may need to be thick or alternatively bone marrow may be used. Later (schizont) stages may be sequestered in deep tissues, so parasites may be deceptively scarce in, or even absent from, the blood. Any case of fever, especially with anemia, splenomegaly or cerebral signs, in a patient who conceivably could have malaria is therefore best treated as malaria. However, the presence of parasites in the blood of an ill patient from an endemic area does not mean malaria is the cause of the illness, since parasitaemia may be asymptomatic. The demonstration of antibody by immunofluorescence or ELISA confirms previous exposure and a predominance of IgM would suggest a recent attack.

Quinine is the drug of choice for life-threatening malaria

The effect of cinchona bark on malaria has been known for 400 years and the active principle, quinine, remains the drug of choice for life-threatening malaria. Complications of quinine treatment include massive intravascular hemolysis ('blackwater fever'). Other major drugs are chloroquine (to which *P. falciparum* is increasingly resistant), and the new Chinese drug quinghaosu (artemisin), with primaquine for preventing relapses.

The most promising forms of prevention are bednets impregnated with mosquito repellents, but drugs such as proguanil or chloroquine are also used. The prospects for a malaria vaccine are discussed in Chapter 31.

Trypanosomiasis
Three species of the flagellated protozoan Trypanosoma cause human disease

The three species are *Trypanosoma brucei gambiense* and *T. b. rhodesiense* (the cause of African trypanosomiasis or sleeping sickness) and *T. cruzi* (the cause of South American trypanosomiasis or Chagas' disease). The diseases differ quite markedly in:

- The nature of the insect vector.
- The habitat of the parasite.
- The effects on the immune system.

African trypanosomiasis
African trypanosomiasis is transmitted by the tsetse fly and restricted to equatorial Africa

The vector of African trypanosomiasis is *Glossina* and there is a reservoir of infection in several domestic and wild animals (cattle, pigs, deer). In man, *T. brucei* remains extracellular, first in the tissues near the insect bite and then in the blood, where it divides rapidly and continuously.

Clinical features of African trypanosomiasis include lymphadenopathy and 'sleeping sickness'

Following an infected bite a swollen chancre develops at the site, with widespread lymph node enlargement, especially in the back of the neck (Winterbottom's sign; *Fig. 25.17a*). The parasite becomes established in the blood where it multiplies rapidly, with fever and splenomegaly, and often signs of myocardial involvement. Within weeks or months the CNS may become involved (more acutely in the East African *T. b. rhodesiense* than the West African *T. b. gambiense*), with the gradual development of headache, psychologic changes ('silent grief'), voracious appetite and weight loss, and finally coma ('sleeping sickness'; *Fig. 25.17b*) and death. Unlike malaria, cured trypanosomiasis can leave the patient with severe residual neurologic and mental disability.

T. brucei evades host defenses by varying the antigens in its glycoprotein coat

The ability of *T. brucei* to survive free in the blood is due to its remarkable degree of antigenic variation, based on switching between some 1000 different genes for the glycoprotein coat.

A high concentration of IgM is found in the blood, and later in the cerebrospinal fluid (CSF), and this is manufactured by the plasma cells (Mott cells), which are a feature of the lymphocytic infiltrate seen as 'perivascular cuffing' around blood vessels in the brain *(Fig. 25.18)*.

African trypanosomiasis is diagnosed by demonstrating parasites microscopically and can be treated with a variety of drugs

T. brucei can be demonstrated in lymph nodes (by puncture) or in late cases in CSF. A raised serum IgM (up to 16-times normal concentration) is highly suggestive of the disease.

Arsenical drugs such as tryparsamide and melarsoprol have been the mainstay of treatment, especially in chronic disease, and several non-arsenicals are used in the acute stages (e.g. suramin, nitrofurazone, pentamidine). Pentamidine is the drug of choice for prophylaxis.

Control of the tsetse fly vector is difficult, though insecticides are widely used. Bed nets are ineffective as the flies feed during daylight hours.

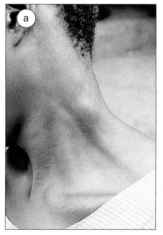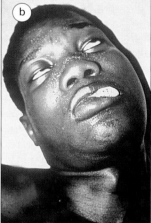

Fig. 25.17 African trypanosomiasis. (a) Enlargement of the lymph nodes in the neck (Winterbottom's sign). (Courtesy of PG Janssens.) (b) Coma (sleeping sickness) due to generalized encephalitis. (Courtesy of ME Krampitz and P de Raadt.)

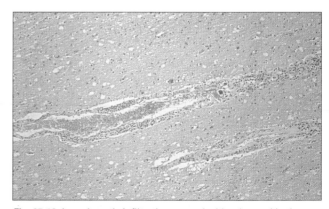

Fig. 25.18 Lymphocytic infiltration around a blood vessel in the brain in *Trypanosoma brucei* infection. (Hematoxylin and eosin) (Courtesy of R Muller and JR Baker.)

Chagas' disease
T. cruzi is transmitted by the reduviid ('kissing') bug

T. cruzi differs from the African trypanosomes in being transmitted by a non-flying vector, the reduviid ('kissing') bug, which restricts the disease to areas of poor housing. Almost all species of mammal can act as reservoirs of infection. In addition, the parasite can infect and inhabit the cells of the host, notably macrophages and cardiac muscle cells.

Chagas' disease has serious long-term effects, which include fatal heart disease

As with African trypanosomiasis, one or more chancres ('chagomas') may develop at the site of infection, with a febrile illness, which is usually transient, but may rarely lead to death by heart failure. Following invasion of the parasites into cells, the disease pursues an extremely slow and chronic course. The two major symptoms, which can take years to appear, involve the heart and the intestinal tract. The major cause of death is myocarditis, with progressive weakening and dilatation of the ventricles due to destruction of cardiac muscle by the parasite *(Fig. 25.19)* and probably also to autoimmune mechanisms induced by cross-reacting antigens. Dilatation of the hollow viscera is due to similar processes in nerve cells and the organs become incapable of proper peristalsis; mega-esophagus and megacolon are the two commonest manifestations.

Chronic Chagas' disease is usually diagnosed serologically

In the acute phase, parasites may be seen in a blood film, but the chronic disease is usually diagnosed either serologically or by 'xenodiagnosis'. The latter involves allowing clean reduviid bugs to feed on the patient and examining the rectal contents 1–2 months later, or homogenizing them and injecting the contents into mice, in which even a single trypanosome will produce a patent infection. In the late stages, muscle biopsy may also be diagnostic.

Chagas' disease is one of the most difficult protozoal infections to cure. Several drugs, including arsenicals, are effective against the blood stage (trypomastigote), but usually fail to eliminate the intracellular stage (amastigote). The role of the physician is chiefly to treat the heart failure and mega-syndromes that accompany this disease.

Prevention is ideally achieved by improved housing and living standards. Vector control by insecticides is difficult and a vaccine, though under investigation, is in practical terms, many years away.

Leishmaniasis
Leishmania are transmitted by sandflies and cause New World and Old World leishmaniasis

Leishmania are related to, and somewhat resemble, trypanosomes, and a variety of species of the parasite cause disease in South and Central America ('New World leishmaniasis') and in India, the Middle East and Africa and on the shores of the Mediterranean (Old World leishmaniasis; *Fig. 25.20*). In the latter areas especially, dogs can act as an important reservoir of infection.

Leishmania is an intracellular parasite and inhabits macrophages

Leishmania avoids elimination in macrophages *(Fig. 25.21)* except when they are strongly activated – for example by interferon-gamma (IFNγ). The two principal sites of parasite growth are:
- The liver and spleen (visceral leishmaniasis).
- The skin (cutaneous leishmaniasis).

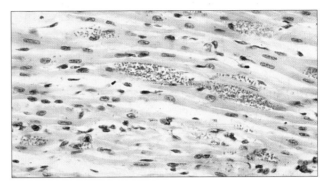

Fig. 25.19 Amastigote forms of *Trypanosoma cruzi* in cardiac muscle in Chagas' disease. (Hematoxylin and eosin) (Courtesy of H Tubbs.)

LEISHMANIA SPECIES AND CLINICAL SYNDROMES		
species	distribution	disease
L. donovani *L. infantum*	Africa, India, Mediterranean	visceral leishmaniasis
L. chagasi	South America	
L. major *L. tropica* *L. aethiopica*	Africa, India, Mediterranean	cutaneous leishmaniasis
L. mexicana *L. braziliensis* *L. peruviana*	South and Central America	

Fig. 25.20 *Leishmania* species – their distribution and clinical syndromes.

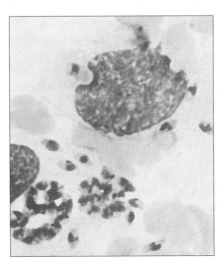

Fig. 25.21 *Leishmania* within macrophages in aspirate from a lesion of New World leishmaniasis. (Courtesy of MJ Wood.)

Untreated visceral leishmaniasis (kala-azar) causes liver failure

Visceral leishmaniasis usually develops slowly, with fever and weight loss, followed months or years later by hepatomegaly and, especially, splenomegaly; the spleen may reach to the right iliac fossa, and the untreated patient will die of liver failure. This form of the disease is known as 'kala-azar'. Skin lesions may appear following treatment; these contain massive numbers of parasites and the syndrome is known as 'post-kala-azar dermal leishmaniasis' (PKDL).

Cutaneous leishmaniasis is characterized by a large ulcer and immunity to reinfection

Classical cutaneous leishmaniasis also progresses insidiously, from a small papule at the site of infection to a large ulcer, which may eventually heal with considerable scarring *(Fig. 25.22)*. Almost alone among protozoal infections, this type of primary lesion leaves the patient relatively immune to reinfection, which has encouraged the hope that an effective vaccine might be produced (see Chapter 31). The cutaneous lesions are known in Old World leishmaniasis as 'Oriental sores' (and also 'Baghdad boil' and 'Delhi sore') and in New World leishmaniasis as 'espundia' (mucocutaneous) and 'chiclero ulcer' (of the ear).

Immunodeficiency is associated with more severe leishmaniasis

Widespread chronic lesions can occur – diffuse cutaneous leishmaniasis – analogous to lepromatous leprosy in immunodeficient patients, while visceral leishmaniasis has become one of the major complications of HIV infection in the tropics.

Leishmaniasis is diagnosed by demonstrating the organism microscopically and is treated with antimonials

Demonstration of the organism in biopsy material – marrow or spleen or skin lesions depending upon the clinical picture – is definitive proof of leishmaniasis. A positive delayed hypersensitivity reaction to leishmania antigens (Montenegro test) can be useful if parasites are not found.

Apart from the simple self-healing cutaneous lesion, leishmaniasis requires prolonged treatment with antimonial compounds (sodium stibogluconate, meglumine antimonate); if these fail, pentamidine or amphotericin B may be successful. If a very large spleen persists after treatment, it is usually removed.

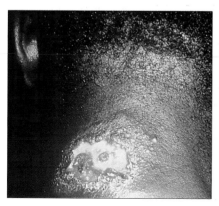

Fig. 25.22
Cutaneous lesion on the neck in *Leishmania braziliensis* infection. (Courtesy of PJ Cooper.)

Impregnated bed nets are effective against the sandfly vector, and the animal reservoir can be eliminated by dog control. As stated above, the prospects for vaccination against the cutaneous disease are quite promising.

Helminth Infections

Schistosomiasis
Schistosomiasis is transmitted through a snail vector

All members of the group to which schistosomes belong (the digenetic trematodes or flukes) must pass through a mollusc intermediate host in order to complete their larval development. However, schistosomes are the only flukes for which larvae penetrate directly into the final host after release from the snail.

The life cycle of schistosomes is illustrated in *Figure 25.23*. Infected snails, which are always aquatic, release fork-tailed larvae into the surrounding water. These penetrate the host's skin, enter the dermis and pass via the blood, through the lungs to the liver, where they mature and form permanent male and female pairs before relocating to their final site:

- The veins surrounding the bladder for *Schistosoma haematobium*.
- The mesenteric veins around the small intestine for *Schistosoma japonicum* and *Schistosoma mansoni*. The cycle is completed when eggs laid by the female worms move across the walls of the bladder or bowel and leave the body.

Clinical features of schistosomiasis result from the host's allergic responses to the different life cycle stages

The stages of skin penetration, migration and egg production are each associated with pathologic changes, collectively affecting many body systems. Penetration can cause a dermatitis, which becomes more severe on repeated reinfection. The developmental stages are associated with the onset of allergic symptoms (fever, eosinophilia, lymphadenopathy, spleno- and hepatomegaly, diarrhea), but the most severe pathology arises following the onset of egg laying. The body becomes hypersensitive to antigens released by the eggs as they pass through tissues to the outside world, or become trapped in other organs after being swept away in the bloodstream:

- In urinary schistosomiasis caused by *S. haematobium*, movement of eggs through the bladder wall causes hemorrhage. With time the bladder wall becomes inflamed and infiltrated, polyps develop, and malignant changes may follow; nephrosis may also occur (see Chapter 18).
- Release of the eggs of *S. japonicum* and *S. mansoni* similarly causes intestinal hemorrhage and inflammation.

A more serious consequence of these infections results from the inflammatory responses to eggs that become trapped in other organs of the body, primarily the liver, but also the lung and CNS. These consequences do not develop in all patients, but if they do, severe disease may ensue (see Chapter 20). Formation of granulomas by delayed hypersensitivity reactions around eggs in the presinusoidal capillaries interferes with blood flow and, together with extensive portal fibrosis

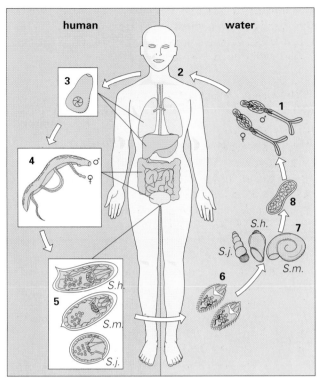

Fig. 25.23 Life cycle of schistosomes. Free-swimming cercariae in water (1) penetrate unprotected skin. (2) During penetration they lose their tails to become schistosomulae. (3) These migrate through the bloodstream via the lungs and liver to the veins of the bladder (*Schistosoma haematobium*) or bowel (*Schistosoma mansoni, Schistosoma japonicum*), where they mature (4) to produce characteristic eggs (5) within 6–12 weeks. The eggs then penetrate the bladder or colon, to be passed in the urine or the feces (6). Eggs released into fresh water are taken up by snail intermediate hosts (7) where they mature into sporocysts (8). These release cercariae (1) into the water to complete the cycle.

(Symmer's pipestem fibrosis), leads to portal hypertension. As a consequence there is hepatosplenomegaly, collateral connections form between the hepatic vessels and fragile esophageal varices develop. The collateral circulation can lead to eggs being washed into the capillary bed of the lungs.

Intense inflammatory reactions are also provoked when worms killed by anthelmintic treatment are carried back from the mesenteric vessels into the liver.

Schistosomiasis is treated with praziquantel
Treatment of individuals with praziquantel removes the worms, but in advanced cases the pathology is irreversible.

Control of infection at a population level is achieved by breaking the transmission cycle, through avoidance of infected water and improvement in sanitation.

Filariasis
The filarial nematodes depend upon blood-feeding arthropod vectors for transmission
The filarial nematodes are characterized by their location in the deeper tissues of the body (see Chapter 3). The most important species in the group can be divided into those located in the

lymphatics (*Brugia, Wuchereria*) and those in subcutaneous tissues (*Onchocerca*). A number of less harmful species also occur. In all species, the female worms release live microfilaria larvae, which are picked up by the vector from the blood (lymphatic species) or skin (*Onchocerca*). Both groups can cause severe inflammatory responses, reflected in a variety of pathologic responses in the skin and lymph nodes, but each is associated with additional and characteristic pathology. Descriptions of the diseases caused by *Onchocerca* are given in Chapters 16 and 23.

Lymphatic filariasis caused by Brugia and Wuchereria, which are transmitted by mosquitoes
The mosquitoes introduce the infective larvae into the skin as they feed. These larvae develop slowly into long thin adult worms (females 80–100 mm × 0.25 mm), which are found in the lymph nodes and lymphatics of the limbs (usually lower) and groin. Infections become patent after about a year, when sheathed microfilariae appear in the blood. Infected individuals may show few clinical signs or have acute manifestations such as fever, rashes, eosinophilia, lymphangitis, lymphadenitis *(Fig. 25.24)* and orchitis. Later chronic obstructive changes, caused by repeated episodes of lymphangitis, may block lymphatics, leading to hydrocele and to the gross enlargement of breasts, scrotum and limbs, the latter condition being known as 'elephantiasis' *(Fig. 25.25)*.

A feature of filarial infections in endemic regions is that not everyone exposed develops symptomatic infections. Many, although microfilaremic, remain asymptomatic, and relatively few show gross pathology *(Fig. 25.26)*. Some individuals develop pulmonary symptoms known as 'tropical pulmonary eosinophilia' (see Chapter 17).

Few drugs are really satisfactory for treating filariasis
Diethylcarbamazine has long been used in treatment, but although this primarily kills microfilariae it can result in a violent allergic response (Mazzotti reaction). Suramin kills adult worms, but is toxic. Ivermectin is currently being used against onchocerciasis with some success and may become the drug of choice for lymphatic filariasis as well.

It is difficult to prevent transmission of filariasis, although this can be minimized by vector control and prevention of biting.

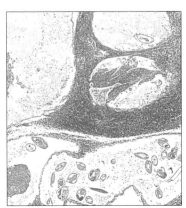

Fig. 25.24 Lymph node containing adult *Wuchereria*, showing dilated lymphatics and tissue reaction in the vessel walls. (Courtesy of R Muller and JR Baker.)

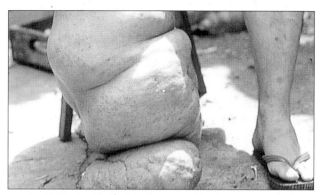

Fig. 25.25 Elephantiasis of the leg, caused by *Brugia malayi*. (Courtesy of AE Bianco.)

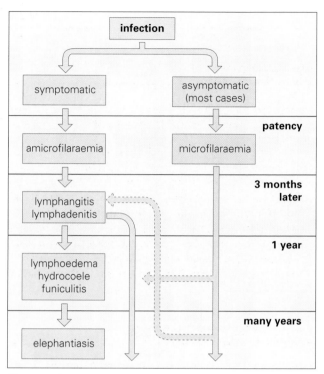

Fig. 25.26 Course of lymphocytic filariasis in symptomatic cases. (Redrawn from Muller and Baker, 1990.)

- Many important infections (arboviruses, rickettsiae, *Borrelia*, protozoa, helminths) are transmitted by insects, ticks or snails.
- Some are chronic (Lyme disease, leishmaniasis, schistosomiasis) or can be lethal (malaria, viral encephalitis).
- Often they are restricted to tropical countries because of the distribution of the vector.
- Strong immune responses are mounted, often leading to immunopathologic complications. Treatment is usually by chemotherapy
- Vector control is difficult, but can lead to disease eradication.
- With very few exceptions (yellow fever), vaccines are not available for this group of diseases.

A 42-year-old businessman is admitted to hospital with a fever, sore throat, chills, headache, muscle aches, abdominal pain, nausea and vomiting. He returned from a three-month trip to Sierra Leone two weeks ago and has taken antimalarial prophylaxis. On examination he has a fever of 38°C, a mildly inflamed pharynx, a regular pulse rate of 100 beats/minute and a blood pressure of 110/70 mmHg. The only other features of note are splenomegaly and a tender, mildly enlarged liver.
1. What differential diagnosis must you consider immediately?
2. What immediate investigations would you perform?
3. How would you manage this patient?

Further Reading

Cook GC ed. *Manson's Tropical Diseases*, 20th edition. London: WB Saunders, 1996.

Fisher–Hoch S. Viral hemorrhagic fever. *Med Int* 1988;**54**:2240–2247.

Greenwood BM, Whittle HC. Immunology of medicine in the tropics. In: *Current Topics In Immunology*, Series. London: Edward Arnold, 1981.

Hoffman SL ed. *Malaria Vaccine Development.* Washington DC: ASM Press, 1996.

Kaslow RA. Current perspective on Lyme borreliosis. *JAMA* 1992;**267**:1381–1383.

Muller R, Baker JR. *Medical Parasitology.* London: Gower Medical Publishing, 1990.

Nimmanitya S. Dengue fever and dengue hemorrhagic fever. *Med Int* 1988;**54**:2247–2251.

Tsai TF. Arboviral infections in the United States. *Infect Dis Clin N America* 1991;**5**:73–102.

Warren KS ed. *Immunology of Parasitic Infections*, 3rd edition. Oxford: Blackwell Scientific Publications, 1992.

Weiss E. The biology of rickettsiae. *Ann Rev Microbiol* 1982;**36**:345–370.

Introduction

Some multisystem infections in man are animal diseases (i.e. zoonoses)
In these infections, a non-human vertebrate host is the reservoir of infection and humans are involved only incidentally. The human infection follows contact with the reservoir host, but is not essential for the microbe's life cycle or for its maintenance in nature. One striking feature of zoonotic infections and of the arthropod-borne infections described in Chapter 25, is that almost none are transmitted effectively from human to human.

Sometimes, however, the zoonotic definition of these infections is less clear. For example, tularemia can be acquired either by direct contact with the reservoir host or from an arthropod vector, and is included in this chapter. Plague is included because it is transmitted from infected rats via the rat flea, although it is also transmissible directly from human to human.

Other zoonoses are dealt with in their relevant chapters (e.g. toxoplasmosis in Chapter 21, rabies in Chapter 22, salmonellosis in Chapter 20, psittacosis in Chapter 17).

Arenavirus Infections

Arenaviruses are transmitted to humans in rodent excreta

Many zoonoses are caused by enveloped single-stranded RNA viruses called arenaviruses. On electron microscopy *(Fig. 26.1)* these pleomorphic virus particles can be seen to contain sand-like granules, giving rise to the name 'arena' (Latin: arena, sand). Arenaviruses are parasites of various species of rodent in which they cause a harmless life-long infection with continuous excretion of virus in urine and feces of apparently healthy infected animals. Humans infected from this source may develop severe and often lethal disease. The arenaviruses and the diseases they cause are included in *Figure 26.2*. As with most zoonoses, infection is not transmitted, or is transmitted with low efficiency, from human to human. However, doctors and nurses have been infected by direct contact with blood or secretions from patients infected with Lassa fever virus. The usual incubation period is 5–10 days.

Arenavirus infection is diagnosed serologically or by virus isolation

Diagnosis by testing for specific antibodies – complement fixation or immunofluorescent tests – or virus isolation can be carried out in special centers. Prevention of infection by reducing exposure to the virus was dramatically illustrated when rodent trapping terminated outbreaks of Bolivian hemorrhagic fever (see panel overleaf). Treatment with the antiviral ribavirin has been successful in Lassa fever, and human immune plasma in Lassa fever and Argentinian hemorrhagic fever.

Lymphocytic choriomeningitis virus occurs worldwide

Lymphocytic choriomeningitis (LCM) has caused sporadic infection in people living in mouse-infested dwellings, and once or twice in children possessing apparently normal, but infected hamsters. There is generally a non-specific febrile illness, but occasionally an aseptic (lymphocytic) meningitis occurs, with recovery.

Lassa fever virus is an arenavirus that infects a bush rat in parts of West Africa

Human exposure to infected rats *(Mastomys natalensis)* or their urine results in a febrile disease, which is generally not very severe. There are about 300 000 cases with 5000 deaths/year, and Lassa fever is the commonest febrile illness in hospitals in parts of Sierra Leone. Transfer of virus from hospital patient to nurse or doctor via blood or tissue fluids often gives rise to a more severe illness. This involves hemorrhage, capillary damage, hemoconcentration and collapse, and was seen when the disease was first recognized in Americans in the village of Lassa in 1969. So far there have been 10 deaths among 21 infected doctors and nurses. The incubation period of 7–18 days would allow an infected individual to carry the disease anywhere in the world. However, person to person transfer via regular routes (e.g. droplets), for instance in aircraft carrying infected patients, does not occur.

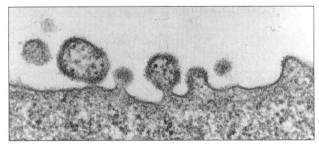

Fig. 26.1 Electron micrograph of lymphocytic choriomeningitis virus budding from the surface of an infected cell. The sand-like granules in the virus particles are characteristic of arenaviruses. (Courtesy of K Mannweiler and F Lehmann–Grübe.)

VIRAL FEVERS AND HEMORRHAGIC DISEASES ACQUIRED FROM VERTEBRATES OR FROM UNKNOWN SOURCES					
virus	virus group	disease	animal of origin	lethality	geographic distribution
lymphocytic choriomeningitis (LCM)	arenavirus	LCM	mouse, hamster	–	worldwide
Lassa fever	arenavirus	Lassa fever	African bush rat (Mastomys natalensis)	+	West Africa
Machupo	arenavirus	Bolivian hemorrhagic fever	bush mouse (Calomys callosus)	+	NE Bolivia
Junin	arenavirus	Argentinian hemorrhagic fever	Calomys spp. mice	+	Argentina
Hantaan	bunyavirus	hemorrhagic fever fever with renal syndrome (Korean hemorrhagic fever) severe pulmonary syndrome	mice, rats	+	Far East, Scandinavia E Europe SW USA
Marburg	filovirus	Marburg disease	unknown	+ +	Africa (lab. infections in Marburg etc.)
Ebola	filovirus	Ebola disease	unknown	+ +	Africa (Sudan, Zaire)

Fig. 26.2 Viral fevers and hemorrhagic diseases acquired from vertebrates or from unknown sources.

Korean Hemorrhagic Fever

The Hantaan virus causes Korean hemorrhagic fever and infects rodents

The Hantaan virus is a bunyavirus that causes a harmless persistent infection in various species of mice and rats. After exposure to the urine of infected animals there is a febrile illness, often with hypotension, hemorrhage and a renal syndrome. Many American soldiers suffered severe infections in Korea, and a milder disease is seen in Eastern Europe and Scandinavia. Related viruses are present in mice and rats in the USA, and in recent outbreaks in SW USA have caused 26 deaths with severe pulmonary disease. Laboratory diagnosis is by the detection of specific IgM or IgG antibody.

Marburg and Ebola Hemorrhagic Fevers

The source of Marburg and Ebola hemorrhagic fevers is unknown

Marburg and Ebola hemorrhagic fevers occur in Central and East Africa and are caused by filoviruses – long filamentous single-stranded RNA viruses. Patients develop fever, hemorrhage, rash, and probably disseminated intravascular coagulation (see Chapter 12). There is no specific treatment and no vaccine, and for both viruses the reservoir of origin and natural cycle of maintenance is unknown.

Infection with Marburg virus was first recognized in 1967 in Marburg, Germany, after exposure of laboratory workers to infected African green monkeys from Uganda. However, these monkeys are not the natural hosts and the ultimate source of the infection is still unknown. Mortality was about 20% and, as with Ebola virus infection, it was noted that semen can remain infected for months after clinical recovery; one patient transmitted the infection to his wife in this way. Altogether 31 infections have been recorded and eight of them have been fatal.

Outbreaks of a similar disease occurred in 1976 in Southern Sudan and in the region of the Ebola river in Zaire. There were more than 500 cases, and person to person transmission took place in local hospitals via contaminated syringes and needles. Overall mortality in this locally terrifying and mysterious outbreak of disease was 70%. Further outbreaks have occurred (1995, 1996) in the same region of Africa. In 1989 monkeys infected with a similar virus were inadvertently imported into the USA from the Philippines, but it failed to cause disease in humans.

Q Fever

Coxiella burnetii, the rickettsial cause of Q fever, is carried by arthropods

The disease Q fever was first recognized in Australia in 1935, but the cause was unknown for several years – hence Q (query) fever. The causative rickettsia, Coxiella burnetii, differs from other rickettsiae (see Chapter 25) in the following ways:
• It is not transmitted to humans by arthropods.
• It is relatively resistant to desiccation, heat and sunlight, and is therefore stable enough to be acquired from infected animals by the airborne route.

Bolivian hemorrhagic fever: A lesson in ecology

In 1962 there was an outbreak of a severe and often lethal infectious disease in the small town of San Joachim, Bolivia. Patients developed fever, myalgia, and an enanthem, followed by capillary leakage, hemorrhage, shock, and a neurologic illness. This disease was termed 'Bolivian hemorrhagic fever' and had a mortality rate of 15%. Extensive investigations failed to incriminate an arthropod vector, but the evidence pointed to a role for mice in the epidemic. Acting on this possibility, hundreds of mouse traps were airlifted to the beleaguered town and it was soon shown that trapping mice had a dramatic effect on the incidence of the disease. The epidemic was completely halted. Quite separately, a virus was isolated from the tissues of a trapped local bush mouse (*Calomys callosus*). The virus was shown to cause a harmless life-long infection in this animal, with continued excretion of virus in urine and feces. The virus (given the name 'Machupo') was an arenavirus, a group that includes lymphocytic choriomeningitis (LCM) virus (infecting mice and hamsters) and Lassa fever virus (infecting an African bush rat). These viruses cause a harmless persistent infection in the natural rodent host, but an often severe disease in humans exposed to infected animals.

This outbreak of Bolivian hemorrhagic fever provided an important lesson in ecology. Because of the high incidence of malaria in the San Joachim area, extensive dichlorodiphenyltrichloroethane (DDT) spraying had been carried out to control mosquitoes. As a result, geckos (small lizards that eat insects) accumulated DDT in their tissues and the local cats that preyed on geckos began to die with lethal concentrations of DDT in their livers. The shortage of cats, in turn, allowed the bush mice to invade human dwellings. The close vicinity of infected mice to humans and human food led to the epidemic (*Fig. 26.3*).

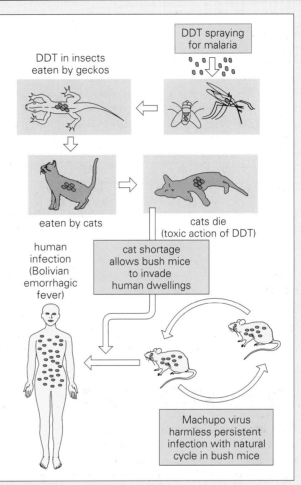

Fig. 26.3 Bolivian hemorrhagic fever – a lesson in ecology. (DDT, dichlorodiphenyltrichloroethane.)

- Its main site of action is the lung rather than vascular endothelium elsewhere in the body, so that there is usually no rash.

C. burnetii is transmitted to man by inhalation

In many countries (e.g. USA) infection of livestock with *C. burnetii* is quite common, but there are few human cases (less than 50/year reported in the USA). People who come into contact with infected animals, especially their placentas, unpasteurized milk and tissue fluids, are most at risk (e.g. veterinarians, farmers, abbatoir workers).

After inhalation, the microbe multiplies in the terminal airways of the lung and about three weeks later the patient develops fever, severe headache, and often respiratory symptoms and an atypical pneumonia. The rickettsia can also spread to the liver, commonly causing hepatitis. Recovery is usually complete in two weeks, but the disease can become chronic. The heart is sometimes involved (endocarditis), with thrombocytopenia and purpura in some patients and this condition is fatal if untreated.

Q fever is diagnosed serologically and treated with an antibiotic

A fourfold or greater rise in complement fixing antibody titer is significant. There are two antigenic forms, phase 1 and phase 2. Antibody to phase 2 is seen in ordinary Q fever, and to both phase 1 and phase 2 in chronic disease. The Weil–Felix test (see Chapter 25) is not used.

The infection is treated with tetracycline or erythromycin, and a killed *C. burnetii* vaccine is available for those at risk. The rickettsia are destroyed when milk is pasteurized.

Anthrax

Anthrax is caused by Bacillus anthracis and is primarily a disease of herbivores

Bacillus anthracis is a large Gram-positive rod and is aerobic and non-motile. Most members of the genus *Bacillus* are saprophytic (see Chapter 3), present in soil, water, air and vegetation. *Bacillus cereus* is a cause of food poisoning, but

B. anthracis is the principal pathogen and is unique in having an antiphagocytic capsule made of D-glutamic acid. It forms spores, which survive for years in soil.

Anthrax is a disease of herbivores such as sheep, goats, cattle and horses, and bacilli are excreted in feces, urine and saliva. It is largely confined to developing countries (parts of Asia, Africa, Middle East), human infection occuring following direct contact with infected animals, or by contact with spores present in animal products. The spores enter the body via the skin or mucous membranes, and sometimes via the respiratory tract. In developed countries, where animal infection is rare, human infection is uncommon and has been due to exposure to contaminated imported goods such as hides, skin, wool, goat hair and bristles, bones and bonemeal in fertilizers.

Anthrax is characterized by a black eschar and the disease can be fatal if untreated

B. anthracis spores germinate in tissues at the site of entry. The bacteria then multiply and produce the anthrax toxin, which consists of an edema factor (an adenylate cyclase), a lethal factor, and a protective antigen. All are plasmid-coded and have been purified and cloned. Host defenses are inhibited by the antiphagocytic capsule surrounding the bacillus (see Chapter 9).

The skin is the usual site of entry. As the toxic material accumulates there is edema and congestion, and a papule develops within 12–36 hours. The papule ulcerates, the center becoming black and necrotic (Greek: anthrax, coal), to form a 'malignant pustule' (although there is no pus) which is painless and is often surrounded by a ring of vesicles *(Fig. 26.4)*. The bacilli spread to the lymphatics and in about 10% of cases reach the blood to cause septicemia. Continued multiplication and production of the toxin causes generalized toxic effects, edema and death.

When the spores are inhaled and enter alveolar macrophages, bacterial growth in the lung leads to pulmonary edema and mediastinal hemorrhage, with spread to the blood and death. Pulmonary anthrax is now very rare in most developed countries, where it was referred to as 'woolsorter's disease'.

Anthrax is diagnosed by culture and treated with penicillin

Films from skin lesions show Gram-positive bacilli, but the diagnosis is confirmed and non-pathogenic bacilli are distinguished after culture on blood agar. Serologic tests are generally not helpful.

Anthrax is successfully treated by penicillin, given early and in large doses. Cutaneous anthrax is fatal in 10–20% of cases when untreated.

Anthrax can be prevented and is now mainly a disease of developing countries

Animals can be protected by vaccination with live avirulent bacteria. Infected animals are isolated, killed, and buried or cremated without autopsy. A vaccine consisting of purified protective antigen is available for humans at high risk.

Human infection is reduced by rigidly controlled disinfection of imported animal products such as hides, hair and wool.

Plague

The plague is caused by *Yersinia pestis*, which infects rodents and is spread to man by fleas

Yersina pestis is a small Gram-negative rod with a surrounding capsule that is associated with virulence. The animal reservoirs are rodents such as rats, squirrels, gerbils and field mice, in which the infection is generally mild, the bacteria being spread between animals by fleas *(Fig. 26.5)*. The bacillus has been endemic in wild rodents in Europe and Asia for thousands of years, and the disease in humans has at times decimated populations and influenced the course of history. In the fourteenth century about 25% of the population of Europe died in plague epidemics (see panel on p. 374). Early in the twentieth century the disease arrived in North America and is at present endemic in wild rodents in western USA. Plague is now extremely rare in Europe and uncommon in the USA.

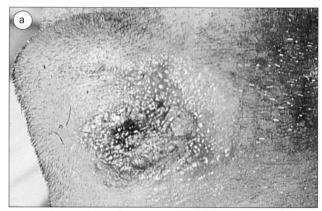

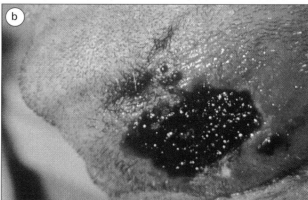

Fig. 26.4 Anthrax. (a) Characteristic black eschar surrounded by a ring of vesiculation. (b) Eight days later, the eschar has enlarged to cover the previously vesicular area, and the surrounding edema has diminished. (Courtesy of FJ Nye.)

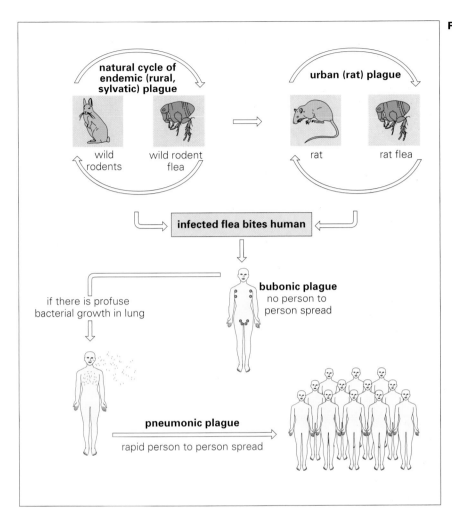

Fig. 26.5 The epidemiology of plague.

Major outbreaks in humans result from exposure to infected rats. The rat flea *(Xeopsylla cheopsis)* carries infection from rat to rat and from rat to human. *Y. pestis* multiplies profusely in the gut of the flea, eventually blocking the lumen so that the flea regurgitates infected material as it attempts to feed. As infected rats sicken, their fleas seek other hosts and may bite nearby humans thus causing 'bubonic' plague. This disease is not generally transmitted from person to person. However, when there is extensive replication of bacteria in the lung, with bronchopneumonia and large numbers of bacteria in the sputum, the infection can spread from person to person by droplets, causing 'pneumonic' plague, with extremely rapid onset.

Plague epidemics are preceded by increased infection in wild rodents and spread to rats. Rodent infection is endemic in India, South east Asia, South Africa, South America, Mexico and the western states of the USA. Sporadic plague continues to occur in these parts of the world, for instance in hunters exposed to infected prairie dogs in the USA and in rural populations elsewhere.

Clinical features of plague include buboes, pneumonia and a high death rate

The infecting bacteria multiply at the site of entry in the skin, and spread via the lymphatics to local and regional lymph nodes. They produce a number of virulence factors, including an antiphagocytic capsular antigen (fraction 1, coded by a plasmid), endotoxin and various other protein toxins. Lymph nodes in the armpit or groin become very tender and enlarge to form 'buboes' (Greek: bubo, groin) *(Fig. 26.7)* with hemorrhagic inflammation 2–6 days after the flea bite. The patient develops fever. In mild forms the infection is arrested

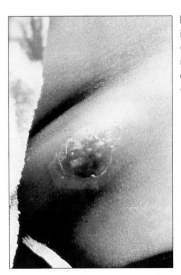

Fig. 26.6 Characteristic inguinal lymphadenitis (bubo) in which the lymph nodes have suppurated and drained spontaneously. (Courtesy of JR Cantey.)

The Black Death in fourteenth century England

For thousands of years, *Yersinia pestis* has been endemic in rodents in the Far East, with occasional epidemic spread into Europe and elsewhere. In January 1348, three galleys laden with spices from the East brought the plague to the port of Genoa, Italy. The disease, which for reasons that are not clear, became known as 'The Black Death' and soon spread to the rest of Europe, arriving in London in December 1348. To the medieval mind, the speed and violence with which the illness passed from person to person (in the pneumonic form in the winter) was its most terrifying feature. The bubonic form *(Fig. 26.6)* was also important, especially in the warmer summer months, there being at least one family of black rats per household and three fleas to a rat.

The disease was attributed to earthquakes, to the movement of the planets, to a Jewish or Arab plot (350 massacres of Jews took place during the Black Death in Europe), and most commonly to God's punishment for human wickedness. You could become infected without touching a plague victim, and to many it seemed that there was something – a miasma or a poison in the air. Physicians wore strange masks and infected houses were labeled and boarded up, together with the inhabitants. But it was impossible to isolate all those who were sick. Rich and poor perished.

The population of England was about four million and over a period of 2.5 years, approximately 35% (more than a million) died. The clergy, for unknown reasons, suffered an even greater mortality of nearly 50%. Altogether in Europe at least 25 million people died. The Black Death was a major human disaster,

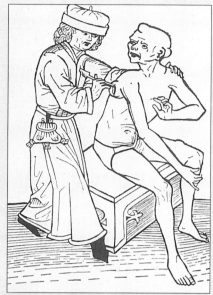

Fig. 26.7
Fifteenth century German woodcut showing incision of a bubo. (Courtesy of The Wellcome Institute Library, London. With permission from Ciba–Zeitschrift, Basel.)

with lasting effects on economic and social structure. There were a further five, less severe, outbreaks in England in the fourteenth century. The epidemic in 1665, the year before the Great Fire of London, was graphically described by Daniel Defoe (who was only five at the time) in his *Journal of a Plague Year in London*. The last pandemic arose in China and reached Hong Kong in 1894, where Yersin and (independently) Kitasato described the causative bacillus.

at this stage, but spread to the blood often occurs, with septicemia, hemorrhagic illness and multisystem involvement (spleen, liver, lungs, CNS).

Common complications are disseminated intravascular coagulation, pneumonia and meningitis. The death rate is about 50% in untreated bubonic plague, and nearly 100% in pneumonic plague. On recovery there is solid immunity and bacteria are eliminated from the body.

Plague is diagnosed microscopically and treated with antibiotic

In pneumonic plague, organisms are found in fluid aspirated from lymph nodes, or from sputum in pneumonic plague. They can be seen in smears after Giemsa, Gram or fluorescent antibody staining (the staining is bipolar) and can also be cultivated.

Streptomycin and/or tetracycline are used in the treatmentof plague.

Plague has been prevented by the following measures:
- Classically, by quarantine measures in ports and on ships. Quarantine – from the Italian 'quarentina' meaning 40 days – refers to the original isolation period for ships suspected of carrying contagion.
- By rodent control, especially of rats (e.g. at the site of entry of ships and aircraft into plague-free countries).
- By strict isolation of patients with plague.
- By chemoprophylaxis (tetracycline) during an epidemic or visit to an affected area.
- By vaccination of military personnel and of certain workers in endemic areas. The vaccine consists of formalin-killed bacteria and gives partial protection.

Yersinia enterocolitica Infection

Yersina enterocolitica is a cause of diarrheal disease (see Chapter 20, *Fig. 20.20*) and is mentioned here because it has a reservoir in rodents and other animals.

Tularemia

Tularemia is caused by Francisella tularensis and is spread by arthropods from infected animals

Tularemia is caused by the small Gram-negative rod *Francisella tularensis*, which was first isolated from rodents in Tulare County, California in 1912 and later shown by Edward Francis to cause human disease. It is present in rodents and in a wide variety of other wild animals in many countries in the northern hemisphere, including the USA (especially Arkansas and Missouri), Russia, Scandinavia and Spain. In the infected animal it causes a plague-like disease and is spread via ticks, mites, lice and biting flies. In *Dermacentor* ticks, the bacteria are transmitted vertically to subsequent generations via the ovum. Human infection is sporadic and follows contact with an infected animal (e.g. skinning of hares, rabbits, muskrats) or with the arthropod vector. There is no spread from person to person.

Clinical features of tularemia include painful swollen lymph nodes

Y. enterocolitica is intracellular, and parasitizes the reticuloendothelial system. It grows at the site of entry, aided by its virulence-associated capsule, and after 3–5 days forms a skin ulcer. There is a febrile illness and lymphatic spread results in swollen painful regional lymph nodes. Blood invasion and involvement of lungs, gastrointestinal tract and liver is not uncommon, with the formation of granulomatous nodules around infected reticuloendothelial cells. There may be a rash. Mortality in untreated patients is 5–15%. The conjunctiva or oral mucosa can be infected via contaminated fingers resulting in ocular or oral manifestations. Infection by inhalation is less common and gives a febrile illness with respiratory symptoms.

Tularemia is diagnosed serologically and treated with streptomycin

Infected tissues can be examined by fluorescent antibody staining, but isolation of bacteria is not often attempted due to the high risk of laboratory infection. Agglutination tests for antibody are more commonly used in diagnosis.

Streptomycin is an effective treatment, and a live attenuated bacterial vaccine is available for people with occupational risk (e.g. fur trappers). Handling animals with gloves gives protection, and contact with ticks should be avoided.

Pasteurella multocida Infection

Pasteurella multocida is part of the normal flora of cats and dogs and is transmitted to man by an animal bite

Pasteurella multocida is an encapsulated Gram-negative rod and is distributed worldwide. It is part of the normal oral flora in cats, dogs and other domestic and wild animals, in whom it can also cause pneumonia and septicemia. It is transmitted to humans by animal bites (especially cat bites), and other types of bacteria including anaerobes are often present in the lesion.

P. multocida infection causes cellulitis, is diagnosed microscopically and treated with penicillin

Local multiplication of bacteria leads within a day or two to cellulitis. Virulence factors include endotoxin and the capsule.

P. multocida can be cultivated and identified in material from the wound.

Penicillin is an effective treatment and ampicillin has been used in prophylaxis after cat or dog bites. Bite wounds should be cleansed and debrided.

Leptospirosis

Leptospirosis is caused by the spirochete Leptospira interrogans, which infects mammals such as rats

Leptospira are tightly coiled spirochetes 5–15 μm long. They show active rotational movement and have two flagellae. Their delicate outline is best seen by dark field microscopy because they are not very well stained by dyes. The ends of the species *Leptospira interrogans* are bent into a quesion-mark-like a hook – hence the name 'interrogans'. This species infects mammals such as rats in various parts of the world (*Fig. 26.8*), causing chronic kidney infection with excretion of large numbers of bacteria in urine. The spirochetes are soon killed on drying, heating and exposure to detergents or disinfectants, but they remain viable for several weeks in stagnant alkaline water or wet soil. Humans are infected by ingestion of, or exposure to, contaminated water or food. The bacteria, aided by their motility, enter through breaks in skin or mucosae, so infection can be acquired by swimming, working or playing in contaminated water (miners, farmers, sewage workers, watersport enthusiasts). There are about 60 cases/year in England and Wales and about 100/year are reported in the USA. Bacteria are excreted in human urine, but person to person transmission is rare. Immunity is serotype specific.

Clinical features of leptospirosis include kidney and liver failure

The bacteria reach the blood and after an incubation period of 1–2 weeks cause a febrile, influenza-like illness. In about 90% of cases this resolves uneventfully, but multiplication can cause:

LEPTOSPIRA INTERROGANS DISEASES			
leptospiral serogroup	animal host	distribution	clinical features
canicola	dog	worldwide	influenza-like illness ('canicola fever', '7-day fever') is the commonest; can progress to aseptic meningitis, liver and kidney damage (Weil's disease)
icterohaemorrhagiae	rat	worldwide	
hebdomadis	mice voles rats cattle	Japan, Europe	

Fig. 26.8 Diseases caused by the three main serogroups of *Leptospira interrogans*. There are 19 different serogroups of this organism, other serogroups including seroja (pigs) and pomona (swine and cattle in USA and Europe). Among the serogroups there are 172 different serotypes.

- Hepatitis, jaundice and hemorrhage in the liver.
- Uremia and bacteriuria in the kidney.
- Aseptic meningitis and conjunctival or scleral hemorrhage in the cerebrospinal fluid (CSF) and the aqueous humor (Fig. 26.9).

The clinical picture depends to some extent upon the particular type of leptospire. Weil's disease, the severe form with hemorrhagic complications and kidney and liver failure, occurs in only 5–10% of patients with leptospirosis.

Leptospirosis is diagnosed microscopically and serologically and treated with antibiotic

There is often a history of exposure. Bacteria can be isolated from blood, CSF and urine and a rise in agglutinating antibody can be demonstrated.

Penicillin and tetracyclines have been valuable in treatment when given within a day or two of the onset of illness, and doxycycline will prevent disease in those exposed to infection.

Measures for prevention include:
- Rodent control.
- Protective clothing.
- Prophylactic penicillin after cuts and abrasions in those at risk (sewer and abbatoir workers).

Rat Bite Fever

Rat bite fever is caused by bacteria transmitted to humans by a rodent bite

This uncommon but worldwide condition is caused by either *Spirillum minor*, a Gram-negative spiral-shaped organism, or by *Streptobacillus moniliformis*, a Gram-negative filamentous bacillus. These bacteria are found in the oropharyngeal flora of 50% of healthy wild and laboratory rats and also in other rodents. Transmission to humans is by biting.

Clinical features of rat bite fever can include endocarditis and pneumonia

After an incubation period of 7–10 days there is an onset of fever, headache and myalgia. Bacteria multiply at the site of the bite, and in the case of *S. moniliformis*, cause an inflamed local lesion. Spread of infection to lymph nodes and the blood leads to lymphadenopathy, rash and arthralgia.

Complications include endocarditis and pneumonia, and there is a mortality of up to 10% in untreated patients.

Rat bite fever is diagnosed by microscopy or culture and is treated with antibiotic

S. moniliformis can be cultured from the wound site, lymph nodes and blood, but *Sp. minor* cannot be cultivated and must be demonstrated in tissues by dark field microscopy.

Penicillin and streptomycin are effective treatments.

Measures for prevention include:
- Rodent control.
- Prevention of rat bites in laboratory workers.

Brucellosis

Brucellosis occurs worldwide and is caused by Brucella species

Brucellae are small Gram-negative non-motile coccobacilli, adapted to intracellular replication. The principal antigens are:
- A *(Brucella abortus)*.
- M *(Brucella melitensis)*.
- An endotoxin, involved in the pathogenesis.

Brucellae are primarily animal pathogens, infecting humans after contact with infected animals or their products (Fig. 26.10). There are three important species, each with a predilection for a certain domestic animal, although capable of infecting a wider range of animals:

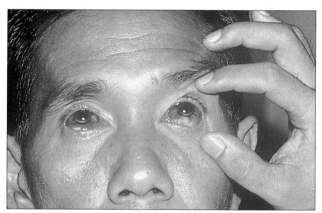

Fig. 26.9 Conjunctival hemorrhages in a jaundiced patient with leptospirosis. (Courtesy of D Lewis.)

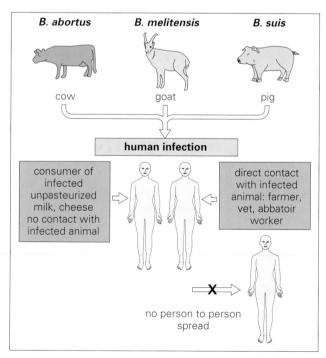

Fig. 26.10 Transmission of brucellosis. Human infection follows contact with infected animals or consumption of infected animal products.

- *B. abortus* infects cows. The distribution is worldwide, but has been eliminated from several developed countries.
- *B. melitensis* infects goats and sheep. It is common in Malta (Latin: melita, honey isle) and other Mediterranean countries, Mexico and South America. It tends to cause more severe disease in humans.
- *Brucella suis* infects pigs. It occurs in the USA where it is the most important cause of brucellosis, and in South America and Southeast Asia.

In cows and goats brucellae localize in the placenta, causing contagious abortion, and also in mammary glands from where they are shed for long periods in milk. They are present in uterine discharges, feces and urine.

Human brucellosis (undulant fever, Malta fever) occurs when the bacteria enter the body via abrasions in the skin, via the alimentary tract or, most commonly, via the respiratory tract. Infection is particularly seen in those who are in close contact with infected animals (farmers, veterinarians, abbatoir workers). Unpasteurized cows' milk (UK, USA), goats' milk or cheese (Mediterranean countries) is a less frequent source of infection. There is no spread from person to person.

Clinical features of brucellosis are immune-mediated and include an undulant fever and chronicity

The infecting bacteria pass from the site of entry into local and regional lymph nodes, reaching the thoracic duct and thus the blood (septicemic phase). Cells of the reticuloendothelial system are then infected (liver, spleen, bone marrow, lymphoid tissues) and it is in these cells and in monocytes and macrophages that the host battles against the parasite. The result is an inflammatory (granulomatous) reaction with epithelioid and giant cells, central necrosis and peripheral fibrosis.

Quite commonly the infection is subclinical. The symptoms of acute brucellosis begin after an incubation period of 1–3 weeks with a gradual onset of malaise, fever, drenching sweats, aching and weakness. A rising and falling (undulant) fever is seen in a minority of patients. Enlarged lymph nodes and spleen may be detected and hepatitis can occur *(Fig. 26.11)*. The bone marrow lesions may progress to osteomyelitis, and cholecystitis, endocarditis and meningitis are occasionally seen. Abortion occurs in infected cows, sows and goats, but not in humans. It is due to the presence in the placenta of erythritol, a sugar compound that stimulates bacterial growth. Erythritol is not present in the human placenta.

The patient generally recovers after a few weeks or months, but a chronic stage (more than one year's illness) can develop with tiredness, aches and pains, anxiety, depression and occasional fever. Relapses and remissions may occur. Brucellae cannot be isolated at this stage, and chronic brucellosis is often a difficult diagnosis. Agglutinin titers are generally high, but antibodies are less relevant than cell-mediated immunity for this intracellular parasite.

Brucellosis is diagnosed serologically and treated with antibiotics

Brucellae can be isolated in some cases from blood cultures (or from bone marrow or lymph nodes), and urine culture may be successful. This takes up to four weeks. Agglutinating antibodies (IgM) are present in acute brucellosis, but not generally in chronic brucellosis. Complement fixation tests and antiglobulin tests are also used, but radioimmunoassay are the most sensitive.

Brucellae are susceptible to tetracycline and streptomycin; cotrimoxazole is also used. The intracellular location of brucellae means that the bacteria are not easily eradicated and so prolonged courses of treatment (three months) are needed.

Brucellae in milk are destroyed by pasteurization. In the USA and UK, brucellosis has gradually declined (about 100 cases/year now reported in the USA) following eradication programs, involving the use of a live attenuated vaccine (S19) in cattle and slaughter of those already infected.

Protective clothing and goggles may be used by those in close contact with infected animals (farmers, veterinarians, abattoir workers) on risky occasions.

There is no satisfactory vaccine available for humans. Indeed veterinarians may develop a mild illness when accidentally infected with the live S19 vaccine.

Helminth Infections

Few helminth infections are true multisystem diseases

The allocation of a particular helminth infection to a chapter on multisystem infection is a somewhat arbitrary decision. Many of the worm parasites that can be acquired from animals, or through the bites of arthropod vectors, have stages that invade a number of the body systems. Others are primarily located in a particular organ, but cause pathologic changes that can be widespread in their effects. Conversely, although stages of certain worms may be widely distributed in the body, their pathologic effects are most commonly associated with a particular organ.

For example:
- The larvae of the pork tapeworm *Taenia solium*, which causes the disease cysticercosis, develop in a variety of

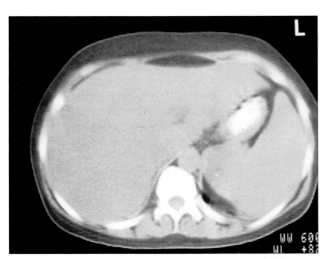

Fig. 26.11 Computerized tomographic scan showing hepatosplenomegaly in *Brucella melitensis* infection. (Courtesy of H Tubbs.)

tissues, including muscle. However, the most serious pathology is caused by larvae found in the CNS. Accordingly, this infection is discussed in Chapter 22.

- After infection with eggs of the dog nematode *Toxocara canis*, larvae migrate throughout the body, causing the condition known as 'visceral larval migrans'. Again, the most serious effects are associated with larvae that localize in the CNS (see Chapter 22) and the eye (see Chapter 16).
- The filarial nematodes that localize in the lymphatics (*Wuchereria*, *Brugia*) or subcutaneous tissue (*Onchocerca*), give rise to lymphangitis, lymphadenopathy and pathologic change in the skin, but their most dramatic pathology is seen as chronic obstructive lymphatic changes (see Chapter 25), and blindness (see Chapter 16), respectively.

However, three helminths can be considered as genuinely multisystem in their effects. These are:

- The tapeworm *Echinococcus granulosus*.
- The nematode *Trichinella spiralis*.
- The nematode *Strongyloides stercoralis*.

Echinococcus
Echinococcus adults are tiny tapeworms in dogs and their larvae cause hydatid cysts in man

The adults of this species live as tiny (3–5 mm long) tapeworms in the intestine of the dog. Eggs laid by the worm leave the dog in fecal material and can survive in the outside world for long periods. If swallowed (under natural conditions by sheep or accidentally by humans), the eggs hatch in the small intestine, releasing larvae which then penetrate the mucosa to enter a blood vessel. The circulating larvae then lodge in a capillary bed, most often in the liver, but also in the body cavity, lung, brain, eye, spinal cord or long bones. Once in the target organ the larvae slowly grow into large, thick-walled, fluid-filled (hydatid) cysts, the pathologic signs being largely due to the mechanical pressure exerted by the cysts *(Fig. 26.12)*.

Echinococcosis (hydatid disease) is diagnosed microscopically and serologically and treated with praziquantel and surgery

Laboratory diagnosis is by finding hooklets and scolices in the cyst fluid and demonstrating specific antibody (enzyme-linked immunosorbent assay, indirect hemagglutination). Although drug treatment (praziquantel) is available, surgical removal, where possible, is the most satisfactory way of dealing with the infection. Great care must be taken during removal to prevent leakage of fluid from the cysts. Not only may this trigger anaphylactic responses in sensitized individuals, but the numerous larvae in the fluid (produced by asexual division) can cause metastatic infections in other sites.

Echinococcus multilocularis closely resembles *E. granulosus*, but results in the formation of a multilocular cyst consisting of hundreds of small vesicles, without a fibrous outer capsule. The parasite generally occurs as a fox–rodent cycle (the fox harbours the adult tapeworm and the rodent the larval stage) in North Europe, Siberia and parts of North America . Hunters or trappers are occasionally infected after ingesting food contaminated by fox feces. Liver involvement leads to jaundice and weight loss, and the condition is usually inoperable.

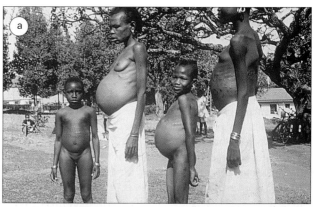
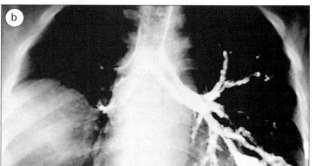

Fig. 26.12 Hydatid cysts. (a) Patients showing marked abdominal swelling caused by hydatid cysts in the liver. (Courtesy of GS Nelson.) (b) Bronchogram showing blockage of a bronchus by a cyst of *Echinococcus granulosus* in the lower left medial region. (Courtesy of RB Holliman.)

Trichinella
T. spiralis is transmitted in undercooked pork and causes the disease trichinosis

T. spiralis is perhaps the most widely distributed of all nematode parasites, being capable of infecting almost any warm-blooded animal. In its natural cycle it is transmitted between predators (e.g. bears, seals) and their prey, and between scavengers and carrion, but a domestic cycle has become established in pigs and rats.

Humans are infected by eating undercooked meat (pork or wild animal) containing the encysted infected larval stages. These larvae mature rapidly into adults in the small intestine, their invasion of the mucosa causing an acute enteritis.

The clinical features of trichinosis are mainly immunopathologic in origin

Female worms release live larvae into the mucosa, and these invade the blood vessels 1–2 weeks after initial infection to become distributed around the body. Bacteremia may occur at this stage. The larvae attempt to invade the cells of many organs (including the heart and CNS), although they can mature only in striated muscles, where they form the characteristic cysts *(Fig. 26.13)*. This stage of infection is associated with a wide spectrum of pathologic signs such as fever, joint and muscle pains, eosinophilia and periorbital edema; myositis, petechial hemorrhage, encephalitis and cardiac abnormalities may also occur. These signs are mainly caused by hypersensitivity and inflammatory responses

Trichinosis is diagnosed microscopically and serologically and treated with anthelmintics and anti-inflammatories

Diagnosis of trichinosis is by muscle biopsy and demonstration of specific antibody. Treatment is possible with anthelmintics (thiabendazole), but symptomatic treatment with anti-inflammatories may also be necessary.

Strongyloides
Strongyloides infections are most often passed between humans, but can develop in animal hosts including dogs

Like *Trichinella*, *Strongyloides* has an intestinal phase, but infection is acquired by the penetration of infective larvae through the skin. The larvae migrate to the lung, enter the alveoli, pass up the bronchi and trachea, and are then swallowed. Only females develop parthenogenetically in the host, and they lay strings of eggs into the intestinal mucosa *(Fig. 26.14)*. The eggs hatch within the intestine to release larvae, which then pass out with the feces. The larvae require warm moist soil, and the geographic distribution of strongyloidiasis is similar to that of hookworm (especially in tropical areas and in rural southern states of the USA).

Strongyloides infection is not strictly a zoonosis as infections are most often passed between humans, but the species can also develop in animal hosts including dogs. It possesses the unusual property that the fecal larval stages may develop directly into the infective stage in a given patient and penetrate the perianal skin to reinfect the host; alternatively, the larvae may complete a free living, sexually reproducing generation in the soil, before once again producing infective larvae. This plasticity of behavior means that the species can undergo complete development within the host (autoinfection).

Strongyloides infections are usually asymptomatic, but can cause disseminated disease in association with T cell deficiencies or malnutrition

Larvae released from eggs laid by females in the intestine can become infective in the bowel and reinvade the body, often in enormous numbers. This is unimportant in immunocompetent hosts and most infected individuals are asymptomatic, though vomiting or diarrhea may occur. However, in those with T cell deficiencies or malnutrition it can lead to the condition known as 'hyperinfection' or 'disseminated strongyloidiasis', the larvae invading almost all organs and causing severe, and sometimes fatal, pathology. Infected patients may show vomiting, abdominal pain, diarrhea with malabsorption and dehydration, eosinophilia, pneumonitis and other 'allergic' signs. Disseminated strongyloidiasis can arise long after initial infection. It has been firmly established that infections can persist for many years (more than 30), being maintained by low level autoinfection until the patient's immune defenses are reduced.

Strongyloides infection is diagnosed microscopically and treated with anthelmintics

Laboratory diagnosis of *Strongyloides* infection depends upon finding the larvae in the feces, and anthelmintics such as thiabendazole or levamisole are used for treatment.

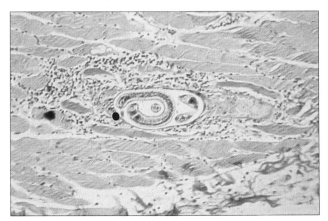

Fig. 26.13 Inflammatory reaction around a cyst containing a coiled larva of *Trichinella spiralis*. Trichrome stain. (Courtesy of IG Kagan.)

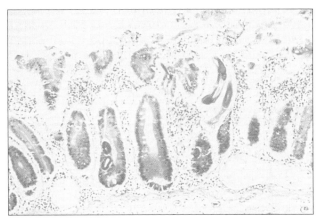

Fig. 26.14 *Strongyloides stercoralis*. Adults and larvae in the mucosa of small intestine, showing disruption of the villous surface.

- The multisystem infections described in this chapter are zoonoses, being maintained naturally in a reservoir of non-human vertebrates.
- Humans are infected incidentally, generally from rodents (arenaviruses, hantaviruses, plague, tularemia, leptospirosis) or from domestic animals (brucellosis, hydatid disease, leptospirosis).
- There is generally no transmission from person to person.
- The nature and the extent of human–animal contact is a determining factor.
- Some of these infections are highly virulent.
- When the reservoir host is common in crowded human communities (e.g. plague), disease epidemics have been major events in history.

- When humans have less extensive contact with the reservoir host, the infection, even when virulent, has less impact (e.g. Lassa fever, Ebola fever).
- Most of these infections are now less frequent in developed countries (e.g. anthrax, brucellosis, hydatid disease), but remain as frequent causes of disease in other parts of the world.
- There are satisfactory antimicrobial agents for most of the non-viral infections, but effective vaccines are generally not available.

A 39-year-old sailor who has just finished a three-month commission in the Far East and then Africa, visits his doctor having felt unwell for the previous month with a fever, headaches, tiredness and sweats. While at sea he had recorded his temperature as 38°C. He has no other symptoms of note. On examination he has a temperature of 39°C. The only other finding is tenderness in the left upper quadrant of his abdomen and one fingerbreadth splenomegaly. His doctor arranges for him to be admitted to hospital where he is investigated. The results of investigations are: hemoglobin 14 g/dl; white cell count 1.8×10^9/l; platelets 250×10^9/l, thick and thin blood film – no malarial parasites seen; erythrocyte sedimentation rate 40 mm/hour,

urea and electrolytes normal; liver function tests normal; chest radiograph normal; blood cultures – no growth after 48 hours; early morning urine – no growth of *Mycobacterium tuberculosis*.

1. This man has a pyrexia of unknown origin and there is a wide differential diagnosis. What further questions would you ask to help you make the diagnosis?
2. He has fever, sweats, malaise and splenomegaly together with leukopenia. What is the most likely diagnosis?
3. How would you investigate him further?
4. How would you manage him?

Further Reading

Evans ME. *Francisella tularensis. Infec Control* 1985;**6**:381–383.

Farr RW. Leptospirosis. *Clin Infect Dis* 1995;**21**:1–8.

Heymann DL, Weisfeld JS, Webb PA *et al.* Ebola haemorrhagic fever: Tandala, Zaire, 1977–1978. *J Inf Dis* 1980;**142**:372.

Howard CR, Simpson DIH. The biology of arenaviruses. *J Gen Virol* 1980;**51**:1.

Kaufmann AF, Boyce JM, Martone WJ. Trends in human plague in the United States. *J Infect Dis* 1980;**141**:522.

Young EJ. Human brucellosis. *Rev Infect Dis* 1983;**5**:821–842.

Introduction

Fever is an abnormal increase in body temperature and may be continuous or intermittent
The homeostatic mechanisms of the body maintain a constant body temperature with daily fluctuations (circadian temperature rhythm) not exceeding ± 1–1.5°C. Although 37°C (98.6°F) is taken as 'normal', individuals vary in their body temperature; in some it may be as low as 36°C, in others as high as 38°C. Fever is defined as an abnormal increase in body temperature – an oral temperature higher than 37.6°C (100.4°F) or a rectal temperature higher than 38°C (101°F), and may be continuous or intermittent:

- In continuous fever the body temperature is elevated over the whole 24-hour period and swings less than 1°C; this is characteristic of, for example, typhoid and typhus fever.
- In an intermittent fever the temperature is above normal throughout the 24-hour period, but swings more than 1°C during that time. A swinging fever is typical of pyogenic infections, abscesses and tuberculosis.

Fever, or 'pyrexia', may be produced in response to:
- Exogenous pyrogen such as endotoxin in Gram-negative cell walls.
- Endogenous pyrogen such as interleukin-1 (IL-1) released from phagocytic cells.

It is thought that fever may be a protective response by the host *(Fig. 27.1)*.

Definitions of Pyrexia of Unknown Origin

Pyrexia (fever) is a common complaint of patients presenting to a doctor. The cause is usually immediately apparent or is discovered within a few days, or the temperature settles spontaneously. If the patient's fever continues for 2–3 weeks or more and the diagnosis is uncertain, despite routine investigations performed during outpatient visits or in hospital, a provisional diagnosis of 'pyrexia of unknown origin' (PUO) – also known as 'fever of unknown origin' (FUO) – is made. This is the classical definition of PUO, but as an increasing number of patients with serious underlying diseases are successfully kept alive by modern medicine, PUO in patients in particular risk groups have also been defined *(Fig. 27.2)*.

Causes of PUO

Infection is the most common cause of PUO
For centuries, fever has been recognized as a characteristic sign of infection, and infection is the single most common cause of PUO, accounting for 30–45% of PUO in adults and up to 50% in children. However, there are important non-infectious causes of fever and the two main non-infectious causes are:
- Malignancies.
- Collagen vascular diseases *(Fig. 27.3)*.

These non-infectious causes need to be differentiated from infections during the investigation of a patient with a PUO. Despite intense and prolonged investigations, however, the cause of fever remains undiagnosed in as many as 10% of patients, and a further 10% may have a factitious fever (one produced artificially by the patient).

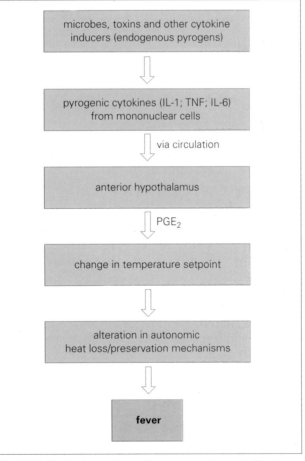

Fig. 27.1 Mechanisms of fever. Fever may be induced either by exogenous pyrogens such as microbes or their toxins or by endogenous pyrogens released in the host, and may have a protective effect. (IL-, interleukin; PG, prostaglandin; TNF, tumor necrosis factor.)

DEFINITIONS OF PYREXIA OF UNKNOWN ORIGIN		
definition	**symptoms**	**diagnosis**
classical PUO	fever (>38.3°C) on several occasions and more than **three weeks'** duration	uncertain despite appropriate investigations after at least **three** outpatient visits or **three days** in hospital
nosocomial (hospital-acquired) PUO	fever (>38.3°C) on several occasions in a hospitalized patient receiving acute care; infection not present or incubating on admission	uncertain after **three days** despite appropriate investigations, including at least **two days** incubation of microbiologic cultures
neutropenic PUO	fever (>38.3°C) on several occasions; neutrophil count <500/mm³ in peripheral blood, or expected to fall below that number within 1–2 days	uncertain after **three days** despite appropriate investigations, including at least **two days** incubation of microbiologic cultures
HIV-associated PUO	fever (>38.3°C) on several occasions; fever of more than **three weeks'** duration as an outpatient or more than **three days'** duration in hospital; confirmed positive HIV serology	uncertain after **three days** despite appropriate investigations, including at least **two days** incubation of microbiologic cultures

Fig. 27.2 Definitions of pyrexia of unknown origin (PUO). The classical definition of PUO requires that the fever is of three or more weeks' duration, but in compromised patients infections frequently progress rapidly because of inadequate host defenses. Consequently the pace of the investigations needs to be rapid if appropriate therapy is to be initiated.

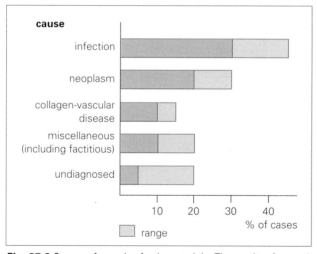

Fig. 27.3 Causes of pyrexia of unknow origin. The results of several retrospective studies show that infection is the single most common cause. In some studies a significant number of fevers remained undiagnosed.

Infective causes of classical PUO

The most common infective causes of classical PUO are shown in *Figure 27.4*. These can be divided into two main groups:
- Infections such as tuberculosis and typhoid fever caused by specific pathogens.
- Infections such as urinary tract infections, biliary tract infections and abscesses, which can be caused by a variety of different pathogens.

Most of these infections are described in detail elsewhere in this book. Bacterial endocarditis is discussed below (p. 000).

Significant infection may be present in the absence of fever in some groups of patients, notably:
- Seriously ill neonates.
- The elderly.
- Patients with uremia.
- Patients receiving corticosteroids
- Those taking antipyretic drugs continuously.

In these people other signs and symptoms of infection have to be sought. This chapter deals only with patients whose presenting complaint is fever.

Investigation of Classical PUO

Steps in the investigative procedure

Because of the many possible causes of PUO, both infectious and non-infectious, it is clearly not practicable to attempt specific investigations for each at the outset. The diagnostic pathway can be divided into a series of stages, each stage attempting to focus the investigation on the likely causes *(Fig. 27.5)*.

Stage 1 comprises careful history-taking, physical examination and screening tests

Careful history-taking is essential and should include questions about travel, occupation, hobbies, exposure to animals and known infectious hazards, antibiotic therapy within the previous two months, substance abuse and other habits. Some of the infections listed in *Figure 27.4* are zoonoses (e.g. leptospirosis, spotted fevers), whereas others are vector-borne

INFECTIVE CAUSES OF PYREXIA OF UNKNOWN ORIGIN	
infection	usual cause
Bacterial	
tuberculosis	*Mycobacterium tuberculosis*
enteric fevers	*Salmonella typhi*
osteomyelitis	*Staphylococcus aureus* (also *Haemophilus influenzae* in young children; *Salmonella* in patients with sickle-cell disease)
endocarditis	oral streptococci, *Staph. aureus*, coagulase-negative staphylococci
brucellosis	*Brucella abortus*, *B. mellitensis* and *B. suis*
abscesses (esp. intra-abdominal)	mixed anaerobes and facultative anaerobes from gut flora
biliary system infections	Gram-negative facultative anaerobes, e.g. *E. coli*
urinary tract infections	Gram-negative facultative anaerobes, e.g. *E. coli*
Lyme disease	*Borrelia burgdorferi*
relapsing fever	*Borrelia recurrentis*
leptospirosis	*Leptospira icterohaemorrhagiae*
rat bite fever	*Spirillum minor*
typhus	*Rickettsia prowazekii*
spotted fevers	*Rickettsia rickettsiae; Rickettsia conori*
psittacosis	*Chlamydia psittaci*
Q fever	*Coxiella burnetii*
Parasitic	
malaria	*Plasmodium* species
trypanosomiasis	*Trypanosoma brucei*
amebic abscesses	*Entamoeba histolytica*
toxoplasmosis	*Toxoplasma gondii*
Fungal	
cryptococcosis	*Cryptococcus neoformans*
histoplasmosis	*Histoplasma capsulatum*
Viral	
infectious mononucleosis	Epstein–Barr virus
hepatitis	hepatitis viruses
cytomegalovirus-infection	cytomegalovirus

Fig. 27.4 Infective causes of pyrexia of unknown origin (PUO). A wide range of infections can present as PUO. Some, such as brucellosis, are zoonoses, and many are vector-borne. Therefore the patient must have had appropriate exposure to contract these infections. For example, there are about 2000 cases of malaria annually in the UK, but all are contracted outside the country. A travel history is therefore very important. (*E. coli*, *Escherichia coli*.)

(e.g. malaria, trypanosomiasis) and/or of limited geographic distribution (e.g. histoplasmosis). Hence the importance of a travel history.

In the light of the history and the differential diagnosis, a complete physical examination of the patient with PUO is essential. In particular:

- The skin, eyes, lymph nodes and abdomen should be examined.
- The heart should be auscultated.

It is also important to confirm that the patient does have a fever. In some series, as many as 25% of patients whose presenting complaint was a PUO did not have a fever, but had a naturally exaggerated circadian temperature rhythm. Up to 10% may have a factitious fever.

Routine investigations such as chest radiography and blood tests should be performed at this stage.

INVESTIGATION OF CLASSICAL PUO	
Stage 1	history physical examination screening tests
Stage 2	review history repeat physical examination specific diagnostic tests non-invasive investigations
Stage 3	invasive tests
Stage 4	therapeutic trials

Fig. 27.5 The diagnostic pathway for the investigation of a patient with pyrexia of unknown origin (PUO) can be divided into several stages.

Stage 2 involves reviewing the history, repeating the physical examination, specific diagnostic tests and non-invasive investigations

A review of the patient's history, particularly after discussion with colleagues and perhaps carried out by a second physician, is valuable to check for omissions such as exposure to particular risk factors in the recent or more distant past. The physical examination should also be repeated because rashes and other signs of infection can be transient.

Clues to the diagnosis elicited by careful history-taking should direct specific investigations. As the most common cause of unexplained fever is infection, collection and careful examination of appropriate specimens are essential. Skin tests may also be appropriate at this stage. The most important specimens include:

- Blood for culture.
- Blood for examination of antibodies. A sample of serum collected when the patient presents should also be stored for comparison with later samples to detect rising antibody titers even if the patient is some weeks into the infection. Serologic tests are helpful, particularly in the diagnosis of cytomegalovirus (CMV) and Epstein–Barr virus (EBV) infection, toxoplasmosis, psittacosis and rickettsial infections. Positive results in syphilis serology should be viewed with caution as other infections can cause biologic false-positives (see Chapter 19).
- Direct examination of blood to diagnose malaria, trypanosomiasis and relapsing fever.

Repeated sampling of blood, urine and other body fluids is often required and the laboratory should be alerted to search for unusual and fastidious organisms (e.g. nutritionally variant streptococci as a cause of endocarditis; see below). If possible, serial cultures should be collected before antimicrobial therapy is commenced.

Technical advances in diagnostic imaging techniques have provided the physician with a wide range of non-invasive investigative methods. Some radiologic procedures such as chest radiographs are considered to be routine in the work-up of patients with PUO (Fig. 27.6), while others such as gallium or technetium scans are applied in the light of the likely diagnosis (Fig. 27.7). Newer imaging techniques involving monoclonal antibodies as markers are being developed.

Stage 3 comprises invasive tests

Biopsy of liver and bone marrow should always be considered in the investigation of classical cases of PUO, but other tissues such as skin, lymph nodes and kidney may also be sampled. It is undesirable or impossible to repeat biopsies and therefore it is important to organize the laboratory examination of material carefully to maximize the information obtained.

Stage 4 involves therapeutic trials

Trials of corticosteroids (e.g. prednisone, dexamethasone) or prostaglandin inhibitors (e.g. aspirin, indomethacin) may be indicated if a non-infectious cause is suspected. There are few indications for empiric antimicrobial or cytotoxic chemotherapy in the management of classical PUO. However, a trial of antituberculous drugs may be advocated in patients with a history of tuberculosis in the absence of supporting microbiological evidence. Infections can progress very rapidly in people who are neutropenic or have AIDS and 'blind' therapy is warranted (see below).

Treatment of PUO

The investigation and management of a patient with PUO requires persistence and an informed and open mind in order to reach the correct diagnosis. As the range of infective causes of PUO is enormous the correct diagnosis is an essential prelude to the choice of appropriate treatment. As soon as the cause has been identified specific therapy, if available, should be given.

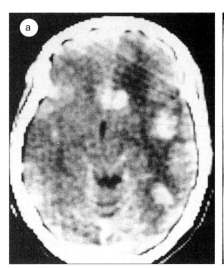
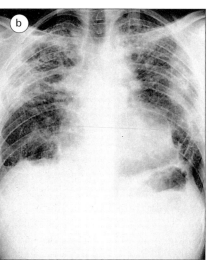

Fig. 27.6 Computerized tomography (CT) scans help in the demonstration of abscesses. The patient in (a) has a tuberculoma of the brain, but the CT appearance is not sufficiently characteristic to distinguish this from a pyogenic abscess or a meningioma. (Courtesy of J Ambrose.) The chest radiograph in (b) shows a patient with sarcoidosis. The differential diagnosis between infective and non-infective causes of granulomas is important, and can be difficult in the early stages of the investigation. (Courtesy of M. Turner–Warwick.)

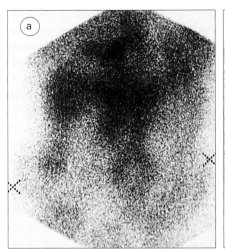

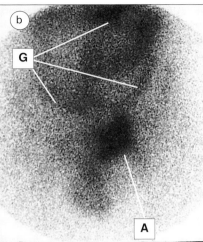

Fig. 27.7 Gallium concentrates in many inflammatory and neoplastic tissues and is a useful non-invasive technique in the investigation of a patient with pyrexia of unknown origin. (a) Retroperitoneal lymphadenopathy of Hodgkin's disease highlighted by a gallium scan. (Courtesy of H Tubbs.) (b) Intra-abdominal abscess shown by a gallium scan. (A, abscess; G, gallium in colon.) (Courtesy of W E Farrar.)

PUO in Specific Patient Groups

The main difference between PUO in these groups and classical PUO is the time course

As mentioned above, an increasing number of people are surviving with severe underlying disease that predisposes them to infection or are receiving treatment such as cytotoxic drugs that compromises their defenses against infection. These groups of patients are discussed in more detail in Chapter 28, but are included here because, in addition to classical PUO, newer classifications of PUO *(Fig. 27.2)* define:

- Nosocomial PUO.
- Neutropenic PUO.
- HIV-associated PUO.

Classically a PUO may exist for weeks or months before a diagnosis is made, whereas for hospital-acquired (nosocomial) PUO and in neutropenic patients the time course is hours to days. The more common infective causes of PUO in these groups are shown in *Figure 27.8*.

Investigation should proceed in the stages listed above, but with the particular emphasis depending upon the patient. In hospital patients the emphasis will depend upon:

- The type of operative procedures performed. Fever is a common complaint in patients who have received transplants and may indicate graft-versus-host disease rather than infection.
- The presence of foreign bodies, especially intravascular devices.
- Drug therapy as drug fevers are a common non-infective cause of PUO.
- The underlying disease and stage of chemotherapy in neutropenic patients.
- The presence of known risk factors such as intravenous drug misuse, travel and contact with infected individuals in patients with HIV. Although the major opportunist infections in people with AIDS are well described (see Chapter 28), common infections can present atypically and new infections continue to emerge.

Infective Endocarditis

Infective endocarditis is an uncommon disease that often presents as a PUO and is fatal if untreated. The infection involves the endothelial lining of the heart, usually including the heart valves. It may occur as an acute rapidly progressive disease or in a subacute form. Approximately 65% of patients have a pre-existing heart defect, either congenital or acquired (e.g. as a result of rheumatic fever), or a prosthetic heart valve *in situ*. However, the patient may be unaware of any defect before the infection.

Almost any organism can cause endocarditis, but native valves are usually infected by oral streptococci

Infection of native valves is most commonly caused by species of oral streptococci such as *Streptococcus sanguis*, *Strep. oralis* and *Strep. mitis*. About 25–35% of cases are caused by staphylococci, although this percentage is higher among intravenous drug misusers, who also have a higher incidence of Gram-negative and fungal endocarditis arising from organisms they inject into themselves. Coagulase-negative staphylococci are common causes of early prosthetic valve endocarditis and are probably acquired at the time of surgery. The species causing late infections – more than three months after cardiac surgery – are more like those causing native valve endocarditis *(Fig. 27.9)*.

Endocarditis is an endogenous infection acquired when organisms entering the bloodstream establish themselves on the heart valves. Therefore, any bacteremia can potentially result in endocarditis. Most commonly streptococci from the oral flora enter the bloodstream, for example during dental procedures or vigorous teeth cleaning or flossing, and adhere to damaged heart valves. It is thought that fibrin–platelet vegetations are present on damaged valves before the organisms implant, and that adherence is probably associated with the ability of the organisms to produce dextran as well as adhesins and fibronectin-

INFECTIVE CAUSES OF PUO IN SPECIFIC PATIENT GROUPS		
category of PUO	**infection**	**usual cause**
nosocomial	vascular-line related	staphylococci
	other device related	staphylococci, *Candida*
	transfusion-related	hepatitis, CMV
	cholecystitis and pancreatitis	Gram-negative rods
	pneumonia (related to assisted ventilation)	Gram-negative rods, including *Pseudomonas*
	postoperative abscesses, e.g. intra-abdominal	Gram-negative rods and anaerobes
	postgastric surgery	systemic candidiasis
neutropenic	vascular-line related	staphylococci
	oral infection	*Candida*, herpes simplex virus
	pneumonia	Gram-negative rods, *Candida*, *Aspergillus*, CMV
	soft tissue, e.g. peri-anal abscess	mixed aerobes and anaerobes
HIV-associated	respiratory tract	Cytomagalovins, *Pneumocystis*, *Mycobacterium tuberculosis*, *M. avium-intracellulare*
	central nervous system	*Toxoplasma*
	gastrointestinal tract	*Salmonella*, *Campylobacter*, *Shigella*
	genital tract or disseminated	*Treponema pallidum*, *Neisseria gonorrhoeae*

Fig. 27.8 Infective causes of pyrexia of unknown origin (PUO) in specific patient groups. Patients who contract their PUO in hospital are most likely to be infected with 'hospital pathogens', either from their own normal flora or from the hospital environment. This also applies to neutropenic patients if they are hospitalized, but some are treated as outpatients and may therefore be exposed to a wider range of pathogens. People with AIDS commonly become infected with opportunist pathogens, though an increasing range of organisms is now implicated. It is important to take a detailed history as latent infections can become florid as the patient's immune status deteriorates.

binding proteins. Having attached themselves to the heart valve, the organisms multiply and attract further fibrin and platelet deposition. In this position they are protected from the host defenses and vegetations can grow to several centimeters in size. This is probably quite a slow process and correspondingly the time period between the initial bacteremia and the onset of symptoms is around five weeks *(Fig. 27.10)*.

A patient with infective endocarditis almost always has a fever and a heart murmur

The signs and symptoms of infective endocarditis are very varied, but relate essentially to four ongoing processes:

- The infectious process on the valve and local intracardiac complications.
- Septic embolization to virtually any organ.
- Bacteremia, often with metastatic foci of infection.
- Circulating immune complexes and other factors.

The patient almost always has a fever and a heart murmur and may also complain of non-specific symptoms such as anorexia, weight loss, malaise, chills, nausea, vomiting and night sweats, symptoms that are common to many of the causes of PUO listed in *Figure 27.4*. Peripheral manifestations may also be evident in the form of splinter hemorrhages and Osler's nodes *(Fig. 27.11)*. Microscopic hematuria resulting from immune complex deposition in the kidney is characteristic (see Chapter 12).

Blood culture is the most important test for diagnosing infective endocarditis

Microbiologic and cardiologic investigations are of critical importance. The blood culture is the single most important laboratory test. Ideally three separate samples of blood should be collected within a 24-hour period and before antimicrobial therapy is administered. Methods for processing blood cultures are described in the Appendix. Isolation of

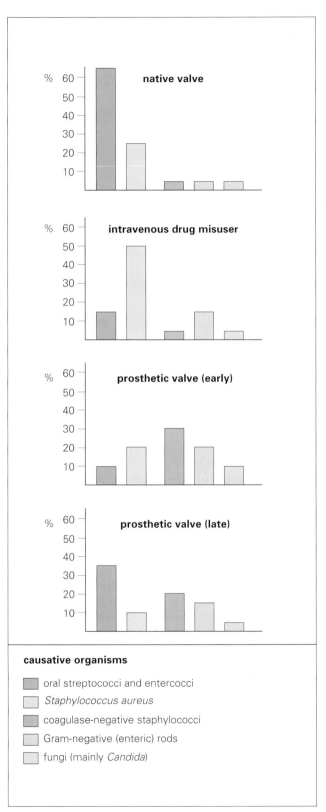

causative organisms

- oral streptococci and entercocci
- *Staphylococcus aureus*
- coagulase-negative staphylococci
- Gram-negative (enteric) rods
- fungi (mainly *Candida*)

Fig. 27.9 Causative agents of endocarditis in different groups of patients. Although almost any organism can cause endocarditis, the majority of cases are caused by a relatively small range of species. The relative importance of these species varies depending upon whether the patient has his/her own heart valves or a prosthetic valve.

the causative organism is essential so that antibiotic susceptibility tests can be performed and optimum therapy prescribed. Nutritionally variant strains of oral streptococci are known to cause infective endocarditis. These may fail to grow in blood culture media unless pyridoxal is added to the broth. Alternatively they grow as satellite colonies around *Staph. aureus* colonies on blood agar.

The mortality of infective endocarditis is 20–30% despite treatment with antibiotics

Although the majority of species causing infective endocarditis are highly susceptible to a range of antibiotics, complete eradication takes several weeks to achieve and relapse is not uncommon. This is probably due to:

- Relative inaccessibility of the organisms within the vegetations both to antibiotics and to host defenses.
- The organism's high population density and relatively slow rate of multiplication.

Before the advent of antibiotics infective endocarditis had a mortality of 100%, and even today despite treatment with appropriate antibiotics, the mortality remains at 20–30%.

The antibiotic treatment regimen for infective endocarditis depends upon the infecting organism

For penicillin-susceptible streptococci, high dose penicillin is the treatment of choice. Patients with a good history of

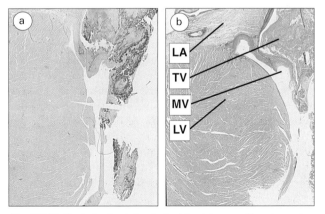

Fig. 27.10 Bacteria circulating in the bloodstream adhere to, and establish themselves on, the heart valves. Multiplication of the microbes is associated with destruction of valve tissue and the formation of vegetations, which interfere with, and may severely compromise, the normal function of the valve. These histologic sections show the virtual destruction of the leaflet at the mitral valve by staphylococci. (a) Gram stain. (b) Eosin-Van Geisen stain. (LA, left atrium; LV, left ventricle; MV, remnant of mitral valve; TV, thrombotic vegetation.) (Courtesy of RH Anderson.)

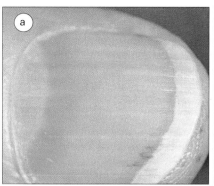
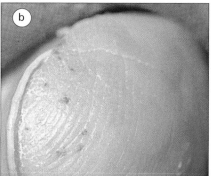
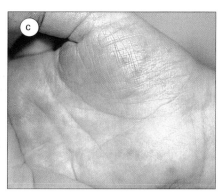

Fig. 27.11 Outward signs of endocarditis may be helpful in suggesting the diagnosis. These result from the host's response to infection in the form of immune complex-mediated vasculitis, focal platelet aggregation and vascular permeability. (a and b, different views) Splinter hemorrhages in the nailbed and petechial lesions in the skin. (c) Osler's nodes. These are tender nodular lesions that tend to affect the palms and fingertips. (Courtesy of H Tubbs.)

penicillin allergy can be treated with clindamycin or with a macrolide, although the latter may be less bactericidal. However, MIC (minimum inhibitory concentration) and MBC (minimum bactericidal concentration) tests (see Chapter 30) should be performed to detect organisms that are less susceptible or tolerant to penicillin (inhibited, but not killed; MBC > 4 × MIC). These organisms and enterococci, which are always more resistant to penicillin, should be treated with a combination of penicillin (or ampicillin) and an aminoglycoside. Combinations such as these act synergistically against streptococci and enterococci (see Chapter 30).

Staphylococcal endocarditis, particularly in prosthetic valve endocarditis when the organisms may be hospital-acquired and consequently often resistant to many antibiotics, often presents a more difficult therapeutic challenge. A β-lactamase stable penicillin such as cloxacillin is often suitable and may be given in combination with an aminoglycoside, rifampicin or fusidic acid. Vancomycin or teicoplanin should be used for penicillin-allergic patients and for treating methicillin-resistant staphylococci. Detailed treatment regimens are published by the American Heart Foundation and the British Society for Antimicrobial Chemotherapy.

People with heart defects need prophylactic antibiotics during invasive procedures

People with known heart defects should be given prophylactic antibiotics to protect them during dental surgery and any other invasive procedure that is likely to cause a transient bacteremia.

Summary

Most people with a PUO have a treatable disease presenting in an unusual manner

The clinical investigation needs to be individualized, but this chapter outlines the essential stages in the investigation of every patient and draws attention to the important infective causes of PUO.

Although classically a patient with PUO presents with a long history (weeks or months of fever), patients also present with fevers that are not immediately diagnosed by routine laboratory investigations. For these groups (nosocomial, neutropenic and HIV-associated), new definitions of PUO have been proposed. The list of pathogens causing fever in these patients is growing.

The clinician's aim in the investigation of every patient with PUO should be to discover the cause, i.e. to change a PUO to a pyrexia of known origin, and to initiate appropriate treatment.

- Pyrexia (fever) is the body's response to exogenous and endogenous pyrogens. It is a common symptom and may have a protective effect.
- The term pyrexia of unknown origin (PUO or FUO) is used when the cause of fever is not obvious, has classically exceeded three weeks' duration, and is not revealed by routine clinical and laboratory investigations.
- The increase in numbers of immunocompromised patients has prompted definition of PUO groups other than classical (i.e. nosocomial, neutropenic and HIV-associated PUO).
- Among the causes of PUO, infection is the most common, but neoplasms and autoimmune diseases are also significant. As many as 20% of cases may remain undiagnosed.
- The list of infective causes is long, therefore the first stage of investigation (i.e. the patient's history and results of physical examination and screening tests) are critical pointers to subsequent specific diagnostic tests.
- Therapeutic trials may be indicated if a diagnosis has not been achieved, but may confuse the results of further tests.
- The correct diagnosis is paramount to direct appropriate specific therapy.
- Infective endocarditis is an uncommon, but classic, example of a PUO. It is usually caused by Gram-positive cocci, the species depending upon the patient's underlying predisposition, and is fatal unless treated.

A 60-year-old woman presents to the clinic with a seven-day history of malaise, nausea and loss of appetite. Ten years previously she had been admitted with an aortic root dissection. This was corrected successfully at operation and her aortic root and valve were replaced. She has been quite well until now, although she is a poor complier and it has been difficult to stabilize her anticoagulant therapy. On examination her temperature is 38°C and she is flushed and unwell. Her pulse rate is 110 beats/min, and her blood pressure is 80/60 mm Hg. A prosthetic valvular click and a systolic murmur are heard on auscultation. Her chest is otherwise clear and abdominal examination is unremarkable. The results of initial investigations are: hemoglobin, 8.3 g/dl normochromic, normocytic film; white cell count, $14.6 \times 10^9/l$ with 60% neutrophils; platelets, $192 \times 10^9/l$.

1. What is the probable diagnosis and what further investigations are critical?
2. What is the most common pathogen responsible for this condition?
3. What are the crucial components of management of this condition?
4. What are the possible complications of this condition?
5. What guidelines are available to reduce the risk of this disease occurring?

Further Reading

Deal WB. Fever of unknown origin: An analysis of 34 patients. *Postgrad Med J* 1971;**50**:182.

Jacoby GA, Swartz MN. Fever of unexplained origin. *New Engl J Med* 1973;**289**:1407.

Larson EB, Featherstone HJ, Petersdorf RG. Fever of undetermined origin: Diagnosis and follow up of 105 cases. 1970–1980. *Medicine* (Baltimore) 1982;**61**: 269.

Petersdorf RG, Beeson PB. Fever of unexplained origin. Report on 100 Cases. *Medicine* (Baltimore) 1961;**40**:1.

Reese RE, Douglas RG eds. *A Practical Approach To Infectious Diseases*. Boston/Toronto: Little, Brown & Co, 1986.

Infections in the Compromised Host

8

Introduction

The human body has a complex system of protective mechanisms to prevent infection, involving both the adaptive (cellular and humoral) immune system and the innate defense system (e.g. skin, mucous membranes). These have been described in detail in earlier chapters (see Chapters 4 and 5). So far we have concentrated on the common and serious infections occurring in people whose protective mechanisms are largely intact. In these circumstances the interactions between host and parasite are such that the parasite has to use all its guile to survive and invade the host, and the healthy host is able to put up a fight against such an invasion. In this chapter we will consider the infections that arise when the host–parasite equation is weighted heavily in favor of the parasite. In other words when the host is compromised.

The Compromised Host

Compromised hosts are people who have one or more defects in their body's natural defenses against microbial invaders. Consequently they are much more liable to suffer from severe and life-threatening infections. Modern medicine has effective methods for treating at least 50% of all serious cancers, has perfected organ transplantation and has developed technology that enables people with otherwise fatal diseases to lead prolonged and productive lives. A consequence of these achievements, however, is an increasing number of compromised people prone to infection. In addition there is a growing population of people with AIDS.

The host can be compromised in many different ways

Compromise can take a variety of forms, falling into two main groups:
- Defects, accidental or intentional, in the body's innate defense mechanisms.
- Deficiencies in the adaptive immune response.

These disorders of the immune system can be further sub-classified as 'primary' or 'secondary' *(Fig. 28.1)*:
- Primary immunodeficiency is inherited or occurs by exposure *in utero* to environmental factors or by other unknown mechanisms. It is rare, and varies in severity depending upon the type of defect.
- Secondary or acquired immunodeficiency is due to an underlying disease state *(Fig. 28.2)* or occurs as a result of treatment for a disease.

Primary defects of innate immunity include congenital defects in phagocytic cells or complement synthesis

Congenital defects in phagocytic cells confer susceptibility to infection, and of these perhaps the best known is chronic granulomatous disease *(Fig. 28.3)*, in which an

WHAT MAKES A HOST COMPROMISED	
factors affecting innate systems	
primary	complement deficiencies phagocyte cell deficiencies
secondary	burns, trauma, major surgery, catheterization, foreign bodies (e.g. shunts, prostheses), obstruction
factors affecting adaptive systems	
primary	T cell defects, B cell deficiencies, severe combined immunodeficiency
secondary	malnutrition, infectious diseases, neoplasia, irradiation, chemotherapy, splenectomy

Fig. 28.1 Factors that make a host compromised.

INFECTIONS THAT CAUSE IMMUNOSUPPRESSION	
viral	**bacterial**
measles	*Mycobacterium tuberculosis*
mumps	*Mycobacterium leprae*
congenital rubella	*Brucella* spp.
Epstein–Barr virus	
cytomegalovirus	
HIV1, HIV2	

Fig. 28.2 Infections that cause immunosuppression.

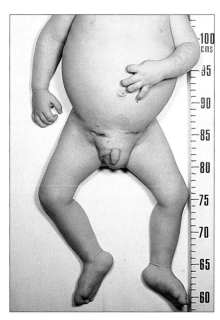

Fig. 28.3 Bilateral draining lymph nodes in an 18-month-old boy with chronic granulomatous disease. Abscesses caused by *Staphylococcus aureus* had developed in both groins and had to be surgically drained. (Courtesy of AR Hayward.)

inherited failure to synthesize cytochrome b_{245} leads to a failure to produce reactive oxygen intermediates during phagocytosis.

The central role of complement in the innate defense mechanisms is undisputed, and inability to generate classical C3 convertase (see Chapter 5) through congenital defects in the synthesis of the early components, particularly C4 and C2, is associated with a high frequency of extracellular infections.

Secondary defects of innate defenses include disruption of the body's mechanical barriers

A variety of factors can disrupt the mechanical non-specific barriers to infection. For example, burns, traumatic injury and major surgery destroy the continuity of the skin and may leave poorly vascularized tissue near the body surface, providing a relatively defenseless site for microbes to colonize and invade. In health, the mucosal barriers of the respiratory and alimentary tract are vital to prevent infection. Damage sustained for example through endoscopy, surgery or irradiation therapy, provides easy access for infecting organisms. Devices such as intravascular and urinary catheters, or procedures such as lumbar puncture or bone marrow aspiration, allow organisms to bypass the normal defenses and enter normally sterile parts of the body. Foreign bodies such as prostheses (e.g. hip joints or heart valves) and cerebrospinal fluid (CSF) shunts alter the local non-specific host responses and provide surfaces that microbes can colonize more readily than the natural equivalents.

The adage 'obstruction leads to infection' is a valuable reminder that the defenses of many body systems work partly through the clearance of undesirable materials (e.g. urine flow, ciliary action in the respiratory tract, peristalsis in the gut). Interference with these mechanisms as a result of pathologic obstruction, central nervous system dysfunction or surgical intervention tends to result in infection.

Primary adaptive immunodeficiency results from defects in the primary differentiation environment or in cell differentiation

The major congenital abnormalities arising in the adaptive immune system are depicted in *Figure 28.4*. A defect in the stromal microenvironment in which lymphocytes differentiate may lead to failure to produce B cells (Bruton-type agammaglobulinemia) or T cells (DiGeorge syndrome).

Differentiation pathways themselves may also be affected. For example, a non-functional recombinase enzyme will prevent the recombination of gene fragments that form the B cell antibody or the T cell receptor variable regions for antigen recognition, with a resulting severe combined immunodeficiency (SCID).

The most common form of congenital antibody deficiency – common variable immunodeficiency – is characterized by recurrent pyogenic infections and is probably heterogenous. Although the number of immature B cells in the marrow tends to be normal, the peripheral B cells are either low in number or in some cases absent. Where present they are unable to differentiate into plasma cells in some cases or to secrete antibody in others.

Transient hypogammaglobulinemia of infancy, characterized by recurrent respiratory infections, is associated with a low serum IgG concentration, which often normalizes abruptly by 3–4 years of age *(Fig. 28.5)*.

Immunoglobulin deficiency occurs naturally in human infants as the maternal serum IgG concentration decays and can become a serious problem in very premature babies.

Causes of secondary adaptive immunodeficiency include malnutrition, infections, neoplasia, splenectomy and certain medical treatments

Worldwide, malnutrition is a common and the most important cause of acquired immunodeficiency. The major form, protein–energy malnutrition (PEM) presents as a wide range of disorders, with kwashiorkor and marasmus at the two poles. It results in:

- Drastic effects on the structure of the lymphoid organs *(Fig. 28.6)*.
- Gross reductions in the synthesis of complement components.
- Sluggish chemotactic responses of phagocytes.
- Lowered concentrations of secretory and mucosal IgA.
- Reduced affinity of IgG.
- In particular, a serious deficit in circulating T cell numbers *(Fig. 28.7)*, leading to inadequate cell-mediated responses.

Infections themselves are often immunosuppressive *(Fig. 28.2)*, and none more so than HIV infection, which gives rise to AIDS (see Chapter 19). Neoplasia of the lymphoid system frequently induces a state of reduced immunoreactivity and splenectomy, for whatever reason, results in impaired humoral responses.

Treatment of disease can also cause immunosuppression. For example:

- Cytotoxic agents such as cyclophosphamide and azathioprine cause leukopenia or deranged T and B cell function.

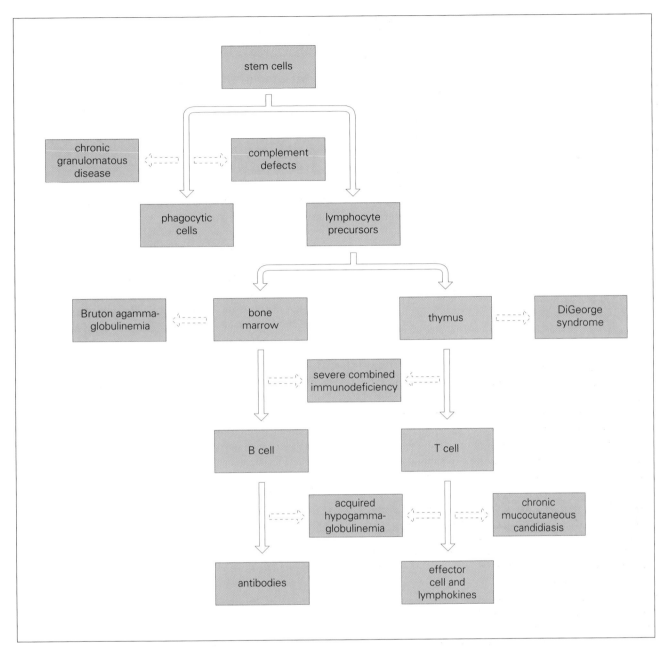

Fig. 28.4 The major primary cellular immunodeficiencies. The deficiency states (shown in purple boxes) derive either from defects in the primary differentiation environment (bone marrow or thymus) or during cell differentiation (shown as dashed arrows derived from the differentiation state indicated).

- Corticosteroids reduce the number of circulating leukocytes, monocytes and eosinophils and suppress leukocyte accumulation at sites of inflammation.
- Irradiation therapy adversely affects the proliferation of lymphoid cells.

Therefore a patient receiving treatment for neoplastic disease will be immunocompromised as a result of both the disease and the treatment.

It is important to recognize immunodeficiencies and to understand which procedures are likely to compromise the natural defenses of a patient. Due to improvements in medical technology, many immune defects (particularly immunosuppression resulting from irradiation or cytotoxic drugs) are transient and patients who survive the period of immunosuppression have a good chance of a complete recovery.

Microbes that Infect the Compromised Host

Compromised people can become infected not only with any pathogen able to infect non-compromised individuals, but also with opportunist pathogens – microbes that are incapable of causing disease in a healthy person, but able to infect when the host's defenses are lowered, often with fatal consequences. Different types of defect predispose to infection with different pathogens depending upon the critical mechanisms operating in the defense against each microorganism *(Fig. 28.8)*. Here we will concentrate mainly on the opportunist infections and refer to other chapters for information about other pathogens.

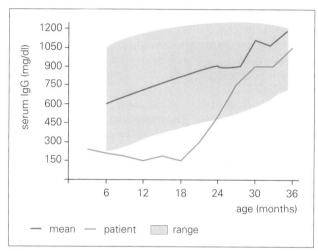

Fig. 28.5 Serum immunoglobulin concentrations in a boy with transient hypogammaglobulinemia compared with the range of normal controls. The patient developed mild paralytic polio when immunized at four months of age with attenuated (Sabin) vaccine.

Deficient Innate Immunity Due to Physical Factors

Burn wound infections

Burns damage the body's mechanical barriers, neutrophil function and immune responses

Burn wounds are sterile immediately after the burn is inflicted, but inevitably become colonized within hours with a mixed bacterial flora. Burn injuries cause direct damage to the mechanical barriers of the body and abnormalities in neutrophil function and immune responses. In addition there is a major physiologic derangement with loss of fluids and electrolytes. The burn provides a highly nutritious surface for organisms to colonize, and the incidence of serious infection varies with the size and depth of the burn and the age of the patient. Modern topical antimicrobial therapy should prevent infection of burns of less than 30% of the total body area, but larger burns are always colonized. Non-invasive infection is confined to the eschar (the non-viable skin debris on the surface of deep burns). It is characterized by rapid separation of the eschar from the underlying tissue and a heavy exudate of purulent material from the burn wound. The systemic symptoms are usually relatively mild. However, organisms can invade from heavily colonized burn eschars into viable tissue beneath and rapidly destroy the tissue, converting partial thickness burns into full skin thickness destruction. From here it is a small step to invasion of the lymphatics and thence to the bloodstream or direct invasion of blood vessels, and to septicemia. Septicemia in patients with burns is often polymicrobial.

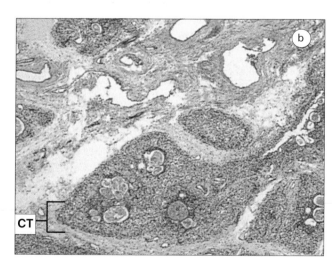

Fig. 28.6 Thymic histology in normal children and children with PEM protein – energy malnutrition. (a) Normal thymus showing well-demarcated cortex and medullary zones. (b) Acute involution in PEM characterized by lobular atrophy, loss of distinction between cortex and medulla, depletion of lymphocytes and enlarged Hassall's corpuscles. (C, cortex; CT, connective tissue; H, Hassall's corpuscle; L, lobule; M, medulla) (Courtesy of RK Chandra.)

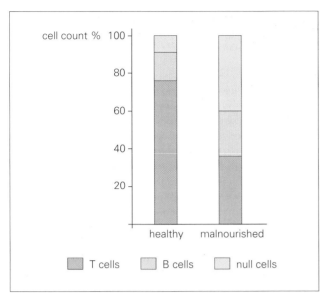

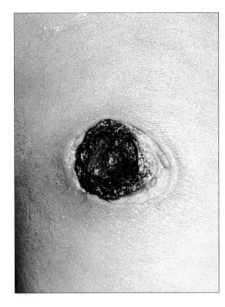

Fig. 28.8 Ecthyma gangrenosum in a child with *Pseudomonas* septicemia associated with immunodeficiency. (Courtesy of H Tubbs.)

Fig. 28.7 The proportion of T cells is decreased in malnourished patients compared with healthy controls. B cell counts are usually unaltered and null cells (non-T, non-B) are increased.

The major pathogens in burns are aerobic and facultatively anaerobic bacteria and fungi

The most important pathogens in burn wounds are:

- *Pseudomonas aeruginosa* and other Gram-negative rods.
- *Staphylococcus aureus.*
- Streptococcus pyogenes.
- Other streptococci.
- Enterococci.

Candida spp. and *Aspergillus* together account for about 5% of infections. Anaerobes are rare in burn wound infections. Viral infections, mostly herpesvirus and cytomegalovirus (CMV), have been reported, but their clinical significance is uncertain.

P. aeruginosa is the most devastating Gram-negative pathogen of burned patients

P. aeruginosa is an opportunist Gram-negative rod that has a long and infamous association with burn infections. It grows well in the moist environment of a burn wound, producing a foul, green-pigmented discharge and necrosis. Invasion is not uncommon and the characteristic skin lesions (ecthyma gangrenosum) that are pathognonomic of *P. aeruginosa* septicemia may appear on non-burned areas *(see Fig. 28.8)*. Host factors predisposing to infection include:

- Abnormalities in the antibacterial activities of neutrophils.
- Deficiencies in serum opsonins.

Added to these are the virulence factors of the organism, which include the production of elastase, protease and exotoxin. This combination makes *P. aeruginosa* the most devastating Gram-negative pathogen of burned patients. Treatment is difficult because of the organism's innate resistance to many antibacterial agents. A combination of aminoglycoside (usually gentamicin or tobramycin) with one of the newer β-lactams (such as azlocillin, ceftazidime or imipenem) is usually favored, but several units have reported strains resistant to these agents.

It is virtually impossible to prevent colonization. Prevention of infection depends largely upon inhibiting the multiplication of organisms colonizing the burn by applying topical agents such as silver nitrate. Both active and passive immunization have been tried, the latter appearing to hold more promise at present.

Staph. aureus is the foremost pathogen of burn wounds

The most important predisposing factor to *Staph. aureus* infection in burns patients appears to be an abnormality of the antibacterial function of neutrophils. Infections follow a more insidious course than streptococcal infections (see below) and it may be several days before the full-blown infection is apparent. The organism is capable of destroying granulation tissue, invading and causing septicemia. *Staph. aureus* infections of skin are discussed in detail in Chapter 23. Treatment with antistaphylococcal agents such as cloxacillin or nafcillin (or a glycopeptide if methicillin-resistant *Staph. aureus* is isolated) should be administered if there is evidence of invasive infection. Every effort should be made to prevent the spread of staphylococci from patient to patient. Although transmissible by both airborne and contact routes, the contact route is by far the most important.

The high transmissibility of Strep. pyogenes makes it the scourge of burns wards

Strep. pyogenes (Group A strep) infections of skin and soft tissue are discussed in some detail in Chapter 23. *Strep. pyogenes* was the most common cause of burn wound infection in the pre-antibiotic era and is still to be feared in burns wards. The infection usually occurs within the first few days of injury and is characterized by a rapid deterioration in the state of the burn wound and invasion of neighboring healthy tissue. The patient may become severely toxic and will die within hours unless treated appropriately. *Strep. pyogenes* rarely infects healthy granulation tissue, but freshly grafted wounds may become infected, resulting in destruction of the graft. Every effort should be made to prevent spread. Penicillin is the drug of choice for treatment, and erythromycin or vancomycin can be used for penicillin-allergic patients.

β-Hemolytic streptococci of other Lancefield groups (notably Group C and G; see Appendix) and enterococci are also important pathogens of burn wounds.

Traumatic injury and surgical wound infections

Both accidental and intentional trauma destroy the integrity of the body surface and leave it liable to infection. Accidental injury may result in microbes being introduced deep into the wound. The species involved will depend upon the nature of the wound, as discussed in Chapter 23.

Staph. aureus is the most important cause of surgical wound infection

Staph. aureus surgical wound infection (see Chapter 34) may be acquired during surgery or postoperatively and may originate from the patient or from another patient or staff member. The wound is less well defended than normal tissue; it may have a damaged blood supply and there may be foreign bodies (sutures). Classic studies of wound infections have shown that far fewer staphylococci are needed to initiate infection around a suture than in normal healthy skin. Wound infections can be severe and the organisms can invade the bloodstream, with consequent seeding of other sites such as the heart valves, causing endocarditis (see Chapter 27) or bones, causing osteomyelitis (see Chapter 23), thereby further compromising the patient.

Infections of plastic *in situ*

The technical developments in plastics and other synthetic materials have enabled many advances in medicine and surgery, but in the process have produced new groups of compromised patients. *Staph. epidermidis* is an important cause of infection of cardiac pacemakers, vascular grafts and CSF shunts.

Catheter-associated infection of the urinary tract is common

Urinary catheters disrupt the normal host defenses of the urinary tract and allow organisms easy access to the bladder. Such catheter-associated infection of the urinary tract is especially common if catheters are left in place for more than 48 hours (see Chapter 18). The organisms involved are usually Gram-negative rods from the patient's own fecal or periurethral flora, but cross-infection also occurs (see Chapter 34).

Staphylococci are the most common cause of intravenous and peritoneal dialysis catheter infections

Intravenous and peritoneal dialysis catheters breach the

integrity of the skin barrier and allow organisms from the skin flora of the patient or hands of the carer easy access to deeper sites. Staphylococci are the most common cause of infection, but coryneforms, Gram-negative rods and *Candida* are also implicated.

Coagulase-negative staphylococci, particularly *Staph. epidermidis*, account for more than 50% of the infections (Fig. 28.9). These opportunists are members of the normal skin flora and for many years were considered to be harmless. However, they have a particular propensity for colonizing plastic and can therefore seed sites adjacent to plastic devices and thence cause invasive infections. Their virulence factors are not well understood, but their ability to produce an adhesive slime material and grow as biofilms on plastic surfaces is likely to be important. Infections are characteristically more insidious in onset than those caused by the more virulent *Staph. aureus*, and recognition is hampered by the difficulty in distinguishing the infecting strain from the normal flora. Treatment is also difficult because many *Staph. epidermidis* carry multiple antibiotic resistances, and agents such as a glycopeptide (vancomycin or teicoplanin) and rifampicin may be required (see Chapter 30). Whenever possible the plastic device should be removed.

Staph. epidermidis is the most common cause of prosthetic valve and joint infections

Patients with prosthetic heart valves or prosthetic joints are compromised by:
* The surgery to implant the prosthesis.
* The continued presence of a foreign body.

Staph. epidermidis is again the most common pathogen, either gaining access during surgery or from a subsequent bacteremia originating from, for example, an intravascular

INFECTIONS INVOLVING *STAPHYLOCOCCUS EPIDERMIDIS*	
infection of:	% of infections caused by *Staph. epidermidis*
prosthetic heart valve early (<2 months postoperatively) late (>2 months postoperatively)	30–70 20–30
Prosthetic hip	10–40
Cerebrospinal fluid shunt	30–65
Vascular grafts	5–20
Peritoneal dialysis related	30
Intravascular catheters	10–50

Fig. 28.9 Percentage of infections caused by *Staph. epidermidis* in patients with plastic *in situ*. (Data from Gemmell and McCartney, 1990.)

line infection. Endocarditis associated with prosthetic heart valves is discussed in Chapter 27.

The most common complication of joint replacement is loosening of the prosthesis, while infection is the second most common complication and is much more likely to lead to permanent failure of the procedure. The difficulties of treatment have been outlined above, but there is understandably great reluctance to remove a prosthetic device, even though it is sometimes the only way to eradicate an infection.

Infections due to compromised clearance mechanisms

Stasis predisposes to infection and in health the body functions to prevent stasis. In the respiratory tract, damage to the ciliary escalator predisposes the lungs to invasion, particularly in patients with cystic fibrosis, who are infected with *Staph. aureus* and *Haemophilus influenzae* and later with *P. aeruginosa* (see Chapter 17).

Obstruction and interruption of normal urine flow allows Gram-negative organisms from the periurethral flora to ascend the urethra and to establish themselves in the bladder. Septicemia is an important complication of urinary tract infection superimposed on obstruction.

Infections Associated with Secondary Adaptive Immunodeficiency

The underlying immunodeficiency state determines the nature and severity of any associated infection and in some cases infection is the presenting clinical feature in a patient with an immunologic deficit. However, septicemia and related infectious complications of immunodeficiency are most commonly encountered in patients hospitalized for chemotherapy for malignant diseases or organ transplantation. In these patients, infection continues to be a major cause of morbidity and mortality *(Fig. 28.10)*. Increasingly these infections are iatrogenic and caused by opportunist pathogens acquired in hospital.

Hematologic malignancy and bone marrow transplant infections

A lack of circulating neutrophils following bone marrow failure predisposes to infection

Susceptibility to infection of patients with leukemia is primarily due to the lack of circulating neutrophils that inevitably follows bone marrow failure. Septicemia may be the presenting feature, but is much more common when the patient has been exposed to chemotherapy to induce a remission of the disease (remission–induction chemotherapy). Neutropenia (defined as a count of less than 0.5×10^9 neutrophils/l) may persist for a few days to several weeks. Similarly, prolonged periods of neutropenia occur after bone marrow transplantation.

The length of time for which the patient is neutropenic influences the nature of any associated infection and the frequency with which it occurs – for example, fungal infections are much more common in patients who are neutropenic for

more than 21 days. Although Gram-negative rods such as *Escherichia coli* and *P. aeruginosa* from the bowel flora have in the past been the most common cause of septicemia in neutropenic patients, Gram-positive organisms – staphylococci, streptococci and enterococci – are gaining in importance. *Staph. epidermidis* septicemia associated with intravascular catheters (see above) is common. Infections caused by fungi are also increasing, partly because more patients are surviving the early neutropenic period with the aid of modern antibacterial agents and granulocyte transfusions. Severe CMV infections are an important feature of bone marrow transplantation due to graft-versus-host reactions as well as immunosuppressive therapy.

OPPORTUNISTIC PATHOGENS IN NEUTROPENIC PATIENTS AND ORGAN TRANSPLANT RECIPIENTS
bacteria
Gram-positive *Staphylococcus aureus* coagulase-negative staphylococci streptococci *Listeria* spp. *Nocardia asteroides* *Mycobacterium tuberculosis* *Mycobacterium avium-intracellulare*
Gram-negative Enterobacteriaceae *Pseudomonas aeruginosa* *Legionella* spp. *Bacteroides* spp.
fungi
Candida spp. *Aspergillus* spp. *Cryptococcus neoformans* *Histoplasma capsulatum* *Pneumocystis carinii*
parasites
Toxoplasma gondii *Strongyloides stercoralis*
viruses
herpesviruses, e.g. HSV, CMV, VZV, EBV hepatitis B hepatitis C polyomaviruses, e.g. BKV, JCV HIV*
* HIV has been transmitted via organ   transplantation and unscreened blood

Fig. 28.10 Opportunistic pathogens in neutropenic patients and organ transplant recipients. (CMV, cytomegalovirus; EBV, Epstein–Barr virus; HSV, herpes simplex virus; VZV, varicella–zoster virus.)

Solid organ transplant infections

Most infections occur within 3–4 months of transplantation

Suppression of a patient's cell-mediated immunity is necessary to prevent rejection of a grafted organ and the cytotoxic regimens used usually suppress humoral immunity to some extent as well. In addition high doses of corticosteroids (to suppress inflammatory responses) are required. The combination of these conditions results in a severely compromised host. Factors that have an effect on infection in recipients of solid organ transplants (e.g. kidney, heart, lung, liver) include:

- The underlying medical condition of the patient.
- The patient's previous immune status.
- The type of organ transplant.
- The immunosuppressive regimen.
- The exposure of the patient to pathogens.

The organisms that cause the most common and most severe infections are shown in *Figure 28.10*.

From 3–4 months after transplantation the risk of infection is reduced, but remains for as long as the patient is immunosuppressed *(Fig. 28.11)*.

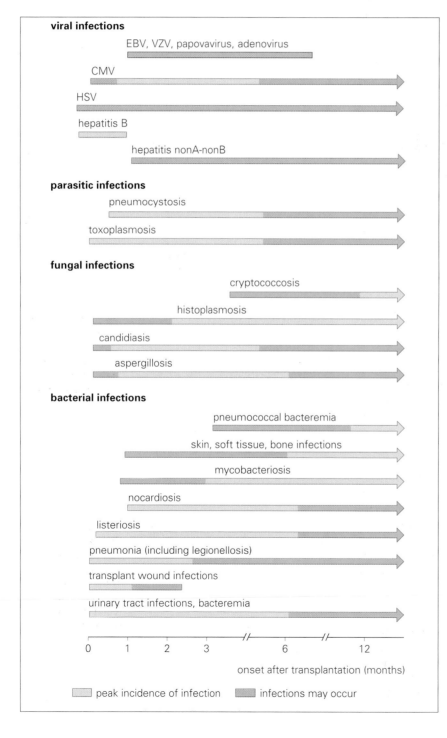

Fig. 28.11 This timetable shows the time of onset and peak incidence of infections in patients after renal transplantation. The patient is at risk of some infections, particularly hepatitis B and wound infections, for a limited period only immediately post-transplant. Other infections may develop after several weeks of immunosuppression, but the majority constitute a risk throughout the period of immunosuppression. Note that *Pneumocystis carinii* (pneumocystosis) is now thought to be a fungus. (CMV, cytomegalovirus; EBV, Epstein–Barr virus; HSV, herpes simplex virus; VZV, varicella–zoster virus.) (Adapted from Reese and Douglas, 1986.)

AIDS infections
The clinical definition of AIDS includes the presence of one or more opportunistic infections

People with AIDS are often infected concomitantly with multiple pathogens, which they fail to eradicate despite prolonged, appropriate and aggressive antimicrobial chemotherapy. Most of the pathogens involved are intracellular microbes that require an intact cell-mediated immune response for effective defense. As the patient progresses from HIV-seropositivity to full-blown AIDS the immunodeficiency deepens and organisms that are usually controlled by cell-mediated immunity are able to reactivate to cause disseminated infections not seen in the immunologically normal individual.

Many of the pathogens that cause infections in the immunocompromised host (see *Fig. 28.10*) are described elsewhere in this book. Other opportunist pathogens are described in more detail below.

Other Important Opportunist Pathogens

Fungi
Candida is the most common fungal pathogen in compromised patients

This yeast is an opportunist pathogen in a variety of patients and in various body sites. It is the cause of:
- Vaginal and oral thrush (see Chapter 19).
- Skin infections (see Chapter 23).
- Endocarditis, particularly in drug addicts (see Chapter 27).
    Candida manifests itself in different ways depending upon the nature of the underlying compromise (see below).

Chronic mucocutaneous candidiasis

This is rare and is a persistent but non-invasive infection of mucous membranes, hair, skin and nails in patients (often children) with a specific T cell defect rendering them anergic to *Candida (Fig. 28.12)*. It may be controlled by intermittent courses of ketoconazole.

Oropharyngeal and esophageal candidiasis

This is seen in a variety of compromised patients, including people with ill-fitting dentures, diabetes mellitus or on antibiotics or corticosteroids, and now characteristically in people with HIV *(Fig. 28.13)*. Treatment with antifungal mouthwashes (nystatin or an azole compound) is recommended, particularly in the immunocompromised in whom the gastrointestinal tract probably serves as one of the routes for disseminated disease (see below).

Gastrointestinal candidiasis

This is seen in patients who have undergone major gastric or abdominal surgery and in those with neoplastic disease. The organism can pass through the intestinal wall and spread from a gastrointestinal focus. Antemortem diagnosis is difficult and as many as 25% of patients do not have any symptoms in the early stages of disease. If there is dissemination

from the gut, blood cultures may become positive and *Candida* antigens may be detectable in the serum. A high index of suspicion is required to initiate antifungal therapy early in these patients, but disseminated disease is often fatal.

Disseminated candidiasis

This is probably acquired via the gastrointestinal tract, but also arises from intravascular catheter-related infections. Patients with lymphoma and leukemia are most at risk. Bloodborne spread to almost any organ can occur. Infections of the eye (endophthalmitis; *Fig. 28.14*) and the skin (nodular skin lesions; see Chapter 23) are important

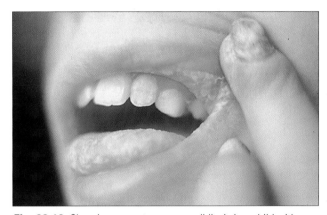

Fig. 28.12 Chronic mucocutaneous candidiasis in a child with impaired T cell response to antigens. (Courtesy of MJ Wood.)

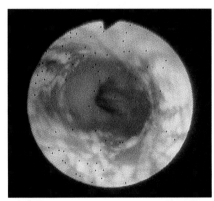

Fig. 28.13 *Candida* esophagitis. Endoscopic view showing extensive areas of whitish exudate. (Courtesy of I Chesner.)

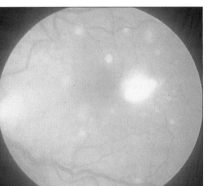

Fig. 28.14 *Candida* endophthalmitis. Fundal photograph showing areas of white exudate. (Courtesy of AM Geddes.)

because they provide diagnostic clues and without these the non-specific symptoms of fever and septic shock make early diagnosis difficult. Immunocompromised patients are often given antifungal therapy 'blindly' if they have a fever and fail to respond to broad-spectrum antibacterial agents *(Fig. 28.15)*.

Cryptococcus neoformans infection is most common in people with impaired cell-mediated immunity

C. neoformans is an opportunistic yeast with a worldwide distribution. It can cause infection in the immunocompetent host, but infection is seen more frequently in people with impaired cell-mediated immunity. The onset of disease may be slow and usually results in lung infection or meningoencephalitis; occasionally other sites such as skin, bone and joints are involved (see Chapter 23).

C. neoformans can be demonstrated in the CSF and is characterized by its large polysaccharide capsule (see *Fig. 22.12*). Rapid identification can be made by antigen detection in a latex agglutination test using specific antibody-coated latex particles. Treatment involves a combination of amphotericin and flucytosine (see Chapter 30) and can be monitored by detecting a fall in CSF antigen concentration.

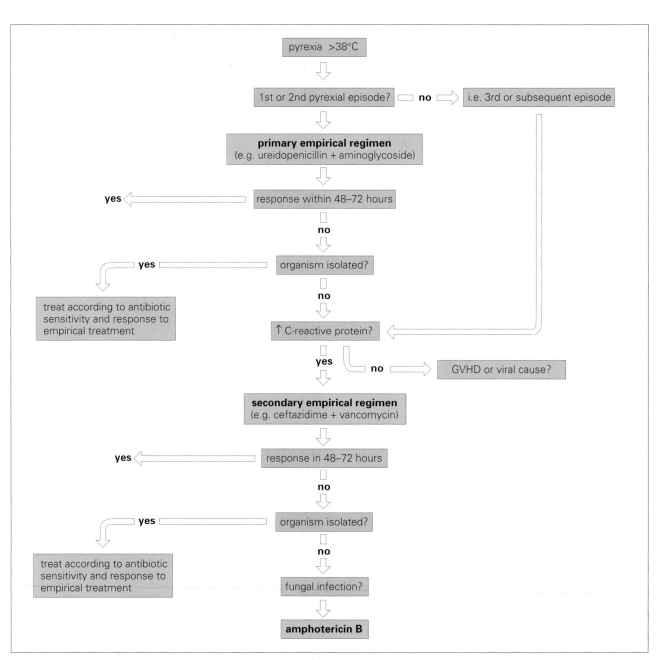

Fig. 28.15 Neutropenic patients succumb very rapidly to infections and decisions to treat have to be made on an empiric basis. This figure shows one example of such a decision-making tree. (GVHD, graft versus host disease.) (Adapted from Rogers, 1989.)

The prognosis depends largely upon the patient's underlying disease and in the severely immunocompromised, mortality is approximately 50%. In patients with AIDS it is almost impossible to eradicate the organism even with intensive treatment.

Disseminated Histoplasma capsulatum infection may occur years after exposure in immunocompromised patients

This is a highly infectious fungus that causes an acute but benign pulmonary infection in healthy people, but can produce a chronic progressive disseminated disease in the compromised host. The organism is endemic only in tropical parts of the world and notably in the so-called 'histo belt' of the central USA, particularly in the Ohio and Mississippi river valleys. The natural habitat of the organism is the soil. It is transmitted by the airborne route and the fungal spores are deposited in the alveoli, from whence the fungus spreads via the lymphatics to the regional lymph nodes. As disseminated disease may occur many years after the initial exposure in immunocompromised patients it may present in patients who have long since left endemic areas. The infection is also seen in people with HIV who have visited endemic areas.

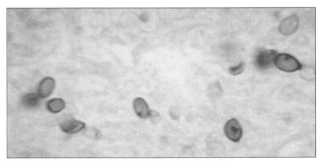

Fig. 28.16 Histologic section of the lung showing yeast forms of *H. capsulatum*. Methenamine silver stain. (Courtesy of TF Sellers, Jr.)

Cultures of blood, bone marrow, sputum and CSF may yield *Histoplasma*, but biopsy and histologic examination of bone marrow, liver or lymph nodes is often required to make the diagnosis *(Fig. 28.16)*. Approximately 50% of cases of progressive disease in the immunocompromised are successfully treated with amphotericin.

Invasive aspergillosis is usually a fatal disease in the compromised patient

The role of *Aspergillus* spp. in diseases of the lung has been outlined in Chapter 17, but this fungus is now increasingly reported as a cause of invasive disease in compromised patients, usually in profoundly neutropenic patients or those receiving high dose corticosteroids *(Fig. 28.17)*. Like *Histoplasma*, aspergilli are found in soil, but have a worldwide distribution. Infection is spread by the airborne route and the lung is the site of invasion in almost every case. Dissemination to other sites, particularly the central nervous system *(Fig. 28.18)* and heart, occurs in about 25% of compromised individuals with lung infection. Because of the ubiquitous nature of the fungus, diagnosis depends upon demonstrating tissue invasion and this usually entails a lung biopsy.

Although invasive aspergillosis is usually fatal in the compromised patient, early diagnosis and institution of treatment – amphotericin is the drug of choice (see Chapter 30) – together with a reduction in corticosteroid and cytotoxic therapy wherever possible, appear to improve the prognosis. Outbreaks of hospital-acquired infection have been reported (see Chapter 34), especially in relation to recent building work.

Pneumocystis carinii only causes symptomatic disease in people with deficient cellular immunity

P. carinii is an organism of uncertain taxonomic status, but is currently considered to be a fungus. It appears to be widespread – a large proportion of the population have antibodies to the organism, but it only causes symptomatic

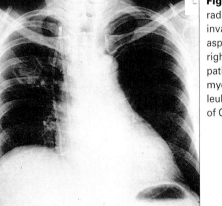

Fig. 28.17 Chest radiograph showing invasive aspergillosis in the right lung of a patient with acute myeloblastic leukemia. (Courtesy of C Kibbler.)

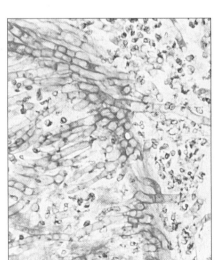

Fig. 28.18 Numerous septate hyphae invading a blood vessel wall in cerebral aspergillosis. Periodic acid–Schiff stain. (Courtesy of WE Farrar.)

disease in people whose cellular immune mechanisms are deficient. There is therefore a high incidence of *P. carinii* pneumonia in patients receiving immunosuppressive therapy to prevent transplant rejection and in people with HIV. It is very rare to find *Pneumocystis* infection in any other site in the body, but the reason for this is unknown.

Diagnosis is not easy and requires a high index of suspicion. The symptoms are non-specific and can mimic a variety of other infectious and non-infectious respiratory diseases. In addition, unlike the other fungi described above, the organism cannot be isolated in expectorated sputum using conventional culture methods, and invasive techniques such as bronchoalveolar lavage or open lung biopsy are required. In samples obtained by these techniques the organism can be demonstrated by silver or immunofluorescent stains *(Fig. 28.19)*. DNA amplification by the polymerase chain reaction improves the sensitivity of the diagnostic tests and has raised doubts that disease results from reactivation of a childhood infection.

Treatment is with high dose cotrimoxazole or pentamidine (see Chapter 30), and cotrimoxazole has been used prophylactically with some success.

Bacteria
Nocardia asteroides is an uncommon opportunist pathogen with a worldwide distribution

The family Actinomycetes, relatives of the mycobacteria, but resembling fungi in that they form branching filaments, contain two pathogenic genera, *Actinomyces* and *Nocardia*. Actinomycosis is discussed in Chapter 20. *N. asteroides* infections have been reported in the immunocompromised, especially in renal transplant patients. The lung is usually the primary site, but infection can spread to the skin, kidney or central nervous system *(Fig. 28.20)*. As with *Aspergillus*, hospital outbreaks of nocardiosis have been described.

Nocardia can be isolated on routine laboratory media, but is often slow to grow and is consequently easily overgrown by commensal flora. Therefore the laboratory staff should be informed if nocardiosis is suspected clinically so that appropriate media are inoculated. The organism is a Gram-negative branching rod and weakly acid fast *(Fig. 28.21)*.

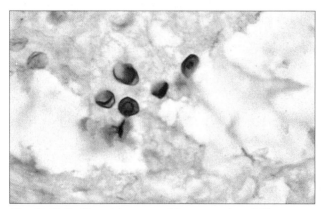

Fig. 28.19 Darkly staining cysts of *Pneumocystis carinii* in an open lung biopsy from an AIDS patient with pneumonia. Grocott silver stain. (Courtesy of M Turner–Warwick.)

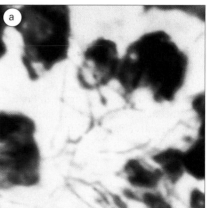

Fig. 28.21 *Nocardia asteroides* in sputum. (a) Acid-fast stain. (Courtesy of TF Sellers, Jr.) (b) Gram's stain. (Courtesy of HP Holley.)

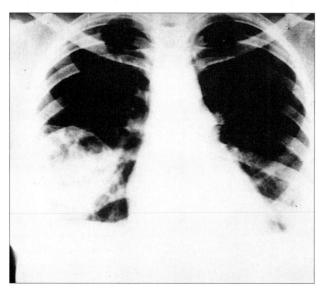

Fig. 28.20 Pulmonary nocardiosis. Chest radiograph showing a large rounded lesion in the right lower zone with multiple cavities. (Courtesy of TF Sellers, Jr.)

Sulphonamides or cotrimoxazole are the drugs of choice, but treatment can be difficult and various other regimens involving tetracycline, aminoglycosides or imipenem have been described.

Mycobacterium avium-intracellulare disease is often a terminal event in AIDS

Although mycobacterial infections are well documented in immunosuppressed patients, it is the association between AIDS and mycobacteria that is now most prominent. This includes disseminated infection with *Mycobacterium tuberculosis* and *Mycobacterium avium-intracellulare* (*Mycobacterium avium* complex or MAC), and these organisms can be isolated from blood cultures from patients with AIDS. *M. tuberculosis* has been described in detail in Chapter 17. *M. avium-intracellulare* belongs to the so-called 'atypical' mycobacteria or mycobacteria other than tuberculosis (MOTT). It resembles *M. tuberculosis* in that it is slow-growing, but it is resistant to the conventional antituberculous drugs. Multidrug therapy with combinations such as clofazimine or rifamycin derivatives together with macrolides (azithromycin or clarithromycin), quinolones, isoniazid, ethambutol, cycloserine or pyrazinamide have been recommended.

Protozoa and helminths
Cryptosporidium and Isospora belli infections cause severe diarrhea in AIDS

Cryptosporidium (Fig. 28.22) is a protozoan parasite that has only recently been recognized as a cause of human disease, although it is well known to veterinarians as an animal pathogen. It causes significant but self-limiting diarrhea in healthy normal people (see Chapter 20), but severe and chronic diarrhea in people with AIDS. Effective treatment is difficult, but the experimental drug spiramycin is currently the first choice (see Chapter 30).

Isospora belli (Fig. 28.23) is a parasite very similar to *Cryptosporidium* and also produces severe diarrhea in people with AIDS. Unlike *Cryptosporidium*, however, it is susceptible to cotrimoxazole.

Immunosuppression may lead to reactivation of dormant Strongyloides stercoralis

Strongyloides stercoralis is a parasitic roundworm that remains dormant for years following initial infection, but may be reactivated to produce massive autoinfection in the immunosuppressed patient. Although rare in the UK and most of the USA, it should be borne in mind in patients who have lived in endemic areas such as the tropics and southern USA, even if this was many years before their immunosuppression.

Viruses
Certain virus infections are more common or more severe in compromised patients

The virus infections that are more common or more severe in the compromised patient (see *Fig. 28.10*) have been described in detail elsewhere in this book. Many of these represent reactivation of latent infections, for example:
- Polyomavirus infection (BK and JC virus) acquired via the respiratory tract and latent in the kidney (see Chapter 18).
- JC virus, which can reactivate and disseminate to cause progressive multifocal leukoencephalopathy in people with AIDS, but is less common than other causes of lesions in the central nervous system (e.g. toxoplasmosis or herpes encephalitis).

Summary

This chapter has attempted to draw together the many different ways in which humans can be compromised in their defense against infection and the enormous variety of microbes that take advantage of the compromised host. Despite therapeutic advances with potent antimicrobial agents many trivial infections become life-threatening in the absence of assistance from the patient's own defense mechanisms.

Early recognition of infections is important because they progress rapidly to a fatal outcome unless antimicrobial therapy is instituted promptly. However, this requires an astute physician and an informed laboratory, as such infections are often

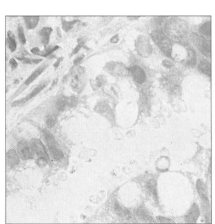

Fig. 28.22 Numerous organisms in the brush border of the intestine in cryptosporidiosis. (Courtesy of J Newman.)

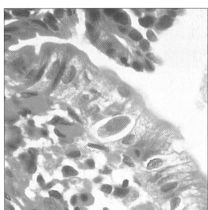

Fig. 28.23 Human coccidiosis, with a single *Isospora belli* organism within an epithelial cell and a chronic inflammatory reaction in the lamina propria. (Courtesy of GN Griffin.)

caused by unusual pathogens and by organisms that may be dismissed as 'harmless' commensals. Reactivation and dissemination of latent infection is also common.

The clinical presentation of infections is often unusual in those who are immunocompromised and is characterized by:

- An absence of the usual signs and symptoms because of the inability of the patient to mount an appropriate immune response.
- Unusual sites of infection.
- Rapid progression to a fatal outcome.

- A compromised person is one whose normal defenses against infection are defective. Immunodeficiences may involve the innate or adaptive immune systems and may be primary or secondary.
- Compromised patients can be infected with any of the pathogens capable of infecting immunocompetent individuals. In addition they suffer many infections caused by opportunist pathogens. The type of infection is related to the nature of the compromise.
- Effective antimicrobial therapy is often difficult to achieve in the absence of a functional immune response, even when the pathogen is susceptible to the drug *in vitro*.
- Important bacterial opportunists include *P. aeruginosa*, especially in neutropenic patients and those with major burns, and *Staph. epidermidis* in patients with plastic devices *in situ*. In AIDS the predominant bacterial opportunists are intracellular pathogens benefiting from the lack of cell-mediated immunity.
- AIDS, and neutropenia (particularly following cytotoxic therapy) predispose to fungal infections (e.g. *Candida*, *Aspergillus* and *Cryptococcus*) especially when the patient has received previous antibacterial therapy.
- Viral infections are more common and severe in immunodeficient patients than in normal patients, particularly reactivation of latent infections (e.g. herpes simplex virus, CMV, JC virus).

A 24-year-old man with HIV visits his doctor with a six-week history of recurrent and worsening headaches. His CD4 count is 80/mm^3 and he has been well since being diagnosed as HIV1 seropositive in 1987. On examination he has no focal neurologic signs and fundoscopy is normal. He has oral candidiasis. A computerized tomographic head scan is normal and a lumbar puncture is performed. The results are: CSF appearance, clear; white cells, 150/mm^3, predominantly lymphocytic; CSF glucose, 2.2 mmol/l; blood glucose, 3.8 mmol/l; protein, 0.4 g/dl.

1. What is the most likely diagnosis and what diagnostic tests would you perform?
2. What other confirmatory investigations might you ask for?
3. How would you manage him?

Further Reading

Brostoff J, Scadding GK, Male D, Roitt IM. *Clinical Immunology*. London: Mosby International, 1991.

Gemmell CG, McCartney AC. Coagulase-negative staphylococci within the hospital environment. *Rev Med Microbiol* 1990;**1**:213–218.

Orr KE, Gould FK. Infection problems in patients receiving solid organ transplants. *Rev Med Microbiol* 1992;**3**:96–103.

Reese RE, Douglas RG, editors. *A Practical Approach To Infectious Diseases*. Baltimore/Toronto: Little, Brown & Co, 1986.

Rogers TR. Management of septicaemia in the immunocompromised with particular reference to neutropenic patients. In: Shanson DC (ed). *Septicaemia and Endocarditis*. Oxford: Oxford Medical Publications, 1989.

5

control

Introduction

Infectious diseases can be controlled by drugs, immunization and a 'healthy' environment
One of the great achievements of applied medical research has been its success in controlling so many infectious diseases; smallpox has even been controlled to the point of eradication. This has been accomplished in three main ways:
- By the use of drugs (chemotherapy).
- By vaccines (immunization).
- By improving the environment (e.g. better sanitation, nutrition) *(Fig. 29.1)*.

These strategies for control will be described individually in the following chapters; here, we will briefly compare and contrast these methods, and evaluate their importance in the control of disease.

Chemotherapy Versus Vaccination

The concept of selectivity – or specificity – is central to both chemotherapy and vaccination

Although they appear so different *(Fig. 29.2)*, both chemotherapy and vaccination developed together from the intensive study that followed the demonstration in the late 1800s that diseases could be caused by microbes. Pasteur (see Fig. 29.4) showed that killed or weakened microbes (e.g. anthrax, rabies) could be used to induce immunity that was specific to one disease, while Ehrlich's work with histologic dyes led him to the idea that specific chemicals ('drugs') might bind to particular microbial structures and damage them (see Chapter 30).

The specificity of an antimicrobial drug resides in its ability to damage the microbe and not the host

In the case of antimicrobial drugs, the drug should ideally bind to a molecule present only in the microbe to ensure specificity for the microbe and not the host. The extent to which this can be achieved varies from microbe to microbe. Bacteria, with their prokaryotic cell structure, are much more remote from humans than fungi, protozoa or worms (which are all eukaryotic). It is not surprising, therefore, that the most effective antibiotics are generally those used against bacteria. There are four major sites in the bacterial cell that are sufficiently different from human cells that they can be targeted by antibacterial agents.

Fig. 29.1 Strategies for controlling infectious diseases.

STRATEGIES FOR CONTROL OF INFECTIOUS DISEASES	
general features	water purification (waterborne diseases) sewage disposal (enteric infections) improved nutrition (host defense) improved housing (less crowding, dirt, etc.)
food	cold storage pasteurization (milk, etc.) food inspection (meat, etc.) adequate cooking
zoonoses and arthropod-transmitted infections	control of vectors (mosquitoes, ticks, lice etc.) control of reservoir animal (rabies, bovine TB)
specific disease treatment or prevention	chemotherapy vaccines
miscellaneous measures	changes in personal habits (reduced promiscuity, use of condoms, improved personal hygiene etc.) control of intravenous drug abuse screening of transfused blood and organs

CHEMOTHERAPY AND VACCINES COMPARED		
	chemotherapy	**vaccination**
specificity	usually high	very high
toxicity	potentially high	usually low
duration of effect	usually short	usually long
duration of treatment	may be prolonged	usually short, but may need boosting
effectiveness	bacteria: high viruses ⎤ fungi ⎬ moderate parasites ⎦	viruses: high bacteria ⎤ low/ fungi ⎬ mode- parasites ⎦ rate

Fig. 29.2 Comparison of chemotherapy and vaccination.

These are:
• The cell wall.
• The bacterial ribosome.
• The nucleic acid synthetic pathway.
• The cell membrane *(Fig. 29.3)*.

What is more surprising, however, is that many antibacterial agents are products of microbes themselves or derivatives of these products. It is presumed that they form part of the self-preservation mechanism by which the microbes prevent overcrowding with their own or other species.

Vaccines avoid host damage by inducing self-tolerance in T and B cells

Vaccine specificity is quite different in that the specific binding molecules already exist in the host, in the shape of the T and B cell receptors, and merely need to be coaxed into action. Host damage is avoided largely, though not entirely, by the induction of self-tolerance in the T and B cells. Therefore a new and untried vaccine is on the whole less likely to be dangerously toxic than a new and untried drug.

The target of both a drug and a vaccine may be the same molecule

Drugs and vaccines do show a certain degree of convergence as the target of both may ultimately be the same molecule. Several parasite enzymes, for example, have been shown to be points of attack both for drugs and for effective vaccine antigens. Perhaps, given enough time, both nature (the evolving lymphocyte repertoire) and the pharmaceutical industry (evolving new drugs) may arrive at vaccines and drugs that recognize one and the same set of microbial targets.

Viruses have been particularly difficult targets for chemotherapy since so much of the viral life cycle uses host components. A few susceptible points do exist, however, and the development of acyclovir for herpesviruses and zidovudine (AZT) for HIV are excellent examples of tailor-made chemotherapy based on a detailed knowledge of the relevant viral enzymes.

Microbe resistance can develop to both drugs and vaccines

The development of resistance is, in effect, a change in balance in favor of the microbe, and affects both drugs and vaccines, though in a variety of different ways. For example:
• Penicillin resistance is often due to the production of an enzyme beta-lactamase by the microbe. This enzyme breaks the penicillin beta-lactam ring.
• Chloroquine resistance in malaria is due to the development of a mechanism that pumps the drug out of the parasite at an increased rate.
• Resistance to the protective effects of vaccination by variants of influenza virus is due to small changes in the surface hemagglutinin and neuraminidase molecules.
• In the African trypanosome, complete replacement of the glycoprotein surface coat reduces both T and B cell recognition.

Clearly, each of these problems has to be approached and dealt with separately.

Usually drugs have to be given regularly, while vaccines often have to be given only once

A major difference between drugs and vaccines is that drugs are designed to treat disease, and have to be given on a regular basis, whereas vaccines are designed to prevent it, and need to be given only a few times, often only once. There are, of course, exceptions to this: passive antibody can be used to treat acute infection just as a drug can, while drugs like pyrimethamine and chloroquine are used for prophylaxis against malaria almost as if they were short-term vaccines. However, in most cases there is a clear-cut distinction between the one- or two-shot vaccine, conferring protection for years, and the daily or twice-daily drug dose. Naturally, patients and doctors favor the former, whereas the

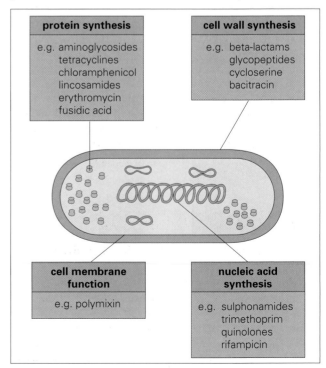

Fig. 29.3 Targets for antibacterial action.

Louis Pasteur (1822–1895)

The science of microbiology was established in the nineteenth century by the work of many distinguished scientists. However one such scientist, Louis Pasteur, may legitimately be regarded as a founding father of this discipline *(Fig. 29.4)*. He, along with Robert Koch, a German doctor (see Chapter 7), was able to show that living organisms or 'microbes' were the cause of disease, and provided a firm scientific basis for their study and control.

Pasteur began work at a time when spontaneous generation was still an accepted explanation for the appearance of microorganisms in decaying material. His elegant experiments showed that sterile organic infusions would not putrify or ferment if there was no subsequent contact with airborne contaminants, proving that spontaneous generation did not occur, and that all microbes must come from pre-existing microbes. This discovery contributed to many fields of science, both basic and applied. Perhaps most important was the contribution Pasteur made to the work of Lister on antiseptics, which revolutionized approaches to surgery.

Pasteur worked in an amazing variety of microbiological fields, from fermentation in the brewing of beers and production of wines, to identification of silk worm diseases, bringing to each a penetrating scientific insight and making discoveries that brought him national and international reknown. His understanding of the roles of organisms in causing diseases, and his acute scientific perception, enabled him to grasp from a series of 'mishaps' with experiments on chicken cholera that attenuated microbes could induce not disease, but immunity from disease. His ideas generated powerful opposition, but his belief then was strong enough to encourage him in 1881 to take part in a public trial of his vaccine against anthrax in domestic animals. Later, he used his insight into rabies, caused by organisms he could not see or culture, to develop an attenuated vaccine made from the dried spinal cords of infected rabbits. This was proven effective in humans in 1885 when Pasteur inoculated Joseph Meister, a nine-year-old boy who had been badly bitten by a rabid dog. Meister survived and Pasteur's views on vaccination became universally accepted.

Pasteur ended his life as a national hero in his native France, and with a worldwide reputation for his work. His name is immortalized not only in the process of sterilization – 'pasteurization' – that he developed, but in the Institut Pasteur in Paris, which remains one of the most important international centers of microbiological work.

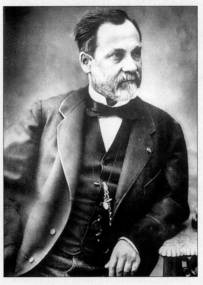

Fig. 29.4 Louis Pasteur (1822–1895).

pharmaceutical industry prefers the latter. Therefore, while drug development is carried out by industry without the need for external encouragement, vaccine development needs an outside stimulus in the form of earmarked funding – a field in which the World Health Organization, in particular, has performed with great distinction.

Epidemiologic Considerations

Epidemiologic studies help in planning control measures

Epidemiology is concerned with the ways in which diseases arise, spread, and die down in the community, and epidemiologic studies can contribute greatly to the planning of control measures (see Chapter 33). For example:

- If it is known that an infectious disease is transmitted by an insect vector, an alternative line of attack is available, namely control of the vector *(Fig. 29.5)*.

- Transmission by the fecal–oral route can be controlled by improvements in the quality of water supplies and sewage disposal.
- If an infection is known to be transmitted by blood products (e.g. HIV, hepatitis), a clear responsibility is placed on transfusion centers to screen for these viruses.
- If it can be demonstrated that an infection is not transmitted by a certain route (e.g. HIV by skin contact) needless restriction can be avoided.

Where person-to-person spread is particularly efficient, eradication of an infectious disease is more difficult. For example, the eradication of smallpox would have been more difficult if it had not been for the relatively poor spreading ability or 'reproductive capacity' of the virus.

Genetic differences between individuals or races are other important factors in the pattern of infectious disease that can influence the success of control measures. Epidemiologists can now generate mathematical models of an individual infection in a particular locality from which highly accurate

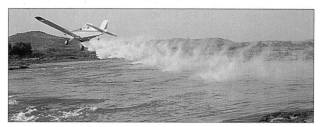

Fig. 29.5 Control of *Simulium* larvae with aerial application of insecticide (temefos) to a river in West Africa. The *Simulium* fly is the most important vector species for human onchocerciasis in Africa. Almost complete control of flies has been obtained in West Africa by the extensive control program, which was begun in 1974. (Courtesy of the World Health Organization.)

FACTORS FAVORING GLOBAL ERADICATION OF AN INFECTIOUS DISEASE	
factor	**rationale**
disease limited to humans	no reinvasion by microbe from animal or arthropod host
no long-term carrier state	no reinvasion by microbe from human carriers
few clinical (unrecognized) cases	surveillance possible
one or few serotypes	a single vaccine is adequate
stable, cheap, effective vaccine available	worldwide program possible
eradication program is cost-effective	program likely to be undertaken

Fig. 29.6 Factors favoring global eradication of infectious disease. Smallpox fitted all categories, whereas some have problems with numbers of unrecognized cases (e.g. polio and rubella) and others with cost-effectiveness (e.g. measles and shigellosis).

- Chemotherapy, vaccination and environmental measures all have their place in the control of infectious disease.
- The most appropriate measure for controlling an infectious disease will depend upon many factors, as described in Chapters 30–34.

1. What are the advantages and disadvantages of chemotherapy compared with vaccination?

predictions can be made of the likely impact of a drug or vaccine campaign; indeed, it would be unwise to embark on an expensive trial without such a prediction (see Chapter 33).

There are, of course, practical limits to the environmental control of disease. Chagas' disease could probably be eliminated by the abolition of slum housing, and schistosomiasis by the universal adoption of Wellington boots, but neither of these seems very likely in practice. Vaccines, and to a slightly lesser extent drugs, have the advantage here, in that they do not depend upon a change in human behavior.

Infection control is particularly important in hospitals

In hospital, patients with a variety of illnesses – some due to infection, some resulting in unusual vulnerability to infection – are crowded together under conditions that favor transmission (see Chapter 34). The acquisition of a drug-resistant infection in hospital is particularly difficult to control, and the physician needs to know what measures are available to prevent this from happening (see Chapter 34).

Control Versus Eradication

What are the chances that other infectious diseases will follow smallpox into oblivion? Various factors are important in determining the effectiveness of any eradication program (*Fig. 29.6*).

Realism is required when considering the long-term aims of control strategies

Hopes raised by the early success of antibiotics were soon dashed by the emergence of resistance, and far from the microbial load borne by the human race being diminished in recent years, it has if anything increased: legionnaires' disease, Lyme disease and AIDS do not feature in older textbooks of microbiology. Control of infectious diseases is therefore a matter of identifying priorities such as:

- Which diseases could, with suitable effort, be eradicated?
- Which diseases need urgent measures to stop them getting worse?
- Which diseases are responsible for the most human suffering and economic loss?

Inevitably, some diseases will not feature strongly on any such list and it must be accepted that they may always be with us.

Introduction

The interactions between host, microbial pathogen and antimicrobial agent can be considered as a triangle, and any alteration in one side will inevitably affect the other two sides *(Fig. 30.1)*. In this chapter two sides of the triangle will be examined in greater detail:
• The interactions between antimicrobial agents and microorganisms.
• The interactions between antimicrobial agents and the human host.
Laboratory aspects of antibiotic susceptibility tests and assays will also be outlined.
The third side of the triangle, the interactions between microorganisms and the human host, have been considered in detail in the preceding chapters. The concluding section of the present chapter will draw together the three sides of the triangle.

Selective Toxicity

The term 'selective toxicity' was proposed by the immuno-chemist Paul Ehrlich (see panel, *Fig. 30.2*). Selective toxicity is achieved by exploiting differences in the structure and metabolism of microorganisms and host cells; ideally the antimicrobial agent should act at a target site present in the infecting organism, but absent from host cells. This is more likely to be achievable in microorganisms that are prokaryotes than in those that are eukaryotes, as they are structurally more distinct from the host cells. (A comparison of the cellular organization of prokaryotic and eukaryotic cells is given in Chapter 1.) At the other end of the spectrum, viruses are difficult to attack because of their obligate intracellular lifestyle – a successful antiviral agent must be able to enter the host cell, but inhibit and damage only a virus-specific target. The desirable features of ideal antimicrobial agents are summarized in *Figure 30.3*.

Discovery and Design of Antimicrobial Agents

Antibiotics are natural metabolic products of fungi, actino-mycetes and bacteria that kill or inhibit the growth of microorganisms. Antibiotic production is particularly associated with soil microorganisms and in the natural environment is thought to provide a selective advantage for organisms in their competition for space and nutrients. Although the majority of antibacterial and antifungal agents in clinical use today are derived from natural products of fermentation, most are then chemically modified to improve their antibacterial or pharmacologic properties. However, some agents are totally synthetic (e.g. sulphonamides, quinolones). Therefore the term 'antibacterial' or 'antimicrobial' agent is often used in preference to 'antibiotic'.

The discovery of new antimicrobial agents used to be entirely a matter of chance. Pharmaceutical companies undertook massive screening programs searching for new soil microorganisms that produced antibiotic activity. In the light of our greater understanding of the mechanisms of action of existing antimi-crobials the processes have become rationalized, searching either for new natural products by target site-directed screening or synthesizing molecules predicted to interact with a microbial target. More recently, genomic approaches to the identification of new (unexploited) targets have been applied. The steps in a rational design program are summarized in *Figure 30.4*.

Ways of Classifying Antibacterial Agents

There are three ways of classifying antibacterial agents:
• According to whether they are bactericidal or bacterio-static.
• By target site.
• By chemical structure.

Some antibacterial agents are bactericidal, others are bacteriostatic

Some antibacterial agents kill bacteria (bactericidal), while others only inhibit their growth (bacteriostatic). Bacteriostatic agents are successful in the treatment of infections because they prevent the bacterial population from increasing and host defense mechanisms can cope with the static population. In immunocompromised patients, bacteriostatic drugs may be less efficacious.

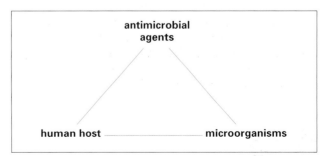

Fig. 30.1 The interactions between antimicrobial agents, microorganisms and the human host can be viewed as a triangle. Any effect on one side of the triangle will have effects on the other two sides.

As a means of classification, the distinction between bactericidal and bacteriostatic agents is blurred because some agents are capable of killing some species, but are only bacteriostatic for others – for example, chloramphenicol inhibits growth of *Escherichia coli*, but kills *Haemophilus influenzae*.

Paul Ehrlich (1854–1915)

Just as Pasteur towers over immunomicrobiology, Ehrlich *(Fig. 30.2)* is the father figure of immunochemistry. His contributions to the science of medicine at all levels are quite extraordinary. He was the first to propose that foreign antigens were recognized by 'side-chains' on cells (1890), a brilliant insight that took 70 years to confirm. He also discovered the mast cell, invented the acid-fast stain for the tubercle bacillus, and devised a method to manufacture and commercialize a strong diphtheria antitoxin. He pioneered the development of antibiotics with his work on '606' (or 'Salvarsan'), a treatment for syphilis, for which he was denounced by the church for interfering with God's punishment for sin.

While working on the treatment of infections caused by trypanosomes he set forth the concept of 'selective toxicity' as illustrated by the following quote: 'But, gentlemen, it should be made clear that in general this task is much more complicated than that using serum therapy. These chemical agents, in contrast to the antibodies, may be harmful to the body. When such an agent is given to a sick organism, a difference must exist between the toxicity of this agent to the parasite and its toxicity to the host. We must always be aware of the fact that these agents are able to act on other parts of the body as well as on the parasites.'

Like Pasteur, he had a grasp of the continuum from the whole body to the cell and the three-dimensional structure

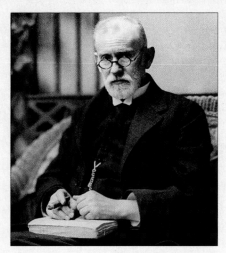

Fig. 30.2 Paul Ehrlich (1854–1915).

of molecules, and throughout his life he stressed the importance of molecular interaction as the basis of all biologic function; this is summed up in his famous maxim 'corpora non agunt nisi fixata' or 'things do not interact unless they make contact'. A Nobel prize winner in 1908, his name was systematically eliminated from the records by the Nazi regimen on account of his Jewish birth, but he was restored to honor by a reconstruction of his laboratory at the Seventh International Congress of Immunology in Berlin in 1989.

DESIRED PROPERTIES OF A NEW ANTIMICROBIAL AGENT
antimicrobial properties
selectivity for microbial rather than mammalian targets broad spectrum of activity cidal activity (antibacterial and antifungal agents)
pharmacological properties
non-toxic to the host long plasma half-life (once-a-day dosing) good tissue distribution including CSF low plasma-protein binding oral and parenteral dosing forms no interference with other drugs

Fig. 30.3 In the design of new antimicrobial agents both antimicrobial activity and pharmacologic properties of the antibiotic for the host have to be considered.

RATIONAL DESIGN OF AN ANTIMICROBIAL AGENT
select an appropriate target
identify a chemical lead (i.e. a new molecule with inhibitory activity on the target)
modify the lead compound to enhance potency
evaluate *in vitro* activity
evaluate *in vivo* activity and toxicity
test in clinical trials and develop

(average 10 years)

Fig. 30.4 The discovery process of new antimicrobial agents has moved away from the random screening of soil microorganisms towards a rational design program. This illustration identifies different steps in this program. From discovery to development and marketing can take at least 10 years and cost up to US$500 million.

There are four main target sites for antibacterial action

A convenient way of classifying antibacterials is on the basis of their site of action. This classification does not allow an accurate prediction of which antibacterials will be active against which bacterial species, but it does help in the understanding of the molecular basis of antibacterial action, and conversely in the elucidation of many of the synthetic processes in bacterial cells. The four main target sites for antibacterial action are:

- Cell wall synthesis.
- Protein synthesis.
- Nucleic acid synthesis.
- Cell membrane function.

These targets differ to a greater or lesser degree from those in the host (human) cells and so allow inhibition of the bacterial cell without concomitant inhibition of the equivalent mammalian cell targets (selective toxicity).

Each target site encompasses a multitude of synthetic reactions (enzymes and substrates), each of which may be specifically inhibited by an antibacterial agent. A range of chemically diverse molecules may inhibit different reactions at the same target site (e.g. protein synthesis inhibitors).

Antibacterial agents have diverse chemical structures

Classification based on chemical structure alone is not of practical use because there is such diversity. However a combination of target site and chemical structure provides a useful working classification and will be used in the later sections of this chapter. Each target site will be considered in turn and the antibacterial agents grouped in families according to their chemical structure.

Resistance to Antibacterial Agents

Resistance to antibacterial agents is a matter of degree. In the medical setting we define a resistant organism as one that will not be inhibited or killed by an antibacterial agent at concentrations of the drug achievable in the body after normal dosage. 'Some men are born great, some achieve greatness, and some have greatness thrust upon them' (William Shakespeare, *Twelfth Night*). Likewise some bacteria are born resistant, others have resistance thrust upon them. In other words some species are innately resistant to some families of antibiotics either because they lack a susceptible target or because they are impermeable to the antibacterial agent. The Gram-negative rods with their outer membrane layer exterior to the cell wall peptidoglycan are less permeable to large molecules than Gram-positive cells. However, within species that are innately susceptible, there are also strains that develop or acquire resistance.

The genetics of resistance

In parallel with the rapid development of a wide range of antibacterial agents since the 1940s, bacteria have proved extremely adept at developing resistance to each new agent that comes along. The rapidly increasing incidence of resistance associated with slowing down in the discovery of novel antibacterial agents to combat resistant strains is now recognized worldwide as a serious threat to the treatment of life-threatening infections.

Resistance may result from a chromosomal mutation

Resistance may arise from:

- A single chromosomal mutation in one bacterial cell resulting in the synthesis of an altered protein, for example streptomycin resistance via alteration in a ribosomal protein or the single amino acid change in the enzyme dihydropteroate synthetase resulting in a lowered affinity for sulfonamides.
- A series of mutations, for example changes in penicillin-binding proteins in penicillin-resistant pneumococci (PBPs).

In the presence of antibiotic, these spontaneous mutants have a selective advantage and survive and outgrow the susceptible population *(Fig. 30.5a)*. They can also spread to other sites in the same patient or by cross-infection to other patients and therefore become disseminated.

Resistance may be acquired from genes on transmissible plasmids

Not content with surviving the antibacterial onslaught by relying on random chromosomal mutation, bacteria are also able to acquire resistance genes on transmissible plasmids *(Fig. 30.5b; see also Chapter 3)*. Such plasmids often code for resistance determinants to several unrelated families of antibacterial agents. Therefore a cell may acquire resistance to many different drugs at once. This so-called 'infectious resistance' was first described by Japanese workers studying enteric bacteria, but is now recognized to be widespread throughout the bacterial world. Some plasmids are promiscuous, crossing species barriers and the same resistance gene is therefore found in widely different species. For example, TEM-1, the most common plasmid-mediated beta-lactamase in Gram-negative bacteria, is widespread in *E. coli* and other enterobacteria and also accounts for penicillin resistance in *Neisseria gonorrhoeae* and ampicillin resistance in *H. influenzae*.

Resistance may be acquired from 'jumping genes'

Resistance genes may also occur on transposons; the so-called 'jumping genes', which are capable of integration into the chromosome or into plasmids. The chromosome provides a more secure position for the genes, but they will be disseminated only as rapidly as the bacteria divide. Transposons moving from the chromosome to plasmids allow chromosomal genes to be disseminated more rapidly. Transposons can also move between plasmids, for example from a non-transmissible to a transmissible plasmid, again accelerating dissemination *(Fig. 30.5c)*.

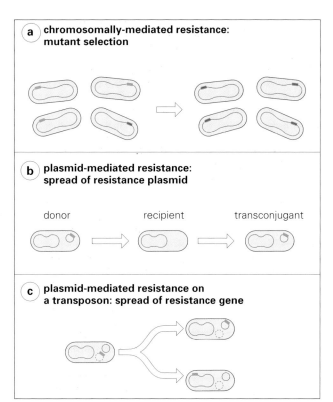

a chromosomally-mediated resistance:
mutant selection

b plasmid-mediated resistance:
spread of resistance plasmid

donor   recipient   transconjugant

c plasmid-mediated resistance on
a transposon: spread of resistance gene

Fig. 30.5 A chromosomal mutation (a) can produce a drug-resistant target, which confers resistance on the bacterial cell and allows it to multiply in the presence of antibiotic. Resistance genes carried on plasmids (b) can spread from one cell to another more rapidly than cells themselves divide and spread. Resistance genes on transposable elements (c) move between plasmids and the chromosome and from one plasmid to another, thereby allowing greater stability or greater dissemination of the resistance gene.

Mechanisms of resistance

Resistance mechanisms can be broadly classified into three main types. These are summarized below and in *Figure 30.6*, and described in more detail where relevant for each antibiotic in later sections of this chapter. Where the mechanisms of resistance in bacteria have been elucidated they appear to involve the synthesis of new or altered proteins and, as mentioned above, the genes encoding these proteins may be either plasmid-mediated or on the chromosome.

The target site may be altered

The target enzyme may be altered so that it has a lowered affinity for the antibacterial, but still functions adequately for normal metabolism to proceed. Alternatively an additional target enzyme may be synthesized.

Access to the target site may be altered (altered uptake)

This mechanism involves decreasing the amount of drug that reaches the target by either:
• Altering entry, for example by increasing the impermeability of the cell wall.
• Pumping the drug out of the cell (known as an efflux mechanism).

RESISTANCE TO ANTIBACTERIAL AGENTS			
antibacterial	mechanism of resistance		
	altered target	altered uptake	drug inactivation
beta-lactams	+	+	++
glycopeptides	+		
aminoglycosides	–	+	++
tetracyclines	–	+	
chloramphenicol		–	+
macrolides	++		
lincosamides	++		
fusidic acid	++		
sulfonamides	++	–	
trimethoprim	++	–	
quinolones	–	+	
rifampicin	++		

– rare; occurs infrequently or only in few species
+ common
++ very common, in many species

Fig. 30.6 Mechanisms of resistance can be classified into three main types. Resistance to some antibiotics is more frequently found through alteration in the target site than other mechanisms. Drug inactivation mechanisms are most important for beta-lactams, aminoglycosides and chloramphenicol.

Enzymes that modify or destroy the antibacterial agent may be produced (drug inactivation)

There are many examples of such enzymes, the most important being:
• Beta-lactamases.
• Aminoglycoside-modifying enzymes.
• Chloramphenicol acetyl transferases.
These will be described in the relevant sections on these antibiotics.

Classes of Antibacterial Agents

The following sections of this chapter deal with groups of antibacterial agents arranged according to their target site and subdivided on the basis of chemical structure. Each section attempts to summarize the answers to the questions set out in *Figure 30.7*, reviewing the interactions between antibacterial agent and bacteria and between the antibacterial and the host, in other words two sides of the triangle (*Fig. 30.1*).

Inhibitors of Cell Wall Synthesis

Peptidoglycan, a vital component of the bacterial cell wall (see Chapter 3), is a compound unique to bacteria and therefore provides an optimum target for selective toxicity. Synthesis of peptidoglycan precursors starts in the cytoplasm; wall subunits are then transported across the cytoplasmic membrane and finally inserted into the growing peptidoglycan molecule. Several different stages are therefore potential targets for inhibition *(Fig. 30.8)* The antibacterials that inhibit cell wall synthesis *(Fig. 30.9)* are very varied in chemical structure. The important groups are the beta-lactams and the glycopeptides; bacitracin and cycloserine have many fewer clinical applications.

Beta-lactams

Beta-lactams contain a beta-lactam ring and inhibit cell wall synthesis by binding to penicillin binding proteins (PBPs)

Beta-lactams comprise a very large family of different groups of compounds all containing the beta-lactam ring. The different groups within the family are distinguished by the structure of the ring attached to the beta-lactam ring – in penicillins this is a five-membered ring, in cephalosporins a six-membered ring – and by the side chains attached to these rings *(Fig. 30.10)*.

PBPs are the carboxypeptidases and transpeptidases responsible for the final stages of cross-linking of the bacterial cell wall structure. Inhibition of one or more of these essential enzymes results in an accumulation of precursor cell wall units, leading to activation of the cell's autolytic system and cell lysis *(Fig. 30.11)*.

Most beta-lactams have to be administered parenterally

Although the majority of beta-lactams have to be administered intramuscularly or intravenously, there are some orally-active agents. Most achieve clinically useful concentrations in the cerebrospinal fluid (CSF) when the meninges are inflamed (as in meningitis) and the blood–brain barrier becomes more permeable. In general, they are not effective against intracellular organisms.

A few of the cephalosporins, notably cefotaxime, are metabolized to compounds with less microbiological activity. All beta-lactams are excreted in the urine and for some, such as benzylpenicillin, this is very rapid – hence the need for frequent doses. Probenecid can be administered concurrently to slow down excretion and maintain higher blood and tissue concentrations for a longer period of time.

Different beta-lactams have different clinical uses, but are not active against species that lack a cell wall

There are more than 40 different beta-lactam antibiotics currently registered for clinical use. Some, such as penicillin, are active mainly against Gram-positive organisms, whereas others have been developed for their activity against Gram-negative rods such as the enterobacteria. Only the more recent beta-lactams are active against innately more resistant organisms such as *Pseudonomas aeruginosa*.

It is important to remember that beta-lactams are not active against species that lack a cell wall (e.g. *Mycoplasma*) or those with very impenetrable walls such as mycobacteria, or

WHAT DO WE NEED TO KNOW ABOUT AN ANTIBACTERIAL AGENT?	
What is it ?	chemical structure natural or synthetic product
What does it do?	target site mechanism of action
Where does it go? (and therefore preferred route of administration)	absorption, distribution, metabolism and excretion of the drug in the body of the host
When is it used?	spectrum of activity and important clinical uses
What are the limitations to its use	toxicity to the human host lack of toxicity, i.e. resistance of the bacteria
How much does it cost?	great variation between agents but cost is a serious limitation on availability of some agents in developing countries

Fig. 30.7 In order to understand the nature and optimum use of an antibacterial agent, the questions listed here must be answered.

intracellular pathogens such as *Brucella*, *Legionella* and *Chlamydia*. The main clinical uses for important beta-lactams are shown in *Figure 30.12*.

Resistance to beta-lactams may involve one or more of the three possible mechanisms

Alteration in target site

Methicillin-resistant staphylococci synthesize an additional PBP, which has a much lower affinity for beta-lactams than the normal PBPs and is therefore able to continue cell wall synthesis when the other PBPs are inhibited. Although the gene coding for the additional PBP is present on the chromosome in all cells of a resistant population, it is only transcribed in a proportion of the cells, resulting in the phenomenon of 'heterogeneous resistance'. In the laboratory, special cultural conditions are used to enhance expression and demonstrate resistance. Methicillin-resistant staphylococci are resistant to all other beta-lactams. The majority of strains also produce beta-lactamase (see below).

Penicillin-resistant strains of *Streptococcus pneumoniae* have multiple changes (arising through mutation) in their PBPs, which seriously diminish the ability of penicillin to bind to the PBPs and variably affect the binding of other beta-lactams.

Alteration in access to the target site

This mechanism is found in Gram-negative cells where beta-lactams gain access to their target PBPs by diffusion through protein channels (porins) in the outer membrane. Mutations in porin genes result in a decrease in permeability of the

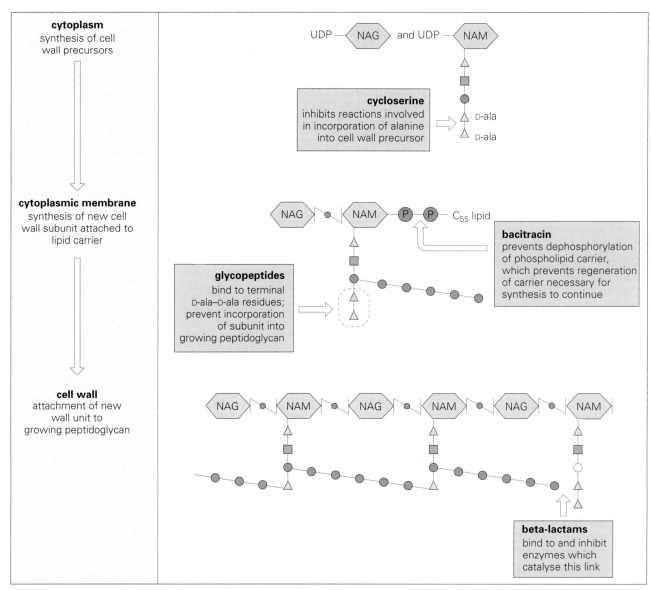

Fig. 30.8 The synthesis of peptidoglycan is a complex process that begins in the cytoplasm, proceeds across the cytoplasmic membrane and leads to the attachment of new wall units to the growing peptidoglycan chain. This synthetic pathway can be inhibited at a variety of points by antibacterial agents. The precise mechanism of inhibition caused by glycopeptides such as vancomycin is unknown, but the mechanism of action of beta-lactams has now been fully elucidated (see below). (NAG, N-acetyl glucosamine; NAM, N-acetyl muramic acid; UDP, uridine diphosphate.)

INHIBITORS OF CELL WALL SYNTHESIS
beta-lactams penicillins, cephalosporins, carbapenems, monobactams
glycopeptides vancomycin, teicoplanin
cycloserine
bacitracin

Fig. 30.9 The beta-lactam group is the largest and most important cell wall synthesis inhibitors. Glycopeptides are active only against Gram-positive organisms. Cycloserine and bacitracin have very limited uses.

outer membrane and hence resistance. Strains resistant by this mechanism may exhibit cross-resistance to unrelated antibiotics that use the same porins.

Production of beta-lactamases
Beta-lactamases are enzymes that catalyze the hydrolysis of the beta-lactam ring to yield microbiologically-inactive products. Genes encoding these enzymes are widespread in the bacterial kingdom and are found on the chromosome and on plasmids.

The beta-lactamases of Gram-positive bacteria are released into the extracellular environment *(Fig. 30.11)* and resistance will only be manifest when a large population of cells is present. The beta-lactamases of Gram-negative cells, however, remain within the periplasm *(Fig. 30.11)*.

There are many different beta-lactamase enzymes with the same function, but differing amino acid sequences and affinities for different beta-lactam substrates. Some beta-lactams (e.g. cloxacillin, ceftazidime, imipenem) are hydrolyzed by very few enzymes (beta-lactamase stable), whereas others (e.g. ampicillin) are much more labile. Beta-lactamase inhibitors such as clavulanic acid *(Fig. 30.13)* are molecules that contain a beta-lactam ring and act as 'suicide inhibitors', binding to beta-lactamases and preventing them from destroying beta-lactams. They have little bactericidal activity of their own.

Toxic effects of beta-lactam drugs include mild rashes and immediate hypersensitivity reactions

Serious allergy to beta-lactam drugs in the form of an immediate hypersensitivity reaction occurs in approximately 0.004–0.015% of treatment courses. Mild idiopathic reactions, usually in the form of a rash, occur more frequently (23% of treatment courses), and especially with ampicillin. Patients who are allergic to penicillin are often allergic to cephalosporins and vice versa, but aztreonam, a monobactam shows negligible cross-reactivity.

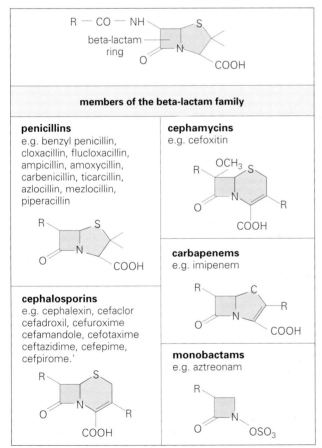

Fig. 30.10 The beta-lactam family. The ring structure is common to all beta-lactams and must be intact for antibacterial action. Enzymes (beta-lactamases) that catalyze the hydrolysis of the beta-lactam bond render the agents inactive. The penicillins and cephalosporins are the major classes of beta-lactam antibiotics, but other members of the family, particularly the carbapenems and monobactams, are the focus of new developments.

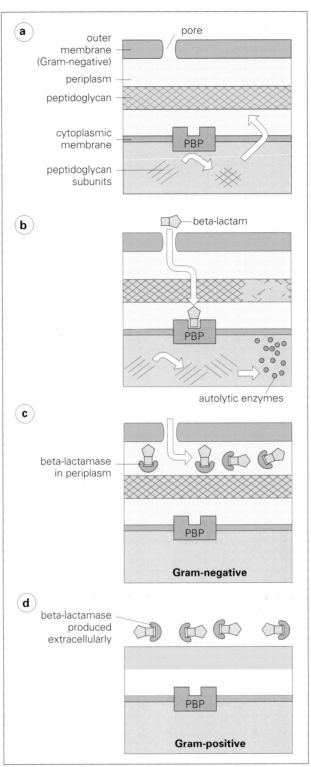

Fig. 30.11 Penicillin-binding proteins (PBPs) play a key role in the final stages of peptidoglycan synthesis. They catalyze the cross-linkage of wall subunits, which are then incorporated into the cell wall (a). Beta-lactams are able to enter the cell through pores in the outer membrane (Gram-negatives) (b), and bind to the PBP. This prevents it from catalyzing the cross-linkage of subunits, leading to their accumulation in the cell and the release of autolytic enzymes, which cause cell lysis. Beta-lactamases (c) and (d) can inactivate beta-lactams before they reach their target PBPs, thereby protecting the cell from the action of beta-lactams.

USES OF BETA-LACTAMS		
beta-lactam class	**examples**	**major clinical use**
penicillins	benzyl penicillin°	bacterial upper respiratory tract infection pneumonia meningitis endocarditis
	cloxacillin flucloxacillin°	skin and soft tissue infection (Gram-positive) osteomyelitis and septic arthritis (Gram-positive)
	ampicillin°# amoxycillin°	urinary tract infection enteric fever ostemyelitis (Gram-negative) meningitis epiglottitis bronchitis
	azlocillin piperacillin #	serious sepsis caused by *Pseudomonas aeruginosa* and other antibiotic-resistant Gram-negative rods (usually in combination with aminoglycoside)
cephalosporins	cephalexin° cefaclor° cefadroxil°	urinary tract infections
	cefuroxime	respiratory tract infections and urinary tract infections
	cefixime° cefpodoxime°	respiratory tract infections
	cefotaxime ceftriaxone	meningitis (in neonates) abdominal sepsis
	ceftazidime cefpirome	serious sepsis caused by *P. aeruginosa* and other antibiotic-resistant Gram-negative rods (usually in combination with aminoglycoside)
cephamycins	cefoxitin	abdominal sepsis
carbapenems	imipenem meropenem	serious sepsis caused by *P. aeruginosa* and other antibiotic-resistant Gram-negative rods (often in combination with aminoglycoside)

Fig. 30.12 Although there are many beta-lactam agents available the most commonly used ones are listed, together with their main indications.
° Oral formulation available.
Can be formulated in combination with beta-lactamase inhibitors (see *Fig. 30.13*).

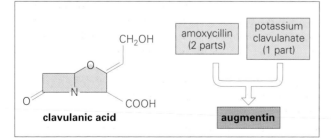

Fig. 30.13 Clavulanic acid, a product of *Streptomyces clavuligerus*, inhibits the most common beta-lactamases (e.g. TEM enzymes) and allows amoxycillin to inhibit cells producing these enzymes. Augmentin is the most widely used of these combination drugs. Other combinations include ticarcillin and clavulanic acid and piperacillin and tazobactam.

Benzylpenicillin can produce neurotoxicity if given in high doses, particularly in patients with renal impairment. This toxicity is manifest as fits, unconsciousness, myoclonic spasms and hallucinations. Carbenicillin can cause platelet dysfunction and sodium overload (because it is given as a sodium salt), especially in patients with liver failure, renal failure and congestive heart failure.

Glycopeptides

Glycopeptides are large molecules and act at an earlier stage than beta-lactams

Glycopeptides include vancomycin and teicoplanin. Both are very large molecules and therefore have difficulty penetrating the Gram-negative cell wall. Teicoplanin is a natural complex of five different but closely related molecules.

Glycopeptides interfere with cell wall synthesis by binding to terminal D-ala–D-ala at the end of pentapeptide chains that are part of the growing bacterial cell wall structure *(Fig. 30.8)*. This binding inhibits the transglycosylation reaction and prevents incorporation of new subunits into the growing cell wall. As glycopeptides act at an earlier stage than beta-lactams it is not useful to combine glycopeptides and beta-lactams in the treatment of infections.

Vancomycin and teicoplanin must be given by injection for systemic infections

Vancomycin and teicoplanin are not absorbed from the gastrointestinal tract and do not penetrate the CSF in patients without meningitis. However, bactericidal concentrations are achieved in most patients with meningitis due to the increased permeability of the blood–brain barrier. Excretion is via the kidney.

Both vancomycin and teicoplanin are active only against Gram-positive organisms

Vancomycin and teicoplanin are used mainly for:
- The treatment of infections caused by Gram-positive cocci and Gram-positive rods that are resistant to beta-lactam drugs, particularly multiresistant *Staphylococcus aureus* and *Staphylococcus epidermidis*.
- For patients allergic to beta-lactams.

Oral administration is used for the treatment of *Clostridium difficile* in antibiotic-associated colitis, although there are now fears that this may be linked to the emergence of glycopeptide-resistant enterococci in the gut flora.

Some enterococci show plasmid-mediated resistance to vancomycin and teicoplanin

Acquired resistance to these agents is extremely rare among bacteria of medical importance, but is now reported with increasing frequency among enterococci, where resistance is plasmid-mediated and transmissible. The mechanism appears to involve a change in the binding of glycopeptide to its target and involves the products of several resistance genes. The fear is that resistance may be transferred from enterococci to staphylococci, thereby rendering some strains of methicillin-resistant staphylococci untreatable with currently-available agents.

The glycopeptides are potentially ototoxic and nephrotoxic

Vancomycin must be given by slow intravenous infusion to avoid 'red-man' syndrome due to histamine release. Blood concentrations should be monitored to achieve peak serum concentrations of 10–40 mg/l. Particular care must be taken to prevent toxic concentrations accumulating in patients with renal impairment. Teicoplanin is less toxic than vancomycin and can be given by intravenous bolus and by intramuscular injection.

Inhibitors of Protein Synthesis

Although protein synthesis proceeds in an essentially similar manner in prokaryotic and eukaryotic cells, it is possible to exploit the differences to achieve selective toxicity. The process of translation of the messenger RNA (mRNA) chain into its corresponding peptide chain is complex and still incompletely understood. A range of antibacterial agents act as inhibitors of protein synthesis, although the full details of their mechanisms of action are not yet known *(Fig. 30.14)*.

Aminoglycosides
The aminoglycosides are a family of related molecules that inhibit and kill organisms

The aminoglycosides contain either streptidine (streptomycin) or 2-deoxystreptamine (e.g. gentamicin; *Fig. 30.15*). The original structures have been modified chemically by changing the side chains to produce molecules such as amikacin and netilmicin that are active against organisms that have developed resistance to earlier aminoglycosides.

Aminoglycosides interfere with the binding of formylmethionyl-transfer RNA (fmet-tRNA) to the ribosome *(Fig. 30.14)* and thereby prevent the formation of initiation complexes from which protein synthesis proceeds. Streptomycin also causes misreading of mRNA codons.

Aminoglycosides must be given intravenously or intramuscularly for systemic treatment

Aminoglycosides are not absorbed from the gut, do not penetrate well into tissues and bone, and do not cross the blood–brain barrier. Intrathecal administration of streptomycin is used in the treatment of tuberculous meningitis, and gentamicin may be administered by this route in the treatment of Gram-negative meningitis in neonates. Aminoglycosides are excreted via the kidney.

Gentamicin and the newer aminoglycosides are used to treat serious Gram-negative infections

Gentamicin, tobramycin, amikacin and netilmicin are important for the treatment of serious Gram-negative infections including those caused by *P. aeruginosa (Fig. 30.16)*. They are not active against streptococci or anaerobes, but are active against staphylococci. Tobramycin is slightly more active than gentamicin against *P. aeruginosa*. Amikacin and netilmicin are both less active, but may be active against strains resistant to gentamicin and tobramycin (see below). Streptomycin is now reserved almost entirely for the treatment of mycobacterial infections. Neomycin is not used for systemic treatment, but can be used orally in gut decontamination regimens in neutropenic patients. Spectinomycin is used to treat beta-lactam resistant *N. gonorrhoeae*.

Production of aminoglycoside-modifying enzymes causes resistance to aminoglycosides

Alteration in the ribosomal target site is not an uncommon mechanism for streptomycin resistance where a single amino acid change in the P10 protein of the 30S subunit prevents streptomycin binding, but is very rare for other aminoglycosides. Resistance may also arise in Gram-negative rods through alterations in cell wall permeability or in the energy-dependent transport across the cytoplasmic membrane.

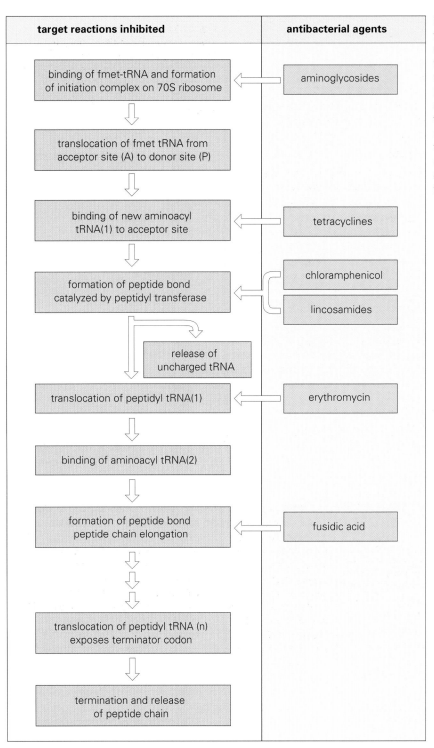

Fig. 30.14 The synthetic pathway leading to the production of new protein in bacterial cells is extremely complicated and still not fully elucidated. A number of different groups of antibacterial agents act by inhibiting proteins with specific reactions in this synthetic pathway. They can be grouped into those that act on the 30S subunit of the ribosome (e.g. aminoglycosides and tetracyclines) and those that act on the 50S subunit (e.g. chloramphenicol, lincosamides, erythromycin and fusidic acid). (fmet-RNA, formylmethionyl-transfer RNA.)

Production of aminoglycoside-modifying enzymes is the most important mechanism of acquired resistance *(Fig. 30.17)*. The genes for these enzymes are often plasmid-mediated and transferable from one bacterial species to another. The enzymes alter the structure of the aminoglycoside molecule, which consequently changes the uptake of drug by the cell. The type of enzyme determines the spectrum of resistance of the organism containing it.

The aminoglycosides are potentially nephrotoxic and ototoxic

The therapeutic 'window' between the serum concentration of aminoglycoside required for successful treatment and that which is toxic is small. Blood concentrations should be monitored regularly, particularly in patients with renal impairment. Netilmicin is reported to be less toxic than the other aminoglycosides.

CHEMICAL GROUPS OF AMINOGLYCOSIDES	
4, 6-disubstituted 2-deoxystreptamines	
Gentamicin*	complex of 3 closely related structures; first aminoglycoside with broad spectrum
Tobramycin**	activity very similar to gentamicin but slightly better against *Pseudomonas aeruginosa*
Kanamycin **	no longer in clinical use
Amikacin	semi-synthetic derivative of kanamycin; active against many gentamicin-resistant Gram-negative rods;
Netilmicin*	activity spectrum similar to amikacin; probably least toxic of aminoglycosides
4, 5-disubstituted 2-deoxystreptamines	
Neomycin**	too toxic for parenteral use but has topical uses in decontaminating mucosal surfaces
streptidine-containing	
Streptomycin**	oldest aminoglycoside; now use restricted to treatment of tuberculosis
others	
Spectinomycin**	important for treatment of beta-lactam resistant *Neisseria gonorrhoeae*
* micins from *Micromonospora* species	
** mycins from *Streptomyces* species	

Fig. 30.15 Aminoglycosides (or more properly aminoglycoside-aminocyclitols) can be classified according to their chemical structure. They are also differentiated by the genus of microorganisms that produces them and this is reflected in the spelling of the names.

INDICATIONS FOR AMINOGLYCOSIDE THERAPY
Basic rule: use only in severe, life-threatening infections
Gram-negative septicemia (including *Pseudomonas*) usually in combination with beta-lactam
Septicemia of unknown* etiology arising from: hospital-acquired infection malignancy immunosuppressive therapy major trauma, major surgery or major burns intravenous catheter urinary catheter extremes of age
Bacterial endocarditis for synergy with penicillin
Staphylococcus aureus septicemia in combination with beta-lactam
Pyelonephritis for difficult cases
Post-surgical abdominal sepsis in combination with anti-anaerobe therapy
* every effort should be made to establish aetiology

Fig. 30.16 Aminoglycosides are valuable additions to the clinician's armamentarium despite their potential toxicity. They are important agents active against Gram-negative facultative bacteria and are often used in combination with beta-lactams to broaden the spectrum to include streptococci and some anaerobes, which are not susceptible to aminoglycosides alone. Resistance to aminoglycosides, particularly among enterobacteria and staphylococci is mediated by the production of aminoglycoside-modifying enzymes, which react with groups on the aminoglycoside molecule to yield an altered aminoglycoside product. This competes with the unmodified aminoglycoside for uptake into the cell and binding to the ribosome.

Tetracyclines
Different tetracyclines differ mainly in their pharmacological properties rather than in their antibacterial spectra

Tetracyclines are a family of large cyclic-structures that have several sites for possible chemical substitutions *(Fig. 30.18)*.

Tetracyclines inhibit protein synthesis by preventing aminoacyl transfer RNA from entering the acceptor sites on the ribosome *(Fig. 30.14)*. However, this action is not selectively toxic for prokaryotes and tetracyclines will also inhibit protein synthesis in cell-free protein synthesis systems

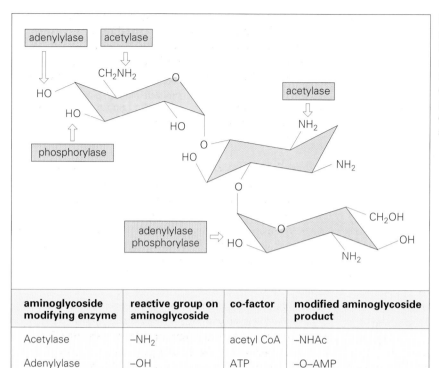

Fig. 30.17 Prototype structure of aminoglycoside consisting of aminohexoses linked via glycosidic linkage to a central 2-deoxystreptamine nucleus. Hydroxyl and amino groups are sites at which these compounds can be inactivated by phosphorylation, adenylation or acetylation catalyzed by enzymes produced by resistant strains.

aminoglycoside modifying enzyme	reactive group on aminoglycoside	co-factor	modified aminoglycoside product
Acetylase	–NH₂	acetyl CoA	–NHAc
Adenylylase (nucleotidyl transferase)	–OH	ATP	–O–AMP
Phosphorylase	–OH	ATP	–O–PO₂–OH

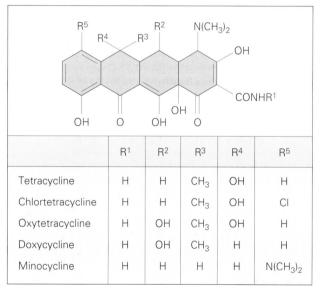

	R¹	R²	R³	R⁴	R⁵
Tetracycline	H	H	CH₃	OH	H
Chlortetracycline	H	H	CH₃	OH	Cl
Oxytetracycline	H	OH	CH₃	OH	H
Doxycycline	H	OH	CH₃	H	H
Minocycline	H	H	H	H	N(CH₃)₂

Fig. 30.18 Tetracyclines are four-ring molecules with five different sites for substitution thereby giving rise to a family of molecules with different substituents at different sites. Members of the family differ more in their pharmacologic properties than in their spectrum of activity.

Tetracyclines are usually administered orally. Doxycycline and minocycline are more completely absorbed than tetracycline, oxytetracycline and chlortetracycline and so result in higher serum concentrations and less gastrointestinal upset because there is less inhibition of normal gut flora. Tetracyclines are well distributed and penetrate host cells to inhibit intracellular bacteria. They are excreted by the kidneys.

Tetracyclines are active against a wide variety of bacteria, but their use is restricted due to widespread resistance

Tetracyclines are used in the treatment of infections caused by mycoplasmas, chlamydiae and rickettsiae. Resistance in other genera is common, due partly to the widespread use of these drugs in humans and also to their use as growth promoters in animal feed. The resistance genes are carried on a transposon and new cytoplasmic membrane proteins are synthesized in the presence of tetracycline. As a result tetracycline is positively pumped out of resistant cells (efflux mechanism).

Tetracyclines should be avoided in pregnancy and in children under eight years of age

Tetracyclines suppress normal gut flora resulting in gastrointestinal upset and diarrhea and encouraging overgrowth by resistant and undesirable bacteria (e.g. *Staph. aureus*) and fungi (e.g. *Candida*).

containing human ribosomes. The selective action of tetracyclines is based on their uptake by bacterial cells, which is much greater than by human cells.

Interference with bone development and brown staining of teeth occurs in the fetus and in children. Systemic administration may cause liver damage.

Chloramphenicol
Chloramphenicol contains a nitrobenzene nucleus and prevents peptide bond synthesis
Chloramphenicol is a relatively simple molecule containing a nitrobenzene nucleus, which is responsible for some of the toxic problems associated with the drug (see below). Other derivatives have been produced, but none is in widespread clinical use.

Chloramphenicol blocks the action of peptidyl transferase, thereby preventing peptide bond synthesis *(Fig. 30.14)*. It inhibits bacterial protein synthesis selectively because it has a much higher affinity for the transferase in the 50S subunit of the bacterial ribosome than it has for the transferase in the 60S subunit of the mammalian ribosome. However, it does have some inhibitory activity on human mitochondrial ribosomes and this may account for some of the dose-dependent toxicity to bone marrow (see below).

Chloramphenicol is well absorbed when given orally, but can be given intravenously if the patient cannot take drugs by mouth. Topical preparations are also available. It is well distributed in the body and penetrates host cells. Chloramphenicol is metabolized in the liver by conjugation with glucuronic acid to yield a microbiologically inactive form that is excreted by the kidneys.

The main indication for chloramphenicol is for Salmonella typhi, though resistance is limiting effectiveness in some areas
Chloramphenicol achieves satisfactory concentrations in the CSF and is a valuable second-line drug in the treatment of bacterial meningitis (particularly *H. influenzae*). Topical preparations are used for eye infections. Chloramphenicol is active against a wide variety of bacterial species, both Gram-positive and Gram-negative, aerobes and anaerobes, including intracellular organisms, but the rare but serious toxic effects (see below) have tended to restrict use of this drug in countries where alternative agents are readily available.

The most common mechanism of resistance involves inactivation of the drug catalyzed by chloramphenicol acetyl transferases produced by resistant bacteria *(Fig. 30.19)*. These plasmid-mediated enzymes are intracellular, but are capable of inactivating all chloramphenicol in the immediate environment of the cell. Acetylated chloramphenicol fails to bind to the ribosomal target. Resistance is becoming increasingly common and this, together with the potential for toxicity, has tended to reduce the use of the drug.

The most important toxic effects of chloramphenicol are in the bone marrow
Nitrobenzene is a bone marrow suppressant and the structurally similar chloramphenicol molecule has similar effects. This toxicity takes two forms:
- Dose-dependent bone marrow suppression, which occurs if the drug is given for long periods and is reversible when treatment is stopped.

- An idiosyncratic reaction causing aplastic anemia, which is not dose dependent and is irreversible. It can occur after treatment has stopped, but is fortunately very rare, occurring in about 1 in 30 000 patients treated.

Chloramphenicol is also toxic to neonates, particularly premature babies whose liver enzyme systems are incompletely developed. This can result in 'gray baby syndrome'. Chloramphenicol serum concentrations should be monitored in neonates.

Macrolides, lincosamides and streptogramins
These three groups of antibacterial agents share overlapping binding sites on ribosomes, and resistance to macrolides confers resistance to the other two groups. The clinically-important drugs are the macrolide erythromycin, and the lincosamide clindamycin; some streptogramins (e.g. pristinamycin) are currently under development.

Macrolides
Erythromycin is the most widely used macrolide and prevents the release of transfer RNA after peptide bond formation
The macrolides are a family of large cyclic molecules all containing a macrocyclic lactone ring *(Fig. 30.20)*. Erythromycin is the best known and most widely used, but some of the newer agents such as azithromycin and clarithromycin with improved activity and pharmacology may substitute erythromycin for

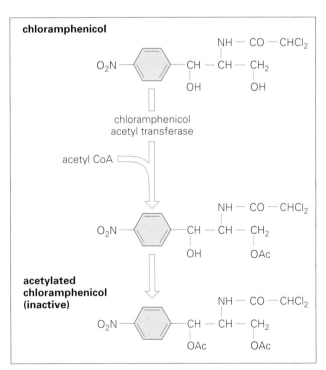

Fig. 30.19 Resistance to chloramphenicol is mediated in some organisms by the production of a chloramphenicol acetyl transferase enzyme, which catalyzes the addition of acetyl groups to the chloramphenicol molecule. This is a two-stage reaction producing acetylated chloramphenicol, which is inactive.

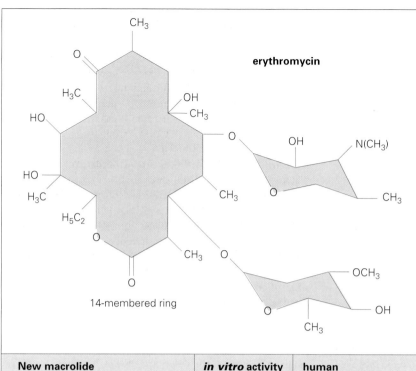

erythromycin

14-membered ring

Fig. 30.20 The macrolides are antibacterial agents composed of large structures, which may be 14-, 15- or 16-membered rings. Erythromycin is the oldest and most widely used of these, but new agents with improved activity and fewer side effects than erythromycin are being developed.

New macrolide	*in vitro* activity compared with erthyromycin	human pharmacokinetics
Roxithromycin (14-membered ring)	comparable	high peak serum concentrations $T\frac{1}{2}$ = 12h
Azithromycin (15-membered ring)	improved against Gram-negative bacteria	high tissue concentrations, once-daily administration
Clarithromycin (14-membered ring)	improved against Gram-positive bacteria and *Legionella* spp.	improved peak serum concentration compared with erythromycin

specific indications. Spiramycin is another macrolide used almost exclusively for the treatment of cryptosporidiosis and in the prevention of congenital toxoplasmosis.

Erythromycin binds to the 23S ribosomal RNA (rRNA) in the 50S subunit of the ribosome and blocks the translocation step in protein synthesis, thereby preventing the release of transfer RNA after peptide bond formation (*Fig. 30.14*).

Erythromycin is usually administered by the oral route, but can also be given intravenously. It is well distributed in the body and penetrates mammalian cells to reach intracellular organisms. The drug is concentrated in the liver and excreted in the bile. A small proportion of the dose is recoverable in the urine.

Erythromycin is an alternative to penicillin for streptococcal infections, but resistant strains of streptococci are common

Erythromycin is active against Gram-positive cocci and is an important alternative treatment of infections caused by streptococci in patients allergic to penicillin. It is active against *Legionella pneumophila* and *Campylobacter jejuni*. It is also active against mycoplasmas, chlamydiae and rickettsiae and is therefore an important drug in the treatment of atypical pneumonia and chlamydial infections of the urinogenital tract.

Resistance is due to alteration in the 23S rRNA target by methylation of two adenine nucleotides in the RNA. The methylase enzyme is plasmid-mediated and inducible. Erythromycin is a better inducer of resistance than the lincosamides, but strains resistant to erythromycin will also be resistant to lincomycin and clindamycin, so-called 'MLS (macrolide lincosamide streptogramin) resistance'. Induction also varies between bacterial species. Resistant strains of Gram-positive cocci such as staphylococci and streptococci are common.

Erythromycin is relatively free of serious toxic side effects

Erythromycin causes nausea and vomiting after oral administration in a significant number of patients. Jaundice is associated with some formulations of the drug.

Lincosamides
Lincomycin and clindamycin inhibit peptide bond formation

Lincomycin and clindamycin are the important lincosamides. Clindamycin is a chlorinated derivative of lincomycin and is more active. It has almost completely superseded lincomycin.

Lincosamides bind to the 50S ribosomal subunit and inhibit protein synthesis by inhibiting peptide bond formation, but the mechanism is incompletely understood *(Fig. 30.14)*. The selectively toxic action results from a failure to bind to the equivalent mammalian ribosomal subunit.

Clindamycin is usually given orally, but can be administered intramuscularly or intravenously. It penetrates well into bone, but not into CSF, even when the meninges are inflamed. Clindamycin is actively transported into polymorphonuclear leukocytes and macrophages. It is metabolized in the liver to several products with variable antibacterial activity and clindamycin activity persists in feces for up to five days after a dose.

Clindamycin has a spectrum of activity similar to that of erythromycin

Clindamycin is much more active than erythromycin against anaerobes, both Gram-positive (e.g. *Clostridium* spp.) and Gram-negative (e.g. *Bacteroides*). However, *Cl. difficile* is resistant and may be selected in the gut causing pseudomembranous colitis (see below). The activity of clindamycin against *Staph. aureus* and its penetration into bone makes it a valuable drug in the treatment of osteomyelitis.

As clindamycin is a less potent inducer of 23S rRNA methylase (see MLS resistance above), erythromycin-resistant strains may appear susceptible to clindamycin *in vitro*. However, resistance will be manifest *in vivo*.

INHIBITORS OF NUCLEIC ACID SYNTHESIS
inhibitors of synthesis of precursors sulfonamides trimethoprim
inhibitors of DNA replication quinolones
inhibitors of RNA polymerase rifampicin

Fig. 30.21 Inhibition of nucleic acid takes place at different stages in its synthesis and function and different groups of antimicrobial agents are involved.

Pseudomembranous colitis caused by Cl. difficile was first noted following clindamycin treatment

Pseudomembranous colitis caused by *Cl. difficile* follows treatment with many antibiotics. The pathogenesis of this complication is described in Chapter 20 and it should be treated with metronidazole or oral vancomycin.

Fusidic acid
Fusidic acid is a steroid-like compound that inhibits protein synthesis

Fusidic acid inhibits protein synthesis by forming a stable complex with elongation factor EF-G (the bacterial equivalent of the human EF-2), guanosine diphosphate and the ribosome.

Fusidic acid can be administered orally or intravenously. It is well-absorbed and penetrates well into tissues and bone, but not into the CSF. Topical preparations are also available, but their use should not be encouraged because of the rapid emergence of resistance (see below). Fusidic acid is metabolized in the liver and excreted in the bile.

Fusidic acid is a treatment for staphylococcal infections, but should be used with other antistaphylococcal drugs to prevent emergence of resistance

Fusidic acid is active against Gram-positive cocci and its most important use is in the treatment of staphylococcal infections resistant to beta-lactams or in patients who are allergic to alternative staphylococcal agents. Fusidic acid should be given in combination with another antistaphylococcal agent (e.g. rifampicin or erythromycin) t`o prevent the emergence of resistant mutants with altered EF-G, which emerge rapidly in staphylococcal populations exposed to the drug.

Fusidic acid has few side effects

Occasionally fusidic acid causes jaundice and gastrointestinal upset.

Inhibitors of Nucleic Acid Synthesis

Antibacterial agents that act as inhibitors of nucleic acid synthesis do so in one of three main ways as shown in *Figure 30.21*. The inhibitory effects may be so fundamental to the cell that protein synthesis and other metabolic pathways also appear to be targets.

Sulfonamides
Sulfonamides are structural analogues of and act in competition with para-amino benzoic acid

This group of molecules are produced entirely by chemical synthesis (i.e. they are not natural products). In 1935, the parent compound sulfanilamide became the first clinically-effective antibacterial agent. The *p*-amino group is essential for activity, but modifications to the sulfonic acid side chain have produced many related agents *(Fig. 30.22)*.

Sulfonamides act in competition with *para*-amino benzoic acid, PABA, for the active site of dihydropteroate synthetase,

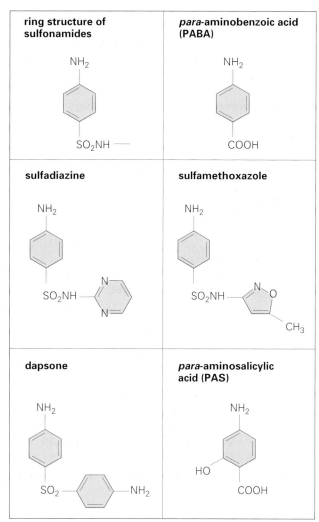

Fig. 30.22 The ring structure of the sulfonamides is very similar to the structure of the normal substrate (PABA) of the dihydropteroate synthetase enzyme, which the sulfonamides inhibit. There are many different sulfonamides available and they differ in their pharmacologic properties more than in their spectrum of activity. Relatively few are now in common clinical use. Dapsone is important in the treatment of *Mycobacterium leprae* and *para*-amino salicylic acid is a second line drug for the treatment of *Mycobacterium tuberculosis*.

an enzyme that catalyzes an essential reaction in the synthetic pathway of tetrahydrofolic acid (THFA), which is required for the synthesis of purines and pyrimidines and therefore for nucleic acid synthesis *(Fig. 30.23)*. Selective toxicity depends on the fact that many bacteria synthesize THFA whereas human cells lack this capacity and depend on an exogenous supply of folic acid. Bacteria that can use preformed folic acid are similarly unaffected by sulfonamides.

Sulfonamides are usually administered orally, often in combination with trimethoprim as cotrimoxazole (see below). Different molecules within the family differ in their solubility and penetrability. Metabolism occurs in the liver and free and metabolized drug are excreted by the kidneys.

Sulfonamides are useful in the treatment of urinary tract infection, but resistance is widespread

The sulfonamides have a spectrum of activity primarily against Gram-negative organisms (except *Pseudomonas*). They are therefore useful in the treatment of urinary tract infections (see Chapter 18). However, susceptibility cannot be assumed as resistance is widespread with plasmid-mediated genes coding for an altered dihydropteroate synthetase. This is essentially unchanged in its affinity for PABA, but has a greatly decreased affinity for the sulfonamide. A resistant cell therefore possesses two distinct enzymes – a sensitive chromosome-encoded enzyme and a resistant plasmid-encoded enzyme.

Rarely, sulfonamides cause Stevens–Johnson syndrome

Sulfonamides are relatively free of toxic side effects, but rashes and bone marrow suppression can occur.

Trimethoprim (and cotrimoxazole)
Trimethoprim is a structural analogue of the aminohydroxypyrimidine moiety of folic acid and prevents the synthesis of THFA

Trimethoprim is one of a group of pyrimidine-like structures analogous in structure to the aminohydroxypyrimidine moiety of the folic acid molecule *(Fig. 30.24)*. Other agents with a similar structure and mechanism of action include the antimalarial pyrimethamine and the anti-cancer drug, methotrexate.

Trimethoprim, like sulfonamides, prevents THFA synthesis, but at a later stage by inhibiting dihydrofolate reductase *(Fig. 30.23)*. This enzyme is present in mammalian cells as well as bacterial and protozoan cells and selective toxicity depends upon the far greater affinity of trimethoprim for the bacterial enzyme.

Trimethoprim is often given in combination with sulfamethoxazole as cotrimoxazole. The advantages of this combination over either drug alone are:
- Mutant bacteria resistant to one agent are unlikely to be resistant to the other (i.e. double mutation).
- The two agents act synergistically against some bacteria (i.e. the action of the combination is greater than the action of either agent alone).

Trimethoprim can be given orally (either alone or as cotrimoxazole) or by intravenous infusion (alone or accompanied by sulfonamide in the same ratio as that given above). Trimethoprim is excreted in urine, and in patients with severe renal failure it is excreted more rapidly than sulfonamide so that the synergistic ratio of the combination may be lost.

Trimethoprim is often given with sulfamethoxazole as cotrimoxazole and both are used for urinary tract infections

Trimethoprim alone is active against Gram-negative rods with the exception of *Pseudomonas* spp. and its main use is in the treatment (and long-term prophylaxis) of urinary tract infection (see Chapter 18). However, it is now used for other Gram-negative infections where cotrimoxazole was used previously.

Cotrimoxazole is active against a wide range of urinary tract pathogens and against *S. typhi*. When given intravenously in high doses, this combination is valuable for the treatment of *Pneumocystis carinii* pneumonia, although pentamidine, another pyrimidine derivative, is probably the preferred alternative (see Chapter 33). Cotrimoxazole is also useful for the treatment of nocardiosis (see Chapter 28) and chancroid (see Chapter 19).

Resistance to trimethoprim is provided by plasmid-encoded dihydrofolate reductases

Plasmid-encoded dihydrofolate reductases with altered affinity for trimethoprim allow the synthesis of THFA to proceed unhindered by the presence of trimethoprim. The 'replacement enzymes' are approximately 20 000-fold less susceptible to trimethoprim while retaining their affinity for the normal substrate. Bacteria that are resistant to sulfonamide and trimethoprim are also resistant to cotrimoxazole.

People with AIDS seem to be more prone to the side effects of trimethoprim and cotrimoxazole

Trimethoprim alone and in combination with sulfamethoxazole can cause neutropenia. Nausea and vomiting may occur.

Quinolones
Quinolones are synthetic agents that prevent supercoiling of the bacterial chromosome

Quinolones form a large family of synthetic agents. Nalidixic acid is one of the earlier prototypes, but the synthesis of fluoroquinolones has led to an enormous number of new chemical derivatives with improved antibacterial activity *(Fig. 30.25)*.

Quinolones act by inhibiting the activity of DNA gyrase and thereby preventing supercoiling of the bacterial chromosome. As a result the bacterial cell can no longer 'pack' its DNA into the cell *(Fig. 30.26)*. The inhibition is specific to bacterial gyrase and does not affect the equivalent topoisomerase enzymes in mammalian cells.

Quinolones are administered orally, are well-absorbed from the gastrointestinal tract and are excreted mostly in the urine, though a small proportion is excreted in the feces. Nalidixic acid does not achieve adequate serum concentrations for systemic therapy, but the newer fluoroquinolones achieve significant serum concentrations after oral dosage and are very well distributed throughout the body compartments.

Quinolones are used to treat urinary tract, systemic Gram-negative, and intracellular infections

Nalidixic acid is only active against enterobacteria and its use is confined to the treatment of urinary tract infections (see Chapter 18).

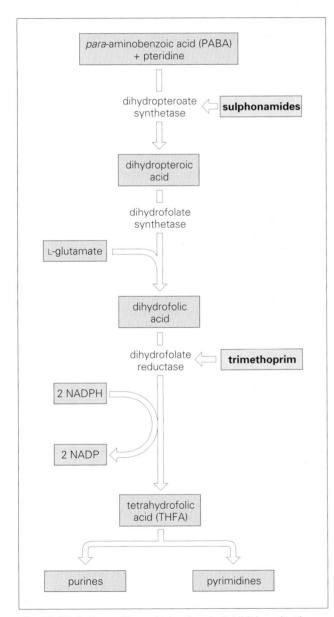

Fig. 30.23 Sulfonamides and trimethoprim inhibit in series the steps in the synthesis of tetrahydrofolic acid by interacting with key enzymes in the pathway.

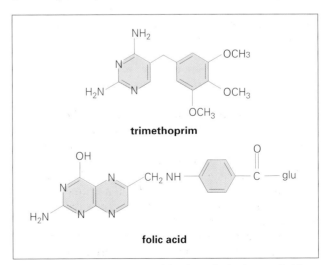

Fig. 30.24 Trimethoprim resembles the aminohydroxypyrimidine moiety of folic acid and in this way antagonizes the enzyme dihydrofolate reductase.

nalidixic acid

norfloxacin   **ciprofloxacin**   **ofloxacin**

Fig. 30.25 The quinolones form a large group of synthetic antibacterial agents. This illustration shows nalidixic acid and only a few of the many new agents that are now available or in development.

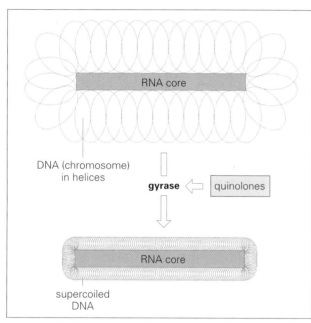

RNA core

DNA (chromosome) in helices

gyrase ⇐ quinolones

RNA core

supercoiled DNA

Fig. 30.26 Quinolones inhibit bacterial gyrase, the enzyme responsible for supercoiling bacterial DNA so that the chromosome can be packed into the bacterial cell.

The newer quinolones such as ciprofloxacin, pefloxacin and norfloxacin have a greater degree of activity than nalidixic acid against Gram-negative rods. Ciprofloxacin is also active against *P. aeruginosa*. In addition to the treatment of urinary tract infections the newer quinolones are useful for systemic Gram-negative infections and in the treatment of chlamydial and rickettsial infections. They are also useful in infections caused by other intracellular organisms such as *L. pneumophila* and *S. typhi*, and in combination with other agents for 'atypical' mycobacteria. They have activity against staphylococci, but are less active against streptococci, while enterococci are resistant.

Resistance to quinolones is chromosomally-mediated

An important feature is that so far there have been no substantiated reports of plasmid-mediated resistance. However, chromosomally-mediated resistance occurs and is exhibited in two forms:

- Changes in DNA gyrase subunit structure resulting in a lowered affinity for the drug.
- Changes in cell wall permeability, resulting in decreased uptake. This mechanism may also lead to cross-resistance to other unrelated agents taken up by the same route.

Fluoroquinolones are not licensed for children due to possible toxic effects on cartilage development

Gastrointestinal disturbances are the most common side effect of quinolones. Neurotoxicity and photosensitivity reactions occur in 1–2% of patients.

Rifamycins

Rifampicin is clinically the most important rifamycin and blocks the synthesis of mRNA

Rifampicin is the most important member of the rifamycin family in clinical use. It is a large molecule with a complex structure. Other family members such as rifabutin and rifapentine are now on the market or in development.

Rifampicin binds to RNA polymerase and blocks the synthesis of mRNA. Selective toxicity is based on the far greater affinity for bacterial polymerases than for the equivalent human enzymes.

Rifampicin is administered orally, is well absorbed and is very well distributed in the body. It crosses the blood–brain barrier and reaches high concentrations in saliva. It also appears to have an affinity for plastics, which can be valuable in the treatment of infections involving prostheses.

Rifampicin is metabolized in the liver and excreted in bile. The compound is red, and urine, sweat and saliva of treated patients turns orange. This is harmless, although disturbing for the patient, but is good evidence of patient compliance.

The newer rifamycins under investigation are excreted more slowly than rifampicin thereby allowing less frequent administration; a feature particularly attractive in the treatment of tuberculosis.

The primary use for rifampicin is in the treatment of mycobacterial infections, but resistance is increasing

Rifampicin is so important in the treatment of mycobacterial infections, that its use in other settings tends to be restricted. It is, however, now the drug of choice for the prophylaxis of close contacts of meningococcal and *Haemophilus* meningitis because of its distribution in the body and because of bacterial resistance to other agents. Short courses only (maximum 48 hours) should be given (see Chapter 22). Staphylococci are extremely susceptible to rifampicin, but rapidly develop resistance. However, the drug can be efficacious if used in combination with another agent, particularly in the treatment of prosthetic valve endocarditis (see Chapter 23).

Resistance is provided by chromosomal mutations that alter the RNA polymerase target, which then has lowered affinity for rifampicin and escapes inhibition. The prevalence of rifampicin-resistant *M. tuberculosis* is increasing, threatening the future of first-line antituberculous therapy.

Rashes and jaundice are side effects of rifampicin treatment.

Intermittent rifampicin can lead to hypersensitivity reactions.

Other Agents That Affect DNA

Nitroimidazoles
Metronidazole is a nitroimidazole with antiparasitic and antibacterial properties

After entry into the microbial cell the molecule is activated by reduction and the reduced intermediate products are responsible for antimicrobial activity, probably through interaction with, and breakage of, the cell's DNA. The reactive intermediates are short-lived and decompose to nontoxic inactive end-products. Metronidazole is active only against anaerobic organisms because only these can produce the low redox potential necessary to reduce the parent drug.

Metronidazole has also been used as a hypoxic cell sensitizer in radiotherapy.

Metronidazole is usually given orally or rectally. It is well absorbed and well distributed in tissues and CSF. The drug is metabolized and most of the parent compound and metabolites are excreted in the urine

Metronidazole was originally introduced for the treatment of the flagellate parasite Trichomonas vaginalis

Metronidazole is also effective against other parasites such as *Giardia lamblia* and *Entamoeba coli*. It is an important agent for the treatment of infections caused by anaerobic bacteria.

Metronidazole resistance is rare and in the few reported cases the mechanism is unclear, but appears to involve either an alteration in uptake or a decrease in cellular reductase activity, thereby slowing the activation of the intracellular drug.

Rarely, metronidazole causes central nervous system side effects

The most serious side effects of metronidazole involve the central nervous system and include peripheral neuropathy. However, these are rare and usually seen only in patients on large doses or prolonged treatment.

Inhibitors of Cytoplasmic Membrane Function

The cytoplasmic membranes that encompass all kinds of living cells perform a variety of vital functions. The structure of these membranes in bacterial cells differs from that in mammalian cells and allows the application of some selectively toxic molecules, but these are few in number compared with those acting at other target sites. The most important are the polymyxins, which act on the membranes of Gram-negative bacteria. The polyene antifungal agents (amphotericin B, nystatin) also act by inhibiting membrane function (see below).

Polymyxins
Polymyxins are cyclic polypeptides and disrupt the structure of cell membranes

The free amino groups of polymyxins act as cationic detergents, disrupting the phospholipid structure of the cell membrane. Colistin (polymyxin E) is the most common member of the family in clinical use.

After oral administration, polymyxins are not absorbed from the gut. In the past they have been used systemically, but have now been superseded by less toxic agents.

Colistin is used for gut decontamination and wound irrigation and as a bladder washout

Colistin is active against Gram-negative organisms except *Proteus* spp. As an oral agent it is used in some gut decontamination regimens for neutropenic patients. Topical uses include wound irrigation and as a bladder washout.

Resistance due to chromosomally-mediated alterations in membrane structure or antibiotic uptake has been reported.

Colistin is nephrotoxic

Colistin is not used systemically because of its nephrotoxicity.

Urinary Tract Antiseptics

Nitrofurantoin and methenamine inhibit urinary pathogens

Nitrofurantoin and methenamine are both synthetic compounds that, when taken orally, are absorbed and excreted in the urine in concentrations high enough to inhibit urinary pathogens. Nitrofurantoin has activity only in acid urine. Methenamine is hydrolyzed at acid pH to produce ammonia and formaldehyde; it is the formaldehyde that has the antibacterial activity. Nitrofurantoin is used to treat uncomplicated urinary tract infection and both agents are used to prevent recurrent urinary tract infections. They have the advantage that resistance rarely develops.

Antituberculous Agents

M. tuberculosis and other mycobacterial infections need prolonged treatment

The treatment of infections caused by *M. tuberculosis* and other mycobacteria presents an enormous challenge to medicine and the pharmaceutical industry because these organisms:

- Have a waxy outer layer that makes them naturally very impermeable and difficult to penetrate with antibiotics.
- Have an intracellular location, often in cells surrounded by a mass of caseous material, that also makes it difficult for antibiotics to get to them.
- Grow and multiply extremely slowly and effective inhibition (and therefore cure) takes weeks or months to achieve. Long-term therapy is therefore a challenge for drug delivery and means that orally-administrable drugs are highly desirable. It also means that the emergence of resistance among the mycobacteria and toxicity in the patient are more likely than with the 'short sharp shock' treatment more often administered for bacterial infections.
- Are common and increasing in the wake of the AIDS epidemic in developing countries, where the cost of drug treatment can be prohibitive.

A number of antituberculous agents are now available. Most are restricted to treating mycobacteria to prevent resistance emerging in other species and potentially being transferred to mycobacteria or because their toxicity makes them unattractive for general use.

In general first-line therapy of tuberculosis is a combination of isoniazid, ethambutol and rifampicin

Treatment regimens vary between countries, but in general first-line (i.e. first-choice) therapy is a combination of isoniazid, ethambutol and rifampicin for 6–9 months. Streptomycin may be added for the treatment of tuberculous meningitis. The structure and mechanism of action of rifampicin and streptomycin have been described in preceding sections.

Isoniazid
Isoniazid inhibits mycobacteria and is given with pyridoxine to prevent neurologic side effects

Isoniazid is isonicotinic acid hydrazide, a compound that inhibits mycobacteria, but does not affect other species of bacteria or humans to any great extent. Despite being used for over 30 years its mechanism of action is unclear, but may involve inhibition of mycolic acid synthesis, which would account for its specificity. It is well absorbed after oral administration and a single daily dose is sufficient, except in the treatment of meningitis or miliary tuberculosis when the frequency of dosage should be increased to three times daily. The main toxic effects in humans are neurologic complications, which can be prevented by the concurrent administration of pyridoxine, and hepatitis.

Ethambutol
Ethambutol inhibits mycobacteria, but can cause optic neuritis

Ethambutol is a synthetic molecule that inhibits, but does not kill, mycobacteria. Its mechanism of action is unknown, but it may interfere with RNA synthesis. It is well absorbed after oral administration and well distributed in the body including the CSF. Resistance appears fairly rapidly if the drug is used alone and it should be combined with other drugs in antituberculous therapy. An important toxic side effect is optic neuritis, and visual acuity should be monitored during therapy.

Second-line therapy for drug-resistant M. tuberculosis includes drugs such as paraminosalicylate, pyrazinamide and thiacetazone

Despite the use of antibiotics in combination, the incidence of resistance among mycobacteria is increasing and a cure may not be achieved by the first-line drugs. Infections with mycobacteria other than *M. tuberculosis* are on the increase as opportunist infections in people with AIDS and these organisms tend to be innately more resistant than *M. tuberculosis*.

The selection and administration of second-line therapy for drug-resistant *M. tuberculosis* requires specialist knowledge.

Treatment of leprosy
Widespread use of dapsone monotherapy for leprosy has led to resistance so it is now often combined with rifampicin

Infection caused by *M. leprae* is characterized by persistence of the organism in the tissues for years and necessitates very prolonged treatment to prevent relapse. For many years dapsone, a sulfone derivative *(Fig. 30.22)* has been used. This drug has the advantages that it is given orally and it is cheap and effective. However, widespread use as monotherapy has resulted in the emergence of resistance and multidrug regimens are therefore preferable. Rifampicin can be combined with dapsone. Alternatively, clofazime, a phenazine compound, is active against dapsone-resistant *M. leprae,* but it is expensive.

Antifungal Agents

In contrast to the antibacterial drugs, the number of antifungal drugs suitable for treatment of infections is very limited. Selective toxicity is much more difficult to achieve in the eukaryotic fungal cells than in the prokaryotic bacteria and although the available antifungals have greater activity against fungal cells than they do against human cells the difference is not as marked as it is for most antibacterial agents. Treatment of fungal infections is further hampered by problems of solubility, stability and absorption of the existing drugs and the search for new agents is a high priority.

Antifungals can be classified on the basis of target site and chemical structure

Antifungals can be classified by the same scheme as that used above for the antibacterials (i.e. on the basis of target site and chemical structure). This immediately reveals a major difference between antibacterial and antifungal agents, with the major antifungals acting on the synthesis or function of the cell membrane. The exceptions are flucytosine (5-fluorocytosine) and griseofulvin. There are currently no inhibitors of fungal protein synthesis that do not also inhibit the equivalent mammalian pathway.

Azole compounds inhibit cell membrane synthesis
Azole antifungals act by inhibiting lanosterol C14-demethylase, which is an important enzyme in sterol biosynthesis. Inhibition of the fungal enzyme in preference to the human one is the key to selective toxicity. Clotrimazole and miconazole are useful as topical preparations. Ketoconazole has become the agent of choice for many serious fungal infections (Fig. 30.27), and fluconazole is increasingly used in the treatment of Candida infections. Further azole compounds are currently under development.

Amphotericin B and nystatin inhibit cell membrane function
Amphotericin B and nystatin are polyenes that act by binding to sterols in cell membranes resulting in leakage of cellular contents and cell death. Their preferential binding to ergosterol over cholesterol is the basis for selective toxicity.

THERAPEUTIC APPLICATIONS OF ANTIFUNGAL AGENTS			
infection	antifungal of choice	route of administration	adverse effects
superficial mycoses			
Ringworm (dermatophytes)	griseofulvin	oral	nil
	ketoconazole	oral	anorexia, nausea vomiting; dose-dependent depression of serum testosterone leading to gynecomastia
Candidiasis	fluconazole	oral	inhibits metabolism of cyclosporin when given at high doses
	nystatin	topical	nil
systemic mycoses			
Histoplasmosis	ketoconazole	oral	see above
Blastomycosis	ketoconazole	oral	see above
Coccidioidomycosis	ketaconazole (amphotericin B for CNS involvement)	oral	do not use ketoconazole and amphotericin B together (some evidence of antagonism)
Paracoccidioidomycosis	ketoconazole	oral	see above
Aspergillosis	amphotericin B	IV (now available in liposomes)	nephrotoxicity and potassium loss; acute reactions within 1/2 - 1 1/2 h of injection include rigors and hypotension
Candidiasis	fluconazole amphotericin B 1 flucytosine	oral IV oral	flucytosine may cause neutropenia and jaundice; emergence of resistant mutants is common if drug is used alone; combination with amphotericin B can be synergistic
Cryptococcosis	amphotericin B 1 flucytosine	IV oral	
Zygomycosis	amphotericin B	IV	

Fig. 30.27 The major therapeutic applications of antifungal drugs. Orally-active agents are important for the treatment of superficial mycoses, which are often minor but troublesome infections and may require prolonged treatment. Amphotericin is the most important agent for the treatment of severe systemic mycoses, but is toxic. The azoles, particularly fluconazole and ketoconazole and some of the newer agents, provide suitable alternative therapy in some instances.

Amphotericin remains the drug of choice for the treatment of serious systemic fungal infections despite its serious toxic side effects. Nystatin is used only in topical formulations.

Flucytosine and griseofulvin inhibit nucleic acid synthesis

Flucytosine (5-fluorocytosine) is taken up by the fungal cell and deaminated to 5-fluorouracil, which inhibits DNA synthesis. Selective toxicity is based on the preferential uptake by fungal cells compared with host cells. Flucytosine is active only on yeasts (e.g. *Candida* spp. and *Cryptococcus*).

Griseofulvin appears to inhibit nucleic acid synthesis and to have antimitotic activity, possibly by inhibiting microtubule assembly. It may also have effects on cell wall synthesis by inhibiting chitin synthesis. In the host, griseofulvin binds specifically to newly-formed keratin and is active *in vivo* only against dermatophyte fungi (see Chapters 3 and 23).

Other topical antifungal agents include Whitfield's ointment, tolnaftate, ciclopirox, haloprogin and naftifine

A variety of other agents such as Whitfield's ointment (a mixture of benzoic and salicylic acids), tolnaftate, ciclopirox, haloprogin and naftifine, are available as creams for the topical treatment of superficial mycoses. These are usually available over the counter and there is little to choose between them.

No single antifungal agent is ideal

The main uses and adverse effects of antifungals are summarized in *Figure 30.27*. Superficial fungal infections are extremely common, but usually mild. Although there are several effective preparations available, some conditions such as ringworm infection of the nails or recurrent vaginal candidiasis are frequently intractable to treatment. The number of antifungal agents for systemic fungal infections is limited and their adverse effects are considerable. Resistance emerges rapidly to flucytosine, which should therefore be used in combination with amphotericin B (whereby it is sometimes possible to reduce the dose of amphotericin B and therefore the toxic side effects). Resistance to the azoles is becoming more widespread and threatens to compromise this group of compounds.

There is an urgent need for safer more efficacious antifungal agents

Systemic fungal infections are relatively uncommon and often present as opportunistic infections in immunocompromised people. However, the incidence of these infections is increasing in parallel with the increasing numbers of such patients and their improved survival due to effective antibacterial therapy. Considerable resources are therefore being channeled into the search for new antifungal agents.

Antiviral Therapy

For most viral infections there is no specific treatment. There are few effective antiviral drugs *(Fig. 30.28)*, in contrast to the great range of successful antibiotics available for bacterial infections. The shortage of antivirals is partly due to the difficulty of interfering with viral activity in the cell without adversely affecting the host. However, the advent of AIDS has stimulated intensive research, and new antiviral drugs will undoubtedly appear. For instance, the protease of HIV is essential for virus assembly and release, and protease inhibitors such as ritonavir show promise in the treatment of AIDS. Virus-specific replication steps can be identified *(Fig. 30.29)* and more of these will doubtless be exploited.

Resistance to antivirals occurs, for example:
- Herpes simplex virus (HSV) to aciclovir.
- HIV to zidovudine.
- Cytomegalovirus (CMV) to ganciclovir.
- Influenza A to rimantadine.

So far, however, the resistant strains have not spread in the community.

There are two other problems with the therapy of virus infections:
- The incubation period is often one week or more and by the time the patient becomes ill most of the viral spread and replication has already taken place (e.g. mumps, polio). Infection cannot be diagnosed during the incubation period and even after the patient becomes ill laboratory diagnosis often takes several days. Some of the rapid (24-hour) diagnostic methods currently being developed will help overcome this problem;
- Viruses that are latent in cells and not actively replicating (e.g. latent herpesviruses) are generally insusceptible to antivirals.

Viruses are resistant to antibacterial antibiotics, although the latter may be needed to control secondary bacterial infection, for instance in influenzal pneumonia.

Aciclovir (acycloguanosine)
Aciclovir inhibits HSV and varicella-zoster virus DNA polymerase

Aciclovir has virtually replaced the other nucleosides in the treatment of herpesvirus infections. It *(Fig. 30.30)* is phosphorylated by the herpesvirus thymidine kinase and the monophosphate is then converted by cellular kinases to the triphosphate, which inhibits the herpesvirus DNA polymerase. Action on cellular DNA polymerase is minimal. The drug is also incorporated into viral DNA, resulting in chain termination. Because aciclovir is inactive until phosphorylated and is efficiently phosphorylated only in infected cells, toxic side effects (neutropenia, thrombocytopenia) are usually not severe. Aciclovir acts on HSV and varicella-zoster (VZV) but is almost inactive against CMV and Epstein-Barr virus (EBV).

Aciclovir is used topically or systemically

Topical aciclovir is used for:
- Primary genital herpes.
- HSV dendritic ulcers.
- Cold sores and zoster, though is less effective than for primary genital herpes and HSV dendritic ulcers.

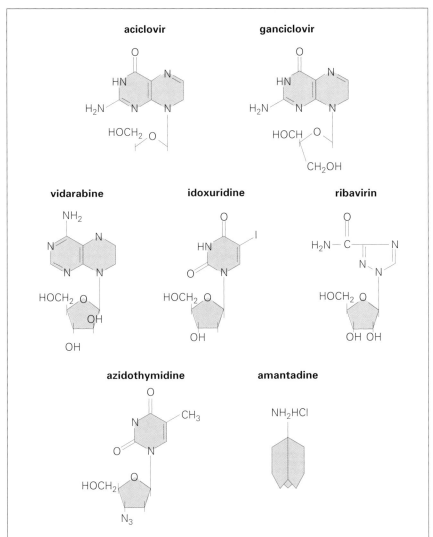

Fig. 30.28 Antiviral agents are few in number and narrow in their spectrum of activity – for example, amantadine is effective against influenza A, but not other myxoviruses, while aciclovir is effective against herpes simplex virus (HSV) and varicella–zoster virus (VZV), but not cytomegalovirus (CMV) or Epstein–Barr virus (EBV).

replication stage	drugs available	
1 Adsorption	none available	
2 Penetration and uncoating	amantadine	
3 Viral DNA/RNA synthesis	idoxuridine vidarabine aciclovir zidovudine ribavirin	
4 Viral protein synthesis	interferons	
5 Assembly	none available	
6 Release	none available	

Fig. 30.29 The site of action of antiviral agents. Resistance to agents is uncommon, but does occur (e.g. cytomegalovirus strains resistant to ganciclovir, herpes simplex virus strains resistant to aciclovir). Adsorption of virus to cell can be blocked by virus-specific antibody.

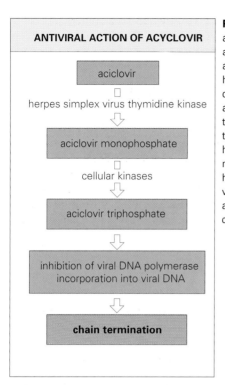

Fig. 30.30 The activity of an antiviral agent against different herpes viruses is correlated with the ability of the viruses to induce a thymidine kinase, hence aciclovir is most active against herpes simplex virus and least active against cytomegalovirus.

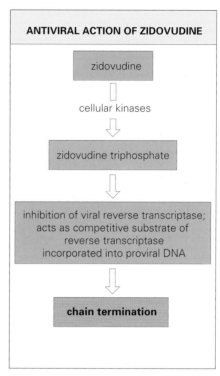

Fig. 30.31 HIV reverse transcriptase is 100 times more sensitive than host cell DNA polymerase to zidovudine triphosphate, but toxic effects are not uncommon.

Systemic aciclovir has revolutionized the treatment of HSV encephalitis, and HSV and VZV infections in immunocompromised patients. In zoster, it accelerates recovery and reduces post-zoster pain. As with HSV, the virus remains latent in ganglia and capable of reactivation. The lack of aciclovir toxicity is illustrated by the fact that it has been given daily for years without side effects to prevent recurrent herpes lesions.

Ganciclovir (dihydroxypropoxy-methylguanine, DHPG)

Ganciclovir is active against CMV and is valuable in disseminated CMV infections and in CMV retinitis in people with AIDS. CMV does not have a thymidine kinase, but the drug is phosphorylated to a greater extent in infected than in uninfected cells. It is toxic to bone marrow.

Idoxuridine (IDU)

This is another nucleoside analogue that is triphosphorylated by cellular kinases and then incorporated into viral DNA. The virus produced is therefore defective. Idoxuridine is also incorporated into cellular DNA, which makes it too toxic to be used systemically. It used to be a treatment for dendritic ulcers.

Foscarnet (phosphonoformate)

This compound attaches to the pyrophosphate-binding site of the herpesvirus and the HIV DNA polymerase, preventing nucleotide binding and therefore inhibiting viral replication. It is used in the treatment of CMV retinitis in AIDS.

Zidovudine (azidothymidine, AZT, 'Retrovir')

Zidovudine is another nucleoside analogue in which the hydroxyl group on the ribose is replaced by an azido group.

After conversion to the triphosphate by cellular enzymes (*Fig. 30.31*) it acts as an inhibitor of, and substrate for, the viral reverse transcriptase. Proviral DNA formation is blocked because the drug is incorporated into the DNA with resulting chain termination. Zidovudine in combination with one of the other nucleoside analogues and a protease inhibitor are currently the most useful drugs for patients with AIDS-related complex (ARC) and AIDS.

Zidovudine is given orally. Toxicity is a problem, with bone marrow suppression (anemia, neutropenia, leukopenia), and less commonly nausea, vomiting, myalgia, malaise. Regular tests are necessary to look out for anemia and myelosuppression. Zidovudine is also very expensive. Drug resistance is beginning to be a clinical problem, and resistant mutants have been isolated in the laboratory.

Deoxycytidine (ddc or zalcitabine) and deoxyinosine (ddi or didanosine)

Like zidovudine, these nucleoside analogues are converted to triphosphates and inhibit the HIV reverse transcriptase. Lamivudine has similar structure and activity. Because the resistant mutant viruses that appear are at the same time less resistant to zidovudine, combinations of lamivudine for instance, with zidovudine have been used with reduction of viral load in the blood, and clinical benefit.

Ribavirin(tribavirin)

This guanosine analogue has various actions including inhibition of production of guanosine triphosphate pools needed for viral nucleic acid synthesis. It is used clinically as an aerosol for severe respiratory syncytial virus (RSV) infection in infants, for severe influenza B and for arenavirus infections such as Lassa fever (see Chapter 26).

Amantidine

It has been known since the 1960s that amantidine specifically inhibits the replication of influenza A viruses, but has no effect on influenza B and other respiratory viruses. It acts by inhibiting the penetration of virus into the cell, or its uncoating. Fusion of the viral envelope with a cell membrane, which normally occurs at a low pH, is prevented. Amantadine raises the pH in intracellular vacuoles and therefore blocks infection. The standard dose (200 mg/day orally) causes minor neurologic side effects such as insomnia, dizziness and headache, especially in elderly patients, and this has discouraged its widespread use. When given prophylactically during community outbreaks of influenza A, amantadine (or rimantidine) is about as effective as influenza vaccine in preventing illness. It can also be used for treatment, and if taken within 48 hours of symptoms there is a reduction in disease severity.

Development of antivirals

A variety of new directions are being taken in the development of antivirals

Directions being taken in the development of new antivirals include:

- Blocking adsorption of virus to the cell by coating the virus with analogues or peptides of the cell receptor molecule (e.g. the CD4 molecule on T cells in the case of HIV) or coating cells with viral attachment proteins (e.g. gp120 in the case of HIV).
- Blocking viral mRNA with short nucleotide sequences that are complementary to viral sequences. These antisense oligonucleotides bind to newly-transcribed viral RNA and block its action. Promising results have been obtained in papillomavirus infections.
- Using compounds that inactivate virus when used topically (e.g. nonoxynol-9 in contraceptive creams inactivates HIV and HSV).

Uses of interferons in human infection

Interferons (IFNs; see Chapter 9) show a dramatic effect on virus replication *in vitro* (at pg/ml of IFN) and are active against certain experimental virus infections. However, their clinical use has been disappointing. One problem has been that their very short half-life in the circulation makes it difficult to deliver adequate amounts to the sites of infection. Very large intravenous doses have an established role in the treatment of chronic hepatitis B and C infection. IFNs have an effect on papillomavirus infections (intralesional injection) and on certain herpesvirus infections, but are not routinely used.

Interferons, especially IFNγ, also have important actions on the immune system and a potential for use as immunomodulators.

Many patients experience flu-like symptoms with IFNs

Flu-like symptoms of fever, myalgia and headache are side effects of IFNs, even with genetically-engineered IFNs. Indeed such symptoms in virus infections have been attributed to the action of endogenously-produced IFNs.

Leukopenia, thrombocytopenia, and central nervous system effects have also been noted with IFN treatment, especially with high-dose treatment.

Antiparasitic Agents

Drugs acting against protozoa are usually inactive against helminths and vice versa

Any consideration of antiparasitic agents must take into account the vast number of different parasites capable of infecting man, the complexities of their life cycles and the differences in their metabolism. Parasites can be divided into two groups – the protozoa and the helminths (see Chapter 3):

- The protozoa are unicellular organisms, often with complicated life cycles.
- The helminths have highly developed internal structures and integuments.

A wide array of different drugs have been developed, and these are summarized in *Figures 30.32* and *30.33*. The problems of finding agents that are toxic to the parasite and not to man are considerable and many of the agents have unpleasant side effects. Some antibacterial agents also have antiprotozoan activity, indicating that their toxicity is not limited to prokaryotic cells.

Laboratory Aspects of Antibacterial Agents

It is clear from the preceding sections of this chapter that although there are certain 'rules of thumb' about the resistance of bacteria to an antibiotic, it is often impossible to do more than guess in the absence of laboratory tests. Susceptibility tests performed in the laboratory examine the interaction between antibiotics and bacteria in an isolated and rather artificial fashion. At best the results are a helpful guide to the likely outcome of therapy, at worst they are misleading. Patient factors such as age, underlying disease, and renal and liver impairment, must be taken into account in the antibiotic management of an infection.

Susceptibility tests

Laboratory tests for antibiotic susceptibility fall into two main categories:

- Diffusion tests.
- Dilution tests.

Diffusion tests involve seeding the organism on an agar plate and applying filter paper discs containing antibiotics

The isolate to be tested is seeded over the entire surface of an agar plate and filter paper discs containing the antibiotics are applied. After overnight incubation the plate is observed for zones of inhibition around each antibiotic disc *(Fig. 30.34)*. The amount of antibiotic in the disc is related to, among other things, the achievable serum concentration and therefore differs for different antibiotics.

\multicolumn{4}{c}{THERAPEUTIC APPLICATIONS OF MAJOR ANTI-PROTOZOAL DRUGS}
disease/site	agent	route of administration	safety
amebiasis			
lumen	diloxanide furoate	oral	safe
tissue	metronidazole	oral	treatment of chronic mild infection and of extra-intestinal infections, all safe
	tinidazole	oral	
	dehydroemetine	IM	treatment of acute and hepatic infections dehydroemetine has some toxicity
	chloroquine	oral	
amebic meningoencephalitis	amphotericin B	IV	nephrotoxic, fever
cryptosporidiosis	spiramycin	oral	experimental, effective agent awaited
giardiasis	metronidazole	oral	safe
	tinidazole	oral	safe
	furazolidone	oral	toxic; hypersensitivity reactions
leishmaniasis	antimonials	IV/IM	toxic
	pentamidine	IM	
	amphotericin B	IV	
malaria pre-erthyrocytic stages	primaquine	oral	radical cure, some toxicity (risk of favism in G6PDH-deficient patients)
blood stages	chloroquine	oral	generally safe
	quinine	oral, IM	some toxicity, used against drug resistant *P. falciparum*
	proguanil	oral	used with chloroquine
	pyrimethamine		used in combination with sulfadoxine
	tetracycline	oral	used against drug resistant *Plasmodium falciparum*
	mefloquine	oral	mild side effects
toxoplasmosis	pentamidine	IM and aerosolized	toxic IM, shock
trichomoniasis	pyrimethamine sulfadiazine	oral	safe, but long-term treatment may produce anemia
	metronidazole	oral	safe
	tinidazole	oral	safe
trypanosomiasis African	suramin	IV	toxic
	pentamidine	IM	toxic
	melarsoprol	IV	toxic, passes blood–brain barrier
	tryparsamide	IV	toxic, passes blood–brain barrier
American	nifurtimox	oral	side effects common
	benznidazole	oral	side effects common

Fig. 30.32 Therapeutic applications of the major antiprotozoan drugs. Several are potentially toxic and must be given under supervision. Some also have antibacterial activity and have been described in detail earlier in the chapter. Drug resistance is a problem, particularly in the treatment of malaria.

THERAPEUTIC APPLICATIONS OF MAJOR ANTHELMINTIC DRUGS		
disease	agent	safety
cestodes (tapeworms)		
adult stage infection	niclosamide	safe
	praziquantel	safe, can prevent cysticercosis following infection with *Taenia solium*
larval stage (e.g. hydatid disease, cysticercosis)	benzimidazole carbonates	safe, but limited use
trematodes (flukes)		
schistosomiasis and intestinal flukes	praziquantel oxamniquine	safe, mild side effects
liver and lung fluke infection	praziquantel	
nematodes (roundworms)		
ascariasis and pinworm infection	mebendazole albendazole flubendazole	all are safe drugs[†], mebendazole drug of choice
	pyrantel pamoate	safe[†], mild side effects, not used in children <1 year
	piperazine	safe[†], except in epilepsy
hookworm infection	mebendazole albendazole flubendazole	all are safe drugs[†] mebendazole drug of choice
	pyrantel pamoate	safe[†], mild side effects, not used or children <1 year
strongyloidiasis	thiabendazole	mild side effects[†]
trichinosis	mebendazole albendazole flubendazole	all are safe drugs[†] mebendazole drug of choice
	thiabendazole	mild side effects[†]
trichuriasis	mebendazole	safe[†]
cutaneous larva migrans (infection with animal hookworm)	albendazole thiabendazole*	safe[†] mild side effects[†]
toxocariasis (visceral larva migrans)	thiabendazole mebendazole	mild side effects[†] safe[†]
lymphatic filariasis	diethyl carbamizine ivermectin	allergic side effects mild side effects
aberrant or unusual species	mebendazole thiabendazole	drugs of choice for majority of infections

* topical administration
† not used in pregnancy

Fig. 30.33 Therapeutic applications of the major anthelmintic drugs. All are administered orally except thiabendazole for larva migrans, which is administered topically. Note that many of these drugs are not safe in pregnancy.

In addition, antibiotics differ in their ability to diffuse in agar, so the size of the inhibition zone (and not simply its presence) is an indicator of susceptibility of the isolate. The zone sizes are compared with those for reference organisms (either tested in parallel or established previously and published in reference tables) and the result recorded as S (susceptible), I (intermediate) or R (resistant). An 'I' result indicates that the isolate is less susceptible than the norm, but may respond to higher doses of antibiotic or in sites where the antibiotic is concentrated (e.g. in urine in the bladder for antibiotics excreted by the kidneys).

A dilution test provides a quantitative estimate of susceptibility to an antibiotic

A more quantitative estimate of the susceptibility of an organism to an antibiotic can be achieved by performing a MIC (minimum inhibitory concentration) test (i.e. a test to find the lowest concentration that will inhibit visible growth of the bacterial isolate *in vitro*). Serial dilutions of the test antibiotic are prepared in broth or agar medium and inoculated with a suspension of the test organism. After overnight incubation, the MIC is recorded as the highest dilution in which there is no macroscopic growth (*Fig. 30.35*). These tests can be performed in a microtiter plate format and form the basis of some automated susceptibility test systems. An alternative approach is the E-test in which a filter paper strip impregnated with a gradient of antibiotic is laid on an agar plate seeded with the test isolate. The concentration on the strip at which growth is inhibited indicates the MIC.

MIC tests are clearly more costly than diffusion tests in terms of time and materials and are not required for every isolate from every patient, but they yield useful information for the management of difficult infections such as bacterial endocarditis or for patients who are failing to respond to apparently appropriate therapy.

An advantage of an MIC test is that it can be extended to determine the MBC (minimum bacterial concentration),

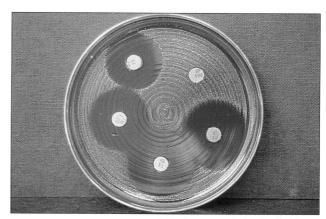

Fig. 30.34 The antibiotic susceptibility of an organism can be tested by the application of filter paper discs impregnated with antibiotic onto a lawn of the organisms seeded on an agar plate. After overnight incubation, during which time the organism grows and the antibiotics diffuse from the discs, a zone of inhibition develops indicating the degree of susceptibility of the organism. This plate shows the antibiotic susceptibility of *Shigella*, indicating sulfonamide resistance. SF100 is the sulfonamide disc. (Courtesy of DK Banerjee.)

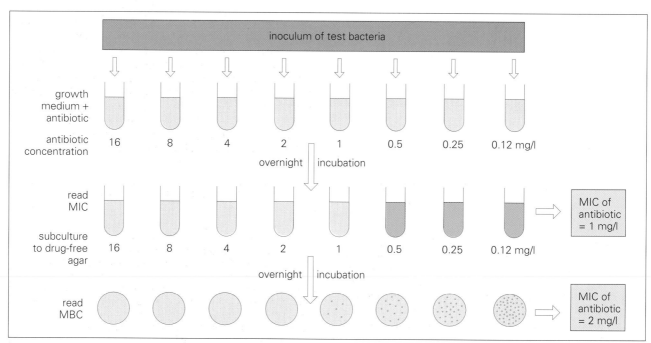

Fig. 30.35 More precise measures of the amount of antibiotic required to inhibit and kill a bacterial population can be estimated by establishing the minimum inhibitory concentration (MIC) and minimum bactericidal concentration (MBC) of the antibiotic. Using the standard method as outlined in this illustration, the MIC result is available after 24 hours and the MBC result after 48 hours. A number of variables such as the inoculum size, the growth medium and the interpretation of the results affect the results of MIC tests.

which is the lowest concentration of an antibiotic required to kill the organism. In order to discover whether the agent has actually killed the bacteria rather than simply inhibited their growth, the test dilutions are subcultured onto a fresh drug-free medium and incubated for a further 18–24 hours *(Fig. 30.35)*. The antibacterial agent is considered to be bactericidal if the MBC is equal to or not greater than four-fold higher than the MIC.

Killing curves provide a dynamic estimate of bacterial susceptibility

One of the disadvantages of MIC and MBC tests is that the result is read at only one point in time. A more dynamic estimate of bacterial susceptibility can be gained by measuring the decrease in viability of the population with time *(Fig. 30.36)*. As with MIC tests, it is not feasible to perform killing curves manually for every test isolate, but they can provide useful information for difficult treatment problems. A number of the automated susceptibility test systems use a measure of bacterial viability (e.g. turbidity, electrical impedance) in the presence of an antibacterial as their indicator system. These machines can produce results more rapidly (within about five hours) than conventional susceptibility tests.

Combinations of Antibacterial Agents

Combining antibacterial agents can lead to synergism or antagonism

Hospital patients frequently receive more than one antibacterial agent and these agents may interact with each other (and also with other drugs such as diuretics).

Antibacterial combinations are described as:
- 'Synergistic', if their activity is greater than the sum of the individual activities.
- 'Antagonistic', if the activity of one drug is compromised in the presence of the other.

Both diffusion and dilution tests allow the action of combinations of antibiotics to be studied. Although synergy can often be demonstrated *in vitro (Fig. 30.37)*, it is difficult to confirm *in vivo*. Cotrimoxazole is an example of a combination that is frequently used (see above). Another example is the combination of penicillin (or ampicillin) with gentamicin in the treatment of endocarditis caused by *Enterococcus* spp. as this combination has been shown to be clearly superior to the effect of the beta-lactam alone *(Fig. 30.38)*.

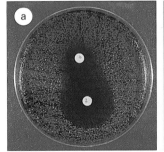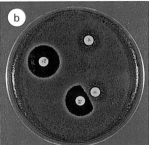

Fig. 30.37 Discs containing sulfonamide and trimethoprim (a) have been placed to demonstrate the synergistic activity of these two agents against *Escherichia coli*. Synergy can be recognized by the fact that the zones of inhibition become continuous between the two discs. Nitrofurantoin is capable of antagonizing the activity of nalidixic acid, as shown (b). When the discs are placed far apart nalidixic acid inhibits the test organism, but when placed close together this inhibition is antagonized by the presence of nitrofurantoin, as evidenced by the foreshortening of the zone of inhibition.

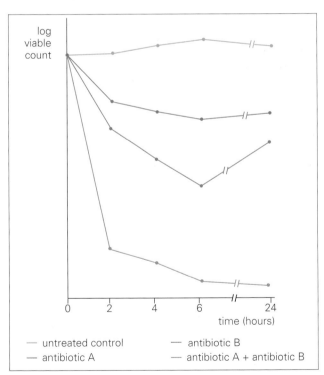

Fig. 30.36 A more dynamic picture of the interaction between an antibiotic and a bacterial population can be gained from producing killing curves. In these experiments a culture of 2×10^6 CFU/ml was treated with antibiotics A and B alone and in combination. Compared with the untreated control both A and B inhibit the growth of the bacterial culture, but B is more active than A. However, in combination, the activity of A plus B is synergistic (i.e. it is more active than the sum of the activities of the two antibiotics alone). The combination also prevents the regrowth seen after 6–24 hours when the antibiotics are used singly.

USE OF ANTIBIOTIC COMBINATIONS
to obtain a synergistic effect e.g. cotrimoxazole
to prevent or delay emergence of persistent organisms e.g. isoniazid, rifampicin and ethambutol for tuberculosis
to treat polymicrobial infections e.g. intra abdominal abcesses where the different microbes have different susceptibilities
to treat serious infections in the stage before the infectious agent is identified

Fig. 30.38 Reasons for using antibiotic combinations. Ideally, single drugs are used, but antibiotic combinations are justifiable under certain circumstances.

Antagonism can be demonstrated between some pairs of antibiotics *in vitro* (Fig. 37.7) but is rarely evident *in vivo*.

Antibiotic Assays

In the preceding sections of this chapter the pharmacokinetic properties (absorption, distribution, excretion) of antibacterial agents have been summarized. Some antibacterials have a narrow 'therapeutic index' – that is, the concentration required for successful treatment and the concentration toxic to the patient are not very different. The concentrations of such antibiotics should be monitored both to prevent toxicity and to ensure that therapeutic concentrations are achieved. Other less toxic agents should be monitored in some circumstances in some patients (Fig. 30.39). Serum concentrations are usually measured, but urine, CSF and other body fluids can be assayed where applicable.

Antibiotic assays can be performed in a manner similar to that described above for diffusion susceptibility tests. The method lends itself to the assay of almost any antibiotic, but it requires technical skill and time before the result is available (about 18 hours). Nowadays most laboratories use automated techniques based on immunologic methods employing labelled antibodies to each antibiotic. Such methods are rapid, require only small volumes of serum, and are highly specific. However, they are available for only a limited range of antibiotics.

Use and Misuse of Antimicrobial Agents

Much has been said in this chapter about the interactions between antimicrobial agents and microbes – the mechanisms of selective toxicity and the defenses put up by resistant organisms. The distribution, metabolism and excretion of agents by the host have been considered briefly, together with the important toxic side effects of the agents. The choice of antimicrobial for treating specific infections is dealt with in the appropriate systems chapter (see Chapters 15–28). Dosage regimens have not been included because they vary with the agent, the infection, the age and the underlying condition of the patient, and sometimes from one country to another. Practitioners should consult appropriate local pharmacy guidelines.

Antimicrobial agents should only be used appropriately for prophylaxis or treatment

In conclusion we should stand back and ask 'Is antimicrobial therapy necessary for this patient, and if so which agent is appropriate?' Antimicrobial agents can be used:
- To help prevent infection (prophylaxis).
- To treat infection.

Prophylactic use of antibiotics is appropriate only in a few clearly defined circumstances and is usually of limited duration (e.g. 1–2 days) (Fig. 30.40). For example, perioperative antibiotic 'cover' for patients with known cardiac defects to prevent endocarditis or in abdominal surgery when the risk of fecal soiling of the peritoneal cavity and the wound is high.

In the community, the main uses are for close contacts of bacterial meningitis or tuberculosis.

Antimicrobial use results in the selection of resistant strains

If antibiotic treatment is necessary several factors must be considered and these are summarized in *Figure 30.41*. It is important to recognize that during treatment not only the infecting microbe, but also the patient and all his or her normal microbial flora are being exposed to the effects of the antimicrobial agent. Use of antimicrobials has been clearly shown to select for resistant strains, both in the individual and in the community, and overuse or inappropriate use only increases this risk. History suggests that microbes will never run out of ways of developing resistance, but we may run out of effective antimicrobials.

Summary

There are now many different antibacterial agents, which can be classified into groups on the basis of their site of action in the bacterial cell and their chemical structure. There are fewer antifungal and antiviral agents and development of further agents in these classes is hindered by the difficulty of discovering and designing agents with appropriate selective toxicity.

Antimicrobial agents are undoubtedly valuable in the treatment and prevention (in well-defined circumstances) of infection. However, their inappropriate use carries with it potential risks to the patient of toxicity and superinfection, and to the community of selection of resistant organisms. Finally, of course, there is also the consideration of cost.

ANTIBIOTIC ASSAYS ARE IMPORTANT
when an antibiotic has a narrow therapeutic index e.g. aminoglycosides
when the normal route of excretion of antibiotic is impaired e.g. in patients with renal failure for agents excreted via the kidney
when the absorption of the antibiotic is uncertain e.g. after oral administration
to ascertain concentrations in sites of infection into which penetration of antibiotic is irregular or unknown e.g. in CSF
in patients receiving prolonged therapy for serious infections e.g. endocarditis
in neonates with serious infections
in patients who fail to respond to apparently appropriate therapy
to check on patient compliance

Fig. 30.39 Assays of antibiotics in clinical practise are particularly important when the antibiotic is potentially toxic, but there is a variety of other situations in which assays are important.

INDICATIONS FOR PROPHYLACTIC USE OF ANTIBIOTICS

patients of normal susceptibility exposed to specific pathogens

rifampicin to eradicate carriage of *Neisseria meningitidis* and *H. influenzae* type b in people who have had close contact with a case of meningitis

isoniazid to asymptomatic contacts of a case of active tuberculosis

patients with increased susceptibility to infection

penicillin (or erythromycin if penicillin-allergic) for patients with damaged or prosthetic heart valves undergoing dental or other operations, to prevent endocarditis

penicillin (long-term) for patients who have had rheumatic fever, to prevent recurrent streptococcal infections

oral, non-absorbable antibiotics (e.g. framycetin and colistin) for neutropenic patients – to reduce aerobic gut flora and help to prevent endogenous Gram-negative bacteraemia

patients undergoing surgery

penicillin or metronidazole for patients having implantation or amputation operations on the lower limbs, to prevent clostridial infection

ampicillin and metronidazole (or other appropriate combination) or cefoxitin (or other broad-spectrum cephalosporin) for patients having abdominal operations when faecal soiling of the peritoneum is likely – to prevent endogenous infection with gut organisms

* cloxacillin and gentamicin for patients having major cardiovascular, orthopedic or neurosurgical operations – to prevent infection particularly with skin organisms

* local antibiotic policies may differ on choice of agents

Fig. 30.40 Antibiotics should not be used indiscriminately with a view to eradicating organisms, but in well-defined situations prophylaxis is valuable and may be life-saving.

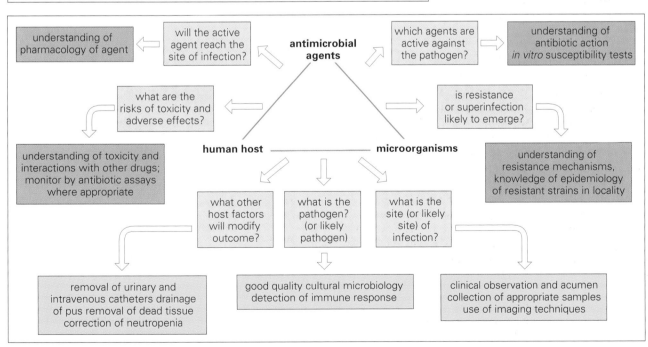

Fig. 30.41 The interactions between antimicrobial agents, microorganisms and the human host can be summarized by examining the answers to several questions affecting each side of the triangle of interaction.

- Infection is unique among the diseases which afflict mankind because it involves two distinct biological systems. Antimicrobial agents are designed to inhibit one system (the microbe) while doing minimal damage to the other (the patient). Antimicrobial agents require selective toxicity.
- Antimicrobial agents are often themselves products of microoganisms (natural products) although most are chemically modified to improve their properties. Other agents are entirely synthetic. Antibacterials are the most numerous; designing antiviral, antifungal and anti-parasitic drugs which are selectively toxic provides much greater challenges.
- Antibacterial are classified by their target site and their chemical family; this helps to understand better their mode of action and the mechanisms of resistance.
- Antibacterials have four possible sites of action in the bacterial cell; cell wall, protein, nucleic acids and cell membrane. The majority act at the cell wall or inhibit protein synthesis. At each site there are many different molecular targets (enzymes or substrates) which can be specifically inhibited.
- Development of resistance is the major limiting factor of antibacterials. It arises through random

- mutation of bacterial chromosomal genes and through acquisition, from other bacteria, of resistance genes on plasmids.
- Mutated or acquired genes confer resistance by altering the target site of the antibacterial, altering the uptake of the drug, or producing drug-destroying enzymes.
- The number of classes of antifungal molecules is very limited. Toxicity (all), difficulty of formulation (polyenes), and emerging resistance (azoles) makes effective treatment of serious fungal infections a real challenge.
- The emergence of AIDS has proved an enormous boost to research in antivirals (especially anti-HIV drugs). Selective toxicity is again a major challenge. Three-drug combinations are beginning to show promise in the treatment of HIV but there is no specific therapy for the majority of viral diseases. Effective antiviral therapy is available for HSV and CMV infections.
- Bacteria can be tested in the laboratory for their susceptibility to antibacterials. The results of well-controlled tests provide a valuable guide to appropriate treatment. *In-vitro* tests with antifungals are less reliable and are rarely performed with anti virals in the clinical laboratory setting.

1. List the main classes of antibacterial agents in clinical use and give an example in each class.
2. List the main mechanisms by which resistance to antibacterials is exhibited and give an example of each.
3. What antimicrobial treatment would you recommend for the following clinical presentations? On what basis have you made these recommendations?

a. Urinary tract infection in an otherwise healthy women;
b. Lower respiratory tract infection in an elderly man (outpatient)
c. Upper respiratory tract infection in an adult
d. Septicaemia in an elderly women.

Further Reading

Baron S, Trying SK, Fleischmann WR Jr, *et al.* The interferons. Mechanisms of action and clinical applications. *JAM Med Assoc* 1991;**266**:1375–1383.

Brock TD. *Milestones in Microbiology*. London: Prentice–Hall International, 1961.

Cohen ML. Antimicrobial resistance: prognosis for public health. *Trends Microbiol* 1994;**2**:422–425.

Dolin R. Antiviral chemotherapy and chemoprophylaxis. *Science* 1985;**227**:1296–1303.

Franklin TJ, Snow GA. Biochemistry of Antimicrobial Action. London: Chapman and Hall, 1989.

Garrod GLP, Lambert HP, O'Grady F. Antibiotic and Chemotherapy. London: Churchill Livingstone, 1992.

Lorian V, ed. Antibiotics in Laboratory Medicine. Maryland: Williams and Wilkins, 1980.

Marriott MS. Rational design of a magic bullet: antifungal drugs. Rev Med Microbiol 1990;1:151–159.

Introduction

Vaccination aims to prime the adaptive immune system to the antigens of a particular microbe so that a first infection induces a secondary response.

'Never in the history of human progress,' wrote the pathologist Geoffrey Edsall, 'has a better and cheaper method of preventing illness been developed than immunization at its best'. It is a sobering thought that the greatest success story in medicine, the elimination of smallpox, began before either immunology or microbiology were recognized as disciplines – indeed before the existence of microbes or the immune system was even suspected. It is in honor of the pioneering work of Jenner with vaccinia (see *Fig. 31.2*) that all forms of specific, actively induced immunity are now referred to as 'vaccination'.

The principle of vaccination is simple: to induce a 'primed' state so that on first contact with the relevant infection a rapid and effective secondary immune response will be mounted, leading to prevention of disease. Vaccination depends upon the ability of lymphocytes, both B and T, to respond to specific antigens and develop into memory cells, and therefore represents a form of actively enhanced adaptive immunity. The passive administration of preformed elements such as antibody is considered in Chapter 32.

The Aims of Vaccination

The aims of vaccination vary from blocking transmission and preventing symptoms to eradication of disease

The most ambitious aim of vaccination is eradication of the disease. Which other diseases will follow smallpox into oblivion depends upon many subtle features of host–parasite balance (discussed in Chapter 32), but there has clearly been a dramatic downward trend in the incidence of most of the diseases against which vaccines are currently in use *(Fig. 31.1)*. However, as long as any focus of infection remains in the community, the main effect of vaccination will be protection of the individual against infection.

In certain cases the aim of vaccination may be more limited; namely, to protect the individual against symptoms or pathology if the simple presence of the microbe is not itself harmful. Diphtheria and tetanus vaccines are examples of 'anti-disease' rather than antimicrobial vaccines.

Finally, in the case of vector-borne diseases with a well-defined infective stage (e.g. malaria), one can visualize a vaccine that will block transmission without benefiting the vaccinated individual at all – the 'altruistic' vaccine.

Requirements of a Good Vaccine

A vaccine should as far as possible be effective, safe, stable and of low cost

To be effective a vaccine must not only induce an adequate response, but the response must also be of the right type. Therefore:

- A purely antibody response is unlikely to be of benefit against tuberculosis.
- A purely cell-mediated response is unlikely to be of benefit against streptococcal pneumonia.
- High levels of serum antibody may be irrelevant to mucosal protection against polio.
- Activation of cytotoxic T cells may be harmful in hepatitis.

The duration of response is of prime importance

For short-term protection (e.g. a tourist about to visit a disease area), the presence of antibody arising from the vaccine itself may be perfectly adequate and memory cells may not be strictly necessary. On the other hand, for protection against exposure at some time in the future, the induction of memory is essential; here the benefit will be correspondingly greater the longer the incubation period of the infection, because the immune system has more time to mount a secondary response. Memory is often naturally boosted by periodic outbreaks of disease in the community (e.g. the annual measles and mumps epidemics), but as diseases gradually die out this can no longer be relied on. Paradoxically, therefore, the less disease there is in the population, the more important it is to be vaccinated – a point that parents often do not appreciate.

In general, living vaccines induce stronger and more lasting immunity than non-living vaccines (see below).

The safety of vaccines is a major consideration

The very high cost of the awards that can follow successful litigation for vaccine-induced damage has been an element in the retreat of several commercial organizations from vaccine production and development, coupled with the fact that vaccination is inherently less profitable than chemotherapy (see below). In addition, vaccines are the only compounds routinely given to healthy people. In fact, considering the enormous number of vaccine administrations (at least 20 000 000/year in the USA alone), the safety record is extremely good. Nevertheless there have been a few serious vaccine accidents, such as the Lubeck disaster of 1926 (see

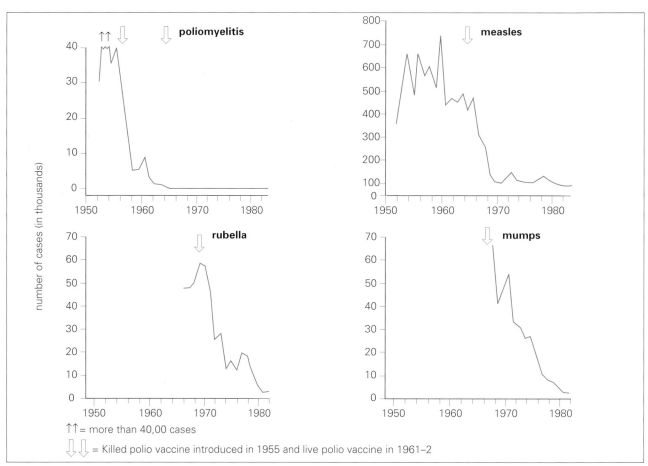

Fig. 31.1 The effect of vaccination on the incidence of various viral diseases in the USA. Most infections have shown a dramatic downward trend after the introduction of a vaccine (arrows). (Redrawn from Mims and White, 1984.)

Chapter 10), and safety testing is now rigorous, requiring extensive quality control and animal trials. The problems encountered in assuring the safety of vaccines are summarized in *Figure 31.3*

Stability is particularly critical with living attenuated vaccines

Stability is a requirement of all compounds destined to remain on the shelf for long periods. Maintenance of the 'cold chain' between the factory and the clinic – which may be a small field hospital thousands of miles away – is not easy, and in one study with measles vaccine in Cameroon, only one dose in six actually reached the patient in an active form. The attenuated polio vaccine has been shown to be stable for one year at 4°C, but for only a few days at 37°C.

The cost of a vaccine is relative, but cannot be high for use in developing countries

One might think that $80 spent on a vaccine that prevented hepatitis B, a potentially fatal infection and one of the major causes of liver carcinoma, is money well spent. However, in terms of the health budget of a typical developing country, such vaccines – and indeed many much cheaper vaccines – are clearly out of reach of the ordinary population. Fortunately the World Health Organization has set up several programs

that specifically direct international funding towards vaccines against diseases of particular importance in the developing world *(Fig. 31.4)*. Whether vaccines made by new technology will cost less or be more expensive is discussed below.

Types of Vaccine

A vaccine should contain some (or at least one) of the protective antigens of the microbe

With the single exception of vaccinia, which is a natural animal ('heterologous') virus sharing antigens with smallpox but of low virulence in man, the vaccines in use today consist of either:

- Microbes for which the virulence has been artificially reduced ('attenuated').
- Killed organisms.
- Subcellular fragments.

  Each type has its merits and drawbacks.

The heterologous vaccine, vaccinia, was in many ways the ideal vaccine

Another equally good heterologous vaccine may one day be found. In animal experiments, for instance, non-virulent

Edward Jenner (1749–1823)

The English physician Edward Jenner *(Fig. 31.2)* is regarded as the founder of modern vaccination, but he was by no means the first to try the technique. The ancient practice of 'variolation' went back to tenth century China, and arrived in Europe in the early eighteenth century by way of Turkey. The technique involved the inoculation of children with dried material from healed scabs of mild smallpox cases, and was a striking foretaste of the principles of modern attenuated viral vaccines. This practice was, however, both inconsistent and dangerous, and Jenner's innovation was to show that a much safer and more reliable protection could be obtained by deliberate inoculation with cowpox (vaccinia) virus. Milkmaids exposed to this infection were traditionally known to be resistant to smallpox and so retained their smooth complexions. In 1796, Jenner tested his theory by inoculating eight-year-old James Phipps with liquid from a cowpox pustule on the hand of Sarah Nelmes. Subsequent inoculation of the boy with smallpox produced no disease. (Note that such an experiment could not even be considered today!) Jenner's book *'An Inquiry into the Causes and Effects of the Variolae Vaccinae, a Disease Discovered in some of the Western Counties of England, particularly Gloucestershire, and Known by the Name of the Cow Pox'*, published in 1798, is a classic of its kind – lively, stylish and well-argued. Although greeted with skepticism at first, Jenner's ideas soon became accepted and he went on to inoculate thousands of patients in a shed in the garden of his house at Berkeley, Gloucestershire. He ultimately achieved world fame, though his fellowship of the Royal Society was conferred for a quite different piece of work on the nesting habits of the cuckoo! His house at Berkeley is now preserved as a museum and is used for small symposia by the British Society of Immunology.

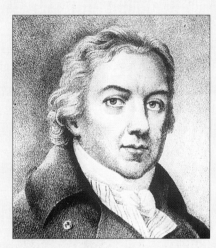

Fig. 31.2
Edward Jenner
(1749–1823).

PROBLEMS WITH VACCINE SAFETY
live attenuated vaccines
insufficient attenuation
reversion to wild type
administration to immunodeficient patient
persistent infection
contamination by other viruses
fetal damage
non-living vaccines
contamination by live organisms
contamination by toxins
allergic reactions
autoimmunity
genetically engineered vaccines
?inclusion of oncogenes

Fig. 31.3 Both living and non-living vaccines require rigorous quality and safety control. Some of the more common problems are listed.

WHO VACCINE-DIRECTED PROGRAMS
special program for research and training in tropical diseases
malaria, trypanosomiasis
leishmaniasis, schistosomiasis
filariasis, leprosy
expanded program on immunization
diphtheria
pertussis
tetanus
measles
poliomyelitis
tuberculosis
program for the control of diarrheal diseases and acute respiratory infections
global program on AIDS

Fig. 31.4 The World Health Organization (WHO) has been responsible for identifying diseases where vaccine research is required, and channels internationally raised funding.

strains of some parasites will induce protection against virulent strains, and several veterinary vaccines are based on the same idea. For example, herpesvirus from turkeys has been used to protect chickens, and monkey and calf-derived rotavirus has been tried with some success in human infants. The ancient Middle Eastern practice of 'leishmanization', in which children are deliberately infected in an inconspicuous skin site with *Leishmania tropica* from a mild case, resulting in a self-healing lesion ('Oriental sore') and subsequent immunity to more widespread disease, could work in the same way. However, an experiment in which volunteers were infected with a squirrel-derived strain of *Leishmania donovani* did not give significant protection against the natural infection.

Live attenuated vaccines make up the bulk of successful viral vaccines

The attenuated virus vaccines in current use have been produced by the selection of mutants induced painstakingly, but ultimately at random – 'genetic roulette' as it has been termed *(Fig. 31.5)*. Two principal methods are used:
- Serial passage in cells cultured *in vitro*.
- Adaptation to low temperatures.

With the development of recombinant DNA technology it is now possible to deliberately induce the required genetic change where this is known. The use of a virus as a carrier of complete genes from another source is considered on p. 448.

The unpredictable character of random mutants is illustrated by the three serotypes of attenuated poliovirus (the 'Sabin' oral vaccine):
- Type 1 contains 57 separate base substitutions.
- Types 2 and 3 contain only a few base substitutions, of which all but two are probably unrelated to the loss of virulence.

This explains why reversion to the wild-type virulent virus is more common with types 2 and 3 (though still rare at less than one per million vaccinations). In this case, attenuation was by passage through monkey kidney cells or human embryo fibroblasts, virulence being checked for by signs of neurotoxicity in monkeys. Analogous methods have been used for measles, rubella, mumps and yellow fever *(Fig. 31.6)*.

Interestingly, the polio and measles vaccines produced in this way turned out to be temperature-sensitive mutant strains. In other cases, temperature sensitivity has been deliberately selected for by the process of cold adaptation, during which the virus is encouraged to grow at low temperatures,

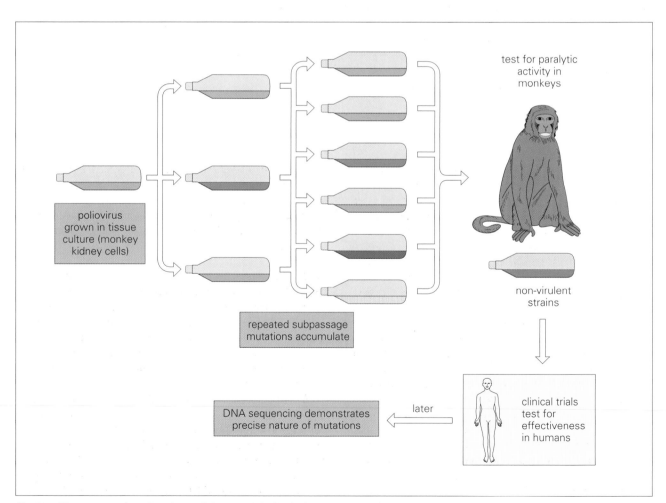

Fig. 31.5 Live attenuated vaccines (e.g. polio) were originally produced by allowing viruses to grow in unusual conditions, and selecting the randomly occurring mutants that had lost virulence.

LIVE ATTENUATED VACCINES	
organism	method of attenuation
viruses	
standard	
poliovirus	passage in monkey kidney, human embryo
measles	passage in human kidney, amnion, chick embryo
rubella	passage in rabbit kidney, human diploid cells
mumps	passage in chick fibroblasts
yellow fever	passage in monkey, mouse, egg
experimental	
influenza	
respiratory syncytial virus	cold adaptation
rotavirus	
cytomegalovirus	
herpesvirus	passage in human embryo fibroblast
varicella	
bacteria	
standard	
Mycobacterium tuberculosis (BCG)	passage for 10 years in glycerol-bile-potato medium
Salmonella typhi	chemical mutagenesis
experimental	
Shigella	chemical mutagenesis
Vibrio cholerae	toxin deleted

Fig. 31.6 Several different approaches are used to produce today's live attenuated vaccines.

for example 25°C, which usually means that it grows less well, if at all, at body temperature. Such a virus might then colonize the upper respiratory tract, but not warmer tissues such as the lungs. An influenza vaccine made in this way has given promising results. However, another temperature-sensitive influenza mutant induced by a chemical mutagen was found to revert rather easily to the wild type, and the same occurred with a respiratory syncytial virus vaccine.

Randomly induced attenuation of bacteria has not been achieved to the same extent, but the development by Calmette and Guérin of an attenuated strain of bovine tuberculosis after more than 10 years (1908–1918) of culture on glycerol–bile–potato medium shows that it is possible. The bacille Calmette-Guérin (BCG) is the one well-established attenuated bacterial vaccine and has not reverted to virulence in over 70 years; in effect it constitutes a new species of mycobacterium. Its effectiveness is, however, still in dispute (see below). A more recent development is the production of an attenuated strain of *Salmonella typhi*, produced by exposure to chemical mutagens, which has proved to be at least as good as the older killed typhoid vaccine.

Genetically engineered or 'site-directed' mutation shows great promise in both viruses and bacteria. The majority are deletion mutants in which a gene related to virulence has been put out of action. Examples range from an experimental poliovirus type 2 strain with a single base change, through *Salmonella* strains with mutations in the aroA or galE enzyme gene, to pseudorabies virus lacking the entire thymidine kinase gene, and cholera organisms lacking the gene for the A toxin subunit.

Killed or 'inactivated' organisms are used where living vaccines are not available

Living vaccines may not be available because attenuation has not been achieved or reversion to the wild type occurs too easily *(Fig. 31.7)*. Killed vaccines have the advantage of non-infectivity and therefore relative safety, but the disadvantage of generally lower immunogenicity and the consequent need for several doses.

A variety of methods are available for inactivation. With the older viral vaccines such as influenza and polio (Salk), formaldehyde was used but, more recently, β-propiolactone and various ethylenimines and psoralens are replacing it (e.g. for the current rabies vaccine). Ultraviolet light is not regarded as fully reliable because it only selectively damages the viral nucleic acid, which can be repaired. Formaldehyde, phenol, acetone or simple heating are all used for bacteria and are equally successful.

INACTIVATED VACCINES	
organism	**method of inactivation**
viruses	
rabies	β-propiolactone
influenza	β-propiolactone
polio (Salk)	formaldehyde
hepatitis A	formaldehyde
bacteria	
Salmonella typhi	heat plus phenol or acetone
Vibrio cholerae	heat
Bordetella pertussis	heat or formaldehyde
E. coli (experimental)	colicin
Yersinia pestis	formaldehyde

Fig. 31.7 Several methods are in use to produce inactivated vaccines. One of the most famous, the rabies vaccine, dates back to the time of Pasteur.

Subcellular fractions can sometimes be used if protective immunity is directed against a particular part of an organism

Established examples of vaccines that are subcellular fractions include the polysaccharide capsules of pneumococci, *Haemophilus*, and meningococci. Also the surface coat of the hepatitis B virus, which is produced by recombinant DNA technology and the fragmented virus or purified surface antigens of influenze virus vaccines. Vaccines based on the protein filaments (pili) used by *Escherichia coli* and *Neisseria gonorrhoeae* to attach to urinary tract epithelium are still experimental. Removal of all live infectious material is obviously a vital element in ensuring the safety of such vaccines.

Toxoids are inactivated bacterial toxins that can induce protective antibody

Bacterial toxins that have been inactivated (usually by formaldehyde) so that they are no longer toxic, but still induce protective antibody, are called toxoids. Two such toxoids – diphtheria and tetanus – are among the most successful and widely used of all vaccines. In combination with killed *Bordetella pertussis*, they constitute the well-known triple vaccine – DPT (diphtheria, pertussis, tetanus). There is some evidence that omission of the pertussis component reduces the antibody response to the two toxoids; thus pertussis acts as an 'adjuvant' as well as a specific vaccine.

With the use of small peptides as potential vaccine antigens (see below), tetanus toxoid has been widely suggested as a useful 'carrier' protein – the idea is that most patients have been previously immunized to the toxoid and therefore possess tetanus-specific T memory cells, which will help the peptide-specific B cells to make antibody. This approach is useful for inducing a good primary response, but less useful for memory responses, in which T cells need to be recalled by the proteins of the infection rather than by those of tetanus.

The same approach led to the development of conjugate *H. influenze* type b (Hib) vaccine. Tetanus and diptheria toxoids are conjugated with capsular polysacchandes of *H. influenze* to improve the immunogenicity of this vaccine in infants and young children.

The other common toxin-inducing bacterium is *Vibrio cholerae*, and vaccines containing the B subunit of cholera toxin plus killed organisms have had some success. Vaccines have also been made against the neurotoxin of *Clostridium botulinum*.

A variety of viruses and bacteria can be used as vectors for cloned genes

The idea of using expression vectors (e.g. *E. coli*, yeast) to clone genes coding for potentially immunogenic proteins is as old as recombinant DNA technology itself. More recently, however, an ingenious modification has been introduced in which the expression vector, complete with inserted gene(s), is itself the vaccine. Following injection into the patient, it will proliferate sufficiently to release an immunizing amount of the foreign protein, but without inducing disease itself.

The first vector to be proposed in 1982 was the vaccinia virus. This had the advantage of being already established as a highly effective vaccine and of possessing a large enough (DNA) genome for insertion of several foreign genes without disrupting virus structure or function. However, it also had the disadvantage that a large proportion of the world's population was immune to vaccinia and would probably eliminate the virus before it had produced the desired amount of foreign gene product. There was also the problem that vaccinia itself could induce complications (principally encephalitis) in about one case in 100 000. Nevertheless, in a pioneer experiment in chimpanzees, vaccinia containing the gene for hepatitis B surface antigen (HBsAg) gave excellent protection against a challenge infection (*Fig. 31.8*), and similarly for influenza and herpes simplex virus (HSV).

Several other viruses have subsequently been considered as vectors, including attenuated yellow fever virus, adenovirus, herpes virus (HSV) and varicella–zoster virus (VZV); successful insertion has been achieved for genes from a variety of viruses including respiratory syncytial virus, Epstein–Barr virus, rabies virus, dengue virus and Lassa fever virus.

Bacteria are also good candidates as vectors, the two leading ones being the attenuated salmonellae mentioned earlier and BCG. *S. typhi* has the advantage of being an intestinal infection so when given orally (with a dose of bicarbonate to prevent inactivation by gastric acid) it will induce mucosal immunity in the gut. Avirulent mutants of *S. typhi* might therefore act as general vectors for vaccines against all enteric diseases – a field in which current vaccines are far from adequate.

BCG is the latest vector to be proposed and the advantages are:

• First, the very large genome.
• Second, the fact that BCG is now the most widely used of all vaccines, being given, usually just after birth, to about 75% of all children in the world.
• Another special merit is that it induces predominantly cell-mediated immunity, both to itself and to other antigens given with it, so it could be the ideal vector for antigens from all persistent intracellular organisms – a large and important category that includes in addition to *Mycobacterium tuberculosis* and *Mycobacterium leprae*,

Brucella, Leishmania, Toxoplasma, Histoplasma, Listeria, rickettsiae and chlamydiae, many viruses, and possibly (in its liver stage) malaria. Perhaps in the future a single vector containing all required antigens may become available (Fig. 31.9).

Gene cloning and peptide synthesis aim to produce immunogenic peptides for use as vaccines

The technologies involved are now reasonably standard, though there is considerable debate about which expression vector to

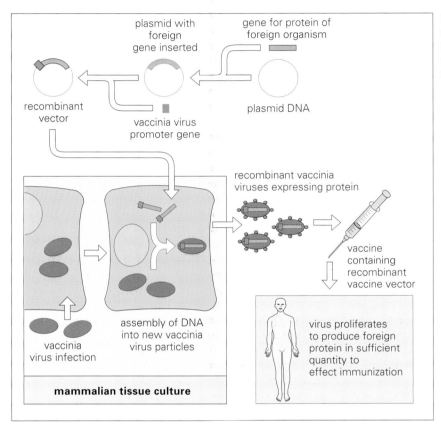

Fig. 31.8 It is now possible to insert genes coding for antigens of one or more microorganisms into a large virus such as vaccinia so that they replicate and are released into the host.

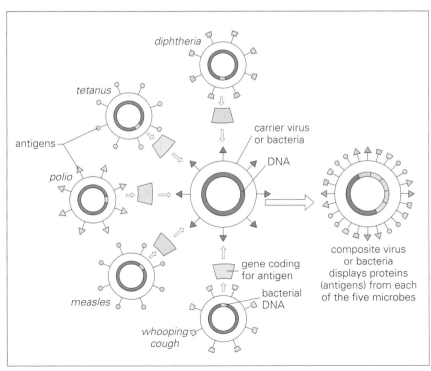

Fig. 31.9 The vaccines of the future may consist of a single viral or bacterial vector containing genes for all required vaccines – the 'one-shot' vaccine. This illustration first appeared in *New Scientist*, London, the weekly review of science and technology.

use for cloning genes. The first successful vaccine made in this way was against foot and mouth disease. First by gene cloning in *E. coli* and soon afterwards by chemical synthesis, it was shown that a 20-amino acid peptide from one of the capsid proteins could protect guinea pigs against infection.

Cloned or synthetic peptides are now available from a wide range of microbes, and there is extensive research into how to select the right peptide and how to make it as immunogenic as possible. One approach is to attach peptides to larger carrier molecules such as tetanus toxin (see above), but whenever possible the attempt is made to include sequences in the peptide that can themselves trigger T cells. These 'T cell epitopes' can to some extent be predicted from the known sequence of the molecule. Where they are not available, the strategy is to construct new sequences including one or more T cell epitopes as well as the epitope against which antibody is required (the 'B cell epitope'). A further refinement has been to couple together several copies of separate T and B epitopes into 'multiple antigen peptides', using a branching core of lysines and up to eight attached peptides – the so-called 'octopus' molecule. In one study, four each of the T cell and B cell epitopes gave the best results. Even then, it has usually been found that an adjuvant is needed to enhance immunogenicity.

Problems with these approaches are:

- The variation in response from patient to patient and the existence of genetic non-responders. The role of major histocompatibility complex (MHC) antigens in this is discussed below.
- Differences in glycosylation in different expression vectors when the carbohydrate portion of glycosylated proteins constitutes part or all of the antigen. *E. coli* is generally

unsuitable. Yeast, insect, and mammalian cells are all used to produce more correctly glycosylated proteins.

Much interest has been generated by the surprising discovery that intramuscular injection of microbial DNA itself, with a suitable promoter, can apparently immunize laboratory animals against infections such as influenza and malaria. It is thought that the corresponding antigen is expressed and presented on muscle cells, but much work is still needed to verify this and to ensure that there is not a risk of side effects such as autoimmunity or microbial tolerance.

Anti-idiotype vaccines are prepared using antibody molecules that are copies of the antigen

The most novel proposal for preparing antigens is to use anti-idiotype molecules. This is possible because antibodies can recognize structures related to each other's combining sites (idiotypes; see Chapter 6), just as they can recognize antigens; thus a first antibody against an antigen can be used to raise second antibodies, some of which will have idiotypes resembling the original antigen (*Fig. 31.10*). Considerable selection is required and monoclonal antibody technology is essential. One advantage of such 'surrogate antigens' is that being large proteins they behave as T-dependent antigens, even when the original antigen was T-independent – a polysaccharide, for example. This strategy has been successfully applied to the vaccination of mice against streptococcal and trypanosomal antigens, and to raise secondary antibody responses to endotoxin. At present it looks as though it could be of value for carbohydrate or glycolipid antigens, which unlike proteins cannot be cloned or synthesized in bulk.

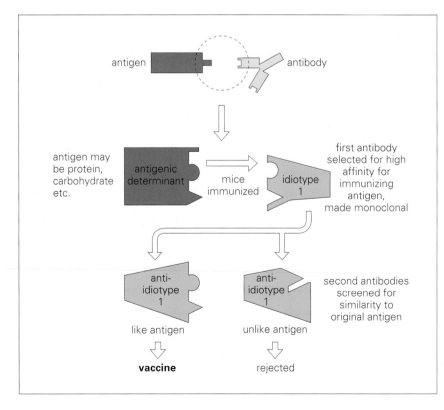

Fig. 31.10 Monoclonal antibody technology and the discovery of the 'idiotype network' has meant that immunoglobulins can now be used as 'surrogate' antigens. In the case of a carbohydrate or lipid antigen, this allows a protein 'copy' to be made, which may have certain advantages as a vaccine.

Special Considerations

Both living and non-living vaccines have advantages and disadvantages

Living versus non-living vaccines is one of the most keenly debated topics in vaccinology and some general points can be made, as well as some that apply specifically to particular vaccines. These are summarized in *Figure 31.11*.

The issue can be appreciated most clearly with those diseases that normally induce good long-term immunity following recovery from infection (e.g. the common childhood viruses). Here, live attenuated vaccines are much more likely to be effective, since they reproduce many of the features of the infection itself, including:

- Replication of the virus.
- Localization to the appropriate part of the body (e.g. gut, lung).
- Efficient induction of cytotoxic T cells, which may be related to the fact that for microbial peptides to become associated with MHC class I molecules it is usually necessary for the peptides to have been synthesized in the cell rather than taken in by endocytosis, as a non-living vaccine antigen would be.

A further theoretic advantage is the possibility that attenuated strains will spread through the population by normal transmission routes protecting those who have not been vaccinated ('herd immunity').

The principal disadvantages of living attenuated vaccines are:

- The possibility of reversion to virulence.
- The danger that they may cause severe disease in immunocompromised patients.

Many natural infections do not leave the patient with solid immunity (e.g. influenza). This can be for a variety of reasons prominent among them being antigenic diversity, antigenic variation, immunosuppression, and the induction of responses that protect the microbe. In such cases the rationale for using a living attenuated vaccine is weaker, and a subcellular component that induces strong immunity, which attacks the microbe at a weak spot (e.g. a polysaccharide capsule or a vital attachment molecule), possibly in the form of a mixture of antigenic types, is more likely to work. The problem of correct localization will then need to be addressed by other means, such as aerosols for the lung and enteric capsules for the gut.

Polio is the only disease at present for which live and killed vaccines compete with approximately equal terms (see poliomyelitis, Chapter 22).

Many polysaccharide antigens fail to stimulate T cells and therefore induce only primary responses

Most complex antigens contain both T and B cell epitopes, so T cells are induced that cooperate with B cells, leading to T and B cell memory, immunoglobulin switching (e.g. IgM→IgG), and affinity maturation – all features of the secondary response, and essential for a vaccine to be effective. Polysaccharide antigens that fail to stimulate T cells (T-independent antigens) induce only primary responses no matter

LIVING VERSUS NON-LIVING VACCINES		
	living	non-living
preparation	attenuation (not always feasible)	inactivation
administration	may be natural route (e.g. oral) may be single dose	injection usually multiple doses
adjuvant	not required	usually required
safety	may revert to virulence	pain from injection
heat lability (for tropical use)	requires cold chain	satisfactory
cost	low	high
duration of immunity	usually years	may be long or short
immune response	IgG, IgA cell-mediated	mainly IgG, little or no cell-mediated

Fig. 31.11 Live and non-living vaccines each have advantages and disadvantages.

how often they are administered. Such antigens are particularly ineffective in children under two years of age. The current strategy is to conjugate the polysaccharide to a suitable protein, preferably from the same microorganism. The results of this are discussed below in relation to pneumococcal and meningococcal vaccines. Another approach to this problem, although still largely experimental, is the use of anti-idiotypic antibody as a 'surrogate' antigen (see above).

MHC class II molecules are needed for T cell responses

Antigens that do stimulate T cells may be less effective in some individuals than in others. This is especially a feature of small peptides and is due to the very precise binding required between the peptide, the MHC class II – human leukocyte antigen (HLA)-D – molecule on the antigen-presenting cell, and the T cell receptor. HLA antigens are extremely polymorphic and it is quite common to find that a particular HLA molecule fails to bind a particular peptide. If none of an individual's available MHC class II molecules (two each of DP, DQ and DR) binds a particular peptide, the individual will be a 'non-responder' and will not mount T cell responses.

It is not known how much MHC restriction contributes to the failure of a certain percentage of individuals to respond well to almost all standard vaccines, and it may be that the problem has been overemphasized even where small peptides are concerned. For example, a 21-amino acid malaria peptide has been found from which peptides of 11–14 amino acids stimulate only T cells from a few DR types, whereas a 15-amino acid sequence stimulates all the DR types tested. This suggests that it may often be possible to confer a broader range of MHC responsiveness by adding a few amino acids to a peptide.

Pathologic consequences of vaccination may be due to the vaccine or the immune response

Vaccine causes of pathologic consequences include:

- Contamination of attenuated viruses with other viruses growing in the same cell lines, particularly since monkey cells are often used and several monkey viruses are lethal for humans.
- Hypersensitivity to egg proteins with living viral vaccines grown in chick embryo cells. Children with a history of egg sensitivity should be skin-tested with diluted vaccine and may have to be immunized in stages with lower than usual doses or, if anaphylaxis is expected, not at all.

A more complicated situation arises where the vaccine antigen itself induces a pathologic response such as hypersensitivity or autoimmunity. Hypersensitivity reactions to the older killed measles vaccines were a stimulus to the development of a living attenuated replacement. It appeared that although the killed vaccine induced good non-neutralizing antibodies to the hemagglutinin, it failed to induce antibody to the fusion (F) protein, which was destroyed by the inactivation process. The F protein is responsible for viral cell to cell spread. As a result, during, infection large amounts of virus were produced together with high titers of non-neutralizing antibody. The resulting immune complexes caused severe type III hypersensitivity during the attack of measles, so the patient's illness was actually made worse. A similar response occurred to the killed respiratory syncytial virus vaccine. The fever and malaise that follow vaccination with killed typhoid organisms is due to the endotoxin, and mediated by cytokines such as interleukin-1 (IL-1) and tumor necrosis factor (TNF).

Autoimmunity during infections can sometimes be traced to antigenic similarity ('mimicry') between host and microbe, and the same is theoretically possible with vaccine antigens. However, this does not seem to have been observed with the present vaccines, but could occur if strong T cell epitopes are conjugated to weak antigens, such as polysaccharides, which might cross-react with host molecules. Where the cross-reacting component can be identified, it should be removed before a vaccine is considered for use; Chagas' disease is a case in point.

Perhaps the most widely publicized complication of vaccination is the occurrence of fits and brain damage, notably after vaccination for pertussis (see Chapter 17). Whether or not this is truly due to the vaccine is discussed below. *Figure 31.12* lists the major reported complications of other vaccines.

Living vaccines should not usually be given to immunocompromised people

The most absolute contraindications to using living vaccine in immunocompromised people are the use of vaccinia or BCG in patients with severe T cell deficiency. Indeed it was the spreading and eventually fatal vaccinia infections that alerted the New York paediatrician Di George to the occurrence of the athymic syndrome that bears his name. However, in less severe T cell deficiency states, including HIV infection, the use of live measles vaccine is now recommended, the risk of complications being on balance less than the risk of death from the natural infection. Measles, mumps and rubella (MMR) vaccine

is generally not advised for other T cell deficiencies of childhood, including those following treatment with glucocorticosteroids or immunosuppressive drugs.

Non-living vaccines are less of a problem in the immunocompromised host since although they may be ineffective they are unlikely to be dangerous. Vaccines aimed specifically at the induction of antibody (e.g. capsular polysaccharides, hepatitis B) are recommended in all but the most severe B cell deficiencies, but the alternative of passive immunization (see Chapter 32) should also be considered.

Adjuvants

Many adjuvants will enhance the immune response when administered with antigen

It has been known since the 1920s that certain substances will enhance the consequent immune response when administered simultaneously with antigen. The first such substances that were shown to be safe, convenient and effective were aluminium salts. These constitute the principal vaccine adjuvants in use today, though numerous other materials are being considered or tried experimentally for clinical use. The word 'adjuvant' is also sometimes used in a slightly different sense to denote a substance that when given alone enhances some immune function such as inhibition of tumor growth or recovery from infection. This type of non-specific immunostimulant is discussed in Chapter 32.

Many years of work in animals have established that a wide range of materials are effective as vaccine adjuvants and these will be briefly described since the clinical adjuvants of the future are likely to be drawn from among them (*Fig. 31.13*).

Alum-precipitated antigens are especially effective at inducing antibody responses, but much less active in inducing cell-mediated immunity

The powerful adjuvanticity of aluminum salts has not been fully explained. Some of it is no doubt due to the formation of small inflammatory lesions, which may progress to granulomas, with consequent trapping of antigen and slow release with exposure to large numbers of macrophages and other antigen-presenting cells. Antigens (e.g. toxoids) were originally

PATHOLOGIC COMPLICATIONS OF VACCINATION	
complication	vaccine

hypersensitivity
  to egg antigens
  to viral antigens
	live measles, mumps
	killed measles, RSV

convulsions, encephalitis	pertussis, measles (1 per million)
meningitis	mumps (1 per million)
arthritis	rubella

Fig. 31.12 Complications are rare with modern vaccines, but the physician must always be aware of the possibility. (RSV, respiratory syncytial virus.)

VACCINE ADJUVANTS
inorganic salts
aluminum hydroxide (alhydrogel)*
aluminum phosphate*
calcium phosphate*
beryllium hydroxide
delivery systems
liposomes**
ISCOMs**
block polymers
slow release formulations**
bacterial products
BCG
Mycobacterium bovis and oil (complete Freund's adjuvant)†
MDP†
*Bordetella pertussis** (with diphtheria, tetanus toxoids)
natural mediators
IL-1
IL-2
IFN-γ
* routinely used in man   ** experimental
† too toxic for human use

Fig. 31.13 A variety of foreign and endogenous substances can act as adjuvants, but only aluminum and calcium salts and pertussis are routinely used in clinical practice. (BCG, bacille Calmette-Guérin; IFN, interferon; IL, interleukin; MDP, muramyl dipeptide; ISCOMs, immune-stimulating complexes)

entrapped in 'floccules' of the salt by adding them during its chemical preparation. Such antigens are described as 'alum precipitated'. Now, however, it is more usual to add the antigen to a preformed gel of aluminum hydroxide or phosphate.

A variety of novel formulations in which antigen is presented on the surface of small spherical structures are also used as adjuvants

A similar 'depot' effect is thought to account for the adjuvanticity of these novel formulations, which include:

- Liposomes, which are single- or multiple-walled phospholipid vesicles.
- ISCOMs (immune-stimulating complexes), which are micelles composed of a saponin derivative, QUIL A, which traps amphipathic proteins.
- Block polymers of polyoxyethylene and polyoxypropylene.

Depending upon the precise formulation and the nature of the antigen used, these have all been shown to be highly effective and many are in veterinary use. It is too early to say which, if any, will become standard clinical adjuvants, and this may depend upon safety testing as much as immunologic efficacy.

Mycobacteria and other bacteria can be effective adjuvants

The adjuvanticity of mycobacteria is remarkable, and was made

use of by Freund in his famous preparation 'complete Freund's adjuvant' (CFA), in which mycobacteria are emulsified with water in an oil vehicle. CFA is particularly effective in boosting cell-mediated immune responses such as delayed hypersensitivity to antigens that are normally weak inducers. Unfortunately, as several accidental injections have shown, CFA is too toxic for use in man, causing chronic non-healing granulomas. The oil-in-water emulsion without mycobacteria is known as 'incomplete Freund's adjuvant' (IFA), and this has been used in man with no apparent undesired side-effects, but without the great potency of CFA for cell-mediated immune responses. An extensive study of the role played by the mycobacteria in CFA has yielded the small water-soluble molecule muramyl dipeptide (MDP), which is claimed to retain most of the benefit of mycobacteria without being so toxic.

Numerous other bacterial derivatives are being investigated as adjuvants and, as already mentioned, the killed pertussis organisms in the 'triple' DPT vaccine appear to act as adjuvants for the diphtheria and tetanus toxoids.

The most recent development in the adjuvant field has been the use of cytokines

It had always been suspected that adjuvants such as CFA and MDP acted partly by inducing cytokines important for lymphocyte triggering differentiation and function such as IL-1, and when purified recombinant cytokines became available it was found that at least three – IL-1, IL-2 and interferon-gamma (IFN-γ) – were indeed effective adjuvants when added to vaccines. IL-1 and IFN-γ have been shown to be particularly useful in cases where the response to a vaccine is impaired (e.g. in hemodialysis patients immunized against hepatitis B).

When to vaccinate
The age of those vaccinated depends upon the age of the vulnerable population

Since most of the diseases that vaccines are designed to prevent affect young children *(Fig. 31.14)*, vaccination is carried out as early as possible, bearing in mind that:

- The presence of maternally-derived antibody reduces the effectiveness of some vaccines, which are therefore usually delayed until the third month of life or later (see Chapter 33).
- Live attenuated vaccines (including vaccinia when it was used) can cause severe disease in immunodeficiency states, which may not be diagnosed immediately after birth.
- If the disease is mainly a risk to the elderly (e.g. pneumococcal pneumonia), vaccination is usually given at a late age.

Figure 31.15 gives the immunization schedule for vaccines in current use. Further details will be found in sections on individual vaccines (see below).

Means of infection control other than vaccines

In the search for new vaccines, we must not lose sight of the fact that some diseases can be controlled equally well by other means. In the developed world, public health measures rather than vaccines (or antibiotics) eliminated malaria and cholera and reduced the incidence of tuberculosis, and it could be argued that tropical diseases such as schistosomiasis or Chagas' disease, could also be controlled by reducing

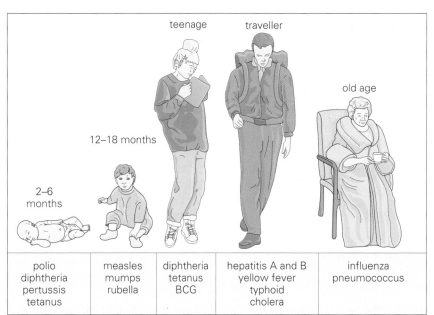

Fig. 31.14 Current vaccine practice. Risk of infection varies with age.

teenage   traveller

old age

12–18 months

2–6 months

| polio diphtheria pertussis tetanus | measles mumps rubella | diphtheria tetanus BCG | hepatitis A and B yellow fever typhoid cholera | influenza pneumococcus |

contact with the snail or insect vector. However, vector control is not easy in practice and like chemotherapy, but unlike vaccination, needs to be maintained more or less indefinitely.

With certain diseases the chance of infection is so slight that a successful vaccine can never justify the cost and effort of producing it, and passive immunization after exposure may be a better approach (e.g. as for snakebite).

Current Vaccine Practice

Vaccines in general use
Diphtheria toxoid is almost universally given with tetanus toxoid and alum, and usually with pertussis vaccine
Although diphtheria toxin loses some antigenicity when converted (by formaldehyde) to the toxoid, it remains a highly effective vaccine. Surprisingly, for a vaccine aimed at the disease rather than the bacterium, it has also reduced the number of carriers of diphtheria, which may imply that the toxin plays a role in the survival or spread of the organism. Diphtheria toxoid is almost universally given with tetanus toxoid and alum, usually with pertussis, in three injections starting at 2–3 months of age plus a later boost. If required, the success of vaccination can be measured by the serum antibody level, or by skin testing. In the Schick test, both toxin and toxoid are injected at different sites: an absent reaction implies a satisfactory level of antibody, an erythematous response to the toxin at 5–7 days indicates inadequate antibody, while an early response at 1–2 days denotes hypersensitivity. Protection is usually 90% or better.

Tetanus toxoid is also highly effective, and is in universal use
However, there are some differences in policy regarding booster injections and the treatment of patients after exposure. In most countries, following the three injections of young children, a booster is given at entry to school, and

another is recommended every 5–10 years. Where exposure is suspected and a booster has not been given within five years, one is given combined with antitoxin if the wound is dirty (see passive immunization, Chapter 32). Reactions to the vaccine are limited to mild hypersensitivity in repeatedly boosted patients, so tetanus toxoid can be considered one of the safest and most effective vaccines.

It is not clear whether pertussis vaccine can cause brain damage, but it does prevent deaths from whooping cough
Mass vaccination against whooping cough was introduced in Britain in 1957, using the whole heat- or formalin-killed vaccine developed during the 1940s. This is given with diphtheria and tetanus toxoid as part of the DTP or 'triple' vaccine, though the later boosts are not given since whooping cough is only a serious disease in young children.

Controversy has surrounded the use of this vaccine. There is no doubt that the incidence of whooping cough has diminished dramatically where the vaccine has been used, but several trials were required to establish statistical evidence for a protective effect. This was partly due to the omission of one of the three serotypes from some batches. In addition, there is no standard vaccine in general use. A more serious controversy concerns undesirable reactions to the vaccine. Mild reactions such as pain, inflammation and fever are quite common, probably due to the endotoxin and other toxins, but in the 1970s studies were published in the UK that claimed that severe screaming attacks, fits and permanent brain damage could follow pertussis vaccination in approximately 1/100 000 injections. The debate still continues about whether this is genuinely cause and effect, but meanwhile the understandable alarm of parents led to a fall of vaccine acceptance to as low as 30%. Predictably, a severe epidemic of whooping cough soon followed in the winter of 1978–1979, with over 100 000 cases and many deaths *(Fig. 31.16)*. This perhaps constitutes the best evidence that the vaccine is in fact effective, but the

ADMINISTRATION SCHEDULE		
vaccine	**UK and USA**	**elsewhere**
'triple' (DTP) vaccine: diphtheria, tetanus, pertussis	primary: given to all at 2–6 months (3 doses at 4-week intervals); booster: 15 months (USA) and 4 years (UK and USA); DT every 10 years (USA)	Japan: primary at 2 years
polio vaccine: Sabin (live, oral)	primary: given to all concomitantly with DTP vaccine; boost: 4 and 16 years (UK), 15 months, 4 years and high-risk adults (USA)	
Salk (killed)	immunocompromised	
'MMR' vaccine: measles, mumps rubella	given to all at 12–18 months; rubella given to seronegative girls at 10–14 years	Africa (WHO program), children at 6 months
BCG: tuberculosis, leprosy*	given to all at 10–14 years (UK); high-risk groups only (USA)	tropics, given at birth
hepatitis B	travellers, high-risk groups (e.g. neonates of carriers, homosexuals, health workers)	Africa and Far East, given to infants
hepatitis A	travellers to endemic areas (e.g. Africa, India, Far East)	
rabies	pre-exposure in high-risk groups (e.g. laboratory, kennel workers); post-exposure in those bitten or licked by animals in endemic areas	
yellow fever typhoid cholera	travellers to endemic areas	tropics, given to infants; yellow fever: boost every 10 years for residents and frequent visitors
meningitis (A+C)	travellers to endemic areas (e.g. parts of Africa, India)	
pneumococcal disease	aged, high-risk groups	
Haemophilus	given to infants at 12 months	
Varicella	given to the immunocompromised and neonates at risk	
influenza	aged, high-risk individuals	

Fig. 31.15 The administration of most vaccines is fairly standard worldwide, but there are important local differences due to variations in risk of infection or in government health policy. (*BCG vaccine also gives some protection against leprosy.) (BCG, bacille Calmette-Guérin; WHO, World Health Organization.)

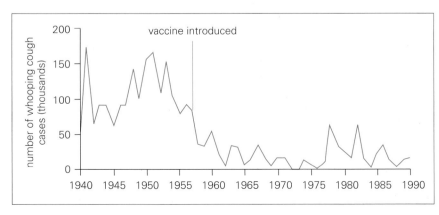

Fig. 31.16 The number of cases of whooping cough notified fell steadily after the introduction of mass immunization in 1958, although epidemics continued to occur at approximately four year intervals. Following the scare about the possible adverse effects of pertussis vaccine, the number of cases rose, and the epidemic in the winter of 1978–1979 was the largest since the introduction of immunization.

controversy undoubtedly damaged the reputation of this vaccine, and of vaccines generally, in the mind of the public.

Not surprisingly, vigorous attempts are now being made to produce a safer vaccine. Among the components of the organism that are considered to be candidates are pertussis toxin (which is responsible for both bacterial adhesion and toxicity) and various other adhesion or toxic molecules, and these are being tried out separately as well as in combination. Some have already come into limited use, for example a two-component vaccine in Japan, which is claimed to be 80–90% effective. Another trial in Sweden has also shown encouraging results. Most recently, a genetically engineered mutant version of the pertussis toxin molecule lacking all toxicity has been proposed as the ideal vaccine, and it seems likely that one or other of these new vaccines will soon be accepted for general use.

Measles is now being considered to be a candidate for worldwide eradication

Live attenuated measles vaccine was introduced in the USA in 1962 and since that time the incidence of the disease, which used to kill over 500 children a year, has shrunk to almost nil. Worldwide eradication could therefore be possible (*Fig 29.6*), but the vaccine would require a considerably better uptake in most other countries than at present.

The principal debate surrounding measles vaccine concerns the best age at which to give the vaccine. Maternal antibody can prevent proper immunization with measles, so it is necessary to wait until at least six months of age. However, even by the age of nine months the vaccine gives only about 80% protection, so in countries where measles is uncommon it is usual to wait until about one year. However, in developing countries, where measles is still widespread, children are likely to be exposed before this age, so the vaccine is generally given at around six months, followed by another dose at one year to protect those who do not respond well to the first. The duration of protection against measles appears to be at least 21 years, though this may be partly due to boosting during natural epidemics, so that as measles disappears from the population, adults may become susceptible again. If so, a logical strategy would be to give a boost as a routine, perhaps at primary or secondary school entry.

Mumps vaccine is most conveniently given with measles and rubella vaccines

What has been said about measles also applies to the live attenuated mumps vaccine. Some countries have questioned the need for a mumps vaccine, but in its absence about 1000 cases per year of mumps meningitis can be expected in the UK, while another calculation predicted 40 deaths and 95 cases of deafness per year in the USA. Mumps vaccine is most conveniently given as part of the MMR vaccine.

Rubella vaccine is given to both boys and girls even though boys do not themselves need such vaccination

Rubella is as relatively mild disease that illustrates vividly the issues that can arise when setting the benefit to the individual against that of the population. In the UK it has until recently been considered that boys do not need vaccinating against rubella and so should not be exposed to the slight risk of vaccine complications; in addition, circulation of wild rubella in the population as a whole is useful in boosting immunity in girls. Therefore the live attenuated vaccine was given only to girls at adolescence to protect them against developing the disease while pregnant and transmitting it to the fetus, resulting in the congenital rubella syndrome.

However, because of its high reproduction rate (see Chapter 32), rubella will maintain its presence in the population indefinitely unless well over 50% of the population are protected. In the USA, therefore, rubella vaccine has been given to boys as well, and this approach (i.e. immunizaton with MMR vaccine at about one year) has recently been adopted in the UK. There is, however, the danger that as the level of infection in the community falls, cases will occur at a later age, therefore actually increasing the chance of fetal damage. Therefore until the disease is eradicated vaccine strategy needs to be carefully tailored to the prevailing situation in each country.

Both oral polio vaccine and inactivated polio vaccine have advantages and disadvantages

The remarkable decline in poliomyelitis is due to the use of one or other of two vaccines:

- The killed virus (Salk 1954).
- The live attenuated virus (Sabin 1957).

Both these vaccines are effective and their advantages and disadvantages are listed in *Figure 31.17*.

The live attenuated oral polio vaccine (OPV) has become the first choice in most countries. Its main advantages are:

- Its lower cost.
- The fact that (as with all live vaccines) immunity is induced in the right place, namely, the mucosal surfaces.
- The prediction that by spreading within the population it will induce 'herd' immunity – this is borne out by the fact that vaccine strains are now more common (e.g. in sewage) in the USA than wild strains.

Against these advantages is the risk of reversion to virulence, particularly by types 2 and 3, which as described earlier, do not differ as much from the wild strains as might be desired. Wild virus has been isolated from the stools within days of vaccination, and there have been several cases of paralytic poliomyelitis, especially in contacts of the vaccine; one estimate put these at 1–2 cases per million. OPV is, of course, not used in immunocompromised patients.

The above considerations have led to the rejection of OPV in favor of an inactivated polio vaccine (IPV) in certain countries, notably Sweden, Finland, Holland and Iceland. Here it is argued that in practice:

- IPV induces equally good immunity.
- IPV might even be more effective in developing countries, where OPV has been somewhat disappointing, presumably because, as was shown for measles, the 'cold chain' between factory and clinic was not adequately maintained.

Surprisingly, the duration of immunity following OPV is not demonstrably longer than with IPV, perhaps reflecting the relatively shorter duration of mucosal than systemic immunity. However, in the absence of substantial herd immunity, a high rate of IPV uptake would be essential for eradication.

ORAL AND INACTIVATED POLIO VACCINES COMPARED		
	inactivated (IPV)	attenuated (OPV)
introduced	Salk 1954	Sabin 1957
in use	Sweden, Finland Holland, Iceland	most other countries
dosage schedule	injection plus alum	oral at 2, 4, 6 months
risks	inadequately killed (very rare) otherwise safe	in immunodeficiency reversion to virulence ?interference by other viruses cold chain failure
advantages	can be added to other childhood vaccines	IgA boosted herd immunity cheaper than Salk vaccine

Fig. 31.17 Poliomyelitis is unusual in that both live attenuated and killed vaccines are available and widely used. Three doses of the attenuated virus vaccine are given as the three types of virus present in the vaccine interfere with each others replication in the intestine. The repeated doses ensure an adequate response to each type. (IPV, inactivated polio vaccine; OPV, oral polio vaccine.)

Clearly, then, although polio vaccination has been highly successful, there is room for further improvements. Two current lines of development are the production of better and cheaper vaccines – both attenuated and inactivated – and the use of combined regimens (e.g. IPV followed by OPV in various sequential combinations).

Calmette and Guérin's attenuated tubercle bacillus (BCG) has been in use for 70 years

However, despite this longstanding use, BCG still inspires fierce debate about its usefulness. This matter is important considering that tuberculosis kills some three million people a year worldwide, and is increasing in countries where AIDS is pandemic.

In its favor is the fact that BCG has given clear protection in controlled trials such as that carried out in the UK (1950) and in the USA on American Indians and Puerto Ricans in the 1970s. Efficacies of 70% or better have also been reported from several South American and African countries. In addition, the same vaccine appeared to be equally effective against leprosy in Uganda and, to a lesser extent, in other countries.

Immunization strategy varies according to the likelihood of infection:

- At birth in high-risk countries.
- At entry to secondary school in the UK and USA (and then only in patients with a negative Mantoux test; see Chapter 9).

One disadvantage of using BCG in countries where tuberculosis is rare is that by causing Mantoux (tuberculin) conversion, it destroys the diagnostic value of this test.

One problem with trials of BCG is the shifting background level of infection, which is dependent upon factors other than vaccination, notably general public health and antituberculous chemotherapy. In countries with a low incidence of disease it would now be impossible to carry out a satisfactory trial based on clinical protection, and there is no rapid test that accurately predicts protection. The tuberculin skin test, widely used as a predictor of protection, has been shown to vary independently of actual protection, and is probably better regarded as a measure of previous exposure rather than immunity.

Another problem is that in other equally well controlled trials, BCG had little or no protective effect. Indeed in two trials, in southern India (1980) and southern parts of the USA, BCG has actually seemed to increase the incidence of tuberculosis. Numerous explanations have been put forward for these extraordinary discrepancies, which are unmatched by any other vaccine. These include differences between vaccine strains (there is no agreed world standard), genetic differences between the human populations, differences in the prevalent clinical pattern of disease, and differences in the type and number of 'environmental' mycobacteria which might modulate the level of immunity in the population.

Quite apart from these debatable effects on tuberculosis, BCG has three other potential uses:

- As an adjuvant for other vaccines.
- As a vector for cloned genes from other organisms (see p. 449).
- As a general non-specific immunostimulant (see Chapter 32).

Vaccines in limited use

Hepatitis B virus vaccine was the first vaccine in human use to be made by recombinant DNA technology

Hepatitis B virus (HBV) vaccine, the most recent vaccine to come into large-scale use, is unusual in several ways. Despite the fact that HBV has not been grown in culture, a non-living antigenic preparation can be derived from the blood of carriers because the surface coat antigen (HBsAg) is over-produced by the virus, and circulates as free non-infectious 22 nm spherical particles (up to 10^{13}/ml of blood; *Fig. 31.18*). When purified and inactivated, so as to be scrupulously free of DNA, these were shown to be at least 95% protective in a controlled trial in American male homosexuals in 1980. The vaccine was licensed for use in the following year, and was given in three doses of 20 mg, at intervals of one and six months. It has three disadvantages:

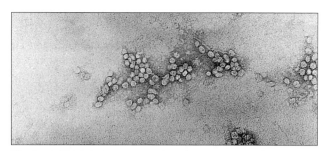

Fig. 31.18 Electron micrograph of purified 22 nm hepatitis B surface antigens expressed in yeast cells. (Courtesy of JR Pattison.)

- Being derived from human blood, it has to be purified with exceptional care because of the risk of transmitting live HBV or other viruses.
- Even after three doses antibody levels start to fall 1–2 years later, so boosting may be necessary. A level of 100 units/l is considered to be protective.
- Finally, it is extremely expensive to make and supplies are limited.

Meanwhile, a second vaccine was produced via recombinant DNA technology – the first such vaccine to go into human use. The same antigen (HBsAg) is involved, the gene being cloned into a yeast vector which produces large amounts of the antigenic protein. Safer and cheaper – about 50% of the cost when introduced, though the plasma-derived vaccine has now come down to the same price – this recombinant vaccine appears to be equally effective. Recent refinements include the insertion of other ('pre-S') genes into the vector, to code for proteins involved in the infectious process. The idea of incorporating HBV genes into a living attenuated vector is also under consideration.

HBV is now clearly a candidate for eventual eradication

Current strategies, however, have to take account of the prevailing level of infection. In the developed world, the vaccines are currently recommended for high-risk groups (*Fig. 31.19*). Since these include a number of likely low- or non-responders (e.g. immunocompromised patients), attention is being directed at the need for further boosts and the use of special adjuvants such as cytokines: both IL-2 and IFN$_\gamma$ have been shown to improve responses to the vaccine in hemodialysis patients.

In Africa, HBV is typically acquired during early childhood, so the vaccine is given at the same time as the usual childhood ones, the major problem being to keep the cost within affordable limits. At present, $1/dose is about the minimum. In the Far East, on the other hand, HBV is commonly transmitted to newborns by mothers who are chronic carriers. Here a course of vaccine injections (at one week, five weeks, nine weeks and one year), is combined with passive immunization with immune globulin. Early results show good protection and it is hoped that the number of carriers will progressively fall, and with it the incidence of liver carcinoma.

Hepatitis A vaccine is available for travellers, but there is no vaccine yet for hepatitis C

Travellers to countries where hepatitis A is endemic can be immunized with a vaccine derived from human diploid cells and formaldehyde inactivated. Until recent years passive immunization with pooled normal human immunoglobulin, which gives good but transient protection, has been the standard method. It is hoped that a vaccine will ultimately be available for the newly discovered hepatitis C virus

Rabies is the only disease where post-exposure vaccination is successful due to its long incubation period

The rabies vaccine is famous for Pasteur's courageous demonstration in 1885 that a desiccated (air-killed) preparation of spinal cord from rabid rabbits would protect humans against rabies, even after infection with the virus (see Chapter 29).

Over one century later, neuro-tissue vaccine (NTV) is still used in some countries, but elsewhere has been replaced by virus grown in human diploid cells, and then inactivated with propiolactone. No safe attenuated virus is yet available, though an attenuated or a genetically engineered vaccine is still a possibility.

For post-exposure cases, a course of 5–6 intramuscular injections, starting as soon as possible, the first combined with an injection of human hyperimmune globulin (20 IU/kg), gives virtually complete protection. Pre-exposure (i.e. for travellers to high-risk areas), 2–3 doses are usually sufficient, with a boost every few years where the risk is maintained (e.g. veterinarians and other animal handlers). Eradication might seem an unattainable goal, but schemes to introduce an attenuated virus to wildlife via infected food bait have been tried out in Switzerland and neighboring countries, as well as Canada, and have had some remarkable success.

Vaccines are available for some arbovirus infections, but notably not for dengue fever

Arbovirus infections are vector-borne fevers and include yellow fever, dengue, south east Asian hemorrhagic fever and Japanese encephalitis. They are among the most virulent virus infections (see Chapter 26), and good vaccines are highly

---

HIGH RISK GROUPS IN WHICH HBsAg VACCINE IS RECOMMENDED

family contacts of known carriers

babies born to HBsAg-positive mothers

medical and nursing staff in high-risk institutes

    e.g. hemodialysis units
           blood banks
           serology laboratories
           dental surgeries
           mental homes

male homosexuals

drug addicts

immunocompromised patients

patients requiring repeated blood transfusion

Fig. 31.19 Hepatitis B vaccines are expensive and are currently recommended only for people at high risk of infection.

desirable. An attenuated yellow fever virus was developed in 1937, and this '17D' strain remains the standard highly effective vaccine for yellow fever. A single subcutaneous dose, with a boost every 10 years for residents in the tropics, or frequent visitors, gives excellent protection and is a requirement for all travellers to endemic countries.

Vaccines are also available against Japanese encephalitis (killed virus), and Rift Valley fever. However, no vaccine is currently available for dengue fever, and this is now recognized as a high priority. One problem is the existence of four serotypes, but a more serious complication is the possibility that one manifestation of the disease may be immunopathologic. This is the 'hemorrhagic shock syndrome' seen in patients infected with a second serotype following earlier exposure to a first. Whatever the mechanism of this condition, there is an obvious possibility that a vaccine that did not protect fully against all serotypes might precipitate the condition.

Vaccines currently used for influenza are only partially effective

Unlike most of the diseases considered so far, influenza does not induce good long-lasting immunity even after recovery from infection in healthy people. This is mainly due to its ability to undergo antigenic 'shift' and 'drift' (see Chapter 17), but also to the curious tendency for responses to different strains to be dominated by antibody against the strain first encountered by the individual ('original antigenic sin'). However, influenza is such an important cause of morbidity and mortality (estimated at 150/million in the USA), that a range of only partially effective vaccines is in use, pending the development of something better.

The most widely used influenza vaccines are formalin- or β-propiolactone-killed viral vaccines, usually including two subtypes of influenza A and one of B, and containing the hemagglutinin (H) and neuraminidase (N) prevalent or anticipated in the population. This vaccine is offered to high-risk groups such as nursing and ancillary staff, the elderly, and patients with chronic respiratory, cardiac, or renal disease, anemia, diabetes mellitus or immunodeficiency. In such patients, efficacy is estimated at about 70% in terms of reducing severity, but only about 30% if total prevention is the criterion. Revaccination in subsequent years is required to maintain antibody levels, but whether with the same or a different strain does not give a further boost of titer.

Trials with live cold-adapted strains have shown some protection, but up to 30% of normal patients may fail to produce antibody and would presumably not be protected. Temperature-sensitive mutants designed to grow in the upper but not the lower respiratory tract have been disappointing, due to reversion to wild type.

An alternative is a recombinant virus containing portions of RNA coding for appropriate H and N antigens. A theoretic advantage of recombinant and other live vaccines would be the induction of cytotoxic T cell memory, which is generally poor or absent with killed viruses. However, viral antigens entrapped in ISCOMs have recently been shown to induce good cytotoxic T cell responses.

A live attenuated VZV vaccine has been shown to be highly protective

Chickenpox, caused by VZV, can occasionally lead to severe complications and is a life-threatening disease in children with leukemia. A live attenuated VZV vaccine has been shown to give up to 95% protection lasting seven years in healthy patients, though considerably less protection in leukemic children on chemotherapy. However, widespread use of VZV vaccine has been discouraged due to:
- Some early cases where severe chickenpox followed vaccination.
- The uncertainty about whether the risk of zoster (shingles) is decreased or even increased.
- The availability of alternative methods of treating chickenpox in children with leukemia (zoster immunoglobulin plus acyclovir).

Nevertheless many authorities consider that it should be added to the triple MMR vaccine for routine use.

Current pneumococcal vaccines contain 23–35 serotypes

Antigenic diversity is a problem with pneumococcal infection. However, since the 84 serotypes of *Streptococcus pneumoniae* are stable in the population and do not show the rapid changes of influenza, it is theoretically possible to produce a complete vaccine containing them all. In practice it has been found that less than half this number is sufficient to protect against the majority of infections.

The antigen used is the capsular polysaccharide prepared from large-scale bacterial culture. The indications for vaccination are similar to those for influenza, and in the USA the vaccine is strongly recommended for the elderly, being appreciably cheaper than the treatment for pneumonia. In children under two, the other main high risk group, the response to the vaccine is generally poor, since the IgG2 class of antibody, which predominates in responses to carbohydrate antigens, develops late and the polysaccharides behave as T-independent antigens.

Conjugation to a protein carrier has been shown to improve the response, presumably by allowing T cells to participate, and trials of protein–polysaccharide conjugates are under way. To conjugate all the available serotypes is, however, a huge task, and it is likely that a smaller number, perhaps about eight, will be used initially.

There is clearly room for improvement, and other approaches are being seriously considered, including protein-based vaccines and the anti-idiotype strategy.

Meningococcal vaccines are only partially effective and only types A and C are used routinely

Here the principle is the same as with the pneumococcus though only three serotypes are needed – types A, B and C. Again the response is less than optimal, particularly in younger children and particularly to the type B polysaccharide, which is a very poor antigen, being largely composed of sialic acid. Current trials of type B conjugated to either tetanus toxoid or to a meningococcal protein (which should theoretically be better) should show how much improvement can be expected.

A problem that has been noted with both pneumococcal and meningococcal vaccines is that other infections, notably even quite mild malaria, interfere with the normal response to the vaccine. Thus it was found in a Nigerian trial that treatment of patients with chloroquine one week earlier improved the anti-polysaccharide responses. This emphasizes the desirability of a malaria vaccine (see below).

Like pneumococcal and meningococcal vaccine, Haemophilus influenzae vaccine is a capsular polysaccharide vaccine

The β serotype of *Haemophilus influenzae* (Hib) is responsible for the most serious disease. Its capsule, a phosphodiester-linked polymer of ribose and ribitol suffers from the same problems as the other polysaccharides – especially low immunogenicity in children under two. Various polysaccharide–protein conjugates are now available, using either tetanus or diphtheria toxoid, given either alone (2–3 doses subcutaneously at 2–6 months) or with the triple DPT vaccine. These appear to induce good antibody and memory responses and, encouragingly, poor initial responders may respond well to later boosting. A large-scale trial in Finland showed 94% efficacy, though this level has not always been achieved elsewhere.

The TY21a strain of typhoid gives 60–90% protection against typhoid lasting at least five years

For nearly a century travellers to the tropics, and particularly military personnel, have been subjected to the 'TAB' vaccine, consisting of heat-, phenol-, alcohol- or acetone-killed whole *S. typhi* and *S. paratyphi* organisms, injected intramuscularly once or twice. Not only is the vaccine fairly unpleasant, with local pain and general malaise due to the endotoxin content, but its efficacy has repeatedly been questioned. In various controlled trials, protection has been estimated at 10–70%, depending partly upon the size of the infecting dose. There is therefore a considerable demand for new and better typhoid vaccines.

Two candidates have emerged:
- A live attenuated organism.
- A capsular polysaccharide.

The first attenuated typhoid bacillus (Ty21a) was produced by random chemical mutagenesis, but current attention focuses on enzyme-deficient strains with mutations in either the galactose epimerase (GalE) or the aromatic aminoacid synthesis pathway (AroA). These mutations allow the bacilli to survive and proliferate for a few days only so that when given orally they induce local immunity in the intestine, but not systemic disease. All these mutant strains appear to be safe and effective, and the latter two have the added advantage of being suitable vectors for inserted genes derived from other organisms. The TY21a strain is given either with a tablet of sodium bicarbonate or in enteric-coated capsules.

The polysaccharide vaccine is composed of purified 'Vi' (virulence) antigen. A single dose of 25 mg has given protection in the 70% range, but as with the other polysaccharides, conjugation to protein is required to induce T-dependent responses and memory.

Current heat-killed V. cholerae vaccines cause unpleasant reactions and give poor protection

Heat-killed whole *V. cholerae* vaccines suffer from the same disadvantages as the older typhoid vaccines – unpleasant reactions and only approximately 50% protection for six months. Vaccination is not recommended, nor legally required for foreign travel. Several replacements are under active study.

Since cholera is essentially a toxin-induced disease, one might expect a toxoid-based vaccine to be sufficient. Some success has been obtained with the B (binding) subunit of the toxin given in combination with whole killed organisms. Another strategy is to construct an attenuated cholera organism with a deletion in the 'A' (toxic) subunit gene. A third idea is to express cholera genes in an attenuated *S. typhi* vaccine which, if it also contained genes from shigellae and *E. coli*, (see below) would constitute a formidable vaccine against enteric bacterial infection. Trials of these different vaccines are under way and should ultimately lead to significantly improved control of cholera.

Experimental vaccines
A live heterologous rotavirus vaccine is a possibility

As mentioned earlier, rotavirus infection might be amenable to a live heterologous vaccine, as was the case with smallpox. Bovine and monkey strains of the virus have been tried as oral vaccines in infants, with 70–80% reported protection. The possibility of using the 'naturally' attenuated human strains that can appear in nurseries is also being explored. Prospects are therefore quite favorable for the eventual availability of a rotavirus vaccine.

A shigella vaccine might be possible using mutated Shigella strains or by inserting shigella antigens into other vectors

Live, randomly attenuated shigella organisms, though fairly effective as oral vaccines, never came into general use because of the short duration of protection and occasional side effects. Current research is concentrated on deliberately mutated strains and on the insertion of shigella antigens into *S. typhi* or other vectors.

A variety of types of E. coli and Mycobacterium leprae vaccines are being investigated

A fully successful vaccine against *E. coli* infection has not yet emerged because of the serotypic diversity of both surface antigens and toxins. However trials have been conducted with toxoids based on the enterotoxins, purified fimbriae, whole killed organisms and live attenuated strains, all of which give some protection. The combined killed cholera/B toxin subunit vaccine mentioned above also gave significant protection against *E. coli* due to cross-reaction between the two toxins.

The effect of BCG in protecting against leprosy (notably in a Ugandan trial) has already been mentioned. Meanwhile trials of combined BCG and killed *Mycobacterium leprae* are under way, and *M. leprae* protein antigens are being cloned for insertion into vectors.

Despite trials there is still no effective malaria vaccine

At the time of writing, several clinical trials of a malaria vaccine have been published, and more will certainly follow. Two were with peptides derived from the major surface protein of the sporozoite (pre-hepatic stage) and others with a hybrid of peptides, mainly from the asexual blood stage. Despite individual cases of protection against a subsequent challenge, the overall results were unimpressive, with marked local variations. Other potential targets for attack within the unusually complex malaria life cycle (see Chapter 25) include the liver stage itself, the merozoite (infective for the red cell), the sexual stages (gametocytes and gametes) and the soluble molecules thought to be responsible for inducing pathology *(Fig. 31.20)*. This wide range of choices clearly increases the chance of success, but each approach has its problems: for example, extensive antigenic variation in the blood stage, and the need for 100% efficacy with the hepatic and prehepatic stages; also the sexual stage vaccines would only block transmission, protecting the community, but not the vaccinee. Each approach has its vigorous proponents, but it seems likely that a successful vaccine will contain antigens from several or all stages.

Three different approaches have given some protection against cutaneous leishmaniasis

These three approaches are:

- 'Leishmanization' with material from active lesions which had some popularity in the former Soviet Union and Israel, but protection is variable and non-virulent disease can never be guaranteed.
- Use of killed promastigotes (the invasive stage), 2–3 times intramuscularly. Up to 80% protection was claimed in a Brazilian trial, but this was of uncertain duration.
- Injection of killed promastigotes plus BCG, which produced the most dramatic results. In a Venezuelan trial over 90% protection was induced, but it is too soon to say for how long this protection lasts.

Vaccines still awaited

There remains a long list of important infectious diseases for which vaccines, although desirable, are not yet available *(Fig. 31.21)*. In some cases it is probably only a matter of time, but in others there are fundamental problems. With the adenoviruses and rhinoviruses, for example, the serotypic diversity (about 40 and 110, respectively) makes it difficult to imagine a

stage		vaccine strategy
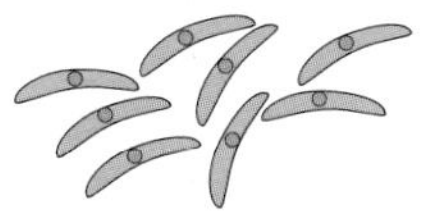	sporozoites	sporozoite vaccine to induce blocking antibody, already field-tested in humans
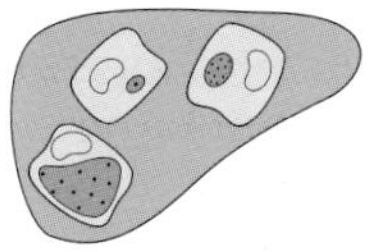	liver stage	sporozoite vaccine to induce cell-mediated immunity to liver stage
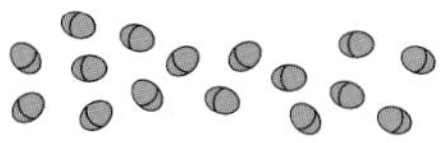	merozoites	merozoite (antigen) vaccine to induce blocking antibody
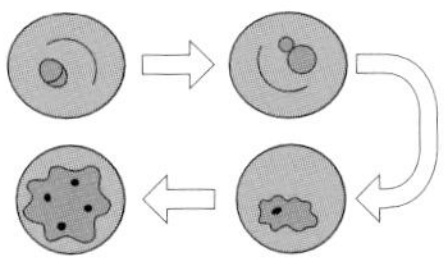	asexual erythrocyte stage	asexual stage (antigen) vaccine to induce other responses to red cell stage, and against toxic products ('anti-disease' vaccine)
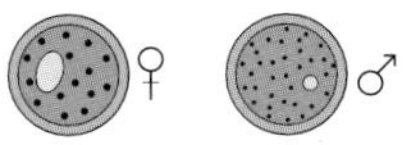	gametocytes	vaccines to interrupt sexual stages – 'transmission blocking' vaccine
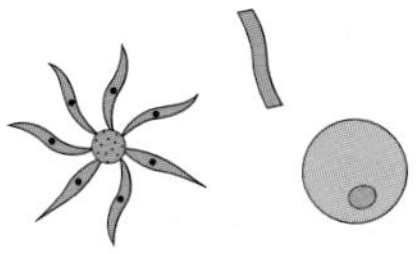	gametes	

Fig. 31.20 Malaria vaccine strategies. A number of different approaches are being investigated, reflecting the complexity of the life cycle and of immunity to this parasite (see Chapter 25).

fully effective vaccine. With the live herpes virus vaccines there is the danger of latency with reactivation, and with the killed vaccines the difficulty of obtaining large amounts of virus (except with herpes simplex). With respiratory syncytial virus, the problem has been reversion of attenuated strains and enhancement of disease by killed vaccines. With the bacterial diseases listed in *Figure 31.21*, it is the lack of convincing immunity following natural infection that is discouraging, syphilis perhaps being the outstanding example. The same applies to the protozoa and helminths, though research is proceeding in a variety of directions, and some quite effective vaccines have been produced for veterinary use (e.g. hookworm in dogs, lungworm in cattle).

The most concentrated effort is probably being directed against HIV, where the production of a vaccine to limit the spread or progression of AIDS is literally a race against time. Most workers have focused on the gp160 molecule by which the virus attaches and fuses itself to cells, and some promising results have been obtained in monkeys with the analogous molecule from simian immunodeficiency virus (SIV), a near relative of HIV2. Several human trials are in progress, but it will be some time before the results are clear, and at present the extraordinarily extensive antigenic variation of this molecule makes success quite problematic.

IMPORTANT INFECTIOUS DISEASES FOR WHICH THERE IS NO SATISFACTORY VACCINE	
organism	**disease**
HIV	AIDS
herpes simplex virus	genital infection
cytomegalovirus	effect on fetus
Epstein–Barr virus	glandular fever
rhinoviruses	common cold
Neisseria gonorrhoeae	gonorrhea
Mycobacterium leprae	leprosy
Treponema pallidum	syphilis
Chlamydia trachomatis	trachoma, urethritis
Plasmodium spp.	malaria
Trypanosoma spp.	trypanosomiasis
Schistosoma spp.	schistosomiasis

Fig. 31.21 Important infectious diseases for which a satisfactory vaccine is not yet available.

- Vaccination aims to prime the adaptive immune system to the antigens of a particular microbe so that a first infection induces a secondary response.
- Vaccines are either live attenuated organisms, killed whole organisms, subcellular fractions or antigens produced artificially by gene cloning or chemical synthesis.
- In general, live vaccines are more effective than other types, but carry the risk of reverting to virulence or inducing disease in immunocompromised patients.
- The details of vaccine choice, route, dose and risks have to be considered for each disease individually, and there is room for considerable improvement in producing safe, effective and affordable vaccines.

1. What are the main safety problems with living vaccines?
2. Which diseases are candidates for elimination by vaccines in the near future?
3. How has recombinant DNA technology contributed to vaccine design?
4. Why is there no vaccine (yet) against the common cold?
5. What are vaccine adjuvants, and why are they needed?

Further Reading

Battle JL, Murphy FL eds. *Vaccine Biotechnology*. London: Academic Press, 1989.

Gregoriadis G, Allison AC, Poste G. Vaccines. Recent trends and progress. *NATO ASI Series A*, volume 215. London: Plenum Press, 1991.

Joint Committee on Vaccination and Immunisation. Immunisation Against Infectious Disease. London: HMSO, 1988.

Mims CA, White DO. Viral Pathogenesis and Immunity. Oxford: Blackwell Scientific, 1984.

Synthetic Peptides as Antigens. CIBA symposium, 1986. 119.

Moxon ER ed, *Modern Vaccines; A Lancet Review*. London: Edward Arnold, 1990.

Introduction

An alternative to vaccination is needed for those who are already infected or are immunodeficient

The most dramatic and successful form of immunotherapy is vaccination, as described in the previous chapter. However, there are some situations where a different approach may be necessary. For instance:

- The patient may already be infected and so a more rapid build-up of immune effector mechanisms than occurs naturally may be needed.
- Alternatively, the patient's immune system may be inadequate and unable to respond either to the infection or to a vaccine, through immunodeficiency or some specially resistant property of the parasite. This chapter deals with such situations.

Passive Immunization with Antibody

Certain diseases are treated by a passive transfer of immunity, which can be life-saving

Before the introduction of antibiotics, acute infectious diseases were often treated by the injection of preformed antibody on the principle that the patient was already ill and it was too late for 'active' vaccination. Indeed, the demonstration that immunity to tetanus and diphtheria could be transferred to mice with serum from vaccinated rabbits was a key experiment in the discovery of antibody in the 1890s. Subsequently, the production of antiserum for the passive treatment of diphtheria, tetanus and pneumococcal pneumonia, and against the toxic effects of streptococci and staphylococci, became an important industry, and generations of horses that had retired from active duty were kept on as the source of 'immune serum'. The introduction of antitetanus serum in the early months of the First World War reduced the incidence of tetanus dramatically by up to 30-fold *(Fig. 32.1)*.

The advent of penicillin and other antibiotics has, of course, changed the picture considerably, and passive immunotherapy is now used for only a select group of diseases *(Fig. 32.2)*. The serum may be specific or non-specific and of human or animal origin.

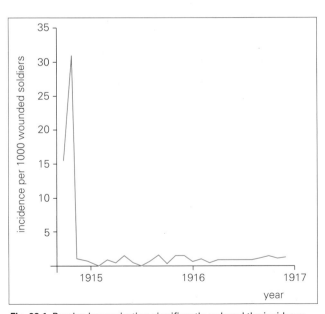

Fig. 32.1 Passive immunization significantly reduced the incidence of tetanus in the early months of the First World War. The figure shows the incidence of tetanus per 1000 wounded soldiers in British hospitals during 1914–1916. There was a dramatic fall after the introduction of antitetanus serum in October 1914.

SPECIFIC PASSIVE IMMUNOTHERAPY WITH ANTIBODY		
infection	**source of antibody**	**indication**
diphtheria	human, horse	prophylaxis, treatment
tetanus	human, horse	
varicella–zoster	human	treatment in immunodeficiencies
gas gangrene	horse	post exposure
botulism		
snake bite scorpion bite		
rabies	human	post-exposure (plus vaccine)
hepatitis B	human	post-exposure
hepatitis A	pooled human immunoglobulin	prophylaxis (travel)
measles		post-exposure

Fig. 32.2 Specific passive immunotherapy with antibody. Although not so commonly used as 50 years ago, passive injections of specific antibody can still be a life-saving treatment.

Specific antibody

The use of antiserum raised in animals can cause serum sickness

The use of antiserum raised in horses or rabbits has largely been abandoned because of the complications resulting from the immune response to the antibody, which is of course a foreign protein. These include progressively more rapid elimination (and therefore reduced clinical effectiveness) and, more seriously, serum sickness due to immune complex deposition in for example the kidney and skin (see Chapter 12), and even anaphylaxis. These complications can be avoided by using human serum taken during convalescence or following vaccination to prevent infection after exposure (e.g. rabies) or to minimize its severity (e.g. varicella in immunodeficient children). However, horse antisera against diphtheria and gas gangrene are still sometimes used.

Theoretically the best form of specific antibody is a monoclonal antibody with a precisely known specificity

In practice, a mixture of several monoclonal antibodies might be required in situations where individual antigens are expressed in low quantities on the microbe or where binding to more than one epitope is required for full effectiveness. Despite some success in animal experiments (e.g. pneumococcal infection in mice and dental caries in monkeys), therapeutic monoclonal antibodies have not yet made a great impact on the treatment of infection. However, a monoclonal antibody against the non-variant lipid portion of Gram-negative bacterial endotoxin is currently undergoing extensive trials for the treatment of septic shock, with some promising results.

INDICATIONS FOR NORMAL IMMUNOGLOBULIN THERAPY
X-linked agammaglobulinemia/hypogammaglobulinemia
common variable deficiency
Wiskott–Aldrich syndrome
ataxia telangiectasia
IgG subclass deficiency with impaired antibody response
chronic lymphocytic leukemia
post-bone marrow transplantation (for CMV)
?AIDS
liver transplant in HBsAg-positive recipients

Fig. 32.3 Indications for normal immunoglobulin therapy. Sufficient antibody to protect immunocompromised patients against common infections can be obtained from pooled normal human plasma. (CMV, cytomegalovirus; HBsAg, hepatitis B surface antigen.)

Non-specific antibody

Antibody in pooled normal serum can provide protection against infection

With common infections, it can be assumed that most normal people have antibody to the pathogen in their serum. The clearest proof of this is that patients with hypogammaglobulinemia can be kept free of recurrent infection by regular injections of IgG from pooled normal serum, and that immunodeficient children can be protected against measles in the same way (Fig. 32.3). Immunoglobulin is prepared from batches of plasma from 1000–6000 healthy donors after screening for hepatitis B and C, and HIV. With improvements in methods of preparation, intravenous injection is now preferred to intramuscular injection in most cases. Dosages for this type of therapy range from 100–400 mg IgG/kg/month.

In healthy individuals the probability of contracting hepatitis A in an endemic area is enormously reduced by a single injection of as little as 5 ml of IgG. The immunity conferred by mothers on their newborn infants by placental transfer of IgG and subsequently by colostral IgA (though the latter is not absorbed, but remains in the intestine) is further evidence for the protective effect of relatively small amounts of antibody.

Non-Specific Cellular Immunostimulation

Cytokines and other molecular mediators stimulate the immune system

The demonstration by William Coley almost one century ago that crude extracts of bacteria could induce remission and sometimes cure cancers indicated the extent to which the immune system can be non-specifically 'overstimulated' with potentially beneficial results. Until recently, many of the compounds used in this way have been of microbial origin, but current interest is directed mainly at cytokines and other molecular mediators, on the principle that their induction was probably the basis of action of the older crude materials (Fig. 32.4).

NON-SPECIFIC IMMUNOSTIMULATORS	
microbial	Coley's toxin (filtered cultures of *Streptococci* and *Serratia marcescens* used against tumors)
	BCG (bacillus Calmette-Guérin)
	Corynebacterium parvum
	endotoxin (lipopolysaccharide)
	streptococcal-derived OK432
endogenous	thymus factors and hormones
	cytokines
	?transfer factor

Fig. 32.4 A variety of foreign and endogenous materials have been used in an attempt to raise the general level of immunologic competence.

Most of the applications of this type of immunostimulation have been in the tumor field, but some infectious diseases respond to treatment with cytokines (*Fig. 32.5*). Foremost among these are the interferons (IFNs), notably IFNα, which is effective in a number of virus infections, though less than might have been predicted from the importance of its normal role in inhibiting viral replication. IFNγ has recently been found to benefit many cases of chronic granulomatous disease (CGD), though the mechanism is unclear. The unpleasant side effects of high-dose therapy with interleukins, IFNs or tumor necrosis factor (TNF) restricts their casual use (*Fig. 32.6*).

There is an interesting 'gray area' where immunostimulation and nutrition overlap

It has been claimed for many years that transfer factor (TF), a dialysed extract of peripheral leukocytes from normal patients, will restore T cell responses in unresponsive recipients, and some dramatic cures (e.g. of chronic mucocutaneous candidiasis) have been reported. Whether this restoration is antigen specific or non-specific has been the subject of great controversy, and in the absence of proper molecular characterization, TF is no longer regarded as an orthodox treatment.

Equally unorthodox, but attracting increasing attention, are a variety of plant products (e.g. saponins, ginseng, Chinese herbal remedies). These substances appear to improve resistance to infection and in some cases also act as adjuvants when combined with vaccines.

Correction of Host Immunodeficiency

Antibody defects are the easiest to treat

This subject is discussed in more detail in Chapter 28, and will only be briefly summarized here:

- Antibody defects are the easiest to treat, since immunoglobulin can be transferred and has a reasonably long half-life (about three weeks for IgG).
- Treatment of T cell defects is much less successful, though thymus or bone marrow grafting has been tried in certain cases (*Fig. 32.7*).
- Phagocytic defects are the most difficult to correct and in practice antibiotics remain the mainstay of therapy, though the future may lie in gene replacement.

Gene defects have recently been identified in certain serious immunodeficiency diseases including hyper-IgM syndrome, CGD and Bruton's agammaglobulinemia.

- Transfer of normal pooled IgG is the most widely practiced type of passive immunotherapy and is used to treat most forms of antibody deficiency.
- Specific antibodies can be used for certain defined conditions.
- Non-specific stimulation of T cell-mediated immunity is still experimental, but cytokines show some promise, particularly IFN for viral infections.

POTENTIALLY THERAPEUTIC CYTOKINES	
IFN-α, IFN-β	hepatitis B (chronic) hepatitis C herpes zoster papillomavirus rhinovirus (prophylactic only) ?HIV warts
IFN-γ	lepromatous leprosy leishmaniasis toxoplasmosis (brain) chronic granulomatous disease
IL-2	leprosy (local treatment to skin lesions)
TNF	anti-TNF in septic shock
IL-1	receptor antagonist in septic shock
IL-10, TGF-β	septic shock
CSFs	bacterial infection due to neutropenia in irradiated patients

Fig. 32.5 Cytokines are increasingly used to improve immunity to infection as well as for some cancers and hematologic disorders. (CSF, colony stimulating factor; IFN, interferon; IL, interleukin; TGF, transforming growth factor; TNF, tumor necrosis factor.)

SOME COMMON SIDE-EFFECTS OF CYTOKINE THERAPY	

interferons	fever
	malaise
	fatigue
	muscle pains
	toxicity to: kidney
	            liver
	            bone marrow
	            heart

IL-2	vascular leak syndrome
	  hypotension
	  edema
	  ascites
	  pulmonary edema
	  renal failure
	  hepatic failure
	mental changes; coma

TNF	shock (as IL-2, with hypotension particularly marked)

Fig. 32.6 Treatment with cytokines, especially if prolonged, can lead to serious side effects. (IL, interleukin; TNF, tumor necrosis factor.)

TREATMENT OF IMMUNODEFICIENCY: AN OVERVIEW				
	B cell defects	**T cell defects**	**phagocyte defects**	**complement defects**
correction of defect	bone marrow graft (SCID)	thymus graft (Di George) ?thymus hormones	?bone marrow graft (CGD)	—
replacement therapy	pooled normal IgG specific IgG	blood transfusion (ADA, PNP deficiency) ?cytokines ??transfer factor	?cytokines	not successful
symptomatic therapy	antibodies	antivirals	antibiotics	antibiotics steroids (for immune complex disease)

Fig. 32.7 The treatment of immunodeficiency depends upon a knowledge of the element at fault, some being more easily restored than others. (ADA, adenosine deaminase; CGD, chronic granulations disease; PNP, purine nucleoside phosphorylase; SCID, severe combined immunodeficiency.)

1. Distinguish between active and passive immunization.
2. What are the common indications for immunoglobulin therapy?
3. Which cytokines are in clinical use?
4. When, if ever, are active and passive immunization used simultaneously?

Further Reading

Allison AC. Immunopotentiation. In: Brostoff J, Scadding GK, Male D, Roitt IM (eds) *Clinical Immunology*. London: Gower Medical Publishing, 1991.

Coley WB. The therapeutic value of the mixed toxins of erysipelas and *Bacillus prodigiosus* in the treatment of inoperable malignant tumours. *Am J Med Sci* 1986;**112**:251.

Parker MT, Collier LH eds. *Topley and Wilson's Principles of Bacteriology, Virology and Immunity,* 9th edition, vol. 1. London: Edward Arnold, 1997.

Epidemiologic Aspects of the Control of Infection and Disease

Introduction

Medical practitioners are primarily concerned with the factors that make each infection unique. However, when considering infection and disease within populations, and their control by vaccination or chemotherapy, a number of general epidemiologic principles emerge. This chapter discusses these principles and explores their relevance to the design of control policies based on vaccination or chemotherapy.

Conflicts between the interests of the individual and those of the community arise in infectious disease epidemiology

This chapter focuses on infection and disease in the community as opposed to in the individual. In most cases what is best for the individual is also best for the community, but this is not always the case. If vaccination carries some risk of inducing serious disease, the optimum policy for the individual is to avoid vaccination while encouraging everyone else to be vaccinated! The resolution of conflicts between the interests of the individual and those of the community is aided by a clear understanding of the precise circumstances in which they arise.

Basic Concepts

Microparasites and macroparasites
Microparasites reproduce directly within the host and are typically transient

'Microparasites' are infectious agents such as viruses, bacteria and some protozoans which reproduce directly – often at very high rates – within the host. They are usually small and have a short generation time. Recovery from infection usually gives immunity against reinfection and, in the case of viral infections, this may be life long. With some important exceptions, the duration of infection is short relative to the life span of the host. Microparasitic infections are, therefore, typically transient.

In defining the epidemiology of these infections it is useful to divide the host population into four classes of individuals:

- Susceptible.
- Infected but latent (i.e. non-infectious); note that this is a different type of latency to that described for persistent infections in Chapter 11.
- Infected and infectious.
- Recovered and immune *(Fig. 33.1)*.

It is also useful to quantify the incubation period (time between infection and disease) and the latent period (time between infection and infectiousness) *(Fig. 33.2)*:

- In some infections (e.g. the herpes viruses), intermittent bouts of infectiousness may occur.
- In other infections (e.g. the AIDS viruses), the degree of infectiousness may vary widely throughout the incubation period. With HIV1, viremia (which is closely correlated with infectiousness) has an early peak a few weeks after infection, followed by a long period of a few to many years of relatively low infectiousness and a final period of very high infectiousness as symptoms of immunodeficiency appear.

The sum of the latent and infectious periods is referred to as the 'generation time' of the infection *(Fig. 33.2)*, a value that helps to determine the frequency with which epidemics may occur (see below). Average latent and infectious periods of some common microparasitic infections are listed in *Figure 33.3*, and distributions of observed incubation periods for hepatitis B virus infection and AIDS in *Figure 33.4*.

Macroparasites do not reproduce directly within the host and are typically not transient

'Macroparasites', such as helminths and arthropods, have no direct reproduction within the definitive host, producing

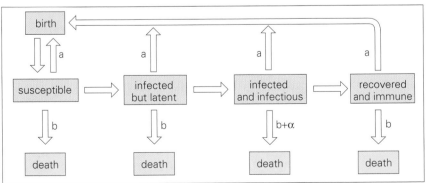

Fig. 33.1 The flow of individuals between susceptible, infected and immune classes in a population exposed to a directly transmitted microparasite. Reproduction at a per capita rate 'a' provides new susceptibles, while death at a per capita rate 'b' removes individuals from the flow. Disease-related death rate 'α' is additional to 'b' in the infectious group. New infections arise as infectious and susceptible individuals mix.

The Science of Epidemiology

Epidemiology is the study of the occurrence, spread and control of diseases. It is based upon the collection of detailed statistical information and can be undertaken at several levels, from the purely descriptive to the analytical and experimental, in which mathematical modelling plays an increasingly important part. Epidemiological data can be used to record the diseases affecting a population and, where infectious, to identify their causes and modes of transmission. They can also be used to predict the future likelihood of infection, to identify risk factors, and to plan control programs.

Like all sciences, epidemiology has its own jargon and specialized use of terms

Infection is the term used to indicate the presence of an infectious organism in an individual or population. The term *disease* is used only when infection has detectable clinical consequences, whether mild or severe. The time interval between exposure to infection and appearance of disease is the *incubation period*. Individuals who are infected and can transmit infection to others are *infectious*. Infectiousness may persist after disease has disappeared, the individuals concerned being known as *carriers*. The carrier state may also occur without disease ever having been apparent. Spread of infection – *transmission* – occurs in many ways, but depends upon direct or indirect contact between infectious individuals and individuals who are susceptible (see Chapter 8).

Infection may lead to an acquired immunity, and immune individuals are then often *resistant* to further infection.

In populations, infection or disease is described as *endemic* if it occurs regularly at low or moderate frequency, or *hyperendemic* if frequency is high. *Epidemics* occur when there are sudden increases in frequency above endemic levels; *pandemics* are global epidemics. *Prevalence* describes the number of cases of infection or disease in members of a population, either at a given point in time (*point* prevalence) or over a given period (*period* prevalence). *Seroprevalence* refers to the number of individuals who are antibody positive for a particular infection. The appearance of such antibodies in individuals is called *seroconversion*. *Incidence* refers to the number of new cases arising in a population over a defined period of time. *Age-specific* prevalence or incidence refers to infection or disease within particular age groups. Prevalence and incidence may show periodic fluctuations or trends over time (often referred to as longitudinal trends). *Secular* trends are long-term changes over periods of years, whereas *periodic* trends are shorter term (months to a few years). *Seasonal* trends are annual or monthly changes, reflecting climatic or behavioral factors, and *acute* trends are those that result in epidemic outbreaks.

Descriptive epidemiologic data can be collected during outbreaks or collected subsequently

The more complete the data, the more fruitful analysis is likely to be. Accordingly, it is necessary to record not only data relating to the infection itself, but also demographic, geographic, climatic, socioeconomic, behavioral and personal data. Division or *stratification* of a population by such parameters is a useful way of seeing whether infection is associated with particular characteristics.

Analytical epidemiology uses two basic approaches, case control and cohort studies

Case control studies are *retrospective*, taking a group in which infection or disease is present and comparing with a matching control group in which it is absent in order to identify cause and effect. Cohort studies are normally *prospective*. They monitor the appearance of infection or disease in carefully defined groups over a prolonged period. Again, comparison with a control group is used to identify cause and effect. A third form of analysis is *epidemiologic investigation*, the study of epidemics as they occur. This involves collection of all relevant data in an attempt to identify the infectious agent and its transmission and to define control measures.

Experimental epidemiology applies epidemiologic methods to experimental systems

Such experimental systems include drug or vaccine trials, in which individuals with or without disease, or exposed or nonexposed to infectious agents, are given specific therapy, and the results compared with individuals given placebos or alternative therapy. Experimental epidemiology requires detailed statistical planning and analysis.

Mathematical modeling is a powerful tool in epidemiology

Mathematical modeling of infection and disease in populations is applied in descriptive, analytical and experimental epidemiology and is a powerful interpretive as well as a predictive tool with very wide applicability to disease control.

Surveillance

In many countries, public health authorities carry out continuing epidemiologic surveys of particular diseases in the national population (e.g. the Centers for Disease Control (CDC) of the US Public Health Service and the Communicable Diseases Surveillance Centres (CDSC) of the Public Health Laboratory Service in the UK). The World Health Organization performs a similar role internationally. At a national level, surveillance is often based on notifiable diseases, practitioners being obliged to report these diseases when they occur in their patients (*morbidity* data). Surveillance records can also be taken from notified causes of death (*mortality* data), from reports sent in by diagnostic laboratories, from population surveys and from detailed case investigations. Such data are then published regularly, for example in the *American Morbidity and Mortality Weekly Report* (MMWR), and the weekly *UK Communicable Diseases Report* (CDR), so that the medical community is alerted to trends in patterns of disease, and recommendations for control are made quickly and efficiently.

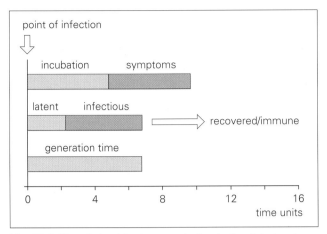

Fig. 33.2 The relationships between the incubation, latent and infectious periods for a hypothetical microparasitic infection. Note that the infectious period and the duration of symptoms of disease are not necessarily synchronous. The generation time is the sum of the latent and infectious periods (see text).

infectious disease	incubation period (days)	latent period (days)	infectious period (days)
measles	8–13	6–9	6–7
mumps	12–26	12–18	4–8
whooping cough (pertussis)	6–10	21–23	7–10
rubella	14–21	7–14	11–12
diphtheria	2–5	14–21	2–5
varicella	13–17	8–12	10–11
hepatitis B	50–110	13–17	19–22
poliomyelitis	7–12	1–3	14–20
influenza	1–3	1–3	2–3

TIME COURSE OF COMMON INFECTIONS

Fig. 33.3 Incubation, latent and infectious periods for a variety of viral and bacterial infections.

transmission stages that pass to the exterior to complete their life cycle. They are typically large and their generation times can often be a significant fraction of the host's life span. Immunity tends to be of a relatively short duration once the parasites are removed, and infections are often persistent, with hosts being continually reinfected. Infections are rarely uniformly or even randomly distributed *(Fig. 33.5)*, most people harboring few parasites and a few harboring many. Models based on dividing populations into susceptible and infected persons are therefore inappropriate. The most useful epidemiologic framework records the prevalence, average intensity and distribution of infection within the population.

Calculating the spread of infection – the basic reproductive rate (R0) and the effective reproductive rate (R)

For a microparasite, R0 is the average number of secondary cases of infection produced by one primary case in a completely susceptible population.

R_0 is also referred to as the 'case reproductive rate' or the 'transmission potential' and this definition of R_0 applies to an idealized situation. However, host populations are rarely, if

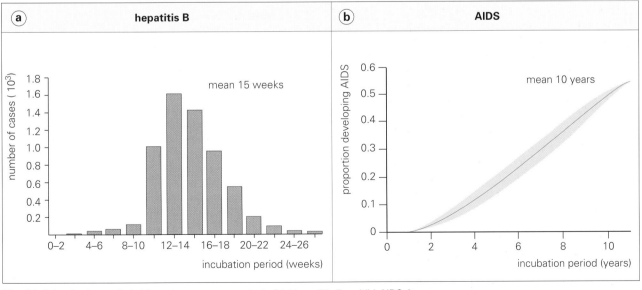

Fig. 33.4 Incubation periods (time since seroconversion) of (a) hepatitis B and (b) AIDS, in sexually active adults. (b) Shows the range of data from different studies in various urban centers in Europe and North America.

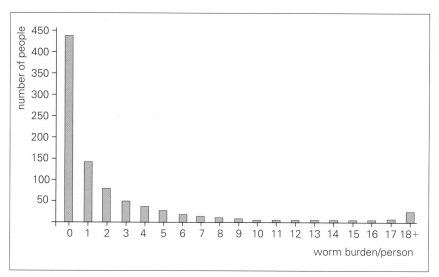

Fig. 33.5 The frequency distribution of the human roundworm *Ascaris lumbricoides* in a rural community in Korea.

ever, completely susceptible as many factors operate to reduce the susceptibility of individuals and the spread of infection is always subject to some constraints. Under these (more realistic) conditions the reproductive rate is best described by the symbol R – the effective reproductive rate. For example, when an infection becomes established in a population and 'herd' immunity develops, the proportion of susceptible individuals will decrease. Eventually some sort of equilibrium is reached (endemic infection), although there may be fluctuations of a seasonal or longer term nature. One example is the seasonal cycle in the incidence of measles, imposed on a regular two-year cycle, which was clearly observable before the introduction of mass vaccination (see *Fig. 33.11*, below).

R = R_0 × the fraction of the community that is susceptible

At equilibrium, the rate at which susceptible individuals are infected is exactly balanced by the rate at which new susceptibles are born into the community, each infection on average producing one secondary case (i.e. the effective reproductive rate is R = 1). In a homogeneously mixed community, R is equal to the basic reproductive rate R_0 discounted by x, the fraction of the community that is susceptible (i.e. $R = R_0x$). Given that at equilibrium R = 1, then $R_0 = 1/x^*$, where x^* is the fraction susceptible at equilibrium. This simple relationship provides a method of estimating the value of R_0 from serologic or other data on age-specific susceptibility.

For a macroparasite, R_0 is the average number of female offspring produced throughout the lifetime of a mature female

Offspring achieve reproductive maturity themselves in the absence of density-dependent regulation. Density-dependent regulation includes competition for space or other resources, and acquired immunity. Theoretically, in the absence of these regulatory mechanisms parasite numbers within the population would grow without constraint, provided $R_0 > 1$. In practise, because of such constraints, macroparasite populations tend to be rather stable.

Other methods of estimating R_0
The initial exponential rise in the proportion of people infected by a micro- or macro-parasite depends upon the magnitude of R_0

We can sometimes observe an infection in its initial phase of invasion, such as with the AIDS virus HIV1 or when macroparasites begin to re-establish themselves after chemotherapy. In both cases the initial exponential rise in the proportion of people infected depends upon the magnitude of R_0. The rate of this rise, Λ, is simply given by $\Lambda = (R_0-1)/D$, where D is the average duration of infectiousness of an individual with a microparasitic infection, or the average life expectancy of an adult macroparasite. This provides a further method of estimating the transmission potential of an infectious agent (R_0).

R_0 can be estimated from serologic surveys by calculating the fraction of the total population susceptible to infection

For most common viral and bacterial infections, serologic tools are available to establish whether or not a person has acquired and recovered from infection at some time in their life. Age-stratified cross-sectional serologic surveys or longitudinal cohort studies provide the best data for estimating the magnitude of R_0 in a given community. *Figure 33.6* shows the decay in maternally-derived antibodies and the subsequent rise in antibody positive individuals due to infection in an unvaccinated population. The magnitude of R_0 can be estimated from this profile by calculating the fraction of the total population susceptible to infection, or equally simply from $R_0 = (L-M)/(A-M)$, where L is life expectancy, M is the average duration of maternal antibody-derived protection (typically six months for many common viral infections such as measles), and A is the average age at infection. The key quantity is A, which can be estimated directly from the serologic profile:

- If A is low, R_0 is large and the infection has high transmission efficiency.
- If A is high, R_0 is small and transmission efficiency is low.

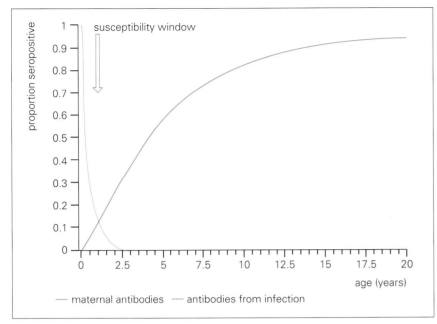

Fig. 33.6 An age-stratified serologic profile recording the presence or absence of antibodies specific to the antigens of a directly transmitted childhood viral infection (average age at infection is five years). There is a susceptibility window between the decay in maternally derived antibody and the rise in seroprevalence due to infection.

Figure 33.7 lists some estimates of A for a variety of common infections in unvaccinated communities. Transmission success can vary widely; in developing countries values of A are typically much lower than those in the UK or the USA.

Serologic surveys provide valuable information about the transmission dynamics of infectious agents

Serologic surveys provide information on:
- The duration of maternally-derived protection.
- The average age at infection.
- The optimum age at which to vaccinate.
- The fraction of the population that should be immunized to block transmission.

However, problems can arise if the duration of measurable antibody production following infection is not life-long, as is the case for many bacterial and protozoan infections, and more sophisticated techniques to detect immunologic markers of past infection are needed.

Behavior influences the spread of infection
For an infection – except an STD – to take hold, the density of susceptible people must exceed a critical value

In the case of a directly transmitted respiratory viral infection, $R_0 = \beta \times D$, where X is the density of susceptible people, β is the transmission coefficient, a composite term defining the rate of mixing and the probability of transmission per contact between susceptible and infectious persons, and D is the average duration of infectiousness. For the infection to take hold R_0 must be equal or greater than 1, which implies that the density of susceptible people must exceed a critical value X_T given by $X_T = 1/(\beta D)$. This concept clarifies the target for mass vaccination programs. To eradicate the infection the density of susceptibles must be reduced below X_T.

R_0 of sexually transmitted diseases depend upon the average rate of new sexual partners

The average rate at which new sexual partners are acquired is usually independent of population size. Sexually transmitted diseases (STDs), which often produce long-lasting infections (e.g. herpes virus, HIV and untreated gonorrhea) are therefore ideally suited to persisting in low density human communities.

AVERAGE AGE AT INFECTION FOR DIFFERENT INFECTIONS IN DIFFERENT LOCALITIES		
infectious disease	average age at infection A (years)	source of data
measles	5–6	USA, 1955–58
	4–5	England and Wales, 1948–68
	1–2	Thailand, 1967
	2–3	India, 1978
rubella	9–10	Sweden, 1965
	9–10	Manchester, UK, 1970–82
	2–3	Gambia, 1976
	6–7	Poland, 1970–88
varicella	6–8	USA, 1921–28
poliomyelitis	12–17	USA, 1955
pertussis	4–5	England and Wales, 1948–68
	4–5	USA, 1920–60
mumps	6–7	England and Wales, 1975–77
	6–7	Netherlands, 1977–79

Fig. 33.7 Average age at infection (A) for different infections at different localities before widescale immunization.

Many behavioral or spatial factors can influence the transmission of infectious agents

Behavioral factors are of particular importance for sexually transmitted infections such as gonorrhea or HIV infection since there is great variability in the rate at which individuals acquire different sexual partners *(Fig. 33.8)*. If sexually active individuals acquire partners in different sexual activity classes in proportion to their representation in the population, then the value of R_0 depends upon the rate at which new sexual partners are acquired multiplied by the probability of transmission at each partner contact multiplied by the average duration of infectiousness. The value of R_0 can be greatly influenced by the variance in sexual activity. Those who have many sexual partners are both more likely to acquire and to transmit infection and therefore play a key role in the persistence of such infections in the community of sexually active individuals, the majority of whom have very few sexual partners *(Fig. 33.8)*.

Transmission between groups

Populations can be stratified using many factors such as age, sex, sexual activity and residence location.

Patterns of population mixing are important in designing policies to control infection

Intensity of transmission will differ within different groupings but, equally importantly, contact between groups can also play a key role in determining patterns of infection and disease. In these circumstances, R_0 will be influenced by both within and between-group transmission rates (i.e. by the likelihood of an individual in one group making contact with someone in the same group or in another group). In the case of STDs, the sexual partner contact pattern may be described as a 'mixing matrix'. The importance of these mixing matrices as determinants of epidemiological trends is illustrated in *Figure 33.9*. This records a simulated epidemic of HIV1 in a male homosexual community in the UK, assuming either random choice of sexual partners or highly assortative choice (like with like) in which those who change partners frequently choose the majority of their sexual partners within their own sexual activity class with all other parameters remaining the same:

- Random choice generates a slowly developing epidemic with wide dissemination of infection within the community.
- In contrast, assortative mixing generates a rapidly growing epidemic, which is of smaller magnitude (largely restricted to the high activity groups) and may show multiple peaks in the incidence of infection, as waves of infection gradually pass from high to lower sexual activity classes.

Different patterns of mixing, whether due to spatial, behavioral or demographic factors, are of great importance in the design of policies for the control of infection.

Patterns of mixing are influenced by the timing of school terms and vacations

For common directly transmitted viral and bacterial infections (measles, rubella, mumps and pertussis), high rates of transmission occur among young children attending primary or secondary schools (5–15 year olds), and this age group serves to seed infection via family contacts in younger and older persons.

Spatial factors are also important. In many developed countries, with a generally high level of vaccination coverage, pockets of infection persist in poor communities or ethnic minorities in major urban centers with low rates of vaccine uptake. Targeting vaccination at children before they enter primary school, and at young children in poor urban centers, is an effective way of minimizing between-group transmission.

People with many sexual partners are an obvious target for treatment and education

For STDs, those who change sexual partners frequently serve as a core group of transmitters who maintain infection in the larger population of sexually active people. This group is an obvious target for treatment (in the case of gonorrhea and syphilis) and education about safer sex practises (most importantly in the case of HIV1).

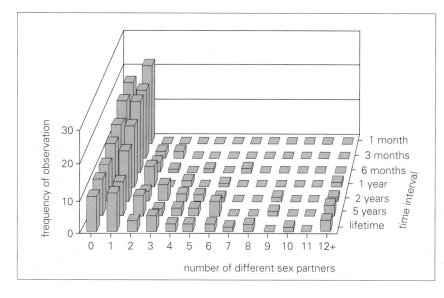

Fig. 33.8 Frequency distribution of claimed number of different sexual partners over various time periods (one month to lifetime) recorded in a survey of male and female students in 1987 in the UK.

Changes in incidence of infection
Many common directly transmitted viral and bacterial infections show regular peaks in incidence

Many countries have public health surveillance systems that record the incidence of certain notifiable diseases. These often extend back to the early part of this century, providing excellent long-term data with which to assess changes in the incidence of particular infections. What can be learned from these notification records? First, they enable one to ask whether observed changes in incidence are more regular than would be expected from chance alone. Long runs of data make it possible to measure the mean inter-epidemic period (the time interval between major peaks in incidence). A striking feature of many common directly transmitted viral and bacterial infections is the regularity of such peaks in incidence. They are usually of two kinds:

- Seasonal (e.g. the effects of school terms and vacations on childhood infections).
- Longer term. Before mass vaccination, the longer term inter-epidemic period for measles in the UK was two years while for pertussis it was 3–4 years (*Fig. 33.10* and see Chapter 31).

These intervals are determined not by chance, but by interactions between the infectious agent and its host. They are generated by fluctuations in the value of R, below and above unity. At the start of an epidemic cycle the infectious agent spreads rapidly. As the epidemic progresses, and the susceptible pool is depleted, more and more contacts are with individuals who are immune and eventually the R falls below unity and incidence begins to decline. This decline continues until the pool of susceptibles is replenished by new births, the density of susceptibles eventually rising to a level sufficient to trigger the next epidemic.

The inter-epidemic period for infections is related to the average age at infection and the duration of the average generation time

Simple theory predicts that the average inter-epidemic period for those infections that induce lasting immunity to reinfection is related to the average age at infection and the duration of the average latent and infectious periods (i.e. the average generation time, *Fig. 33.2*). This theoretical prediction agrees with observed trends for a wide variety of infections and emphasizes two important general points:

- First, the average age at infection is inversely related to the transmission potential of the organism concerned (the value R_0), hence infections with high transmission potential have short inter-epidemic periods and vice versa.
- Second, infections with short generation times will have short inter-epidemic periods if they also have high transmission success, and vice versa (*Fig. 33.10*).

These factors, combined with the ability to induce lasting immunity in those who recover from infection, determine whether or not an infectious disease will exhibit longer term fluctuations in incidence. Infectious diseases like gonorrhea will not (apart from seasonal fluctuations) because of their inability to induce lasting immunity. The same is true for AIDS, but this disease has an additional factor that mitigates against recurrent epidemics, namely a very long incubation period (an average period of at least 10 years, *Fig. 33.4*).

The transmission success of an infection is inversely measured by the average age at infection

The transmission success of an infection will vary between communities because of differences in demographic parameters (net birth rate) and behavioral factors (patterns of mixing). For example, the inter-epidemic period for measles

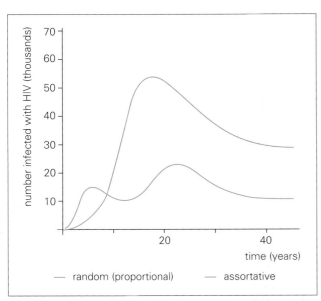

Fig. 33.9 Influence of the sexual partner mixing matrix (preferences) on the predicted changes with time in the number of HIV1 infected individuals in a population of homosexual men. One trajectory assumes random (proportional) mixing between the different sexual activity classes (defined according to rates of sexual partner change) while the other assumes assortative (like with like) mixing; all other parameters were kept the same.

INTER-EPIDEMIC PERIOD OF SOME COMMON INFECTIONS		
infectious disease	inter-epidemic period T (years)	source of data
measles	2 1 1	England and Wales, 1948–68 Yaounde, Cameroun, 1968–75 Ilesha, Nigeria, 1958–61
rubella	3–5	Manchester, UK, 1961–83
mumps	3	England and Wales, 1960–80
poliomyelitis	3–5	England and Wales, 1948–82
pertussis	3–4	England and Wales, 1948–85

Fig. 33.10 Inter-epidemic period (T) of some common infections, at different localities.

in large urban centers in Africa or India before the introduction of mass vaccination was often one year. In contrast, in the UK and the USA the period was typically two years. The difference is a direct reflection of difference in the average age at infection *(Fig. 33.7)*.

Mass vaccination reduces transmission success

It therefore acts to increase the average age at infection. The implications of this are discussed on pages 474 and 475, but one consequence is an increase in the inter-epidemic period *(Fig. 33.11)*. Therefore mass vaccination not only alters the incidence of infection, but affects the age distribution of cases and the temporal pattern of fluctuations.

Community-Based Control by Vaccination

Different vaccination coverage is needed to eradicate different infections

Other things being equal, the larger the value of R_0, the harder it will be to eradicate an infection by mass vaccination from the community in question. In a 'homogeneously mixing' population, eradication will be achieved if the proportion successfully immunized, p, exceeds a critical value, p_c, where $p_c = (1-1/R_0)$, so that too few susceptibles remain to perpetuate transmission (i.e. $X < X_T$ or $x < x^*$). Therefore, the larger the value R_0 the higher the coverage (p_c) needed to eliminate infection. p_c values for various vaccine-preventable childhood viral and bacterial infections are listed in *Figure 33.12*.

Global eradication of measles, with its R_0 of 15–17 and p_c of 92–95%, will almost certainly be more difficult than the eradication of smallpox (R_0 2–4). In the USA, where measles/mumps/rubella (MMR) vaccination is essentially compulsory before entry to primary school (see Chapter 31),

the average age at infection for rubella before immunization was about nine years, compared with around five years for measles. The R_0 value for rubella is roughly half that for measles, and rubella has been effectively eradicated by the vaccination program. The incidence of measles on the other hand has declined more slowly and continues to show local flare-ups in poor urban centers with low vaccine uptake.

Average age at vaccination must be less than average age at infection for eradication

Much depends upon the influence of maternally-derived antibodies against the infectious agent, and on the likelihood that vaccination will give good protection. For most live vaccines (e.g. MMR) efficacy is reduced if high titers of maternal antibodies are present. These typically decay to undetectable levels at around six months to one year *(Fig. 33.6)*. The subsequent rise in seropositivity in an unvaccinated community reflects immunity acquired via natural infection. The trough in seropositivity at about one year is obviously the optimum age to vaccinate, but high efficacy or high potency vaccines, such as those recently developed against measles and mumps, allow effective vaccination at younger ages when maternal antibodies are still present. This is particularly important in high transmission areas in developing countries, where the susceptibility age window for vaccination may be very narrow *(Fig. 33.6)* and, more importantly, where the fraction susceptible to infection at this age may be less than the critical proportion of infants that must be immunized to block transmission.

When vaccination does not take place soon after birth or when a broad age range of children is immunized, the estimation of the critical fraction to be immunized to eliminate infection must take account of the average age at vaccination. For eradication to be possible the average age at vaccination must be less than the average age at infection, and cohort vaccination should therefore focus on young infants, taking account of vaccine performance in those with maternal antibodies.

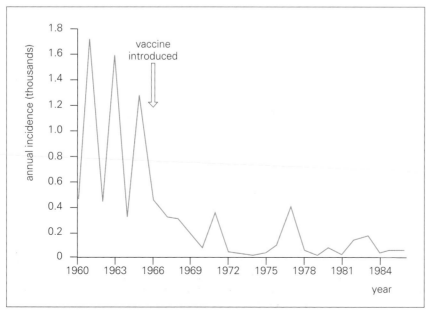

Fig. 33.11 Annual measles notification in an urban population over the period 1960–1985. Before mass vaccination two-year cycles are clearly apparent in the fluctuations in incidence. The introduction of measles vaccination in 1966, combined with high levels of vaccine uptake among young children, resulted in a significant increase in the period between epidemics. (Data from the Office of Population Censuses and Surveys, UK.)

A two-stage vaccination program can eradicate certain infections

There are difficulties in eradicating infections such as measles in major urban centers in some developing countries where the average age at infection is often between 1–2 years *(Fig. 33.7)*. To block transmission, more than 97% of infants would have to be effectively immunized before their first birthday. In practise this is impossible. An alternative approach is a two-stage vaccination program, for example, targeted at infants around one year of age and then young children at around 2–3 years of age:

* The first stage acts to reduce transmission efficacy (but not to block transmission) and hence widens the age window of susceptibility in which vaccine can be administered.
* The second stage attempts to block transmission via the creation of very high levels of herd immunity.

100% vaccination coverage is not needed to eradicate infection

Immunization has both a direct and an indirect effect. The direct effect protects those successfully immunized and results in fewer infected individuals to transmit infection to those still susceptible. The latter therefore benefit indirectly from those who have been immunized. The effective proportion of susceptibles will eventually fall below the level required to maintain $R_0 > 1$ ($X < X_T$), even though immunization coverage is less than 100%.

Mass immunization at levels below those needed to block transmission obviously reduces the incidence of infection. Surprisingly, it has little impact on the total number of individuals remaining susceptible *(Fig. 33.13)*. As long as the infection remains endemic the fraction remaining susceptible depends only on R_0, and not on whether those

CRITICAL VACCINATION COVERAGE TO BLOCK TRANSMISSION OF CERTAIN CHILDHOOD INFECTIONS			
infectious disease	average age at infection before immunization* (years)	case reproductive rate (R_0)	critical vaccination coverage (p_c)
measles	4–5	15–17	92–95%
pertussis	4–5	15–17	92–95%
mumps	6–7	10–12	90–92%
rubella	9–10	7–8	85–87%
diphtheria	11–14	5–6	80–85%
poliomyelitis	12–15	5–6	80–85%
* in developed countries			

Fig. 33.12 Estimates of vaccination coverage necessary to block transmission of certain vaccine-preventable childhood viral and bacterial infections.

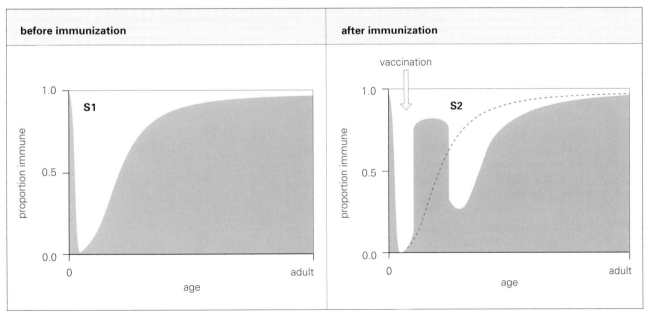

Fig. 33.13 Predicted impact of mass immunization against a typical childhood viral or bacterial infection on the age distribution of susceptibility in a population. Before immunization there is a 'valley' of susceptibility (S1) in the young age classes. Vaccination reduces the rate of transmission, creating an upward shift in the age at which susceptibles acquire natural infection. Paradoxically, mass childhood vaccination does not alter the fraction of the population that is susceptible (i.e. area S2 = S1).

losing susceptibility did so as a result of immunization or natural infection.

Mass vaccination can have indirect effects

Mass vaccination at below eradication levels reduces the probability of an unimmunized individual acquiring infection. In consequence, infection tends to be acquired at an older average age than before vaccination *(Fig. 33.13)*. If the risk of disease associated with infection increases with age, a program of immunization at levels below that required to block transmission (i.e. below p_c) can have perverse complications. The outcome depends upon precisely how the risk of serious disease per case of infection changes with age *(Fig. 33.14)*. For example measles can lead to encephalitis in a small fraction of those infected. The risk increases with age at infection, but all levels of vaccination coverage reduce both the incidence of infection and the incidence of disease. Rubella and mumps are different since mass vaccination at certain levels of coverage will reduce the incidence of infection, but increase the incidence of serious disease.

Mass vaccination can increase the risk of serious disease associated with rubella or mumps

Rubella can damage babies whose mothers are infected in the first trimester of pregnancy. The risk of this damage is therefore proportional to the age-specific fertility profile for a given country *(Fig. 33.14a)*. Vaccinating, say, 50% of all two year olds would reduce the total number of cases of rubella but push the average age of the small number who become infected towards the childbearing years. If very high levels of coverage can be attained (under a compulsory program, as in the USA, or a highly coordinated system of recall, incentives and surveillance, as in the UK), eradication can be achieved by vaccinating successive cohorts of 1–2 year olds. If levels of vaccine uptake under a voluntary scheme only reach 60–70% (as in the UK earlier in the rubella vaccination campaign), vaccination should be confined to early teenage girls before they join the 'pregnancy' age classes, so that infection can spread and confer immunity at younger ages. How can we tell at what level of coverage to switch from one strategy to the other? Epidemiologic calculations suggest that a switch to the mass cohort strategy (where MMR is offered to 1–2 year olds) is advisable provided that more than 70% of boys and girls can be immunized by two years of age. A two-stage program of adding vaccination of 1 to 2-year-old boys and girls to an existing strategy focused on teenage girls would have little effect on disease, provided uptake in 12 to 13-year-old girls was high (80–90%) before MMR was added to the program. Some benefit will accrue over 10 years or more once the uptake of MMR in 1–2 year olds reaches very high levels (90%).

Mumps can lead to complications *(Fig. 33.14b)* such as meningitis and/or encephalitis, which occur in approximately 10% of all diagnosed cases, and orchitis, which occurs in about 27% of clinical cases in postpubertal males. Case complication rates are age- and sex-related. Inclusion of the mumps vaccine in the child immunization program in the UK began in October 1988 with the introduction of MMR. Analysis shows that the incidence of serious disease will

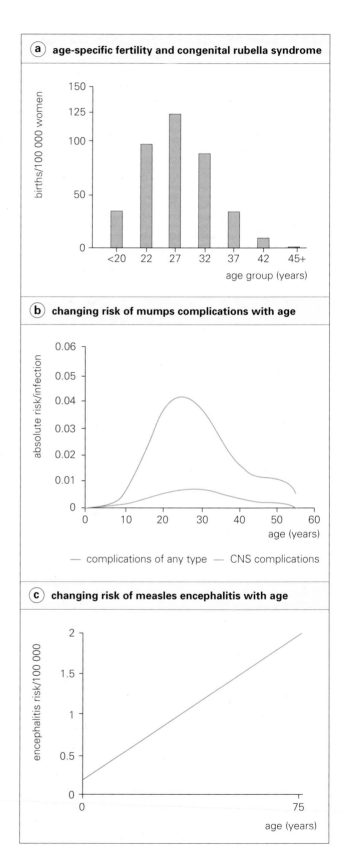

Fig. 33.14 Age-dependent risk of complications from infection. (a) Age-specific fertility of women, as shown, directly influences the risk of congenital rubella syndrome in infants. (Data for the UK.) (b) Changes in the absolute risk of complications from mumps infection in the UK relative to age. (c) Changes with age in the risk of measles encephalitis in the USA.

increase if vaccine uptake levels are less than approximately 60–70% of 1–2 year olds. Higher levels of uptake, as have now been achieved, should reduce both the incidence of infection and infection-related complications.

Abrupt introductions or changes in immunization programs perturb the nature of herd immunity in the population because of sudden reductions in the transmission potential of the infectious agent. As stated above, the fraction susceptible remains the same, it is simply the distribution of susceptible individuals across age classes that changes.

Factors Influencing the Success of Vaccination

Vaccine success is influenced by population density

The design of immunization programs, particularly in developing countries, is influenced by variations in population density. In small villages in rural areas, population density and the associated net birth rates may be too low for the endemic maintenance of infections such as measles or pertussis (see Chapter 8). However, people living in these regions are at risk from contact with large urban centers. One solution is to target vaccination coverage in relation to group size, with dense groups receiving the highest levels of coverage. In some circumstances transmission can be blocked by high levels of mass immunization in the urban centers alone, since they provide the reservoir of infection for the low density rural regions.

High vaccine coverage in infants and children, particularly in poor communities, must be a central aim in national immunization programs

Programs in developed countries may be influenced by regional variation in vaccine uptake. In the USA, poor and ethnic minorities in large urban centers create pockets of susceptibility (due to low vaccine uptake) that prevent the virtual elimination of infections such as measles and pertussis. Serologic surveillance, in both urban and rural areas, is a key component in the identification of weaknesses in current programs.

The rate at which susceptibles acquire many common vaccine-preventable childhood infections varies with age

For many common vaccine-preventable childhood infections, such as measles, mumps and rubella, the per capita rate at which susceptibles acquire infection varies with age. For rubella *(Fig. 33.15)* the rate changes from a low level in the 0–4 year olds via a high level in the 5–15 year olds back to a lower level in adults. This reflects social patterns of behavior, the high rates in the 5–15 year olds reflecting frequent and intimate contact within school environments. These age-dependent variations can reduce the predicted level of cohort vaccination required to block or eliminate transmission. This is because immunization increases the average age at infection (see above). Susceptibles who avoid vaccination and infection may move from an age class with a high rate of infection to an older one with a lower rate.

The risks of infection must outweigh any risk associated with vaccination

Most vaccines have some small risk of inducing serious complications. Any assessment of the benefit from an immunization program must therefore include a comparison of the number of cases of serious disease prevented by mass vaccination with the number of cases due to vaccination itself. Such calculations are not straightforward because they depend upon the interrelation between various factors such as:

- Vaccine efficacy and safety.
- Proportion of each cohort of children immunized.
- Average age of immunization.
- Indirect effects of mass vaccination on the rate of transmission of the infectious agent.

Typically, the risks from infection and from vaccination change as vaccination coverage increases. When infection is common and vaccination rare, the risks due to the former are invariably greater, often by many orders of magnitude. When infection is very rare as a result of vaccination, the reverse may be true. Ultimately, the risk of vaccination will always be greater once vaccination has eliminated infection.

The new, more immunogenic vaccines provide better protection, but may be less safe

A factor relevant to concerns about vaccine-associated complications is the development of high potency live virus vaccines, which provide protection for the vast majority of those immunized and allow vaccination at an age (around six months) when maternally derived antibodies are still present. Although the new, more immunogenic vaccines provide better protection, their use may be associated with increased reactogenicity or lower safety, exacerbating the conflict between individual and community interests. Are there circumstances in which a higher efficacy vaccine should be used,

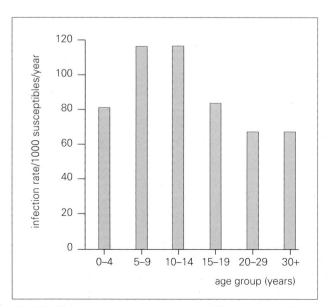

Fig. 33.15 Age-related changes in the rate of infection with the rubella virus.

even though it may lead to more cases of vaccine-associated disease? In the case of mumps, for example, the high potency 'Urabe Am 9' vaccine is estimated to have an efficacy of approximately 98% while the lower potency 'Jeryl Lynn' vaccine has an efficacy of around 94%, and evidence suggests higher complication rates with the former. At levels of vaccine coverage high enough to block transmission, the sensible option is to use the lower potency vaccine. However, if high uptake cannot be achieved then the total incidence of serious disease (both vaccine- and infection-produced) is reduced to a greater extent by the high potency vaccine.

Control of AIDS and HIV infection

Estimation of R_0 for HIV is fraught with problems, but approximate values can be obtained

Typical epidemiologic surveys record prevalence through time in specified risk groups such as male homosexuals, female prostitutes or pregnant women *(Fig. 33.16)*. By ignoring differences in the transmission probability from men to women and women to men (twice as likely from men to women) a rough guide to the magnitude of R_0 can be obtained in the early stages of the epidemic from a simple relationship that relates the magnitude of R_0 to the doubling time of the epidemic.

A doubling time in the prevalence of infection within a cohort of pregnant women of roughly two years *(Fig. 33.16)* and an average infectious period of 10 years, gives an R_0 value of approximately 2.5 in the urban heterosexual population in some of the worst afflicted regions in Africa. The aver-

age infectious period may be somewhat less than the average incubation period; virologic data suggest that viremia (and therefore infectiousness) fluctuates widely over the period. Furthermore, the genetic constitution of both host and viral populations may influence susceptibility, pathogenesis and infectiousness. The average incubation period may also be less than 10 years in developing countries, where continuous exposure to a wide range of infectious diseases may speed the development of severe immunodeficiency. If this is the case, the estimate of R_0 is reduced. However, taking the pessimistic view that R_0 is around 2–3 (one primary case generating 2–3 secondary cases) then the target of education programs is to reduce the combined influence of epidemiologic and behavioral parameters by at least 50–65%.

Reducing the rate of, and variation in, sexual partners is particularly important in the control of HIV infection

Control options include the use of condoms to reduce the probability of transmission, and behavioral changes to reduce both the rate of, and the variation in, sexual partner change in the population. The latter factor is of particular importance, since variance in sexual partner change rates is usually much greater than the mean value *(Fig. 33.8)* because of the small fraction of individuals who change sexual partners frequently. These individuals are also likely to experience higher than average levels of infection with other STDs, such as genital ulcers and gonorrhea. These may act as cofactors to enhance the likelihood of HIV transmission, and contribute disproportionately to transmission within a community, underlining

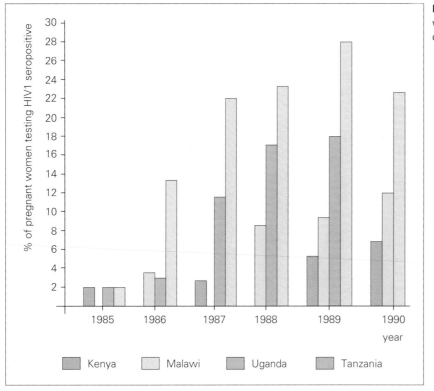

Fig. 33.16 The spread of HIV1 in pregnant women from urban centers in various African countries over the period 1985–90.

further the importance of targeted control measures. Enhanced STD control in general, particularly if targeted at this group, is therefore likely to slow the spread of HIV.

In developed countries, drugs are used to delay the onset of symptoms of AIDS. However, this may, under certain circumstances, have negative effects:

- First, widespread use by asymptomatic individuals at low dosage levels may promote the spread of drug resistant strains of HIV.
- Second, and more importantly, it may prolong the period of infectiousness and could enhance the net rate of transmission.

Treatment might therefore be good for the individual, but detrimental to the community at risk.

Summary

The development of a safe, effective and cheap vaccine or drug is only the first step – albeit a vital one – towards the control of an infectious disease within a community. The interaction between a population of hosts and an infectious agent is inherently non-linear. For example, when population density doubles the prevalence of many directly transmitted viral and bacterial infections may increase more than two-fold. Complex patterns of change in the incidence of infection can arise when immunization programs with partial coverage are initiated. The many variables that influence rates of transmission often hinder the assessment of the likely impact of a given control program. Epidemiologic analysis at the level of the population biology of the interaction between host and infectious agent is critical for the development of community-based programs. Appreciation of the components that determine the transmission potential of an infectious agent, as measured by the basic or case reproductive rate R_0, is vital.

In the design of control policies, most attention is presently directed towards what is best for the individual to be treated or vaccinated. However, what is best for the individual is not always best for the community and there can be genuine tensions between the interests of these two that are not easily resolved. However, the resolution of these tensions is eased greatly by a clear understanding of the precise circumstances that generate such conflicts.

- Epidemiology contributes to an understanding of infection and disease in populations and assists approaches to treatment and control.
- Each pathogen has a characteristic basic reproductive rate (R_0) that determines its ability to spread in fully susceptible populations.
- R_0 is constrained by many factors, which determine the actual (effective) reproductive rate R.
- Knowledge of the values for R_0 and R allow predictions about the spread of epidemics, the effectiveness of control measures and the implementation of vaccination program.
- Different epidemiological approaches are needed when dealing with infections caused by microparasites (e.g. viruses) and macroparasites (e.g. worms) and for diseases that are sexually transmitted.

1. Define the terms epidemic, endemic, hyperendemic and pandemic.
2. How is the R_0 of an infectious disease measured?
3. How do the differences in transmission of infections such as measles and HIV affect their epidemiology and control?
4. What is the relationship between the basic reproductive rate (R_0) of an infection and the percentage of the population that must be vaccinated to prevent transmission?
5. What can be the indirect effects of mass vaccination against measles, rubella and mumps?

Further Reading

Anderson RM, May RM. *Infectious Diseases Of Humans: Dynamics and Control*. Oxford: Blackwell Scientific Publications, 1992.

Giesecke J. *Modern Infectious Disease Epidemiology*. London: Edward Arnold, 1994.

Gordis L. *Epidemiology*. Philadelphia: W.B. Saunders, 1996.

Scott ME, Smith G. *Parasitic and Infectious Diseases. Epidemiology and Ecology*. New York: Academic Press, 1994.

Hospital Infection, Sterilization and Disinfection

Introduction

A nosocomial infection is any infection acquired while in hospital

Amassing a large number of sick people together under one roof has many advantages, but some disadvantages, notably the easier transmission of infection from one person to another. Hospital infection – also known as nosocomial infection – is defined as any infection acquired while in hospital. Most of these infections become obvious while the patient is in hospital, but some (as many as 25% of postoperative wound infections) are not recognized until after the patient has been discharged. The number of these unrecognized infections may increase as earlier discharges are encouraged to reduce costs, although a shorter preoperative stay reduces the chance of acquiring hospital pathogens (see below).

Hospital infection may be acquired from:

- An exogenous source (e.g. from another patient – cross-infection – or from the environment).
- An endogenous source (i.e. another site within the patient – self or auto-infection) *(Fig. 34.1)*.

An infection that is incubating in a patient when he or she is admitted into hospital is not a hospital infection. However, community-acquired infections brought into hospital by the patient may subsequently become hospital infections for other patients and hospital staff.

Many hospital infections are preventable

In 1850, Semmelweiss demonstrated that many hospital infections are preventable when he made the unpopular suggestion that puerperal fever (an infection in women who have just given birth, see Chapter 21) was carried on the hands of physicians who came directly from attending an autopsy to the delivery ward, without washing. A death rate of 8.3% was reduced to 2.3% by introducing the simple measure of hand-washing before and after any clinical examination. Extensive studies in the USA in the 1970s showed that the direct costs arising from hospital infection were around one billion dollars/year and that about 35% of all infections acquired in hospital could be prevented.

Common Hospital-Acquired Infections

Urinary tract infections are the most common hospital-acquired infections

The infections most commonly acquired in hospitals are:

- Surgical wound infections.
- Respiratory tract infection.
- Urinary tract infection (UTI).
- Bacteremia.

The relative frequencies of these infections are illustrated in *Figure 34.2*. Each may be acquired from an exogenous or endogenous source, and even the 'self-source' may be

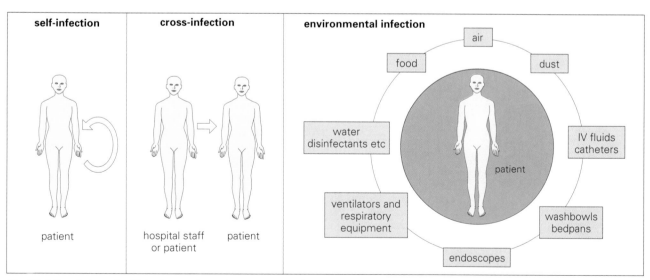

Fig. 34.1 Hospital-acquired infection can be endogenous (i.e. self-infection from another site in the body) or exogenous (i.e. from another person or from an environmental source). The sorts of organisms acquired from environmental sources depend upon the nature of the source, for example moist areas tend to be colonized with Gram-negative rods (e.g. *Escherichia coli, Klebsiella, Pseudomonas*) whereas air and dustborne organisms are those that can withstand drying (e.g. streptococci, staphylococci, mycobacteria and *Acinetobacter*). (IV, intravenous.)

derived from outside by the patient who becomes colonized with pathogens during his or her stay in hospital. Bacteremia may arise from a variety of sources and may be:

- Primary – due to the direct introduction of organisms into the blood from, for example, contaminated intravenous fluids.
- Secondary to a focus of infection already present in the body (e.g. UTI).

Other infections that may cause outbreaks in the hospital setting include gastroenteritis and hepatitis.

Important Causes of Hospital Infection

Escherichia coli and Staphylococcus aureus are the most common causes of hospital-acquired infection

Almost any microbe can cause a hospital-acquired infection, though protozoal infections are rare. The pattern of hospital infection has changed over the years, reflecting advances in medicine and the development of antimicrobial agents. In the pre-antibiotic era the majority of infections were caused by Gram-positive organisms, particularly *Streptococcus pyogenes* and *Staphylococcus aureus*. With the advent of penicillin and other antibiotics active against staphylococci, Gram-negative organisms such as *Escherichia coli* and *Pseudomonas aeruginosa* emerged as important pathogens. More recently, the development of more potent and broad-spectrum antimicrobials and the increase in invasive medical techniques has been accompanied by an increase in the incidence of:

- Antibiotic-resistant Gram-positive organisms such as *Staph. epidermidis*, enterococci and methicillin-resistant *Staph. aureus* (MRSA).
- *Candida*.

Many of these organisms are considered as 'opportunists' – microbes that are unable to cause disease in healthy people with intact defense mechanisms, but can cause infection in

compromised patients or when introduced during the course of invasive procedures. Currently *E. coli* accounts overall for more hospital infections than any other single species, but *Staph. aureus* is a close second *(Fig. 34.3)*.

Viral infections probably account for more hospital-acquired infections than previously realized

The most important hospital-acquired viruses are:

- Respiratory viruses, especially influenza and respiratory syncytial virus (RSV).
- Viruses acquired by the respiratory route such as measles and rubella.
- Herpes viruses, especially varicella–zoster virus (VZV).
- Rotavirus.
- Hepatitis viruses.
- HIV in countries where blood and blood products are not screened.

The risks of viral infections in hospital are summarized in *Figure 34.4*.

Sources and Routes of Spread of Hospital Infection

Sources of hospital infection are people and contaminated objects

As stated above, the source of infection may be:

- Human – from other patients or hospital staff, and occasionally visitors.
- Environmental, from contaminated objects ('fomites'), food, water or air *(see Fig. 34.1)*.

The source may become contaminated from an environmental reservoir of organisms, for example contaminated antiseptic solution distributed for use into sterile containers *(Fig. 34.5)*. Eradication of the source will also require eradication of the reservoir.

Human sources may be:

- People who are themselves infected.
- People who are incubating an infection.
- Healthy carriers.

The time period for which a human source is infectious varies with the disease (see Chapter 33). For example, some infections can be spread during their incubation period, others in the early stages of clinical disease, while others are characterized by a prolonged carrier state even after clinical cure (e.g. hepatitis B, typhoid fever) *(Fig. 34.6)*. Carriers of virulent strains of, for example, *Staph. aureus* or *Strep. pyogenes* may act as sources of hospital infection, although they themselves do not develop clinical disease. The carrier state may persist for a long time and go unnoticed unless there is an outbreak of infection that is traced to the carrier.

Hospital infections are spread in the air and by contact and common vehicle

The important routes of spread of infection in hospitals are those common to all infections – airborne, contact and

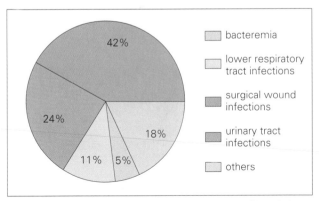

Fig. 34.2 The relative frequencies of different kinds of hospital infection vary in different patient groups, but overall urinary tract infections are the most common hospital-acquired infections.

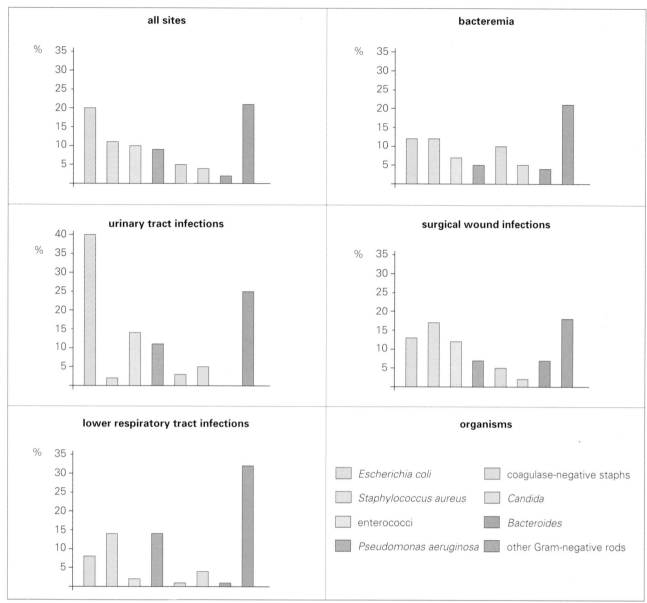

Fig. 34.3 Although a few species are the most important in all kinds of hospital infection, the rank order of their importance varies in different infections. *Staphylococcus aureus* is very important in surgical wound infections and bacteremia, but much less important in urinary tract infections. The importance of Gram-negative rods has increased since the advent of broad-spectrum antibiotics because these organisms often carry multiple antibiotic resistances.

common vehicle. Examples of organisms spread by these routes in hospitals are illustrated in *Figure 34.5*. Although theoretically possible, vector-borne spread is very unusual in the hospital setting, as is sexually-transmitted infection. It is important to remember that the same organism may be spread by more than one route. For example, *Strep. pyogenes* can be spread from patient to patient by the airborne route in droplets or dust, but is also transmitted by contact with infected lesions, for example on a nurse's hand.

Host Factors and Hospital Infection

Underlying disease, certain treatments and invasive procedures reduce host defenses

Host factors play a fundamental role in the infection equation, particularly in hospitals because of the high proportion of hospital patients with compromised natural defenses against infection. The spread of an infectious agent to a new host can result in a spectrum of responses from

VIRUSES AS CAUSES OF HOSPITAL-ACQUIRED INFECTION			
virus	**transmissibility**	**susceptibility of other patients and staff**	**resultant risk of hospital infection**
influenza	++	+/–*	++
respiratory syncytial virus	++	++*	++
parainfluenza adenovirus rhinovirus	+	+*	+
varicella–zoster	++	–*	–
varicella–zoster (localized)	+	– –	– –
cytomegalovirus	–	+	– –†
rubella	++	+**	++
measles	++	– –	– –
exotic viruses (Lassa, Marburg, Ebola, rabies)	– –	++	– –
rotavirus	++	+	+
enteroviruses	+	+	+
hepatitis A	+	+	+
gepatitis B	++§	++	++
HIV (in countries where not screened)	++‡	++	++

*   high in pediatric age group   ** decreased since immunization program initiated

†   except for blood transfusion and organ transplantation   § from needle-stick injuries   ‡ from blood or blood product

Fig. 34.4 Viruses are probably more important causes of hospital infection than generally recognized. The risk of hospital infection is a sum of the transmissibility of the virus and the susceptibility of the patient group. Some viruses, such as varicella–zoster, are of low risk in general, but very important in pediatric units and particularly in immunocompromised children.

colonization, through subclinical infection, to clinically apparent disease, which may be fatal. The degree of host response differs in different people depending upon their degree of compromise. The very young are particularly susceptible because of the immaturity of their immune system. Likewise, the elderly suffer a greater risk of infection because of predisposing underlying disease, impaired blood supply and immobility, which contribute to stasis and therefore to infection in, for example, the lungs. In all age groups, underlying disease and the treatment of that disease (e.g. cytotoxic drugs, steroids) may predispose to infection (*Fig. 34.7*), while invasive procedures allow organisms easier access to previously-protected tissues (*Fig. 34.8*). The important host factors to be considered in hospital infection are summarized in *Figure 34.9*. Infections in the compromised host are discussed in more detail in Chapter 28.

A variety of factors predispose to wound infection

Wound infection or wound sepsis is characterized by the presence of inflammation, pus and discharge in addition to the isolation of organisms such as *Staph. aureus*. Extensive studies of postoperative wound infection have identified a number of predisposing factors:

- Prolonged preoperative stay increases the opportunity for the patient to become colonized with antibiotic-resistant hospital pathogens.
- The nature and length of the operation also have an effect (*Figs 34.10, 34.11*; see also Chapter 23).
- Wet or open wounds are more liable to secondary infection.

From these studies it has been possible to identify the patients and operations with greatest risk and apply preventive measures such as prophylactic antibiotic regimens and ultra-clean air in orthopedic operating theaters (see below).

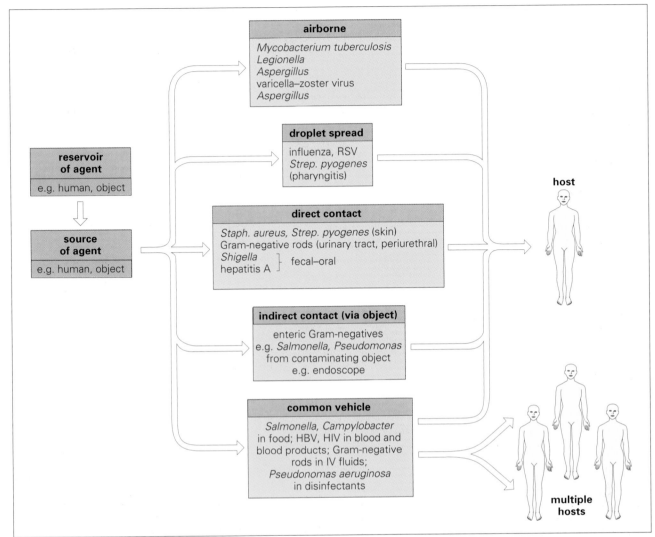

Fig. 34.5 Hospital infections are spread by the same routes as infections spread in the community. The reservoir and the source of infection may be human or inanimate and may be one and the same (e.g. a nurse with an infected skin lesion). If the reservoir and source are distinct (e.g. contaminated distilled water supply used to prepare a variety of pharmaceuticals), both must be eliminated if the spread of infection is to be halted, otherwise the reservoir may continue to contaminate new sources. (HBV, hepatitis B virus; IV, intravenous; RSV, respitory syncytial virus.)

The Consequences of Hospital Infection

Hospital infections affect both the patient and the community

Hospital infection may result in:

- Serious illness or death.
- Prolonged hospital stay, which costs money and results in a loss of earnings and hardship for the patient and his or her family.
- A need for additional antimicrobial therapy, which is costly, exposes the patient to additional risks of toxicity, and increases selective pressure for resistance to emerge among hospital pathogens.
- The infected patient becoming a source from which others may become infected, in hospital and in the community.

Prevention of Hospital Infection

There are three main strategies for preventing hospital infection

For the reasons outlined above, the prevention of hospital infection deserves a very high priority and the three main strategies are:

- Excluding sources of infection from hospital the environment.
- Interrupting the transmission of infection from source to susceptible host (breaking the chain of infection).
- Enhancing the host's ability to resist infection.

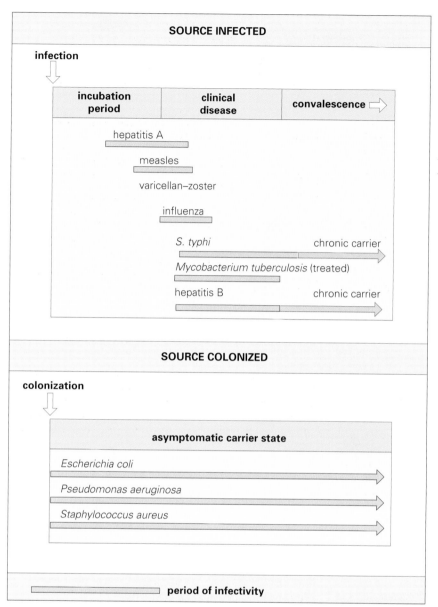

SOURCE INFECTED

infection

incubation period	clinical disease	convalescence

hepatitis A

measles

varicellan–zoster

influenza

S. typhi   chronic carrier

Mycobacterium tuberculosis (treated)

hepatitis B   chronic carrier

SOURCE COLONIZED

colonization

asymptomatic carrier state

Escherichia coli

Pseudomonas aeruginosa

Staphylococcus aureus

period of infectivity

Fig. 34.6 Pathogens differ in the time periods for which they can be disseminated from an infected person. For some it is during the incubation period when infected people may not realize they are ill and infectious. Some people continue to carry organisms such as *Salmonella typhi* and hepatitis B virus long after they have recovered from the clinical disease. Opportunist pathogens are often members of the normal flora and may therefore be carried for long periods without the host experiencing any adverse effects.

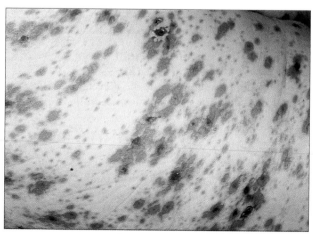

Fig. 34.7 Varicella in a patient with chronic myeloid leukemia resulting in purpuric confluent lesions on the trunk. (Courtesy of GDW McKendrick.)

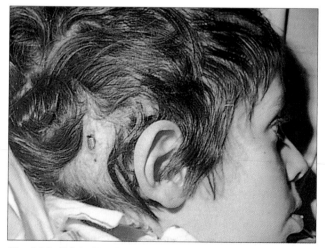

Fig. 34.8 Child with infected Spitz–Holter valve used to relieve hydrocephalus. (Courtesy of JA Innes.)

FACTORS WHICH PREDISPOSE PATIENTS TO HOSPITAL INFECTION	
Age	patients at extremes of age are particularly susceptible
Specific immunity	patient may lack protective antibodies to e.g. measles, chicken pox, whooping cough
Underlying disease	other (non-infectious) diseases tend to lead to enhanced susceptibility to infection, e.g. hepatic disease, diabetes, cancer, skin disorders, renal failure, neutropenia (either as a result of disease or of treatment)
Other infections	HIV and other immunosuppressing virus infections, patients with influenza prone to secondary bacterial pneumonia, herpes virus lesions may become secondarily infected with staphylococci
Specific medicaments	cytotoxic drugs (including post-transplant immunosuppression) and steroids both lower host defenses, antibiotics disturb normal flora and predispose to invasion by resistant hospital pathogens
Trauma accidental	burns, stab or gunshot wounds, road traffic accidents
intentional	surgery, intravenous and urinary catheters, peritoneal dialysis

(Trauma rows bracketed:) disturb natural host defense mechanisms

Fig. 34.9 Hospital patients are not all at equal risk of infection. Some factors that predispose to infection can be influenced by, for example, treating underlying disease, improving specific immunity and avoiding inappropriate use of antibiotics. Other factors such as age are unalterable.

RISK FACTORS FOR POSTOPERATIVE INFECTIONS	
Length of pre-operative stay	longer stay – more likely to become colonized with virulent and antibiotic-resistant hospital bacteria and fungi
Presence of intercurrent infection	operating on an already infected site more likely to cause disseminated infection
Length of operation	longer – greater risk of tissues becoming seeded with organisms from air, staff, other sites in patient
Nature of operation	any operation which results in fecal soiling of tissues has higher risk of infection (e.g. postoperative gangrene), 'adventurous' surgery tends to carry greater risks
Presence of foreign bodies	e.g. shunts, prostheses, impairs host defenses
State of tissues	poor blood supply encourages growth of anaerobes, inadequate drainage or presence of necrotic tissue predisposes to infection

Fig. 34.10 The risks of infection after surgery have been studied in considerable detail and as a result surgeons are much more aware of the problems. However, 'high-tech' surgery is often long and difficult and predisposes the patient to postoperative infection.

Fig. 34.11 Postoperative gangrenous cellulitis. There is a huge area of ulceration filled with gangrenous skin, with sloughing adjacent to the wound and surrounding cellulitis. (Courtesy of MJ Wood.)

Exclusion of sources of infection
Exclusion of inanimate sources of infection is achievable, but it can be difficult to avoid contamination by humans

Exclusion of inanimate sources of infection is both desirable and to a large extent achievable. For example the provision of sterile instruments and dressings, sterile medicaments and intravenous fluids and the use of blood and blood products screened for infectious agents, clean linen and uncontaminated food. However, many of the sources of infection are human or are objects that become contaminated by humans, in which case exclusion is more difficult. Hospitals must attempt to prevent patient contact with staff who are carriers of pathogens. The problem is the identification of staff who are carriers of pathogens and their relocation to less hazardous positions. Staff must undergo health screening before employment and should have regular health checks (see Fig. 34.12). They should also be encouraged to report any incidences of infection (e.g. an infected cut or a bout of diarrhea). Appropriate immunizations should be offered and in some instances made mandatory. Work restrictions for personnel with selected infectious diseases are summarized in *Figure 34.12*. However, healthy carriers of, for example, virulent staphylococci are difficult to identify unless bacteriologic screening is undertaken, which is not feasible on a routine basis. In addition, staff are sources of opportunist organisms such as coagulase-negative staphylococci or enterobacteria, which are part of their normal flora and cannot be excluded.

Breaking the chain of infection

There are two elements to be considered in breaking the chain of infection: the structural and the human. The structure of the hospital and its equipment can play a role in preventing airborne spread of infection and in facilitating aseptic practices by the staff, but this is of no avail if staff do not use the facilities correctly and do not themselves act positively to prevent the spread of infection.

Control of airborne transmission of infection
Ventilation systems and air flow can play an important role in the dissemination of organisms by the airborne route

Wards comprising separate rooms have been shown to afford some protection against airborne spread and rooms with controlled ventilation are even better. However, neither prevent the carriage of organisms into the room on staff and their clothing, and some studies suggest that this is a more important route of infection than airborne spread. There is no doubt, however, that *Legionella* infection is acquired by the airborne route, and air conditioning systems throughout the hospital should be maintained so as to prevent the multiplication of these organisms (see Chapter 17). Hospital-acquired *Aspergillus* infection has been attributed to dissemination of the spores in hospital air, especially when building work is ongoing in the locality.

Ventilation systems in operating theaters must be properly installed and maintained to prevent the ingress of contaminated air and to minimize air currents carrying organisms from the staff in the operating room to the operation site. 'Ultra-clean' air is air passed through high-efficiency filters to remove bacteria and other particles and has been shown to contribute positively to a reduction in the number of postoperative wound infections developing after long orthopedic operations.

Airborne transmission of infection can be reduced significantly by isolating patients

Patient isolation may be carried out:

- To protect a particularly susceptible patient from exposure to pathogens (i.e. protective isolation).
- To prevent the spread of pathogens from an infected patient to others on the ward (i.e. source isolation).

Isolation also helps to prevent the transmission of infection by other routes by limiting access to the patient and reminding staff of the importance of contact in the spread of infection.

Protective isolation

Protective isolation can be provided by a single room on a ward or by enclosing the patient in a plastic isolator. With appropriate positive pressure ventilation, air should flow from the 'clean' patient area out of the room or isolator. Staff entering the room or in contact with the patient should wear sterile gowns, gloves and masks to prevent organisms they are carrying or have picked up from other patients from coming in contact with the patient.

Source isolation

Source isolation is ideally arranged by accommodation in an isolation unit in a separate building, thus the tuberculosis sanatoria of the past. In a general, hospital isolation is more often arranged in a separate ward or in side rooms off the main ward. To prevent airborne transmission of organisms from the patient's room to the ward, air should flow from the ward to the isolation room. In practice it is difficult to maintain the correct air flows without sophisticated designs, including double doors and air locks.

Facilitation of aseptic behavior

A general state of cleanliness throughout the hospital is essential and the design of hospital facilities affects the ease with which the environment can be kept clean and the staff can practise good techniques.

Bacteriologically effective handwashing is one of the most important ways of controlling hospital infection

The hands of staff convey organisms to patients from septic lesions and healthy carrier sites of other patients, from

INFECTIOUS DISEASES WHERE STAFF CONTACT WITH PATIENT SHOULD BE AVOIDED
diarrhea
hepatitis A
herpes simplex on hands (herpetic whitlow)
Streptococcus pyogenes infections
Staphylococcus aureus skin lesions
measles
mumps
whooping cough
rubella
varicella–zoster infections
upper respiratory tract infections (high-risk patients)

Fig. 34.12 Recommended work restrictions for staff with infectious diseases. In the event of a member of staff becoming infected either in the hospital or outside, he or she should be relieved from direct contact with patients. Kitchen staff should also be relieved from duty if they are suffering from diarrhea or hepatitis A, or have infected lesions on their hands.

equipment contaminated by these sources and from carrier sites of the staff themselves (*Figs 34.13, 34.14*).

Staff should therefore wash their hands:

- Before any procedure for which gloves or forceps are necessary.
- After contact with an infected patient or one who is colonized with multiply resistant bacteria.
- After touching infective material.

Soap and water are adequate in most circumstances, but when dealing with infected patients disinfectant soaps are recommended. Drying hands after washing is important. A more prolonged and thorough scrub is required before commencing surgery.

The design of taps, soap dispensers and other washing facilities, including bedpan washers has reached a high degree of sophistication. However, human behavior can be influenced by architectural design only to a limited degree and there is often a disappointingly low compliance with the simple technique of handwashing. Therefore training and regular reinforcement in appropriate behavior is essential.

Enhancing the host's ability to resist infection
Host resistance can be enhanced by boosting immunity and reducing risk factors

Although attempts can and should be made to control and prevent hospital infection by removing sources of infection and preventing transmission from sources to susceptible hosts, neither of these strategies is failsafe. In addition, they do not protect the host from endogenous infection. A way of tipping the balance in favor of the host is to enhance his or her ability to resist infection, both by boosting specific

immunity and by reducing personal risk factors. The following aspects should be considered:

- Boosting specific immunity by active or passive immunization.
- The appropriate use of prophylactic antibiotics.
- Care of invasive devices that breach the natural defenses (e.g. urinary catheters, intravenous lines).
- Attention to the risks predisposing to postoperative infection.

Boosting specific immunity
Passive immunization provides short-term protection

Boosting specific immunity by immunization has been discussed in Chapter 32. The problem for the immunocompromised patient is that he or she may not be able to mount an antibody response. Passive immunization can afford short-term protection, for example in patients who are neutropenic as a result of cytotoxic therapy and whose white cell count should recover after successful treatment. With the advent of efficacious hepatitis B vaccines it is recommended that all seronegative patients in dialysis units (and all staff in such units) should be immunized. Other immunizations for protecting hospital patients are summarized in *Figure 34.15*.

Appropriate use of prophylactic antibiotics
There are well-documented uses for prophylaxis, but antibiotics tend to be misused

This is discussed in Chapter 30. There are several well-documented uses for prophylactic antibiotics in 'dirty' surgery and

CONTACT SPREAD OF OPPORTUNIST PATHOGENS		
patient	nursing activity	number of klebsiellae recovered per hand*
A	physiotherapy	10–100
	taking blood pressure and pulse	100–1000
	washing patient	10–100
	taking oral temperature	100–1000
B	taking radial pulse	100–1000
	touching shoulder	1000
	touching groin	100–1000
C	touching hand	10–100
D	extubation	100–1000
	touching tracheostomy	1000
*control hand washings taken prior to procedure yielded no klebsiellae		

Fig. 34.13 Nursing procedures involving skin contact resulting in contamination of staff hands. These data are derived from experiments performed during an outbreak of *Klebsiella* infection among urology patients. (Data from Casewell and Phillips, 1977.)

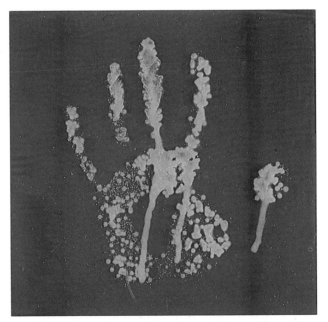

Fig. 34.14 Gram-negative rods are not usually part of the resident skin flora except in moist environments, but are readily carried on hands and can be transferred from a source to a susceptible patient. This picture shows an impression of a hand that was inoculated with approximately 1000 *Klebsiella aerogenes*.

BOOSTING SPECIFIC IMMUNITY OF PATIENTS		
patient group	immunization	
	active	passive
elderly (especially those with multisystem disease)	influenza vaccine	–
pre-splenectomy pre-renal or bone marrow transplant	pneumococcal vaccine	–
hemodialysis patients	pneumococcal vaccine	–
infants born to HBs Ag positive mothers	hepatitis B vaccine	–
immunocompromised: exposed to varicella–zoster virus (VZV)	live attenuated VZV vaccine in trials	zoster immune globulin within 3 days prevents severe disease
exposed to measles	–	normal human immune globulin within 5 days

Fig. 34.15 Many patients will have been protected against some infections by routine immunization during childhood, but sometimes it is helpful to boost specific immunity by immunization of patients at particular risk of infection.

when the consequences of infection would be disastrous (e.g. in cardiac, neuro- and transplant surgery). However, there is a tendency to misuse antibiotics:

- First, by using them too often or for too long, thereby increasing the selection pressure for the emergence of resistant organisms.
- Second, by choosing inappropriate agents.

Treatment (as opposed to prophylaxis) of patients and staff who are carriers of pathogens such as *Staph. aureus* or *Strep. pyogenes* has been used successfully to prevent endogenous infection and to control outbreaks of infection with these organisms. Topical preparations of antibiotics such as bacitracin, neomycin and fucidin have been used, but there is no doubt that the emergence of resistance is a problem. Pseudomonic acid (mupirocin), a fermentation product of *Pseudomonas fluorescens*, has been shown to be efficacious. It is unrelated to any other class of antibiotic in clinical use – therefore diminishing concern over the emergence of resistant strains with cross-resistance to other agents – and it is very active against Gram-positive cocci. In recent years it has played an important role in eradicating carriage of MRSA, but resistance is now beginning to emerge.

Gut decontamination regimens and selective bowel contamination aim to reduce the reservoir of potential pathogens in the gut

Gut decontamination regimens to reduce the aerobic Gram-negative flora of neutropenic patients has been practiced for

some time. More recently the use of selective bowel decontamination (SBD) in intensive care unit (ICU) patients has become fashionable in some centers. The aim is to reduce the reservoir of potential pathogens in the gut by oral administration (or via a nasogastric tube) of a high concentration of a mixture of antibiotics (polymyxin plus tobramycin plus amphotericin, or a similar combination) to ICU patients throughout their stay in the unit. At the present time there is still controversy about the efficacy and safety of SBD.

Care of invasive devices
Care of invasive devices is essential to reduce the risk of endogenous infection

It is essential to take care of intravascular devices to reduce the risk of endogenous infection from skin organisms, and of catheters to reduce the risk of endogenous infection from the periurethral flora causing infection of the bladder in catheterized patients. Guidelines for the care of urinary catheters are discussed in Chapter 18.

Up to 35% of hospital-acquired bacteremias and the majority of candidemias are infusion-related

These infusion-related bacteremias and candidemias derive mainly from vascular catheters. Most bacteremias associated with invasive devices are caused by the patient's own skin flora, although this may be a more resistant flora acquired during the patient's stay in hospital replacing his or her 'community-acquired' flora. *Staph. epidermidis* accounts for more than 50% of infections, but other aerobic bacteria including *Staph. aureus*, enterococci, coryneforms, various Gram-negative rods, and *Candida* are also implicated. These infections are largely preventable if appropriate steps are taken. The sources of infection and measures for prevention are shown in *Figure 34.16*.

Reducing the risks of postoperative infection
Prevention of postoperative infection involves minimizing the risks

Reducing the risks of postoperative infection involves an understanding of the risks and the ways in which they can be circumvented. For example:

- The preoperative length of stay in hospital should be kept to a minimum.
- Intercurrent infections should be treated appropriately before surgery whenever possible (e.g. treatment of UTI before resection of the prostate).
- Operations should be kept to the minimum duration consistent with good operating technique.
- Adequate debridement of dead and necrotic tissue is essential, together with adequate drainage and maintenance or re-establishment of a good blood supply to provide the body's natural defenses with optimum working conditions.
- Prevention of pressure sores and stasis to minimize the risks of developing respiratory tract infection or UTI by good nursing techniques and active physiotherapy.

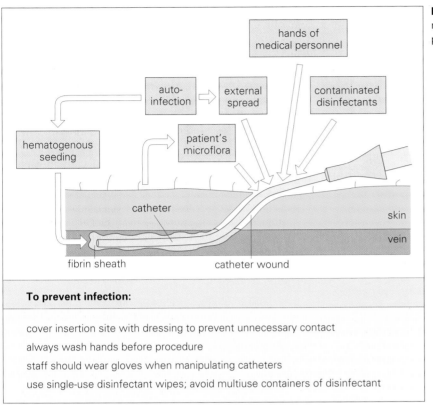

Fig. 34.16 Sources of intravascular device-related infection and opportunities for the prevention of infection.

hands of medical personnel

auto-infection

external spread

contaminated disinfectants

hematogenous seeding

patient's microflora

catheter

skin

vein

fibrin sheath

catheter wound

To prevent infection:

cover insertion site with dressing to prevent unnecessary contact

always wash hands before procedure

staff should wear gloves when manipulating catheters

use single-use disinfectant wipes; avoid multiuse containers of disinfectant

Investigating Hospital Infection

In many hospitals the responsibility for investigating hospital infection falls on the infection control committee, which includes an infection control officer (who may be a physician or microbiologist) and at least one nurse. The roles of the infection control committee include:
- The surveillance of hospital infection.
- The establishment and monitoring of policies and procedures designed to prevent infection (e.g. catheter care policy, antibiotic policy, disinfectant policy).
- The investigation of outbreaks.

Surveillance
Surveillance allows early recognition of any change in the number or type of hospital infections
Although hospital infection has been recognized for many years, accurate records of its incidence and prevalence were not initiated until the late 1950s. Since 1960 several surveys carried out nationally and internationally have highlighted the prevalence and importance of hospital infection. By maintaining surveillance, the infection control team can establish the normal trends in their hospital and therefore recognize any change in the number or type of infections early. Sources of surveillance data are:
- Microbiology laboratory reports. These can be used for general surveillance or for monitoring 'alert' organisms

such as *Staph. aureus*, *Strep. pyogenes*, *M. tuberculosis*, salmonellae and shigellae.
- Ward rounds. New cases of infection can be identified by direct inspection and previously identified cases of infection can be followed up. Surveys can also be carried out on the wards (e.g. of wound infections after different practises or procedures).
- Other sources such as autopsy reports, staff health records and surveys of patients after discharge from hospital.

Investigation of outbreaks
When an outbreak (or epidemic) occurs or when routine surveillance highlights an increase in the incidence of infection, the control of infection team should initiate an investigation. There is no universally-applicable routine for finding the cause of an outbreak, but in principle each investigation has an epidemiological element and a microbiological element.

There must be a definition of any outbreak in epidemiological terms
Such an epidemiological definition involves answering a variety of questions such as:
- How many people are infected?
- When were they admitted?
- When did they develop their infection?
- Are they all on the same ward?
- Are they all treated by the same medical or surgical team?

The causative organism needs to be isolated in all patients in the outbreak

It is the role of the microbiology laboratory to attempt to isolate the causative organism and to show that all patients in the outbreak are infected with the same strain (i.e. strains that are indistinguishable; see below). The identity of the infecting organism provides clues to the possible source; for example, an outbreak of wound infection with *Staph. aureus* is likely to be associated with contact spread from staff in theater or on the ward, whereas an outbreak of salmonella gastroenteritis is more likely to originate in the kitchen.

While the investigation is proceeding, efforts are needed to contain the outbreak and prevent spread to other patients. Infected patients must be isolated and treated appropriately, and staff who are found to be infected or carriers must be suspended from duty until they have been treated. At the end of the investigation the relevant procedures must be reviewed to try and prevent a similar outbreak occurring again.

Epidemiological typing techniques
A variety of phenotypic and genotypic characters are used to 'fingerprint' strains for epidemiological purposes

In epidemiological studies of the spread of infections, and in the investigation of outbreaks both in hospital and in the community, it is necessary to compare bacterial isolates to determine whether they belong to the same species, and if so, whether they are distinct or of the same strain – in fact it is not possible to say that two organisms are the same, only that they are indistinguishable. If the species is a regular member of the normal human flora or is found frequently in the environment, it is necessary to distinguish the 'outbreak' strain from other strains of the same species not involved in the outbreak, but that may also be isolated during the course of the investigation.

A good typing technique must:
- Be discriminatory (i.e. able to show differences between strains of the same species).
- Be reproducible (i.e. the same strain gives the same result when tested on different occasions and in different places).
- Have a high degree of typability (i.e. capable of assigning a type to all strains).

Antibiotic susceptibility patterns and simple biotyping can be carried out in most routine diagnostic laboratories, whereas the specialized typing techniques are based in reference laboratories. This has the advantage that quality assurance can be optimized, but also means that there is an inevitable delay in reporting the results and therefore in learning whether an outbreak of hospital infection is caused by a single strain.

Antibiotic susceptibility patterns and simple biotyping
Antibiotic susceptibility patterns are performed readily in the diagnostic laboratory

These tests are performed readily in the diagnostic laboratory (see Chapter 30) and are useful as a preliminary clue as to whether two isolates are indistinguishable. However, dis-crimination is poor, many susceptibility patterns are common and quite different strains may have the same pattern. Conversely, during an outbreak, strains may gain or lose plasmids carrying antibiotic resistance markers.

Biotyping involves typing organisms by their ability to grow on different substrates or produce different enzymes

Ideally the biochemical test employed in a biotyping scheme should differ from those used to identify the organisms. Identification tests are chosen because they 'lump' similar organisms together; biotyping tests are chosen because they 'split' species into distinct strains. However, diagnostic laboratories often use the profiles from miniaturized multi-test identification systems as biotypes *(Fig. 34.17)*.

Specialized typing techniques
Serotyping distinguishes between strains using specific antisera

This classical technique distinguishes between strains by a difference in their antigenic structure, which is recognized by reaction with specific antisera. The 'O' somatic antigens and 'H' flagellar antigens are therefore used to divide salmonellae into types (sometimes referred to as species; see Chapter 20). *Strep. pneumoniae*, *Neisseria meningitidis* and *Klebsiella aerogenes* can be typed on the basis of their capsular (K) antigens and *Strep. pyogenes* on their M and T cell wall proteins. The established schemes use polyclonal antisera, but newer schemes based on monoclonals are being developed. Serotyping requires the production and maintenance of appropriate banks of antisera, which is both time-consuming and costly. It is therefore usually restricted to reference laboratories.

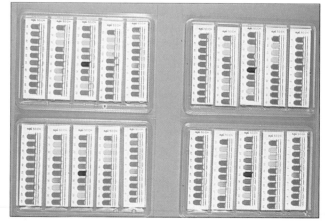

Fig. 34.17 Biotyping isolates of *Bacillus cereus* from an outbreak of infection in an intensive care unit. Biotyping schemes are based on the ability of different strains within a species to metabolize and grow on different substrates. Commercially-available multi-test systems are designed primarily for identification purposes, but can also be used for biotyping. The strips contain a series of different biochemical tests. The isolate is inoculated into each well and, after incubation, a positive result is indicated by a color change. (Courtesy of S Dancer.)

Bacteriophage (phage) typing is used to type Staph. aureus, Staph. epidermidis and Salmonella typhi

This technique compares the pattern of lysis obtained when isolates (grown as lawns on agar plates) are exposed to a standard series of phage suspensions *(Fig. 34.18)*. This method is important for typing *Staph. aureus, Staph. epidermidis* and *Salmonella typhi*, but has been applied to other species such as *P. aeruginosa*. As with serotyping, phage typing requires the production, maintenance and testing of the standard phage suspensions and is usually carried out in reference laboratories rather than in the hospital diagnostic laboratory.

Bacteriocin typing has been most successfully applied to P. aeruginosa and Shigella sonnei

Bacteriocins are small protein molecules produced by species of bacteria and lethal to other strains of the same or closely related species. The production of bacteriocins by the test strain produces a pattern of inhibition of growth of a standard set of indicator strains, which can be used to assign the test strain to a type *(Fig. 34.19)*. The method is potentially applicable to any species that produces bacteriocins (and most do). It has been most successfully applied to *P. aeruginosa* (pyocine typing, from the old name for the organism; *Pseudomonas pyocyaneus*) and *Shigella sonnei* (colicine typing, so-named because the species is genetically very similar to *E. coli* and sensitive to bacteriocins called colicines produced by that species).

Molecular typing techniques involve characterizing an organism's DNA

With the development of techniques in molecular biology, there has been a trend away from the classical phenotypic methods towards characterization of an organism's DNA – either chromosome or plasmid or total protein profile (i.e. all of the proteins in the cell encoded by the DNA). Plasmid profiles are only useful for species that carry a variety of plasmids and they suffer from the drawback that what is actually being characterized is the plasmid and not the organism containing it. Different Gram-negative rods may acquire the same plasmids by conjugation between different species. However, this method has also been used to advantage to map the spread of antibiotic resistance plasmids among hospital pathogens *(Fig. 34.20)*.

The advantage of DNA techniques for epidemiological fingerprinting is that all isolates can be typed

The total DNA of a cell can be analysed by extracting it and digesting it with restriction endonucleases. These enzymes cut the DNA at specific sites producing many short lengths of DNA, which can be separated on a gel to give a pattern characteristic of the organism and the restriction enzyme (because different restriction enzymes cut the DNA at different sites they produce different fragment lengths from the same DNA). Comparison of the DNA from different isolates of the same species cut by the same restriction enzyme will show whether the isolates have the same pattern of bands and by implication, indistinguishable DNA *(Fig. 34.21)*.

DNA techniques allow typing of all isolates (i.e. typability is 100%) and with the choice of restriction enzyme, discrimination is also high. However, the band patterns are fairly complex and isolates need to be run on the same gel for comparisons to be valid. Simpler patterns can be obtained by using DNA probes to identify gene sequences in isolates. Ribotyping (i.e. probing for the

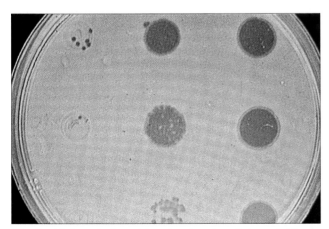

Fig. 34.18 Bacteriophage (phage) typing of staphylococci. After seeding the surface of an agar plate with the organism to be typed, suspensions of different phages are dropped onto the surface and the plate incubated. Phages that are able to lyse the strain will produce zones of clearing of the bacterial lawn. The patterns of lysis obtained with the same set of bacteriophages on different isolates of *Staph. aureus* collected, for example during an outbreak of wound infections, can be compared.

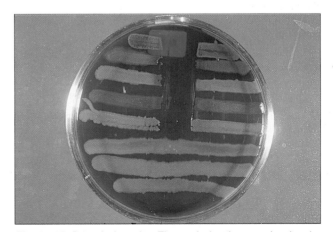

Fig. 34.19 Bacteriocin typing. The test isolate is grown in a band across the agar plate and during this time bacteriocins produced by the isolate diffuse into the agar. After overnight incubation, the macroscopic growth is removed and the surface of the plate exposed to chloroform to kill remaining organisms (bacteriocins are resistant to the action of chloroform). Indicator strains are streaked across the plate at right angles to the original line and the plate incubated a second time. The pattern of inhibition of growth of the indicator is recorded and the strain assigned to a type.

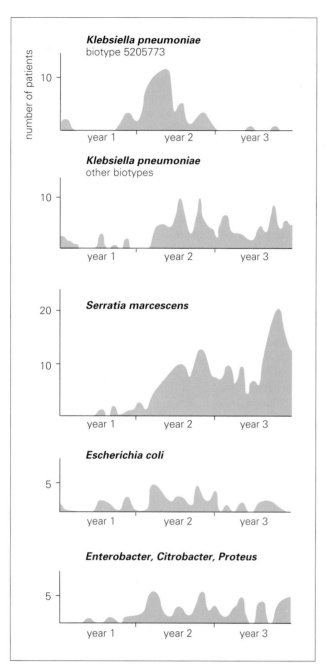

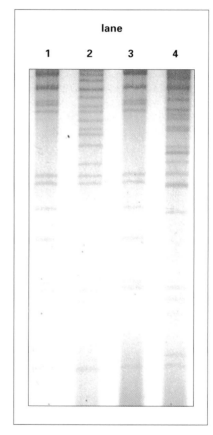

Fig. 34.20 Dissemination of a single resistance plasmid into several different strains and species of enterobacteria in one hospital. In year 1 in this hospital there were very few isolates of gentamicin-resistant enterobacteria. In the first four months of year 2, there was an outbreak of infection with a gentamicin-resistant *Klebsiella pneumoniae* belonging to a single biotype. Although this outbreak was contained, over subsequent months the same plasmid coding for the same aminoglycoside-modifying enzyme was found in other biotypes of the *Klebsiella* and in other Gram-negative species. (Adapted from O'Brien *et al*, 1980.)

Fig. 34.21 DNA typing. The illustration shows DNA from isolates of *Enterococcus faecalis* from four patients on the same ward. The DNA was extracted from each isolate and digested with the restriction endonuclease Sst1. After digestion the DNA fragments are separated by gel electrophoresis and stained with ethidium bromide. Comparison of the pattern of bands shows that isolates in lanes 1 and 3 are indistinguishable and different from those in lanes 2 and 4. (Courtesy of L Hall.)

genes that encode ribosomal RNA) has been applied successfully to type some species. However, discrimination between strains of the same species may be less because the ribosomal RNA genes tend to be highly conserved. Again, for valid results, the isolates that are to be compared should be run on the same gel.

Sterilization and Disinfection

It is clear that the prevention of hospital infection depends in part upon the availability of clean, and where necessary, sterile equipment, instruments and dressings, isolation facilities and the safe disposal of infected material. Sterilization and disinfection are often talked about by microbiologists in relation to the production of sterile culture media and other laboratory activities, but it must be stressed that the concept of sterility is central to almost all areas of medical practice. An understanding of the rationale of sterilization and disinfection will aid intelligent use of the range of sterile equipment (from needles to protheses) and techniques (from surgery to handwashing) employed in medical practice.

Definitions

Sterilization is the process of killing or removing all viable organisms

An item that is sterile is free from all viable organisms – in this sense viable means capable of reproducing. Sterilization is achieved by physical or chemical means, either by the removal of organisms from an object or by killing the organisms *in situ*, sometimes leaving toxic breakdown products (pyrogens) in the object.

Disinfection is a process of removing or killing most, but not all, viable organisms

Disinfection employs either:

- A chemical 'disinfectant', which kills pathogens but may not kill viruses or spores.
- A physical process such as boiling water or low pressure steam, which reduces the bioburden (i.e. the load of viable organisms).

Antiseptics are used to reduce the number of viable organisms on the skin

Antiseptics are a particular group of disinfectants. Some act differentially, destroying the transient flora but leaving the normal skin flora deep in the skin pores and hair follicles untouched *(Fig. 34.22)*. It is impossible to sterilize the skin (except by burning!), but thorough washing with antiseptic soaps can reduce the numbers of organisms on the surface considerably and therefore reduce contact spread of infection (see above). However, the resident bacteria in the hair follicles and ducts of sweat glands can recolonize the skin surface within hours.

Pasteurization can be used to eliminate pathogens in heat sensitive products

Pasteurization reduces the total numbers of viable microbes in bulk fluids such as milk and fruit juices without destroying flavor and palatability. It does not affect spores, but is effective against intracellular organisms such as *Brucella* and mycobacteria and many viruses.

Since recorded history, various other techniques have been used to prevent the multiplication of microorganisms such as drying and salting of food.

Deciding Whether Sterilization or Disinfection Should Be Used

Sterilization and disinfection processes are costly and so it is important to choose the appropriate method and the one that causes the least damage to the material involved. A variety of considerations influence the choice of method. The detailed mechanisms of the death process of microorganisms may vary with the sterilizing technique used, but the net effect is similar in that essential cell constituents (nucleic acids or proteins) are inactivated.

It is easier to sterilize a clean object than a physically dirty one

This is because organic matter protects microbes and hinders penetration of heat or chemicals and may inactivate certain chemicals. In other words, a low bioburden is a prerequisite for cost-effective sterilization.

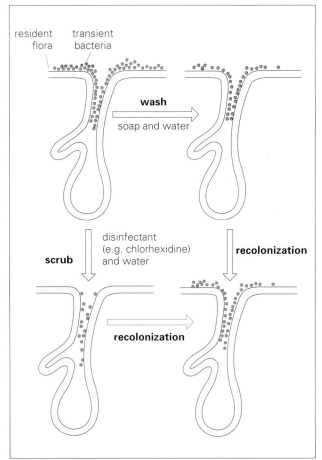

Fig. 34.22 Normal skin is colonized with bacteria both on the surface and deep in the pores and ducts of the sweat and sebaceous glands. In addition, bacteria may be carried transiently on the skin surface and may be transmitted from a contaminated source to a susceptible patient. Careful handwashing with soap and water removes the transient flora and some of the superficial resident flora. Scrubbing the hands with disinfectants removes more of the resident flora, but the skin surface is recolonized within hours from the normal flora deep in the skin pores.

The rate of killing of microorganisms depends upon the concentration of the killing agent and time of exposure

The number of survivors can be expressed by the equation: N is proportional to $1/CT$, where N is the number of survivors, C is the concentration of agent and T is time of exposure to the agent. If a population of microbes is exposed to a sterilizing technique and the number of survivors expressed as a logarithm is plotted against time, the slope of the graph defines the death rate *(Fig. 34.23)*. These lines may be sigmoid or have shoulders, indicating that individual cells respond slightly differently, some being killed more easily than others. In the case of bacteria, the physiologic state of the organisms influences the shape of the killing curve; young, replicating cells are usually more vulnerable than stationary or decline-phase organisms or those that are sporing. Graphs like those shown in *Figure 34.23* can be used to predict the conditions necessary to achieve sterility. However, these experimental data are usually based on pure cultures in the laboratory (bacterial spores are often used as model systems) whereas in real life the bioburden is mixed. Therefore predictions from such data may be inappropriate for mixed populations.

Techniques for Sterilization

Sterilization may be achieved by:
- Heat.
- Irradiation (gamma and ultraviolet).
- Filtration.
- Chemicals in liquid or gaseous phase.

Other techniques of doubtful efficiency include freezing and thawing, lysis, dessication, ultrasonication and the use of electrical discharges, but these are not applied in hospital practise.

Ultraviolet irradiation is inefficient as a sterilant and its important uses in the hospital setting are in inhibiting growth of bacteria in water in complex apparatus such as auto-analyzers and in air in safety hoods in virology laboratories. The potential for damage to the cornea and skin precludes wider use of ultraviolet irradiation. It should be remembered that the agents of Creutzfeldt–Jakob disease (CJD), bovine spongiform encephalopathy (BSE) and scrapie are highly resistant and are not completely inactivated by formalin, ultraviolet irradiation, ionizing radiation or regular autoclaving. Sterilization can be achieved by autoclaving at a higher temperature for a longer period than usual (134°C for 18 min), but obviously this technique cannot be applied to living tissues or materials that are damaged at high temperatures.

Heat

Heat, as a way of transferring energy, is the preferred choice for sterilization on the grounds of ease of use, controllability, cost and efficiency.

Dry heat sterilizes by oxidation of the cell components

Incineration and the use of the laboratory Bunsen burner are examples of sterilization by dry heat. Glassware can be sterilized in a hot air oven at 160–180°C for one hour.

The most effective agent for sterilization is saturated steam (moist heat) under pressure

This can be achieved using an autoclave. Steam under pressure aids penetration of heat into the material to be sterilized (such as dressings) and there is a direct relationship between temperature and steam pressure. Steam under pressure has a temperature in excess of 100°C, which results in increased killing of microbes.

Sterilizing efficiency is improved by evacuating all of the air from the autoclave chamber. The subsequent introduction of high pressure steam rapidly penetrates to all parts of the chamber and its load, and results in predictable rises in temperature in the center of articles to be sterilized. The length of an autoclave cycle is determined

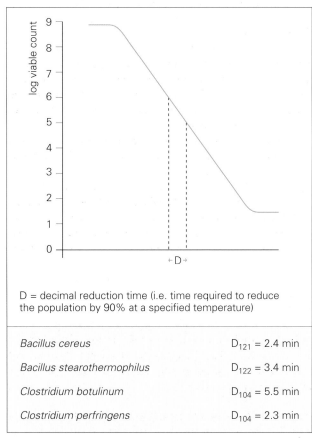

D = decimal reduction time (i.e. time required to reduce the population by 90% at a specified temperature)

Bacillus cereus	$D_{121} = 2.4$ min
Bacillus stearothermophilus	$D_{122} = 3.4$ min
Clostridium botulinum	$D_{104} = 5.5$ min
Clostridium perfringens	$D_{104} = 2.3$ min

Fig. 34.23 Theoretically there is a straight line relationship between the log viable count of a bacterial population and time when the population is exposed to a lethal temperature. In practise these lines are usually sigmoid. The D value is the time required to reduce the population by 90% at a specified temperature. *Bacillus stearothermophilus* spores are used as biologic indicators of effective heat sterilization by including filter paper strips carrying a standard number of spores into the autoclave cycle. The strips are then incubated to attempt to recover viable organisms. The usual autoclave cycle of 121°C for 15 minutes is adequate to kill *B. stearothermophilus* with a margin of safety.

by the holding time plus a margin of safety, and is derived from the thermal death curves for heat-resistant pathogens such as clostridia. Therefore the usual cycle of 121°C for 15 minutes is sufficient to kill the spores of *Cl. botulinum* with an adequate margin of safety. However, the spores of some bacterial species, especially soil organisms, are able to withstand this temperature. The safety margin is reduced in the presence of large numbers of organisms because there is a greater probability of more heat-resistant individuals existing in a large population and hence the importance of cleaning instruments whenever possible, before sterilization.

Moist heat in an autoclave is used to sterilize surgical instruments and dressings and heat-resistant pharmaceuticals. A method for the sterilization of heat-sensitive instruments such as endoscopes uses a combination of low temperature (subatmospheric) steam and formaldehyde.

All of these processes need to be carried out in a suitable pressure vessel and are therefore usually available in the hospital central sterile supply department.

Immersion in boiling water for a few minutes can be used as a rapid emergency measure to disinfect instruments

Immersion in boiling water for a few minutes will kill vegetative bacteria and many, but not all, spores. The addition of 2% sodium carbonate to the water potentiates the sporicidal effect.

Pasteurization uses heat at 62.8–65.6°C for 30 minutes

This technique was devised by Pasteur to prevent the spoilage of wine by heating it to 50–60°C. It is now used for fluids such as milk to reduce the number of bacteria. This helps to eliminate pathogens present in small numbers and to improve the shelf-life of milk. The fluid is held at a temperature of 62.8–65.6°C for 30 minutes or may be 'flash' pasteurized at 71.7°C for 15 seconds. After either process the fluid should be kept at a temperature below 10°C to minimize subsequent bacterial growth.

Irradiation
Gamma irradiation energy is used to sterilize large batches of small volume items

The use of gamma irradiation energy is now the method of choice for sterilizing large batches of small volume items such as needles, syringes, intravenous lines, catheters and gloves. It can also be used for vaccines and to prevent food spoilage. Although the capital cost of the equipment is high, the process is continuous and 100% efficient. Articles are sterilized sealed in their final packaging without any heat gain. The process must be conducted in a suitably constructed building, usually at a location distinct from the hospital and usually outside the hospital administration. It is not a technique applicable to 'one-off' use. The killing mechanism involves the production of free radicals, which break the bonds in DNA. Irradiation kills spores, but at a higher dose than vegetative cells because of the relative lack of water in spores. The recommended dose is 4.5 megarads.

Sterilization using ultraviolet irradiation is discussed above.

Filtration
Filters are used to produce particle- and pyrogen-free fluid

Solutions that are heat-sterilized will contain pyrogens. These heat-stable breakdown products of microbes are capable of inducing fever and are therefore undesirable in products such as intravenous fluids. Filtration or separation of the product from the contamination has a long history in the clarification of water and wine. Modern filters are composed of nitrocellulose and work by electrostatic attraction and physical pore size to retain organisms or other particles. The resulting fluid should be particle-free. Filtration is used in some parts of the world to purify drinking water.

Filtration techniques are also used to recover very small numbers of organisms from very large volumes of fluid (e.g. *Legionella* from cooling tower water) and can be used as a method for quantitating bacteria in fluids.

Chemical agents
The gases ethylene oxide and formaldehyde kill by damaging proteins and nucleic acids

The need for sterilization by gaseous chemicals has been greatly reduced by the success of gamma irradiation (see above), but two alkylating gases, ethylene oxide and formaldehyde, are still used:

- Ethylene oxide is used in some centers to sterilize single-use medical requisites such as heart valves. However, it is toxic and potentially explosive.
- Formaldehyde is not explosive, but has an extremely unpleasant odor and is an irritant to mucous membranes. It is used as a disinfectant to decontaminate rooms (such as isolation rooms) and in the laboratory to disinfect exhaust-protective cabinets. A high relative humidity is essential for effective killing.

The liquid glutaraldehyde is used to disinfect heat-sensitive articles

Glutaraldehyde is less toxic than formaldehyde and can be stabilized in solution to remain active for up to four weeks at in-use concentration. It is used for the disinfection of, but does not sterilize, heat-sensitive articles such as endoscopes and for inanimate surfaces.

Many different antimicrobial chemicals are available, but few are sterilant

Some, like the derivatives of pine and turpentine, have been known since ancient times, and chloride of lime and coal tar fluids were in use before the germ theory of disease was established. Most fall into the category of disinfectant or antiseptic, but a few are capable of rendering articles sterile. Factors that affect their efficacy include:

- Physical environment (e.g. porous or cracked surfaces).
- Presence of moisture.
- Temperature and pH.
- Concentration of the agent.

- Hardness of water.
- The bioburden on the object to be disinfected.
- The nature and state of the microbes in the bioburden.
- The ability of the microbes to inactivate the chemical agent.

It is obvious that the above factors are difficult to control in every circumstance. The main groups of chemical agents are shown in *Figure 34.24*. They act by causing chemical damage to proteins, nucleic acids or cell membrane lipids. The activity of a given disinfectant may result from more than one pathway of damage.

Controlling Sterilization and Disinfection

In general it is preferable to control the process rather than the product

This means that it is better to run checks on the technique while it is in operation rather than attempting to recognize process failure by isolating microorganisms from the product. Trying to discover whether one or a few viable organisms remain is analogous to trying to find a needle in a haystack. It is known that damaged bacteria can recover given time and special nutrient recovery media, but it may not be feasible to

DISINFECTANTS FOR HOSPITAL USE		
group	**examples**	**advantages and disadvantages**
Phenolics	clear-soluble phenolic compounds, white fluids	good general-purpose disinfectants, not readily inactivated by organic matter, active against wide range of organisms including mycobacteria, not sporicidal
	chloroxylenols	inactivated by hard water and organic matter, *Pseudomonas* grows readily in chloroxylenol solutions, limited activity against other Gram-negatives
Halogens	hypochlorites (chloramine)	cheap, effective, act by release of free chlorine, active against viruses and therefore recommended for disinfection of equipment soiled with blood (because of hepatitis risk), inactivated by organic material, corrode metals
	iodine and iodophors	useful skin disinfectants, sporicidal
Other heavy metals	mercuric chloride	used as topical skin preparation
Quaternary ammonium compounds	benzalkonium chloride, cetavlon	have detergent properties, activity against Gram-negative << Gram-positive, improved by combination with diguanide, e.g. chlorhexidine, useful as skin disinfectants, inactivated by hard water and organic materials, contamination of stock solutions with Gram-negative rods can be a problem
Diguanides	chlorhexidine	useful disinfectant for skin and mucous membranes, inactivated by many materials and too expensive for environmental use, alcoholic solutions are less easily contaminated, combinations of chlorhexidine and detergent highly effective for disinfection of hands
Alcohols	ethyl alcohol, isopropyl alcohol	good choice for skin disinfection and for clean surfaces, sometimes used in combination with iodine or chlorhexidine (see above), water must be present for bacterial killing (i.e. 70% ethanol best), isopropyl preferred for skin and articles in contact with patient
Aldehydes	formaldehyde/formalin	too irritant for use as general disinfectant
	glutaraldehyde	kills vegetative organisms, including mycobacteria, slowly but effectively, more active, less toxic than formaldehyde, sporicidal (within 6 hours when fresh), slightly irritant, used in alkaline solution which is stable for 1–2 weeks, expensive, limited use, e.g. disinfection of endoscopes
Hexachlorophane		activity against Gram-positive >> Gram-negative, used in soap or dusting powder as skin disinfectant (use restricted after potentially toxic blood levels found in infants who had hexachlorophane emulsion spread over whole body)
		introduced as substitute for hexachlorophane in soap, considerable antibacterial effect on repeated use

Fig. 34.24 Disinfectants for use in hospitals. Note that no one group of disinfectant has all the properties desirable for use both on skin and on inanimate surfaces.

hold back a batch of product for such tests. In addition, how many samples of the product should be tested? If too few are examined, the likelihood of missing a failed sample is high; if too many are examined, too much of the batch is used up in quality control to be economically sensible.

The usual process controls are either physical or chemical checks on the technique, for example tests that show that the autoclave reached the desired temperature for the desired time. They do not show that there are no viable organisms remaining after the process, but this is assumed if the process satisfies the controls. However, the stringency of the controls can be altered intentionally or accidentally to give either an undersensitive or oversensitive test.

- Any infection acquired in hospital is a hospital-acquired or nosocomial infection.
- Most common hospital-acquired infections are UTIs, respiratory tract infections, surgical wound infections and bacteremia (septicemia).
- The most important bacterial causes are Gram-positive cocci (staphylococci and streptococci) and Gram-negative rods (e.g. *E. coli, Pseudomonas*). Multiply antibiotic-resistant organisms are common. *Candida* is the significant fungal cause and viruses probably cause more hospital-acquired infections than previously recognized.
- Infecting organisms originate from the patient's own flora (endogenous infection) or from other human or inanimate sources (exogenous or cross-infection). Airborne and contact spread are the most important routes of transmission.
- Host factors are of critical importance in determining susceptibility to infection.
- Surveillance should be an ongoing activity to facilitate early recognition of outbreaks of infection. Investigation of outbreaks involves both epidemiologic and microbiologic expertise. Techniques to 'fingerprint' the causative organism are becoming increasingly sophisticated.
- Prevention of hospital-acquired infections by excluding sources, interrupting transmission and enhancing the patient's resistance is fundamental to improving patient care and reducing costs.
- Sterilization and disinfection are key processes in the control and prevention of hospital-acquired infections as well as being central to many areas of medical practice.

Disinfectants can be monitored by microbiological 'in-use' tests

These tests involve challenging the solution with a bacterial suspension and withdrawing samples, which are then treated to prevent carryover of the disinfectant and cultured. However, these tests are rarely performed in the hospital setting where the use of disinfectants is guided largely by the manufacturer's recommendations.

Summary

Hospital infections often have serious consequences for the individual, for the hospital community and for the community at large. They may be caused by almost any organism, but a few species cause the vast majority of infections. In addition the hospital environment favors the survival of resistant strains and therefore infections are often caused by organisms with limited antibiotic susceptibility. In view of the serious consequences of infection, control and prevention of infection should have a high priority and depend upon the education of staff in proper procedures as well as the provision of a clean environment and sterile equipment. Sterility cannot be demonstrated unequivocally (i.e. it is not possible to prove that no viable organisms remain). Nonetheless it is a cornerstone upon which much modern medicine and surgery depends.

As a surgeon you are called by the nurses to see a patient who has developed a fever. Three days ago he underwent a colonic resection for carcinoma of the colon. The operation went smoothly, and he was progressing well on the ward. His past medical history before admission was unremarkable, although he is noted to be a smoker. On examination his temperature is 37.8°C, he is slightly dyspneic at rest and there are a few basal crackles in his chest at both bases. His abdominal wound is dressed and you are reluctant to disturb the dressings.

1. What are the common causes of postoperative infections in patients and what steps can be taken to reduce these problems?
2. What investigations would you order?
3. How would you treat him?

Further Reading

Bennet JV, Brachman PS, eds. *Hospital Infections*. Baltimore/Toronto: Little Brown & Co, 1986.

Casewell MW, Phillips I. Hands as route of transmission for *Klesiella* sp. *Br Med J* 1977;**2**:1315.

Department of Health and Public Health Laboratory Service Report. *Hospital Infection* Control. London: Department of Health and Public Health Laboratory Service, 1995.

Lowbury EJL, Ayliffe GAJ, Geddes AM, Williams JD, eds. *Control of Hospital Infection*, 3rd edition. London: Chapman and Hall, 1992.

Maurer IM. *Hospital Hygiene*. London: Edward Arnold, 1974.

O'Brien TE, Ross DG, Guzman MA, *et al*. Dissemination of an antibiotic resistance plasmid in hospital patient flora. *Antimicrob Ag Chemother* 1980;**17**:537.

Williams REO, Blowers R, Garrod LP, Shooter RA. *Hospital Infection*. London: Lloyd Luke, 1966.

A

appendix

VIRUSES

PARVOVIRUSES

Characteristics	Virus family	Type	Envelope	Shape	Size (nm)	Nucleocapsid
	Papovaviridae	ssDNA	–	Icosahedral	22	Icosahedral

The family contains human parvovirus B19 (single serotype), and the adeno-associated viruses (four serotypes). The latter are defective, requiring concurrent infection of the cell with 'helper' adenovirus or herpes virus; positive DNA strands and negative DNA strands are carried in separate particles. The former are autonomous, but require mitotically active cells.

Replication   Occurs in the nucleus. Viral DNA replication takes place only when cell DNA replication is occurring (i.e. during the S phase of the cell cycle). Cellular transcriptase forms a cDNA strand to give dsDNA, and transcripts produce mRNAs.

Laboratory identification   Detection of parvovirus-specific IgM antibody or viral nucleic acid sequences.

Diseases   B19 parvovirus causes a mild disease, erythema infectiosum, in children, with a 'slapped cheek' rash. Aplastic crisis may occur in those with sickle cell anemia. Arthropathy common in infected adults. Intrauterine infection may result in fetal death with hydrops fetalis. The adeno-associated viruses are not known to cause disease.

Transmission   Via respiratory droplets.

Pathogenesis   Virus spreads from respiratory tract and can infect hemopoietic cells in bone marrow.

Treatment and prevention   There is no specific treatment and no vaccine.

PAPOVAVIRUSES

Characteristics	Virus family	Type	Envelope	Shape	Size (nm)	Nucleocapsid
	Papovaviridae	dsDNA (circular)	–	Icosahedral	45–55	Icosahedral

Replication   Virus attaches via unknown receptor to epithelial cell; viral mRNA is transcribed in the nucleus by a cellular transcriptase; early gene products initiate viral DNA replication, transcription, transformation; late gene products are structural proteins. Only the early genes (for T antigens) are expressed in transformed cells. The papovaviridae include **pa**pillomaviruses, **po**lyomaviruses and simian **va**cuolating viruses (e.g. SV40), with at least 65 types of human papillomavirus and two polyomaviruses (BK and JC). These viruses persist in latent form and can reactivate.

Laboratory identification   Serologic methods are unsatisfactory. Vacuolated or inclusion-bearing cells (koilocytosis) seen on Papanicolaou staining; virus particles visible (urine or tissues) by electron microscopy. Virus culture either difficult (polyomaviruses) or impossible (papillomaviruses). In special laboratories viral antigens or viral DNA sequences (southern blotting, *in situ* hybridization, polymerase chain reaction) can be tested for.

Diseases   Papillomaviruses cause warts on skin and genital regions. Sexually transmitted warts can cause laryngeal papilloma in children (infected via birth canal) and types HPV16, HPV18 strongly associated with carcinoma of cervix [also carcinoma of penis, vulva, rectum. Polyomaviruses on primary infection cause mild upper respiratory illness. In immunocompromised patients JC virus causes progressive multifocal leukoencephalopathy (PML), and BK virus is excreted in urine, but only rarely with pathologic consequences.

Transmission	Papillomaviruses: from skin to skin by direct or indirect contact, and between mucosae by sexual intercourse. Polyomaviruses: from the upper respiratory tract by droplets and perhaps by contact with infected urine.
Pathogenesis	Papillomavirus infection of epithelial cells and local multiplication results in a wart after an incubation period of up to 1–2 months. The wart regresses over the course of many months; there is no spread to deeper tissues, but viral DNA remains in basal epithelial cells and can reactivate. When genital warts undergo malignant change, viral genome remains in cell; cofactors are involved. Polyomaviruses spread from the upper respiratory tract and localize in tubular epithelium in the kidney (excretion in urine) or in oligodendrocytes to cause PML.
Treatment and prevention	No effective antivirals or vaccines available. Skin warts can be destroyed by freezing (liquid nitrogen) and areas of cervical dysplasia (genital warts) by laser treatment. Many slower methods are used (podophyllin, salicylic acid). Preventive measures include shoes for plantar warts and condoms for genital warts.

HERPESVIRUSES

Characteristics	Virus family	Type	Envelope	Shape	Size (nm)	Nucleocapsid
	Herpesviridae	dsDNA	+	Icosahedral	180–200	Icosahedral

Replication	Virus attaches to specific receptor on cell and enters by fusion of envelope with plasma membrane. Nucleocapsid moves to nucleus; viral DNA is uncoated at nuclear pores and then transcribed by cellular RNA polymerase so that the five sets of viral genes are sequentially activated. 'Immediate–early' gene products stimulate synthesis of second wave of 'early' gene products that are involved in genome replication and include the DNA polymerases. After DNA replication the remaining 'late' gene products are expressed and are involved in assembly. In the nucleus viral DNA is inserted in capsids and resulting nucleocapsids attach to sites on inner nuclear membrane where envelope proteins are present and budding takes place between inner and outer nuclear membranes. Enveloped virus particles are transported through the cytoplasm and released by reverse phagocytosis. Replication cycle about 36 h. Generally persist for long periods in body, often in latent form (in neurones, monocytes, T cells, B cells), and can reactivate.
Laboratory identification	Isolation of virus in cell culture – herpes simplex virus (HSV), cytomegalovirus (CMV); multinucleated cells – HSV, varicella–zoster virus (VZV) or intranuclear inclusions (CMV) in smears, tissues. Rise in antibody titer (all). Lymphocytosis, atypical lymphoyctes, and heterophil antibody (Monospot) for EBV.

Diseases	**Type**	**Clinical features**
	HHV1 (HSV1)	Gingivostomatitis, cold sores, encephalitis
	HHV2 (HSV2)	Genital herpes, cutaneous herpes, encephalitis, meningoencephalitis
	HHV3 (VZV)	Varicella, zoster
	HHV4 (EBV)	Mononucleosis (glandular fever), hepatitis, encephalitis, BL, NPC
	HHV5 (CMV)	Mononucleosis, hepatitis, pneumonitis, congenital CMV
	HHV6	Exanthem subitum, mild febrile illness
	HHV7	Exanthem subitum, mild febrile illness
	HHV8	Associated with Kaposi's sarcoma

Transmission	HSV: saliva, vesical fluid, sexual contact, birth canal in neonate.
	VZV: respiratory droplets, vesical fluid.
	EBV: saliva.
	CMV: saliva, urine, semen, cervical secretions, milk; also via transplanted tissues and across placenta.
	HHV6, 7: saliva
	HHV8: semen

Pathogenesis	HSV: vesicular lesions on mouth, skin, genitals; axonal travel to latency sites in sensory ganglia; reactivation (cold sores).
	VZV: respiratory infection, systemic spread to skin, axonal travel to latency sites sensory ganglia; reactivation (zoster).
	EBV: pharyngeal infection, systemic spread, latency in B cells, epithelium; subclinical reactivation.
	CMV: pharyngeal infection, systemic spread, latency in mononuclear cells; reactivation.
	HHV6, 7: present in T cells.
	HHV8: infects endothelial cells in Kaposi's sarcoma.
Treatment and prevention	Aciclovir (HSV, VZV); ganciclovir (CMV).
	Varicella–zoster immune globulin (VZIG) is used to prevent disease when immunocompromised are exposed to infection.
	No vaccines yet available for herpes viruses.

ADENOVIRUSES

Characteristics	Virus family	Type	Envelope	Shape	Size (nm)	Nucleocapsid
	Adenoviridae	ds DNA	–	Icosahedral	70–90	Icosahedral

42 types, sharing a common group-specific antigen. Rod-like structures (fibers) topped with knobs project from the vertices of particles, and function by attaching virus to the cell.

Replication	After attachment, endocytosis and uncoating, viral DNA is transcribed within the nucleus by cellular DNA-dependent RNA polymerase. RNA transcripts corresponding to several genes (less than the whole genome) undergo cleavage and splicing to form monocistronic mRNA. Early mRNA codes for enzymes needed for replication; late mRNA (after viral DNA synthesis) for structural proteins. Particles are assembled in the nucleus and released from the damaged cell.
Laboratory identification	Rise in complement fixing antibody titer. Demonstration of the virus in samples such as mouthwashings, throat swabs, feces, using human embryo lung (HEL) or Hela cells and looking for cytopathic effect (cpe), for antigen by fluorescent antibody (FA) staining, or for virions by electron microscopy.
Diseases	Cause pharyngoconjunctival fever; epidemics of acute respiratory disease, including pneumonia (especially types 3, 4, 7, 14, 21); intestinal illness (mesenteric adenitis, intusussception); keratoconjunctivitis. Very occasionally cause hemorrhagic cystitis or CNS disease. Some are oncogenic in laboratory animals, but not in humans.
Transmission	Via respiratory droplets, via feces, and sometimes from eye to eye via for example contaminated hands, towels, or eye drops.
Pathogenesis	Adenoviruses infect epithelium of respiratory tract and eyes, and probably intestine. Spread to involve lymphoid tissues and can persist for long periods in tonsils and adenoids of children (types 1, 2, 5, 6). Viral proteins interferes with immune defences (eg. block action of interferon and Tc cells).
Treatment and prevention	No specific treatment. Live oral vaccine (types 3, 4, 7 in enteric-coated capsules) has been used in military recruits.

HEPADNAVIRUSES (HEPATITIS B)

Characteristics	Virus family	Type	Envelope	Shape	Size (nm)	Nucleocapsid
	Hepadnaviridae	ds DNA (circular)	+	Spherical	42	Icosahedral

Particles consist of an envelope (HBs antigen) surrounding a core containing HBc (core antigen) and HBe antigen. Infected blood contains 22 nm particles of HBs, outnumbering by at least 100 to one the 42 nm infectious (Dane) particles. One serotype (minor antigenic variants such as adn, adw, give complete cross-protection). Virus encodes a reverse transcriptase.

Replication

After attachment to hepatocytes, particles are endocytosed and uncoated. In the nucleus, viral DNA polymerase converts viral DNA into a complete circular dsDNA. Negative strand DNA is transcribed by cellular RNA polymerase to form a single positive RNA strand, which moves to the cytoplasm, is translated into protein, and is then encapsulated into cores together with viral DNA polymerase. The positive RNA strand is then used to synthesize negative-strand DNA (reverse transcriptase activity). A small fragment from the 5' end of the positive RNA strand primes synthesis of all but about one-third of the positive DNA strand. Hence complete particles contain dsDNA with a ssDNA region. Release from cell is by budding. Viral DNA can be integrated into host DNA.

Laboratory identification

The virus cannot be grown in cell culture. HBs antigen in blood (detectable during incubation period) indicates either acute or persistent infection. Presence of HBe antigen means blood is highly infectious. Presence of anti-HBs, anti-HBc (latter occurs early in the disease before anti-HBs), and anti-HBe indicates recent or past infection and immunity.

Diseases

Causes hepatitis, often severe in adults; important immunopathologic contribution to disease. Incubation period 10–12 weeks. Persistent infection common, especially after infection in infancy or early childhood, when blood remains infectious, possibly for life; this can lead to chronic hepatitis, cirrhosis, liver cancer. 350 million carriers worldwide – up to 0.5% of population in developed countries.

Transmission

Spread via blood (e.g. contaminated needles), by sexual routes and from mother to offspring.

Pathogenesis

Virus spreads via blood to liver; replicates in hepatocytes. Immune complex formation can cause initial rash, arthritis; hepatitis is probably largely due to immune destruction of infected liver cells.

Treatment and prevention

No specific treatment. Carriage of virus can be terminated by massive doses of alpha and beta interferon. The excellent vaccine consists of genetically engineered HBs antigen. Post-exposure treatment is possible with human hyperimmune immunoglobulin.

POXVIRUSES

Characteristics

Virus family	Type	Envelope	Shape	Size (nm)	Nucleocapsid
Poxviridae	ds DNA	+/–	Brick or ovoid	200–300	Complex structure

The largest viruses; dermatotrophic, causing 'pocks' on the skin.

Replication

Takes place in the cytoplasm (unlike other DNA viruses) and viral DNA-dependent RNA polymerase is used to synthesize mRNA. Transcripts are translated directly into proteins, some of which undergo post-translational cleavage to give functional molecules. After assembly, infectious virions are released as the cell disintegrates, some of them acquiring an envelope in the Golgi complex.

Laboratory identification

Characteristic poxvirus particles are seen on electron microscopic examination of scrapings or biopsies of the skin lesions. Neither cell culture methods for virus isolation nor antibody tests are routinely available.

Diseases

Molluscum contagiosum causes a mild infection with nodular skin lesions. Cowpox or milkers' nodules virus lesions on cow udders can cause vesicular lesions on the skin of milkers. Orf virus is responsible for contagious pustular dermatitis in sheep, and those in contact with infected animals (e.g. shepherds) may develop vesicular skin lesions. After exposure to monkeys infected with monkeypox virus (monkeys are a favorite food in some parts of the

Ivory Coast), humans develop a smallpox-like disease, which is distinguishable from smallpox by laboratory tests.

Transmission	By direct contact with virus from skin lesions. Molluscum contagiosum is transmitted between humans, but monkeypox, cowpox, orf, and milkers' nodules viruses are zoonoses, transmissible from the animal host to humans. Smallpox was eradicated in 1979.
Pathogenesis	Infection generally initiated in skin with local replication to form virus-rich vesicles; limited spread to local lymph nodes. Smallpox, however, infected via respiratory tract, and spread via blood to cause severe disease with disseminated skin and mucosal lesions.
Treatment and prevention	In the past methisazone was used to treat the serious side effects very occasionally caused by vaccination against smallpox with live vaccinia virus. Vaccination was the principle method used to eradicate smallpox, but is no longer necessary. Vaccinia was the first virus to be used as an expression vector for live recombinant vaccines (see Chapter 31).

PICORNAVIRUSES

Characteristics	Virus family	Type	Envelope	Shape	Size (nm)	Nucleocapsid
	Picornaviridae	ssDNA +ve sense	–	Icosahedral	25–30	Icosahedral

Replication	Virus binds to cell via receptor molecule intercellular adhesion molecule-1 (ICAM-1), resulting in endocytosis and uncoating. The positive-sense viral ssRNA acts as mRNA, which is translated into a single polyprotein, cleaved by virus-coded protease into separate proteins. These include the RNA polymerase that makes negative-strand cRNA, which in turn acts as template for positive strands of viral RNA. RNA and capsid proteins assemble in the cytoplasm to form nucleocapsids, which are released on death of the cell. General features: four viral capsid proteins (VP1–VP4). There is no envelope.
Laboratory identification	Rhinoviruses cannot be routinely cultivated. Enteroviruses recoverable from for example throat, feces, cerebrospinal fluid by cultivation in monkey kidney or human embryo lung cells, where they cause cytopathic effect and cell death. Significance of isolations need thought because these viruses are ubiquitous in children. Tests for antibody not useful in view of multiple serotypes, but rise in titer to specific serotype (e.g. coxsackievirus B in myocarditis) may be useful.
Diseases	Rhinoviruses: more than 100 serotypes; common cold viruses. Enteroviruses: • Polioviruses, types 1–3; aseptic meningitis, paralytic poliomyelitis. • Echoviruses (enterocytopathic human orphans): 32 types; aseptic meningitis, rashes. • Coxsackieviruses: 29 types; aseptic meningitis, herpangina, myopericarditis (coxsackievirus B). • Enteroviruses 68–72: conjunctivitis (enterovirus 70), polio-like illness (enterovirus 71), hepatitis type A (enterovirus 72).
Transmission	Respiratory (droplet) spread for rhinoviruses and certain group A coxsackieviruses. Other enteroviruses fecal-oral spread.
Pathogenesis	Rhinoviruses (acid-labile, optimal growth 33°C) replicate in upper respiratory tract. Enteroviruses (resist pH 3.0–9.0) replicate in pharynx and gastrointestinal tract, often with spread to lymph nodes and blood, and then to CNS (e.g. polio, echoviruses), heart and muscle (coxsackie B), or liver (hepatitis A).
Treatment and prevention	No specific treatment. Poliomyelitis prevented by vaccination with live attenuated (Sabin) or killed (Salk) vaccine. Hepatitis A prevented by immunoglobulins or inactivated virus vaccine. No vaccines for other picornaviruses.

ORTHOMYXOVIRUSES (INFLUENZA VIRUSES)

Characteristics	Virus family	Type	Envelope	Shape	Size (nm)	Nucleocapsid
	Orthomyxoviridae	ssRNA, linear eight segments –ve sense	+	Spherical	80–120	Helical

Envelope glycoproteins: hemagglutinin (H) attaches virus to sialic acid-containing receptor on cell and (after exposure to endosomal acid) acts as fusion protein; neuraminidase (N) cleaves sialic acid from glycoproteins and is involved in release of virus from cell surface.
Influenza A: widespread in birds, horses, pigs, humans. Genetic reassortments between animal and human strains produce subtypes with novel combinations of H and N genes (i.e. antigenic 'shift'); new strains can cause pandemics. Antigenic 'drift' also occurs (i.e. point mutations occur in H to generate new strains). Influenza B: occurs only in humans; undergoes antigenic drift and can cause epidemics. Influenza C: of doubtful pathogenicity in humans.

Replication Virus binds to cell via its H, enters a vesicle, its envelope fusing with vesicle wall. After uncoating, viral polymerase transcribes genome into eight mRNAs, which are translated in the cytoplasm. Progeny RNA synthesized in nucleus and nucleocapsids assembled in cytoplasm. Viral matrix protein joins nucleocapsid to viral envelope components in the cell wall and maturation takes place by budding.

Laboratory identification Serology: complement fixing tests with S (soluble) antigen, and H inhibition tests. Isolation of virus in monkey kidney cells. Detection of viral antigen by immunofluorescence.

Diseases Incubation period 1–2 days. Fever, myalgia, malaise, nasal discharge, sore throat, cough, pneumonia.

Transmission Via respiratory droplets.

Pathogenesis Infection limited to respiratory tract. Cytokines contribute to symptoms and secondary bacterial infection quite common.

Treatment and prevention Amantadine can be used (also in prophylaxis). A killed vaccine containing current A and B strains prevents disease in susceptible individuals (e.g. the elderly)

PARAMYXOVIRUSES (E.G. MEASLES, MUMPS)

Characteristics	Virus family	Type	Envelope	Shape	Size (nm)	Nucleocapsid
	Paramyxoviridae	ssRNA non-segmented –ve sense	+	Pleomorphic	45–55	Helical

Envelope glycoproteins are H (hemaglutinin), N (neuraminidase), F (fusion), and G. H and N are combined (HN) in paramyxoviruses (mumps, parainfluenza 1–4), morbillivirus (measles) has H and pneumovirus (respiratory syncytial virus, RSV) has G (no H or N).

Replication Virus particle binds via its attachment protein (HN, H or G) to cell surface, penetrates and is uncoated. Viral polymerase transcribes genome into mRNAs, which are translated into viral proteins. Nucleocapsid is assembled and matrix protein joins it to the envelope proteins forming on the plasma membrane of the infected cell. Release then occurs by budding.

Laboratory identification Serology of limited value for parainfluenza, measles; complement fixing tests for RSV, mumps. Demonstration of viral antigen by immunofluorescence in nasal aspirates (RSV, measles). F protein of measles forms multinucleated giant cells (syncytia).

Diseases	Measles: fever, nasal discharge, rash (very rarely encephalitis, subacute sclerosing panencephalitis); incubation period 10–14 days. Mumps: parotitis, aseptic meningitis (rarely orchitis, encephalitis); incubation period 18–24 days. Parainfluenza viruses: common cold; bronchiolitis, pneumonia; incubation period 3–6 days. RSV: common cold (adults), bronchiolitis, pneumonia (infants); incubation period 2–8 days.
Transmission	Respiratory droplets.
Pathogenesis	Initial infection via respiratory tract. RSV and parainfluenza virus infections: local replication and disease. Measles and mumps: no lesions at site of initial infection, spread to local lymph nodes, blood and invasion of skin and mucosa (measles) or salivary glands, CNS (mumps).
Treatment and prevention	Aerosolized ribavirin for infants with severe RSV infections. Nil available for other paramyxoviruses. Measles and mumps prevented by live attenuated virus vaccines. No vaccines in routine use for RSV and parainfluenza viruses.

TOGAVIRUSES (E.G. RUBELLA, YELLOW FEVER)

Characteristics	Virus family	Type	Envelope	Shape	Size (nm)	Nucleocapsid
	Togaviridae	ssRNA +ve sense	+	Spherical	60–70	Icosahedral

	Human togaviruses include rubella (genus *rubivirus*), and more than 80 serologically distinct arthropod-transmitted viruses (arboviruses). The latter occur in all parts of the world, often have exotic names (Kyasanur Forest disease virus, India; Omsk hemorrhagic fever virus, Russia), and replicate in the arthropod vector as well as in the vertebrate host. Most have animal reservoirs. The alphaviruses responsible for western equine encephalomyelitis (WEE), eastern equine encephalomyelitis (EEE), Ross River Virus are distinguished from the flaviviruses (yellow fever, dengue, St Louis encephalitis). Hepatitis C is a flavivirus.
Replication	The positive strand RNA is translated into structural and non-structural proteins, the latter including the RNA-dependent RNA-polymerase, which replicates the viral genome by directing the formation of a negative-strand template and thus giving rise to positive-strand progeny. Full length and subgenomic length RNA is formed (full length only in flaviviruses*, with rapid cleavage of the polyprotein that is formed). After assembly, the virus exits from the cell, budding from the plasma membrane (or endoplasmic reticulum in the case of flaviviruses*).
Laboratory diagnosis	Rubella can be isolated in cell culture and specific IgM antibody – H inhibition, enzyme-linked immunosorbent assay (ELISA) – indicates recent infection. Serologic methods and to a lesser extent virus isolation are used to diagnose the arthropod-borne togavirus infections.
Diseases	Rubella causes a mild exanthematous disease, in adults sometimes complicated by arthralgia, and in pregnant women by fetal infection, with congenital malformations. The remaining togaviruses cause febrile illnesses, which may be severe when there is involvement of liver (yellow fever) or CNS (equine encephalitides), or when there are immunopathologic complications (dengue hemorrhagic fever).
Transmissions	Rubella is transmitted between humans by the respiratory droplets; the rest are transmitted by the bite of infected arthropodes, but not directly from human to human.
Pathogenesis	Initial infection via respiratory tract (rubella) or skin (arthropod-borne viruses) causes no detectable local lession. Virus spreads to local lymph nodes and blood, multiplying in respiratory tract, placenta and fetus (rubella), liver (yellow fever), or CNS (equine encephalitides). Mononuclear cells often infected (rubella, dengue). Immunopathology important in dengue hemorrhagic fever and probably in the equine encephalitides. In mosquitoes, ingested virus infects gut epithelium, spreads to salivary glands, and multiplies there.

*Flaviviruses are now placed in a separate group, but are included with togaviruses for convenience. Arboviruses include not only togaviruses, but bunyaviruses (Californian encephalitis, Rift Valley fever virus) and reoviruses (Colorado tick fever virus).

Treatment and prevention

There is no antiviral therapy. A live attenuated virus vaccine prevents rubella and congenital rubella, a live attenuated (17D) vaccine is highly effective against yellow fever, and there is a live attenuated vaccine for Japanese encephalitis. Vaccines are not available for the other arthropod-transmitted togaviruses, but horses can be protected from WEE and EEE with veterinary vaccines.

RETROVIRUSES

Characteristics

Virus family	Type	Envelope	Shape	Size (nm)	Nucleocapsid
Retrovidae	ssRNA diploid +ve sense	+	Spherical	80–120	Icosahedral

Family includes HVI1,HIV2 (lentiviruses); HTLV1, HTLV2 (oncoviruses); human foamy virus (spumavirus), which causes foamy change in cells, but little else known; endogenous retroviruses, which exist as sequences in human genome.

Replication

HIV: binds to CD4 on cell surface, enters and is uncoated. Virion RNA-dependent DNA polymerase (reverse transcriptase) transcribes viral genome into dsDNA (provirus), which is then integrated into host cell DNA by viral integrase. Transcription is by host RNA polymerase; genomic and viral mRNA are formed, and translated into structural and regulatory proteins. Viral genes *gag, pol, env* code for structural proteins and (in the case of HIV) five other gene products have regulatory functions. Nucleocapsids assemble in cyoplasm and released by budding.

Laboratory identification

HIV: antibodies to envelope antigens gp120 (CD4-binding), gp41 (fusion protein), p24 (group-specific antigen in core) are tested by enzyme-linked immunosorbent assay (ELISA), latex agglutination, western blotting (similar tests for HTLV1 antibodies); p24 antigen may be detected in serum. Virus isolation in cultured T cells, but only in specialized laboratories.

Diseases

HIV: mild early illness with mononucleosis; sometimes aseptic meningitis; later 1) often after many years progessing to AIDS, with multiple opportunistic infections, Kaposi's sarcoma, 2) HIV-specific CNS disease (AIDS neuropathy, AIDS-related dementia), 3) intestinal syndrome, with diarrhea, weight loss ('slim' disease in Africa). HTLV1: tropical spastic paraparesis, T cell leukemia. HTLV2: hairy cell leukemia.

Transmission

HIV: via blood, semen, transplacental transfer. HIV1 worldwide, HIV2 mainly West Africa. HTLV1: via milk and blood; occurs in certain islands in Caribbean and Japan, and in parts of South America, Africa. HTLV2: via blood.

Pathogenesis

HIV: initial entry via mucosal route with infection of CD4-positive cells (helper T cells, dendritic cells, monocytes, macrophages). Spread through body including CNS, placenta. Action on immune cells results in severe immunosuppression leading to opportunist infections and reactivations (viral, bacterial, protozoal). Also Kaposi's sarcoma associated with presence of HHV8. HTLV1: pathogensis of CNS disease not clear. Leukemia (mean 30 years after infection) results from multistage process initiated by *tat* gene product in infected T cells stimulating transcription of host genes that control cell division.

Treatment and prevention

HIV: zidovudine inhibits virus replication and arrests disease progress without eliminating virus from body (viral DNA transcripts remain in infected cells). Treatment of opportunist infections. Various vaccines are undergoing clinical trials. Prevention by avoiding bloodborne virus (e.g. needle exchange programs, treatment of blood and blood products) and practising safe sex (e.g. education, condoms). HTLV1 and 2:zidovudine presumably effective.

RHABDOVIRUS (RABIES)

Characteristics

Virus family	Type	Envelope	Shape	Size(nm)	Neucleocapsid
Rhabdoviridae	ss –ve sense RNA	+	Bullet shaped	180	Helical

Replication	Viral G protein attaches to acetylcholine receptor or other molecules on cell; virus is endocytosed and uncoated. Virion RNA polymerase synthesizes five mRNAs, and virus-coded RNA polymerase replicates viral RNA. After assembly of nucleocapsid the envelope is acquired by budding from the plasma membrane without detectable cell damage. Rabies virus can infect all mammals. Present in wild animals in all continents except Australia and Antarctica. Only one serotype.
Laboratory identification	Brain tissue (at autopsy), corneal scrapings, biopsy of hair-bearing skin, examined for presence of inclusions (Negri bodies) or rabies antigen (by fluroresent antibody (FA) staining). Virus isolation is not necessary.
Diseases	Incubation period 2–10 weeks. CNS symptoms and signs (excitement, confusion, lethargy, hydrophobia), progression to seizures, paralysis, coma and death.
Transmission	Via bite of infected dog, cat, skunk, racoon, bat. Human to human transmission not a feature.
Pathogenesis	Virus replicates at site of bite, ascends axons to CNS where it spreads, and then descends down peripheral nerves to skin, salivary glands.
Treatment and prevention	No specific treatment. Post-exposure prophylaxis by washing wound, giving human rabies-specific immune serum and vaccine. Disease prevented by inactivated vaccine produced in human diploid cells.

ARENAVIRUSES (LCM, LASSA FEVER)

Characteristics	Virus family	Type	Envelope	Shape	Size (nm)	Nucleocapsid
	Arenaviridae	ssRNA –ve sense	+	Spherical	50–300	Helical

	Virions are pleomorphic containing two circular RNA segments, one negative and one ambisense, and in addition host ribosomes, visible as granules inside the envelope (Latin *arena*, sand).
Replication	Viral RNA-dependent RNA polymerase produces positive strand RNA, which is translated to form a nucleoprotein and two glycoproteins. Maturation by budding with no cytopathic effect on the cell.
Laboratory identification	Detection of specific antibody – complement fixation, enzyme-linked immunosorbent assay (ELISA), immunofluorescence tests – or (in special laboratories) virus isolation.
Diseases	Febrile illness, sometimes complicated by aseptic meningitis (lymphocytic choriomeningitis: LCM), or by severe hemorrhagic disease (Lassa fever, Argentinian and Bolivian hemorrhagic fevers).
Transmission	Cause inapparent persistent infections in the natural rodent host and spread (as zoonoses) to humans via contact with rodent excreta. LCM virus occurs worldwide, comes from mice and hamsters; Lassa fever virus in West Africa from the bush rat *Mastomys natalensis;* Junin and Machupo viruses from bush mice (*Calomys* spp.) in South America causing Argentinian and Bolivian hemorrhagic fevers).
Pathogenesis	Natural rodent host is infected *in utero* or neonatally, and virus (noncytopathic) remains in all tissues throughout life. In human host, virus spreads systemically causing meningitis or hemorrhagic disease by local or general replication plus immunopathology.
Treatment and prevention	Ribavirin may be useful in Lassa fever and the South American hemorrhagic fevers. Vaccines for routine use are not available.

REOVIRUSES (COLORADO TICK FEVER, ROTAVIRUSES)

Characteristics	Virus family	Type	Envelope	Shape	Size (nm)	Nucleocapsid
	Reoviridae:	dsRNA, 10 (reo) or 11 (rota) segments	–	Icosahedral	75	Icosahedral (double layered)

Replication	Virion resists acid pH, drying, detergents. Host protease (in intestinal phagolysosme) cleaves outer capsid protein to produce a fully infectious particle, which binds to cell membrane via receptor. Core enters cytoplasm, viral RNA-dependent RNA polymerase (one molecule for each genome segment) synthesizes 10–11 mRNAs (not polyadenylated), which direct synthesis of proteins, one of which is an RNA polymerase. The latter produces negative-strand viral RNA; positive strands are formed, and the assembled virus is released by cell lysis.
Laboratory identification	Detection of antibody rise, or of antiviral IgM (Colorado tick fever). Serology not useful for rotaviruses. Virus particles visible in stool by electron microscopy (rotaviruses). Detection of viral antigens by immunofluorescence (on erythrocytes, Colorado tick fever) or by enzyme-linked immunosorbent assay (ELISA), latex agglutination (feces, rotaviruses). Virus isolation not generally used.
Diseases	Orthoreovirus (three types): few if any symptoms; the word reovirus derives from respiratory enteric orphan virus (orphan because initially not associated with any disease). Rotaviruses (types A–D): diarrheal illness, especially in infancy and childhood, and sometimes respiratory symptoms. Colorado tick fever virus (orbivirus group): acute febrile illness.
Transmission	Orthoreoviruses: fecal-oral and possibly respiratory spread. Rotaviruses: fecal-oral spread (virus survives drying and stomach acid). Colorado tick fever virus: by bite of an infected tick.
Pathogenesis	Orthoreoviruses: entry via respiratory or gastrointestinal tract (M cells) and spread to local lymphoid tissue. Rotaviruses: infection of enterocytes with no spread to deeper tissues; causes gastrointestinal illness (shortening of villi, interference with transport mechanisms). Colorado tick fever: virus enters skin via tick bite, spreads to local lymph nodes and blood, infects erythrocytes, and causes febrile illness.
Treatment and prevention	No antiviral agents and no vaccines routinely available. Rotavirus diarrhea (prevented by improved hygiene) is treated by replacing water and electrolytes. Antitick measures protect against Colorado tick fever.

CORONAVIRUSES

Characteristics	Virus family	Type	Envelope	Shape	Size (nm)	Nucleocapsid
	Coronaviridae	ssRNA +ve sense	+	Spherical (corona)	80–160	Helical

Replication	Viral RNA-dependent RNA polymerase uses genomic positive-strand to produce negative-strand RNA, which acts as template for new positive strands. Nucleocapsids bud into endoplasmic reticulum from which they are released by exocytosis.
Laboratory identification	Antibody tests, electron microscopic examination (clubs project from envelope and form 'corona'), and viral isolation (difficult) are not routinely available and rarely necessary.
Diseases	Common cold-type illness (possibly gastroenteritis).
Transmission	Respiratory droplets.
Pathogenesis	Replication in cells lining upper respiratory tract. Optimum growth temperature 33–35°C.
Treatment and prevention	No antivirals or vaccines available.

BUNYAVIRUSES

Characteristics	Virus family	Type	Envelope	Shape	Size (nm)	Nucleocapsid
	Bunyaviridae	ssRNA –ve sense	+	Helical	90–100	Icosahedral

Contains more than 100 different viruses. Bunyamwera is a locality in Africa where the prototype virus was isolated. Important human members are the hantaviruses (Southeast Asia, USA), Rift Valley Fever (RVF, Africa) virus, and La Crosse (Californian encephalitis) virus.

Replication	After attachment to cell receptors and endocytosis, nucleocapsid enters cytoplasm by fusion with endosomal membranes; the three segments of RNA are transcribed into mRNA and translated. Virus RNA is then transcribed, replicated. Glycoproteins are synthesized and glycosylated in endoplasmic reticulum, entering the Golgi where budding takes place, with release by exocytosis or lysis of the cell.
Laboratory identification	Rises in antibody titer by enzyme-linked immunosorbent assay (ELISA) or neutralization tests. Virus isolation only in special centers.
Diseases	Cause febrile viremic illnesses; generally mild. RVF can cause hemorrhagic phenomena, sometimes with a lethal outcome; La Crosse virus can cause encephalitis, and hantaviruses, renal disease (Korean hemorrhagic fever) or a severe pulmonary syndrome.
Transmission	With the exception of the hantaviruses, which are acquired from urine of infected rodents, bunyaviruses are transmitted by mosquitoes (or ticks or sandflies), and there is a bird or mammal reservoir.
Pathogenesis	After reaching the blood, virus disseminates to the CNS, liver, kidney, multiplies in vascular endothelium (hantaviruses).
Treatment and prevention	Prevention is by avoiding contact with arthropod vector (RVF virus, La Crosse virus) or with infected rodents (hantaviruses). Vaccines have been developed for RVF.

SCRAPIE-TYPE AGENTS

Characteristics	Not viruses. Prototype agent (scrapie) causes CNS disease in sheep. Structure and mode of replication unknown. Contain little or no nucleic acid. Host-coded prion protein in slightly altered form (protease-resistant) is closely associated with infectivity. Highly resistant to heat (special autoclaving procedures required for destruction), chemical agents, and irradiation. Very slow replication, very long incubation period (up to 20 years in humans). Infect a variety of mammals and can be transmitted to cows, mink, cats and mice for example when food contains infected material.
Laboratory identification	Intracellular vacuoles (spongiform change) visible histologically in brain. Altered prion protein detectable in brain, but test not routinely available. Isolation of agent requires experimental animals and is lengthy, difficult and not undertaken. No specific immune (e.g. antibody) responses.
Diseases	'Spongiform encephalopathies', 'prion diseases'. Kuru: fatal neurologic diseases in Papua New Guinea, no longer seen. Creutzfeldt–Jakob disease (CJD): rare chronic encephalopathy, occurs worldwide; 10% cases familial with mutated prion protein gene. Gerstmann–Straussler–Scheinker syndrome (GSS). Fatal familial insomnia.
Transmission	Kuru: from infected human brain by cannabalism. CJD: in most cases unknown; occasionally transmitted from infected human brain by medical and surgical procedures; familial cases genetically transmitted. Newtype CJB from consumption of BSE (bovine spongiform encephalopathy) contain infected food.
Pathogenesis	Infectious agent replicates inexorably in lymphoid tissues, and then in brain cells, where it produces intracellular vacuoles and deposition of altered host prion protein. Uniformly fatal if host lives long enough.
Treatment and prevention	No treatment or vaccine. Kuru died out when cannbalism ceased. Iatrogenic transfer of CJD preventable (e.g. when genetically engineered growth hormone became available).

BACTERIA

GRAM-POSITIVE COCCI

GENUS *Staphylococcus*

Genus contains at least 15 different species, of which three are of medical importance: *Staph. aureus, Staph. epidermidis, Staph. saprophyticus.*

Major distinguishing features of medically important staphylococci	Test	*Staph. aureus*	*Staph. epidermidis*	*Staph. saprophyticus*
	Coagulase production*	+	–	–
	Protein A on cell surface	+	–	–
	Production of recognized exotoxins	+	–	–
	Hemolysin production	+**	–**	+
	Resistance to novobiocin (5μg)	***	–	+

* Note that the coagulase-negative species *Staph. epidermidis* and *Staph. saprophyticus* and other less commonly isolated coagulase-negative species are often referred to simply as 'coagulase-negative staphylococci' without further identification.

** Usual result, but not for all strains.

*** Useful for distinguishing between *Staph. epidermidis* and *Staph. saprophyticus.*

Staphylococcus aureus

Characteristics	Gram-positive coccus; cells in clusters (reflecting ability to divide in more than one plane); individual cells approximately 1 μm in diameter. Some strains produce capsules. Non-fastidious; capable of aerobic and anaerobic respiration.
Laboratory identification	White or golden colonies on blood agar. Catalase positive, coagulase positive; most strains ferment mannitol anaerobically. Kits available for biochemical characterization.
Diseases	Boils; skin sepsis; postoperative wound infection; scalded skin syndrome; catheter-associated infection; foodborne infection; septicemia, endocarditis; toxic shock syndrome; osteomyelitis; pneumonia.
Transmission	Normal habitat: humans (and animals associated with them); skin, especially nose and perineum (carriage rates higher in hospital patients and staff). Spread is by contact and airborne routes. Organism survives drying; tolerant of salt and nitrites.
Epidemiological markers	Bacteriophage typing.
Pathogenesis	Virulence multifactorial and most factors shown below are present in some strains. Present in all strains: • Mucopeptide. • Coagulase. Present in some strains: • Cell-associated – capsule, protein A*, fibronectin-binding protein, collagen-binding proteins. • Extracellular products – enterotoxins, epidermolytic toxin, toxic shock syndrome toxin, membrane-damaging toxins (hemolysins), leukocidin, staphylokinase. * Many strains have protein A bound to the mucopeptide of the cell wall. This protein interacts nonspecifically with host IgG antibodies reducing opsonization and causing local activation of complement.
Treatment and prevention	Antibiotics of choice are beta-lactamase stable penicillins (over 80% of hospital isolates are beta-lactamase producers). Methicillin resistance is a local problem and vancomycin is indicated. Mupirocin can be used for topical treatment of carriage. Prevention of spread by isolation and/or treatment of carriers in high risk areas in hospital. No vaccine available.

Staphylococcus epidermidis

Characteristics	As for *Staph. aureus*.
Laboratory identification	White colonies on blood agar; catalase positive, coagulase negative, mannitol not fermented anaerobically. Kits available for biochemical characterization.
Diseases	Opportunist pathogen associated with device-related sepsis (e.g. catheter-related sepsis; prosthetic valve endocarditis; infection of artificial joints; shunt infections); urinary tract infection; sternal wound osteomyelitis.
Transmission	Normal habitat: skin (carriage rate approximately 100%). Spread by contact with self, other patients or hospital personnel. Almost all infections acquired in hospital, but may be endogenous. Survives drying; salt tolerant.
Epidemiologic markers	Bacteriophage typing.
Pathogenesis	Extracellular slime production thought to be marker of virulence and may account for ability to colonize plastic implants (e.g. intravenous catheters and prostheses).
Treatment and prevention	Antibiotic resistance: often multiresistant (including penicillin and methicillin). Prevention of infection: catheter care; no vaccine available.

Staphylococcus saprophyticus

Characteristics	As for *Staph. aureus*.
Laboratory identification	White colonies on blood agar; catalase negative, coagulase negative, mannitol not fermented anaerobically. Kits available for biochemical characterization.
Diseases	Urinary tract infection in previously healthy women (associated with intercourse).
Transmission	Normal habitat: skin, and genitourinary mucosa. Endogenous spread to urinary tract in colonized women.
Epidemiologic markers	None in common use.
Pathogenesis	Virulence factors unknown, but organism has the ability to colonize periurethral skin and mucosa.
Treatment and prevention	Urination after intercourse helps to wash organisms out of the bladder and prevent infection.

GENUS *Streptococcus*

A large group of Gram-positive cocci distributed widely in man and animals, mostly forming part of the normal flora, but some species responsible for some major infections. Individual cells 0.5–1 μm in diameter and because they divide in one plane only, occur in pairs and chains. The medically significant streptococci may be conveniently divided on the basis of either hemolysis on blood agar (complete hemolysis – beta; partial hemolysis – alpha; no hemolysis – gamma) or by the presence or absence of a group-specific carbohydrate antigen (i.e. the Lancefield Group labelled alphabetically A to S).

BETA-HEMOLYTIC STREPTOCOCCI

Streptococcus pyogenes (GROUP A STREPTOCOCCUS)

Characteristics	Gram-positive cocci in chains, cells less than 1 μm diameter, non-motile, non-sporing.
Laboratory identification	Grown on blood agar. Pronounced hemolytic activity (enhanced anaerobically). Catalase negative. Bacitracin (0.04 units) used as an identifier; all strains are susceptible.
Lancefield grouping	Acid extraction of antigen from cell wall reacting with specific antisera (rabbit) either in a precipitin or latex agglutination reaction. In addition to this group-specific polysaccharide, type-specific M and T antigens can be detected and are used as a typing scheme for epidemiologic purposes.
Diseases	Infections of upper respiratory tract and of skin and soft tissue (e.g. pharyngitis, cellulitis, erysipelas, lymphadenitis). Toxic manifestations include scarlet fever. Non-suppurative sequelae (acute glomerulonephritis and rheumatic fever) important complications of both skin and throat infections.
Transmission	Normal habitat is the human upper respiratory tract and skin. Spread by airborne droplets and by contact. Survival in dust may be important. Epidemiologic typing of strains based on M and T proteins (see above) useful in outbreaks.
Pathogenesis	*Strep. pyogenes* elaborates many enzymes and exotoxins, which may play a role in infection: erythrogenic toxin (lysogenic phage mediated); streptolysins; streptokinase A and B (therapeutic applications); deoxyribonuclease; hyaluronidase ('spreading factor').
Treatment and prevention	Penicillin is drug of choice. Vaccines not available. Erythromycin is an alternative for penicillin-allergic patients, but resistance to erythromycin is increasing.

Streptococcus agalactiae (GROUP B STREPTOCOCCI)

Characteristics	Gram-positive cocci in chains.
Laboratory identification	Beta-hemolytic on blood agar; colonies larger than *Strep. pyogenes* frequently pigmented after anaerobic incubation on Columbia agar (Islam's medium). Grow in the presence of bile on MacConkey agar. Biochemical tests include hippurate hydrolysis (positive), aesculin hydrolysis (negative). Possess Group B Lancefield capsular antigen.
Diseases	Neonatal meningitis and septicemia. Mastitis in bovines.
Transmission	Normal habitat; gut and vagina. Babies acquire organism from colonized mother at birth or by contact spread between babies in nursery after birth.
Pathogenesis	Virulence factors not clearly identified.
Treatment and prevention	Susceptible to penicillin, but less so than *Strep. pyogenes*; combination of penicillin and gentamicin for serious infections. Screening pregnant women not reliable, but prophylactic antibiotics may be given to babies (especially prematures) of carriers.

OTHER BETA-HEMOLYTIC STREPTOCOCCI OF MEDICAL IMPORTANCE

Streptococci of Lancefield Groups C and G may sometimes cause pharyngitis; Group D streptococci are now reclassified in the genus *Enterococcus* (see below).

Streptococcus milleri

A microaerophilic streptococcus that often forms small colonies and carries Lancefield Group F or G antigen. Has a propensity for abscess formation (especially in liver and brain).

ALPHA-HEMOLYTIC STREPTOCOCCI

Streptococcus pneumoniae

Characteristics	Gram-positive coccus characteristically appearing in pairs (diplococci) in Gram films. Cells approximately 1 μm, often capsulate. Requires blood or serum for growth. Capable of aerobic and anaerobic respiration; growth may be enhanced in CO_2.
Laboratory diagnosis	On blood agar alpha-hemolytic 'draughtsman' colonies that may autolyse within 48 h at 35°C. Catalase negative. Susceptible to bile (bile solubility test) and optochin (ethyl hydrocuprein hydrochloride; available in paper discs). Polysaccharide capsules can be demonstrated by appropriate staining techniques. They are antigenic and in the presence of specific antiserum appear to swell (quellung reaction).
Diseases	Pneumonia, septicemia and meningitis. Otitis and related infections in children. Capsular type III frequently associated with pneumonia.
Transmission	Normal habitat is the human respiratory tract; up to 4% of population may carry in small numbers. Transmission via droplet spread.
Pathogenesis	Capsule protects the organism from phagocytosis. Pneumolysin may have a role as avirulence factor, but to date no known exotoxins. Splenectomy appears to predispose to infection. Viral infection may be a precursor to pneumonia.
Treatment and prevention	Penicillin remains the antibiotic of choice, but resistance is increasing rapidly in some countries and susceptibility test results should be used to guide therapy.

ORAL STREPTOCOCCI

There are several other species of alpha-hemolytic streptococci that in the past have been lumped together under the colloquial heading 'viridans streptococci'. These and some of the non-hemolytic streptococci have now been reclassified. Most species are commensals in the mouth. *Strep. mutans* is strongly associated with dental caries. Several species are capable of causing bacterial endocarditis. They are all susceptible to penicillin. It is important to distinguish these streptococci from *Strep. pneumoniae* in cultures from the respiratory tract.

GENUS *Enterococcus* (FECAL STREPTOCOCCI)

Formerly classified in the genus *Streptococcus* with which they share many characteristics; there are currently 15 species of which two, *E. faecalis* and *E. faecium* are of medical importance and are considered together.

Characteristics	Gram-positive cocci, cells often in pairs and chains; more ovate appearance than streptococci. Non-fastidious; capable of aerobic and anaerobic respiration.
Laboratory dentification	On blood agar may produce alpha, beta or no hemolysis. Bile tolerant (grow on MacConkey agar and in 40% bile); relatively heat tolerant (grow at 45°C), and salt tolerant (grow in 6.5% NaCl). Hydrolyze aesculin and arginine. Kits available for complete biochemical identification. Carry Lancefield's Group D antigen, but extraction of the antigen is more difficult than with streptococci (it is teichoic acid rather than polysaccharide).
Diseases	Urinary tract infection; endocarditis; infrequent, but severe septicemia after surgery and in the immunocompromised.
Transmission	Normal habitat is the gut of humans and animals. Most infections thought to be endogenously acquired, but cross-infection may occur in hospitalized patients.

Pathogenesis	No toxins or other virulence factors convincingly demonstrated. Plasmid-mediated hemolysin may play a role.
Treatment and prevention	Susceptible to penicillins, but less than streptococci. Penicillins used in combination with aminoglycosides for synergy in severe infections. Resistant to cephalosporins and incidence of resistance to vancomycin increasing. Patients with known heart defects should be given prophylactic antibiotics to prevent endocarditis before dentistry or surgery on gut or urinary tract.

GRAM-POSITIVE RODS

GENUS *Corynebacterium*

This genus contains many species, is widely distributed in nature, and is part of a spectrum, with *Mycobacterium* and *Nocardia*, of similar cell wall structure containing mycolic acids. The species of major importance is *C. diphtheriae*. This and other pathogens within the genus need to be distinguished from commensal corynebacteria.

Corynebacterium diphtheriae

Characteristics	Gram-positive, non-capsulate, non-sporing, non-motile rods, 2–6 μm in length. In Gram-stained films cells arranged as 'Chinese letters' or pallisades and showing irregular staining or granule formation are characterisitic. Non-fastidious, but growth enhanced by inspissated serum (Loeffler medium). Capable of aerobic and anaerobic respiration.
Laboratory diagnosis	Grows on blood agar, but identification aided by a selective medium (e.g. blood tellurite) on which characteristic black colonies form within 48 h at 35°C (but many other organisms may produce black colonies). Three biotypes of *C. diphtheriae* are recognized: *mitis*, *intermedius* and *gravis*, and they have characteristic colony morphology. *C. diphtheriae* is catalase positive and reduces nitrate. Species identification on the basis of carbohydrate fermentation tests should be performed in serum base not peptone. Toxin production is demonstrated by the Elek test. (Important to demonstrate toxigenicity to confirm a diagnosis of diphtheria because non-toxigenic strains may be carried as part of the normal skin or throat flora).
Diseases	Diphtheria caused by toxigenic strains of *C. diphtheriae*. Focus of infection may be the throat or, increasingly commonly, the skin.
Transmission	Normal habitat: usually nasopharynx, occasionally skin of humans. Infection is usually spread by aerosol. Patients may carry toxigenic organisms for up to 2–3 months after infection.
Pathogenesis	Disease is due to production of diphtheria toxin controlled by the *tox* gene, which is integrated into the bacterial chromosome on a lysogenic phage. When concentration of exogenous inorganic iron (Fe^{3+}) is very low, toxin production is maximal; the selective advantage to the organism is unknown. The mode of action of the toxin is to block protein synthesis of the host cells by inactivating an elongation factor.
Treatment and prevention	Urgent supportive therapy to maintain airway essential in throat diphtheria. Antitoxin neutralizes toxin, penicillin kills organisms; antibiotics have little effect since diffusion of toxin not influenced by inhibition of organisms at local site. In outbreak, carriers treated with penicillin or erythromycin. Immunization effective in prevention of diphtheria; in areas where immunization rates reach 85%, herd immunity sufficient to protect whole population. Circulating antibody after immunization neutralizes test dose of standardized toxin (Schick test). Positive result equates with insufficient antibody. Babies acquire immunity from immune mothers for a few months.

OTHER CORYNEBACTERIA

C. ulcerans has been found in diphtheria-like disease. It produces two toxins, one of which is neutralized by diphtheria antitoxin, the other is similar to that produced by *C. pseudotuberculosis*. *C. jeikeium* is being isolated increasingly from blood cultures and wounds in immunosuppressed patients. It is usually detected by its relative resistance to all antibiotics other than vancomycin and teicoplanin. *C. pseudotuberculosis* is a significant pathogen of horses and sheep. *C. xerosis* and *C. pseudodiphtheriticum* are skin inhabitants and many other coryneforms may also be found on skin. These, and other related genera such as *Brevibacterium* and *Rhodococcus*, are lipophilic and require lipids for optimal growth.

GENUS *Bacillus*

This genus contains nearly 50 species, most of which are soil organisms. There are two species of major medical importance: *B. anthracis* and *B. cereus*.

Bacillus anthracis

Characteristics	Large (4–10 μm) Gram-positive spore-forming encapsulated rods. Spores are formed only after the organism is shed from the body. Respires aerobically.
Laboratory identification	In smears of body fluids the capsule can be stained with polychrome methylene blue (McFadyean reaction). This is diagnostic of *B. anthracis*. The species is non-fastidious; grows well on simple media. Characteristic colonies (Medusa head) are probably related to chaining of the long rods. Non-hemolytic on horse blood agar (many of the other species are hemolytic). Growth in CO_2 encourages the formation of the capsule and smooth colonies. Biochemical reactions are unhelpful except in expert hands.
Diseases	Anthrax is a significant disease in both domesticated and wild animals. It is a zoonosis and humans are usually infected by contact with infected hides or bones. Woolsorters' disease i.e. respiratory or inhalation anthrax, is now rare. Intestinal anthrax is rare in humans, but remains a possibility that attracts interest as an aspect of biological warfare.
Transmission	Soil organisms; *B. anthracis* can survive in competition with other organisms for many years depending on the temperature and humidity. The carcasses of animals dying with anthrax are buried six feet deep to prevent organisms being carried to the surface. Humans are accidental hosts and infection is usually acquired when spores enter abrasions on the skin or are inhaled.
Pathogenesis	The polyglutamic acid capsule is antiphagocytic. In addition an exotoxin encoded on a temperature-sensitive plasmid is produced. Toxin has three components: edema factor, lethal factor and protective antigen. Individually the components have no biologic effect, but toxicity is produced by either of the first two factors together with the antigen. The toxin acts locally in the skin and lung. Pasteur used heat attenuation to produce a virulent strain that could be used as an attenuated vaccine.
Treatment and prevention	Penicillin is the drug of choice. Prevention includes control measures such as formalin disinfection of hides, strict control of infected domestic animals, and the immunization of veterinarians and laboratory workers at risk.

Bacillus cereus

Characteristics	Large Gram-positive spore-forming rod. This and many other *Bacillus* species are similar to *B. anthracis* in many respects except most are motile and non-capsulate. Respires aerobically.
Laboratory identification	Non-fastidious. Produces hemolysis on horse and sheep blood agar. Lecithinase production and inability to utilize mannitol are used as distinguishing features on a specially-designed selective medium.
Diseases	*B. cereus* causes food poisoning, the commonest association being with reheated cooked rice and pulses. Two different syndromes are recognized, due to different toxins (see below). The organism is also a rare cause of bacteremia in immunocompromised hosts.

Transmission	*B. cereus* spores are found on many foods, especially rice, pulses and vegetables. Infection is acquired by ingestion of organisms or toxin.
Pathogenesis	Some strains produce heat-stable toxin in food associated with spore germination; this gives rise to a syndrome of vomiting within 1–5 h of ingestion. Others produce a heat-labile enterotoxin after ingestion, which causes diarrhea within 10–15 h.
Treatment and prevention	The majority of illness is short-lived and self-limiting and antibiotic treatment is not indicated. Bacteremia in immunocompromised patients should be treated promptly with penicillin or vancomycin. As with other foodborne infections, hygienic preparation of food is paramount. Cooked food should be stored in a refrigerator and re-heated thoroughly before serving.

GENUS *Listeria*

These organisms were included with the genus *Corynebacterium* in earlier classifications. They also share antigenic relationships with enterococci and lactobacilli. *L. monocytogenes* is the species of major medical importance.

Listeria monocytogenes

Characteristics	Short Gram-positive rods, often coccobacillary in clinical material (must avoid confusion with streptococci in chains); frequently Gram variable. Motile at 25°C with a characteristic 'tumbling' movement; non-motile at 37°C.
Laboratory identification	Hemolytic on sheep or horse blood agar. Selective medium aids recovery of these organisms, especially from food samples (fish, chicken and cheeses). Cold enrichment at +4°C for several weeks is also an effective selective technique. On translucent, non-blood containing agar colonies appear green-blue in oblique light. Catalase-positive, nitrate reduction negative; coupled with motility at room temperature these results are useful identifying features.
Diseases	Meningitis and sepsis in neonates. Infections in the immunocompromised (particularly meningitis) and in pregnant women.
Transmission	Widely distributed in nature, survives well in cold. Reaches food chain via silage as well as more directly via for example vegetables. Excreted in large numbers in cows' milk. Humans may carry *Listeria* in gut as normal flora. Infection may be acquired by ingestion or transplacentally to the baby *in utero*. Serotyping has been used to investigate outbreaks, but not practicable except for reference laboratories. Many serotypes exist, but 4b appears to be associated with outbreaks.
Pathogenesis	Virulence factors unknown, but organism can survive in phagocytes.
Treatment and prevention	Treatment with penicillin or ampicillin, often in combination with gentamicin. Widespread distribution of organism in nature makes prevention of acquisition difficult. Pregnant women have been advised against eating uncooked food thought to be of particular risk (e.g. coleslaw, paté, soft cheese, unpasteurized milk).

GENUS *Clostridium*

This genus contains many species of Gram-positive anaerobic spore-forming rods; a few are aerotolerant. Widely distributed in soil and in the gut of man and animals. The spores are resistant to environmental conditions. The major diseases associated with species of the genus are gangrene, tetanus, botulism, food poisoning and pseudomembranous colitis. In each of these the production of potent protein exotoxins is an important cause of pathology and in several species the genes encoding toxins are carried by plasmids or bacteriophages.

Clostridium perfringens

Characteristics	Anaerobic Gram-positive rods; spore-forming, but spores rarely seen in infected material. More tolerant of oxygen than other clostridia.

Laboratory diagnosis	Hemolytic colonies on blood agar incubated anaerobically. Identification confirmed by demonstration of alpha-toxin (lecithinase) production in the Nagler's test. Heat resistant spores may be responsible for food poisoning (see Specimen Processing Section, p. 548). Five types of *Cl. perfringens* (A–E) identified on the basis of toxins produced; type A strains can be further divided into several serotypes.
Diseases	Gas gangrene resulting from infection of dirty ischemic wounds. Food poisoning following ingestion of food contaminated with enterotoxin-producing strains.
Transmission	Spores and vegetative organisms widespread in soil and normal flora of man and animals. Infection acquired by contact; may be endogenous (e.g. wound contaminated from patient's own fecal flora) or exogenous (e.g. contamination of a wound with soil, ingestion of contaminated food).
Pathogenesis	In ischemic wounds, production of various (at least 12) toxins and tissue-destroying enzymes allows organism to establish itself and multiply in wound. Local action of toxins produce necrosis thereby further impairing blood supply and keeping conditions anaerobic, and aiding spread of organism into adjacent tissues. Food poisoning results from the ingestion of large numbers of vegetative cells, which sporulate in the gut and release enterotoxin.
Treatment and prevention	Gangrene requires rapid intervention with extensive debridement of the wound. Penicillin or metronidazole are the antibiotics of choice. Anti-alpha-toxin may be given. The role of hyperbaric oxygen treatment is debated. Food poisoning does not usually require specific treatment.

Clostridium tetani

Characteristics	Gram-positive spore-forming rod with terminal round spore (drumstick). Strict anaerobe.
Laboratory identification	Grows on blood agar in anaerobic conditions as a fine spreading colony; 'ground glass' appearance (hand lens inspection of all cultures essential). Has very little biochemical activity useful for identification purposes. Demonstration of toxin in a specimen is possible in a two-mouse model in which one animal is protected with antitoxin, the other unprotected. Injection of suspect material is via the root of the tail.
Diseases	Tetanus (lockjaw). Severe disease characterized by tonic muscle spasms and hyperflexia, trismus, opisthotonos and convulsions.
Transmission	Organism widespread in soil. Acquired by man by implantation of contaminated soil into wound. Wound may be major (e.g. in war, in road traffic accident) or minor (e.g. a rose thorn puncture while gardening). No person-to-person spread.
Pathogenesis	Tetanus results from neurotoxin (tetanospasmin) produced by organisms in wound. Toxin genes are plasmid-encoded. The organism is non-invasive, but the toxin spreads from site of infection via bloodstream and acts by binding to ganglioside receptors and inhibiting release of inhibitory neurotransmitter glycine. Causes convulsive contractions of voluntary muscles.
Treatment and prevention	Antitoxin is available (hyperimmune human gamma globulin). Penicillin and spasmolytic drugs indicated. Prevention readily available and effective in form of immunization with toxoid. Usually given in childhood, but if immunization status of injured patient is unknown, toxoid is given in addition to antitoxin.

Clostridium botulinum

Characteristics	Anaerobic Gram-positive rods. Not easily cultivated in competition with other organisms. Produces most potent toxins known to man. Eight immunologically-distinct toxins (A, B, Cα, Cβ, D, E and F) produced by different strains of *Cl. botulinum*. Three are most commonly associated with human disease: serotypes A and B associated with meat, E with fish.

Laboratory identification	Requires strictly anaerobic conditions for isolation. Grows on blood agar, but very rarely isolated from human cases of disease. Detection of the toxin in the food or serum from the patient is the way of confirming the diagnosis.
Diseases	Major pathogen of birds and mammals, but very rare in humans. Botulism acquired by ingesting preformed toxin. Disease entirely due to effects of toxin. Infant botulism results from ingestion of organisms and production of toxin in infant's gut. Associated with feeding honey contaminated with spores of *Cl. botulinum*. Extremely rare. Wound botulism: toxin produced by organisms infecting a wound. Extremely rare.
Transmission	Soil is the normal habitat. Intoxication most often by ingestion of toxin in foods that have not been adequately sterilized (e.g. home-preserved foods) and improperly processed cans of food. Toxin is associated with germination of spores. There is no person-to-person spread.
Pathogenesis	Toxin released from organism as inactive protein and cleaved by proteases to uncover active site. It is acid stable and survives passage through stomach. Taken up through stomach and intestinal mucosa into bloodstream. Acts at neuromuscular junctions inhibiting acetylcholine release. Results in muscle paralysis and death from respiratory failure.
Treatment and prevention	Supportive therapy is paramount. Antitoxin is available from reference centers. In the rare cases of infant and wound botulism (i.e. when the organism is growing *in vivo*), penicillin is effective. Prevention relates to good manufacturing practice. The toxin is not heat stable, therefore adequate cooking of food before consumption will destroy it.

Clostridium difficile

Characteristics	Slender Gram-positive anaerobic rod; spore-former; motile.
Laboratory identification	Difficult to isolate in ordinary culture because of overgrowth by other organisms; selective medium containing cefoxitin, cycloserine and fructose is effective. The mere presence of this organism is not indicative of infection, but a marker to note. Diagnosis by detection of toxin in feces is practicable.
Diseases	Pseudomembranous colitis (antibiotic-associated diarrhea). Can be rapidly fatal especially in the compromised host.
Transmission	Component of normal gut flora; flourishes under selective pressure of antibiotics. May also be spread from person to person by the fecal-oral route.
Pathogenesis	Toxin-mediated damage to gut wall. More than one toxin involved; at least one is a cytotoxin.
Treatment and prevention	Oral vancomycin or metronidazole. Other antibiotics should be withheld if possible. Prevention of cross-infection in hospitals depends upon scrupulous attention to hygiene.

GENUS *Mycobacterium*

Mycobacteria are widespread both in the environment and in animals. The major human pathogens are *M. tuberculosis* and *M. leprae*, but awareness of the importance of other species is increasing with their recognition as pathogens in AIDS patients.

Characteristics	Aerobic rods with a Gram-positive cell wall structure, but stain with difficulty because of the long-chain fatty acids (mycolic acids) in the cell wall. Acid fastness can be demonstrated by resistance to decolorization by mineral acid and alcohol (Ziehl–Neelsen stain). Mycobacteria grow more slowly than many other bacteria of medical importance, but the genus can be divided into: rapid growers (form visible colonies within seven days); slow growers (form visible colonies only after 14 or more days' incubation).

Laboratory identification	Staining and microscopic examination of specimens for acid-fast rods is important because of the time required for culture results. All species except *M. leprae* can be grown in artificial culture, but they require complex media. Identification is based on rate of growth (rapid or slow), optimum temperature of growth and pigment production. Scotochromogens produce pigment in the absence of light whereas photochromogens require exposure to light before pigment becomes apparent. Further biochemical tests are required for full specification. Polymerase chain reaction methods and DNA probes are available for identification purposes.
Diseases	*M. tuberculosis* causes tuberculosis in humans and animals. *M. leprae* is restricted to man and causes leprosy. Mycobacteria other than tuberculosis (MOTT) are associated with a range of conditions, usually in immunocompromised hosts. The *M. avium-intracellulare* complex has important associations with AIDS patients.
Transmission	Droplet spread aided by ability of organisms to survive in the environment (*M. tuberculosis, M. leprae*). Milkborne spread of *M. tuberculosis* to humans from infected cattle has been important in the past. Social and environmental factors and genetic predisposition all have a role. Leprosy requires close and prolonged contact for spread.
Pathogenesis	Both *M. tuberculosis* and *M. leprae* are intracellular parasites surviving within macrophages. They give rise to slowly developing, chronic conditions in which much of the pathology is attributable to host immune responsiveness rather than to direct bacterial toxicity.
Treatment and prevention	Prolonged treatment with combinations of antimycobacterial drugs is required. Bacille Calmette–Guérin (BCG) vaccination is valuable for prevention (in people who are not environmentally exposed to heavy loads of mycobacteria early in life). Isoniazid prophylaxis used for contacts of cases of tuberculosis. Pasteurization of milk and improvement of living conditions have played a major role in prevention.

GENUS *Actinomyces*

The actinomycetes are true bacteria, although they have in the past been considered to resemble fungi because they form branching filaments. They are related to the corynebacteria and mycobacteria in the chemical structure of their cell walls and some are acid fast. It is important to differentiate them from fungi because infections with actinomycetes should respond to antibacterial agents whereas similar clinical presentations caused by fungi are resistant to antibacterials (and extremely refractory to treatment by antifungal agents). This genus contains many species, some of which are important to man as producers of antimicrobial agents. A few are pathogenic to man and animals; *A. israelii* causes actinomycosis.

Actinomyces israelii

Characteristics	Gram-positive anaerobic filamentous branching rods. Non-sporing, non-acid fast.
Laboratory identification	Forms 'sulphur granules' composed of a mass of bacterial filaments in pus. These can be identified by washing pus, squashing granules and observing in stained microscopic preparations. Gram-positive branching rods also visible in stained pus. Forms characteristic breadcrumb or 'molar tooth' colonies on blood agar after 3–7 days anaerobic incubation at 35°C
Diseases	Actinomycosis follows local trauma and invasion from normal flora. Hard non-tender swellings develop which drain pus through sinus tracts . Cervicofacial lesions are most common, but abdominal lesions after surgery and infection related to intrauterine contraceptive devices also occur.
Transmission	*A. israelii* is part of normal flora in mouth, gut and vagina. Infection is endogenous. There is no person-to-person spread.
Pathogenesis	Virulence factors not described.
Treatment and prevention	Penicillin is the drug of choice. Prolonged treatment is required, accompanied by surgical drainage.

GENUS *Nocardia*

Characteristics	Aerobic Gram-positive rods that form thin branching filaments. Widespread in the environment. *N. asteroides* is the important human pathogen, although other species can cause infection.
Laboratory diagnosis	Gram stains of pus may reveal Gram-positive filaments or rods. Sulphur granules not seen. Grow as 'breadcrumb' colonies on blood agar within 2–10 days' incubation. Often acid fast.
Diseases	*N. asterioides* is an opportunist pathogen infection in immunocompromised patients; primarily a pulmonary infection, but secondary spread to form abscesses in brain or kidney is common. *N. brasiliensis* is the cause of actinomycetoma in Central and South America.
Transmission	Infection is acquired from the soil by the airborne route. Outbreaks of infection in renal transplant units have been associated with local building work. Actinomycetoma is acquired by implantation of organisms into wounds and progressive destruction of skin, fascia, bone and muscle.
Pathogenesis	Appears to be related to oranisms's ability to survive the host's inflammatory responses. Infection is controlled by cell-mediated immunity, but this may be defective in immunocompromised patients.
Treatment and prevention	Nocardiosis is often difficult to treat, but most regimens include sulfonamides as the drug of choice.

GRAM-NEGATIVE RODS

ENTEROBACTERIACEAE

Most numerous facultative anaerobes in the human gut, comprising approximately 10^9/g of feces. Outnumbered only by Gram-negative anaerobes (e.g. *Bacteroides*), which are present in numbers approximately ten times those of the enterobacteria. Genera of the family Enterobacteriaceae share features that distinguish them from other families; can be distinguished from each other by biochemical tests.

GENUS *Escherichia*

Genus contains only one species of medical importance: *E. coli*.

Escherichia coli

Characteristics	Gram-negative rod; motile; with or without capsule; non-fastidious, facultative anaerobe; bile tolerant; capable of growth at 44°C.
Laboratory identification	Grows readily on routine laboratory media and on bile-containing selective media. Lactose fermenter. Kits available for full identification.
Diseases	Urinary tract infection; diarrheal diseases; neonatal meningitis; septicemia.
Transmission	Normal habitat is gut of man and animals; may colonize lower end of urethra and vagina. Spread is by contact and ingestion (fecal-oral route); may be food-associated; may be endogenous. Possesses O (somatic), H (flagellar), K (capsular) and F (fimbrial) antigens, which can be used to characterize strains by serotyping. Colicin (bacteriocin) typing also available.
Pathogenesis	A variety of virulence factors have been identified, particularly in strains associated with diarrheal disease: • Endotoxin: present in all strains. • Adhesins – p fimbriae associated with urinary tract infection; colonization factors (e.g. CFA I and II, K88, K99) associated with gastrointestinal tract infection in humans and animals. • Capsule present in some strains; may be associated with adhesion. K1 capsular type associated with neonatal meningitis.

- Enterotoxins associated with diarrheal disease: ETEC (enterotoxigenic *E. coli)* produce cholera-like heat-labile (LT) toxin; EIEC (enteroinvagive *E. coli*) produce shiga-like cytotoxin; EHEC (enterohemorrhagic *E. coli*) produce verotoxin – associated with hemolytic uremic syndrome.

Treatment and prevention	Wide range of antibacterial agents potentially available, but incidence of resistance variable and often plasmid-mediated; must be determined by susceptibility testing. Specific treatment of diarrheal disease usually not required. No currently available vaccine.

GENUS *Proteus*

Genus contains several species, of which two are of medical importance: *Pr. mirabilis* and *Pr. vulgaris.*

Characteristics	Gram-negative rod; non-fastidious; facultative anaerobe; bile tolerant; likes alkaline pH; characteristic unpleasant odor; highly motile and swarms on some media.
Laboratory identification	Lactose non-fermenter; produces urease; kits available for full identification. Species can be distinguished by indole test; *Pr. mirabilis,* indole-negative; *Pr. vulgaris,* indole-positive. O (somatic) and H (flagellar) antigens characterized. *Pr. vulgaris* strains OX-19, OX-2 and OX-K share antigens with rickettsiae in the typhus and spotted fever groups and are agglutinated by antibodies produced by patients with these rickettsial infections (Weil–Felix test). Serologic response to *Proteus* infection not useful diagnostically.
Diseases	Urinary tract infection; hospital-acquired wound infection, septicemia, pneumonia in the compromised host.
Transmission	Normal habitat is human gut, soil and water. Contact spread; infection often endogenous.
Pathogenesis	Characterized virulence factors include endotoxin, urease; possible role for bacteriocins.
Treatment and prevention	Range of agents available, but *Pr. vulgaris* usually more resistant to antibacterials than *Pr. mirabilis.* Prevention is by good aseptic technique in hospitals. No vaccine available.

GENUS *Klebsiella* and related ENTEROBACTERIA *Serratia* and *Enterobacter*

Unlike *E. coli,* species of the genera *Klebsiella, Serratia* and *Enterobacter* are rarely associated with infection except as opportunists in compromised patients.

Characteristics	Gram-negative rods, sometimes capsulate (usual for *Klebsiella*), non-fastidious growth requirements. Capable of aerobic and anaerobic respiration.
Laboratory identification	Lactose-fermenting, bile-tolerant organisms. Grow readily on routine laboratory media. Oxidase negative. Full identification based on bicohemical reactions (commercial kits available).
Diseases	Opportunist infections in the compromised (usually hospitalized) host. Urinary and respiratory tracts most common sites of infection. Distinction between colonization and infection can be difficult.
Transmission	Normal habitat is gut of man and animals and moist inanimate environments, especially soil and water. Infection may be endogenous or acquired by contact spread. *Klebsiella* have remarkable capacity for survival on hands. Various methods of epidemiologic fingerprinting available for investigation of outbreaks of hospital-acquired infection.
Pathogenesis	All possess endotoxin and fimbriae or other adhesins. Capsules, where present, are important in inhibiting phagocytosis.
Treatment and prevention	Multiple antibiotic resistance, usually plasmid-mediated, is common, and susceptibility must be determined by laboratory tests if treatment is indicated. Prevention depends upon scrupulous attention to aseptic techniques and to handwashing in hospitals.

Salmonella and shigella

Unlike other members of the Enterobacteriaceae, *Salmonella* and *Shigella* are not normal inhabitants of the human gut (except in post-infection carriers). Both genera are responsible for diarrheal disease, which may be severe; *Salmonella typhi* is also invasive and gives rise to systemic infection.

GENUS *Salmonella*

Has been classified into over 2000 species on basis of serologic differences; more recent studies suggest such divisions are below the level of species and that three, or fewer, species exist. Distinction on basis of infection is between *S. typhi* (also *S. paratyphyi* A and B), which cause enteric fevers and *S. enteritidis* (many other serotypes), which cause diarrheal disease.

Salmonella TAXONOMY

Kauffmann–White classification recognizes each serologically distinct salmonella (of which there are over 2000) as a species. These are then arranged in groups. Ewing classification restricts genus to three species only. Further serologic distinctions recognized as subtypes. Recently proposed that genus contains only a single species, *S. enterica,* within which six subgroups can be distinguished. Future DNA hybridization studies may reveal yet different groups.

Kauffmann–White classification	Group	Name*	Somatic (O) antigen	Flagella (H) antigen Phase I	Flagella (H) antigen Phase II
	A	*S. paratyphi*	A, 1,2, 12	a	–
	B	*S. paratyphi* B	1,3,5,12	b	1,2
		S. typhimurium	1,4,5,12	i	1,2
	C1	*S. paratyphi* C	6,7, Vi	c	1,5
		S. cholerae-susi	6,7	c	1,5
		S. virchow	6,7	r	1,2
	D	*S. typhi*	9, 12, Vi	d	
		S. enteritidis	1,9,12,	g,m	–

* examples of a few important species only

Ewing classification (three species)	*S. cholerae-suis* (one serotype)
	S. typhi (one serotype)
	S. enteritidis (over 2000 serotypes)

Characteristics	Gram-negative, motile non-sporing rods. All except *S. typhi* are non-capsulate. Capable of aerobic and anaerobic respiration.
Laboratory identification	Bile tolerant. Non-fastidious. Oxidase negative. Lactose non-fermenters. Produce acid and gas from glucose (except *S. typhi,* which is anaerogenic). Combination of biochemistry (commercial kits available) and serotyping required for full identification; important to distinguish enteric fever salmonellae from others. Detection of circulating antibody (Widal test) may aid diagnosis of enteric fevers. Serotyping (and phage typing of most important serotypes) useful for investigation of outbreaks.
Diseases	Vast majority cause diarrheal disease; very occasionally invasive (particularly *S. cholerae-suis*). Sickle cell disease predisposes to osteomyelitis. *S. typhi* and *S. paratyphi* cause systemic disease, typhoid and paratyphoid (enteric fevers).
Transmission	Widespread in animals; encountered in food chain (especially in poultry, eggs, meat, milk and cream). Acquired by ingestion of contaminated food or person to person via fecal-oral route. *S. typhi* human pathogen only. Spread via fecal-oral route, usually via contaminated water or food. Carriers are important source of organisms.
Treatment and prevention	*S. typhi* and *S. paratyphi* infections should be treated with systemic antibiotics. Antibiotic resistance is an increasing problem in many countries (important implications for travellers).

Salmonella diarrhea should not be treated with antibiotics unless there is evidence of invasive disease. Prevention depends upon interrupting fecal-oral transmission and on eliminating opportunities for transmission via the food chain. Effective vaccines are available to protect against *S. typhi* and *S. paratyphi*.

GENUS *Shigella*

Contains four species of importance to man as causes of bacillary dysentery: *Sh. dysenteriae, Sh. boydii, Sh. flexneri* and *Sh. sonnei* (in descending order of severity of symptoms).

Characteristics	Gram-negative rods. Non-motile (in contrast to salmonellae). Non-capsulate. Capable of aerobic and anaerobic respiration.
Laboratory identification	Non-fastidious, bile-tolerant. Lactose non-fermenters. Full identification requires use of biochemistry (commercial kits available) and serologic tests for O antigens. (Serodiagnosis of disease not applicable.
Diseases	Bacillary dysentery. Very rarely invasive.
Transmission	Human pathogens spread by fecal–oral route, especially in crowded conditions. Small infective dose.
Pathogenesis	Invasion of ileum and colon causes damage, which results in diarrhea. Intense inflammatory response involving neutrophils and macrophages characteristic. Enterotoxins have not been identified, but *Sh. dysenteriae* produces a neurotoxin.
Treatment and prevention	Antibiotic therapy should be avoided if possible; usually not required and many strains carry multiple antibiotic resistances, usually on plasmids. Prevention depends upon interrupting fecal-oral spread; hand hygiene important. No vaccine available.

GENUS *Pseudomonas*

This genus contains a large number of species, a few of which are human pathogens, some are animal pathogens and others are important pathogens of plants. Species also widely distributed and may contaminate the hospital environment and cause opportunist infections. Most important species in humans are *P. aeruginosa* (important opportunist in compromised patients) and *Pseudo. mallei* (cause of melioidosis, a disease of restricted geographic distribution).

Pseudomonas aeruginosa

Characteristics	Aerobic Gram-negative rod, motile by means of polar flagella. Able to utilize a very wide range of carbon and energy sources and to grow over a wide temperature range. Does not grow anaerobically (except when nitrate is provided as a terminal electron acceptor).
Laboratory identification	Grows readily on routine media including bile-containing selective media. Produces irregular irridescent colonies and a characteristic smell. Most strains produce a blue-green pigment (pyocyanin; unique to *P. aeruginosa*). and a yellow-green pigment (pyoverdin). Pigment production is enhanced on special media (King's A and B). Oxidase positive and oxidative in the Hugh and Liefson test.
Diseases	*P. aeruginosa* is an opportunist pathogen that can infect almost any body site given the right predisposing conditions. It causes infections of skin and burns, it is a major lung pathogen in cystic fibrosis and can cause pneumonia in intubated patients. It can also cause urinary tract infections, septicemia, osteomyelitis and endocarditis.
Transmission	Carriage as part of the normal gut flora occurs in a small percentage of normal healthy people and in a higher proportion of hospital inpatients. Thus endogenous infection may occur in compromised patients. *P. aeruginosa* is widespread in moist areas in the environment; patients usually become infected by contact spread, directly or indirectly, from these environmental sites.

Pathogenesis	A number of virulence factors have been identified, including endotoxin and exotoxin A, which acts as an inhibitor of elongation factor in eukaryotic protein synthesis. Extracellular slime (particularly massive amounts of alginate produced by strains specifically in cystic fibrosis patients) helps to prevent phagocytosis. Pigments may have a role in pathogenicity and pyoverdin acts as a siderophore.
Treatment and prevention	Resistant to antibacterial agents; *P. aeruginosa* is susceptible only to aminoglycosides and some cephalosporins and imipenem. Strains within the species may also acquire resistance to these agents. Immunotherapy with anti-endotoxin monoclonal antibodies may have a role in the future in severe infections. Prevention depends upon good aseptic practice in hospitals, avoidance of unnecessary or prolonged broad-spectrum antibiotic treatment and prophylaxis. Experimental vaccines have been tested in burned patients, but have doubtful usefulness.

CURVED GRAM-NEGATIVE RODS

There are several genera of curved Gram-negative rods that contain species that occur in humans as pathogens or as part of the normal flora:
* *Vibrio*: aerobic.
* *Wolinella*: anaerobic.
* *Anaerobiospirillum*: anaerobic.
* *Campylobacter*: microaerophilic.
* *Helicobacter*: microaerophilic.

Aerobes and microaerophiles cause infection of gastrointestinal tract; anaerobic curved rods form part of normal flora of mouth and vagina. Role in endogenous infection unclear; unusual growth requirements (for formate and fumarate) means they often fail to grow in reoutine culture conditions.

GENUS *Vibrio*

Most important species, *V. cholerae*, causes cholera. *V. parahaemolyticus* also causes diarrheal disease.

Characteristics	Curved Gram-negative rods, highly motile by means of single polar flagellum. Capable of aerobic and anaerobic respiration. Many species salt (NaCl) tolerant; some salt-requiring.
Laboratory identification	Grow in alkaline conditions (can be selected from other gut flora in alkaline peptone water). Oxidase positive. Grow on thiosulfate citrate bile salts sucrose (TCBS) medium to form yellow colonies *(V. cholerae)* or green colonies (other species). *V. cholerae* susceptible to O129 (vibriostatic agent), *V. parahaemolyticus* usually resistant. Biochemical tests and use of specific antisera required for complete identification.
Diseases	Cholera caused by *V. cholerae*. *V. parahaemolyticus* causes diarrheal disease. Other species (e.g. *V. vulnificus, V. alginolyticus)* may cause wound infections.
Transmission	*V. cholerae* is a human pathogen; no animal reservoir, but El Tor biotype survives better in the inanimate environment than classicial *V. cholerae*. Infection is acquired from contaminated water (usually) or food (sometimes). *V. parahaemolyticus* infection acquired from consumption of contaminated fish and seafood.
Pathogenesis	*V. cholerae* possesses several virulence factors (e.g. motility, mucinase, adhesins, and most importantly, enterotoxin). Chromosomally-encoded subunit toxin produced after cells bind to enterocytes, enters cells and binds to ganglioside receptors, activating adenylyl cyclase and causing fluid loss, resulting in massive watery diarrhea. *V. parahaemolyticus* produces a cytotoxin (which also hemolyzes human red blood cells – the Kanagawa test).
Treatment and prevention	For cholera, fluid replacement (oral rehydration therapy: ORT) of prime importance. Tetracycline shortens symptoms and duration of carriage. Specific treatment not indicated for *V. parahaemolyticus* diarrhea. Prevention of cholera depends upon provison of a clean (chlorinated) water supply and adequate sewage disposal. A whole cell vaccine is available, but of limited use (new vaccines are under development). *V. parahaemolyticus* infection can be prevented by adequate cooking of seafood.

GENUS *Campylobacter*

Curved Gram-negative rods, once classified as vibrios. More recently *C. pylori* the organism associated with gastritis and duodenal ulcers, has been moved into a new genus as *Helicobacter pylori*. Campylobacters are primarily pathogens of animals, but several species also cause infections in man. The most important is *C. jejuni*.

Campylobacter jejuni

Characteristics	Slender curved (seagull-shaped) Gram-negative rods. Motile by means of a polar flagellum at one or both ends. Microaerophiles. Do not utilize carbohydrate.
Laboratory identification	Require enriched media and moist microaerophilic environment (10% O_2) for growth. Incubation at 42°C for 24–48 h. Colonies resemble water drops. Full identification by biochemical tests and antibiotic susceptibility pattern.
Diseases	Diarrhea. Can invade to give septicemia.
Transmission	Animal reservoir. Organisms acquired from contaminated food and milk (but do not multiply in these vehicles). Person-to-person spread rare.
Pathogenesis	Little known, but cytotoxin implicated. Also invasion and local destruction of gut mucosa.
Treatment and prevention	No specific treatment necessary for diarrhea. Erythromycin for invasive disease. Prevention depends upon good food hygiene. No vaccine.

GRAM-NEGATIVE NON-SPORING ANAEROBES

Historically, all short Gram-negative anaerobic rods or coccobacilli have been classified in the genus *Bacteroides* and longer rods with tapering ends in the genus *Fusobacterium*. Recent applications of new techniques to the *Bacteroides* have resulted in the definition of two additional genera: *Porphyromonas* and *Prevotella*. The genus *Bacteroides* is now restricted to species found among the normal gut flora. *Prevotella* contains saccharolytic oral and genitourinary species, including *Pr. melaninogenica* (formerly *Bacteroides melaninogenicus*), which produces a characteristic black–brown pigment. The genus *Porphyromonas* contains assacharolytic pigmented species, which form part of the normal mouth flora (*P. gingivalis*) and may be involved in endogenous infection within the oral cavity. Most important non-sporing anaerobe causing infection is *Bacteroides fragilis* although others are much more common (e.g. in gingivitis and other endogenous oral infections).

Bacteroides fragilis

Characteristics	Small pleomorphic Gram-negative rod. Capable only of anaerobic respiration. Non-spore forming, non-motile.
Laboratory identification	Grows on blood agar incubated anaerobically and in other media designed for isolation of anaerobes. Plates may require up to 48 h. Incubation at 35°C for colonies to become visible. Cultures have a foul odor due to the fatty acid endproducts of metabolism. These can be used as identifying characteristics by analysis of culture supernates by gas–liquid chromatography (GLC). The major products of *Bacteroides* are acetate and succinate. Full identification in the diagnostic laboratory is based on biochemical tests and antibiogram. Commercial kits are available.
Diseases	Intra-abdominal sepsis; liver abscesses; aspiration pneumonia; brain abscesses; wound infections. Infections often mixed with aerobic and microaerophilic bacteria.
Transmission	Endogenous infection arising from contamination by gut contents or feces is most common route of acquisition.
Pathogenesis	Little is known about the virulence factors of *B. fragilis*. A polysaccharide capsule and production of extracellular enzymes are probably important features. An anaerobic environment is essential and in mixed infections growth of aerobic organisms probably helps the growth of *Bacteroides* by using up available oxygen.

| Treatment and prevention | Metronidazole well-established as the drug of choice for *Bacteroides* infections licensed for this indication in USA. Many strains produce beta-lactamases and thus susceptibility to penicillin and ampicillin is unreliable. Augmentin or cefoxitin are beta-lactams in common use. Chloramphenicol used for treatment of abscesses as it penetrates very well. Prevention of endogenous infection difficult; good surgical technique and appropriate use of prophylactic antibiotics important in abdominal surgery. |

GRAM-NEGATIVE COCCI

GENUS *Neisseria*

This genus contains several more or less fastidious species of which two, *N. gonorrhoeae* and *N. meningitidis* are important human pathogens.

Characteristics	Non-motile Gram-negative diplococci with fastidious growth requirements: capnophilic; *N. meningitidis* is capsulate, *N. gonorrhoeae* is not.
Laboratory identification	Gram stains of pus or cerebrospinal fluid may reveal Gram-negative kidney-shaped diplococci, often intracellular (in polymorphs). Require supplemented media for growth (chocolate agar). *N. gonorrhoeae* easier to isolate on enriched media containing antibiotics to inhibit other organisms of normal flora from sample sites. The two species are differentiated by sugar utilization pattern.
Diseases	*N. gonorrhoeae*: gonorrhea, and pelvic inflammatory disease and salpingitis in females; ophthalmia neonatorum in infants born to infected mothers. *N. meningitidis:* meningitis; occasionally septicemia in absence of meningitis.
Transmission	Human pathogens; no animal reservoir. *N. gonorrhoeae* may be carried in genital tract, nasopharynx and anus. Spread by sexual or intimate contact. *N. meningitidis* carried in pharynx. Carriage rate in population increases during epidemics. Droplet spread. *N. meningitidis* has several immunologically distinct capsular types (A, B, C).
Pathogenesis	Several virulence factors have been identified. *N. gonorrhoeae:* pili or fimbriae act as adhesins; endotoxin; outer membrane proteins; protease production; resistance to lytic activity of serum; IgA proteases. *N. meningitidis:* the polysaccharide capsule is antiphagocytic; endotoxin and IgA protease also implicated.
Treatment and prevention	*N. gonorrhoeae:* resistance to first-line drugs now widespread; usual choice is beta-lactamase stable cephalosporin. Spectinomycin for beta-lactam resistant strains. *N. meningitidis:* penicillin or cefotaxime (or equivalent cephalosporin); can be combined with chloramphenicol. Prevention of gonorrhea requires education, contact tracing. No vaccine available. Rifampicin is used for prophylaxis of close contacts of *N. meningitidis* meningitis. Vaccine is available for types A and C, but ineffective in preventing infection with type B strains.

GENUS *Branhamella (Moraxella)*

Branhamella catarrhalis, now reclassified by some into the genus *Moraxella,* is a Gram-negative coccus morphologically similar to *Neisseria,* but with less fastidious growth requirements. Formerly regarded as a commensal in the respiratory tract, it has been associated with severe infections including endocarditis. The majority of strains produce beta-lactamase and may be involved in the 'protection' of more obvious pathogens, especially in the respiratory tract, by destroying penicillin or ampicillin administered as treatment.

GENUS *Haemophilus*

The genus contains many species: *H. influenzae* and *H. ducreyi* are of medical importance.

Haemophilus influenzae

| Characteristics | Small Gram-negative rods, frequently coccobacillary. Non-motile. Fastidious, capnophilic, facultative anaerobe. May be capsulate when isolated from site of infection. |

Laboratory identification	Requires both hematin (X factor) and NADP (V factor) for growth (other species require one factor only). Grows on blood containing enriched media. Larger colonies around colonies of other organisms that secrete V factor (e.g. *Staph. aureus*) (satellitism). Dependence on X and V used as indicator of identity. *H. influenzae* can also be distinguished from other species by its inability to produce porphyrin. Six antigenically distinct capsular types recognized (a–f) of which type b is most frequently found in disease. Capsulate organisms can be agglutinated by specific antisera and detected directly (e.g. by latex agglutination) in specimens.
Diseases	Capsular type b *H. influenzae* causes meningitis, osteomyelitis, epiglottitis, otitis. All are more common in children than older age groups. Non-capsulate strains associated with acute exacerbations of chronic bronchitis.
Transmission	Normal habitat is upper respiratory tract in humans and associated animals. Transmitted from person to person by airborne route. Osteomyelitis probably follows septicemia from respiratory focus.
Pathogenesis	Polysaccharide capsule is important virulence factor. Outer membrane proteins and endotoxin may play a part, but no known exotoxin.
Treatment and prevention	Ampicillin (or amoxycillin) if non-beta-lactamase producing strain. Third-generation cephalosporin (e.g. cefotaxime, ceftriaxone or cefixime) or chloramphenicol are usual alternatives. All children should be immunized with Hib vaccine. Rifampicin prophylaxis recommended for close contacts of *Haemophilus* meningitis.

Haemophilus ducreyi

Cause of the genital tract infection 'soft chancre'. Slender Gram-negative rods appearing in pairs or chains. Direct microscopic examination of smear from chancre can be diagnostic. Organism very susceptible to dehydration; inoculate plates in clinic. Requires enriched medium (as for *H. influenzae*, but with addition of antibiotics to inhibit growth of other genital tract organisms).

GENUS BORDETELLA

There are three species, of which one, *B. pertussis* is of medical importance.

Characteristics	Small Gram-negative rod. Slow growing and fastidious in its growth requirements.
Laboratory identification	Requires enriched medium (e.g. Bordet–Gengou or blood charcoal agar). Intolerant of fatty acids in medium. Fails to grow on routine blood agar (i.e. 5–7% blood). Requires 3–5 days incubation in moist atmosphere. Irridescent bisected pearl colony type characteristic on Bordet–Gengou. Further identification by reaction with specific antisera.
Diseases	Whooping cough (pertussis).
Transmission	Human pathogen spread by airborne route from cases of disease (healthy carriage not documented).
Pathogenesis	Tracheal cytotoxin, fimbrial antigen and endotoxin all implicated as virulence factors. Stimulates a lymphocytic response.
Treatment and prevention	Erythromycin is the drug of choice for cases and close contacts of whooping cough. Antibacterial therapy has little effect on clinical course, but may reduce infectivity and incidence of superinfection. Whole cell inactivated vaccine administered to young children in three doses together with diphtheria and tetanus toxoids. New subunit vaccines currently undergoing trials.

GENUS *Brucella*

There are several species of the genus *Brucella*, each characteristically associated with an animal species. Three species: *B. abortus* from cattle, *B. suis* from pigs, and *B. melitensis* from goats are the species most often found causing human zoonotic infections.

Characteristics	Small Gram-negative rods. Intracellular pathogens. Growth enhanced by erythritol in placenta of animals (not in man).
Laboratory identification	Some strains slow-growing and fastidous, requiring complex growth media. Isolation from blood cultures improved by use of biphasic systems (e.g. Castenada bottles). Usually require 3–5 days' incubation in CO_2-enriched environment, but some strains of B. abortus may take up to four weeks – important in investigation of pyrexia of unknown origin (PUO). Identification is by biochemical reactions, patterns of resistance to certain dyes, and serologic tests. The disease may be diagnosed by examination of patient's serum for antibodies.
Diseases	Undulant fever (brucellosis). Patients frequently present with PUO. Infection may become chronic if not adequately treated.
Transmission	Zoonotic infections transmitted to man through consumption of contaminated milk or other unpasteurized dairy products (increasingly seen in 'health freaks' who prefer untreated products) and by direct contact (occupational hazard for veterinarians, abbatoir workers and farmers).
Pathogenesis	Virulence associated with ability to survive intracellularly, especially in bone marrow, liver and spleen, and thus 'hide' from host defences. Erythritol is a growth stimulant for the organism in animals and accounts for the tropism of the organisms to the placenta and fetus. This is not true in humans.
Treatment and prevention	Erythromycin or tetracycline; the latter may not be tolerated during long treatment courses required. Recrudescence of infection is common. Prevention depends upon eliminating the disease from domestic animals by vaccination (SV19 live attenuated vaccine) and pasteurization of milk. Vaccination is available for persons at risk in some countries, but is not used in USA and UK.

GENUS *Legionella*

A relatively recent discovery in microbiology history. Originally demonstrated by techniques used for virus isolation (e.g. growth in embryonated hens' eggs). In free-living state can grow in water, but difficult to cultivate on routine laboratory media. Large number of species (distinguished mainly on the basis of their DNA restriction patterns), but *L. pneumophila* is the pathogen of greatest medical importance.

Legionella pneumophila

Characteristics	Gram-negative rods, but stain poorly with Gram's stain (and therefore easily missed). Fastidious growth requirements in laboratory.
Laboratory identification	Direct fluorescent antibody tests performed on sputum samples have the advantage of specificity, distinguishing *L. pneumophila* from environmental contaminants. However relatively few organisms may be present in expectorated sputum. Silver staining techniques better than standard Gram staining method. Require enriched media containing iron and cysteine and absorbents to remove fatty acids. Most require incubation for 3–5 days for growth. Produces tenacious colony. Further identification based on requirement for cysteine and serologic characteristics. Diagnosis is often based on antibody detection rather than culture.
Diseases	Legionnaires' disease; one of the causes of atypical pneumonia. Pontiac fever which may be caused by other species is a less severe flu-like illness.
Transmission	Environmental saprophyte acquired by inhalation of contaminated water from showers, air conditioning systems, cooling towers.
Pathogenesis	Virulence factors unclear, but intracellular survival in alveolar macrophages important. Host prediposition (e.g. immunocompromise, chronic lung disease) important.

| **Treatment and prevention** | Erythromycin (may be combined with rifampicin or ciprofloxacin). No vaccine available; prevention depends upon maintenance of hot water and air conditioning systems, particularly in large buildings such as offices, hospitals and hotels. |

SPIRAL BACTERIA

There are three genera of medical importance: *Treponema*, *Leptospira* and *Borrelia*.

GENUS *Treponema*

Regularly coiled spirochetes with a longer wavelength than *Leptospira*. Several species and subspecies important human pathogens; others are members of the normal flora, especially in the mouth. *T. pallidum* and its subspecies *pertenue* and *T. carateum* are most important species.

Characteristics	Individual cells too small to visualize by direct light microscopy; can be seen with dark ground illumination or after silver impregnation or immunofluorescent staining. Cells are actively motile by means of flagella contained within the periplasmic sheath.
Laboratory identification	*T. pallidum* and closely related species cannot be grown in artificial media; diagnosis of infection depends upon microscopic examination of fluid from primary lesions and on serology.
Diseases	*T. pallidum*: syphilis. *T. pallidum-pertenue* and *T. carateum*: the non-sexually transmitted treponematoses, yaws and pinta.
Transmission	Very susceptible to heat and drying, so successful transmission depends upon very close contact. *T. pallidum* is spread by close sexual contact and may also be vertically transmitted *in utero*. Yaws and pinta spread by direct contact from infected skin lesions. No animal reservoir.
Pathogenesis	Study of virulence factors hampered by the inability to grow *T. pallidum* in artificial culture media. Disease presents characteristically in three phases: after local primary infection, organisms widely disseminated in the body and may become quiescent for months or years. Immunopathology plays a major role in causing damage to the host particularly in the tertiary stage of disease.
Treatment and prevention	Penicillin is the treatment of choice for syphilis. Tetracycline may be given to penicillin-allergic patients. Prevention depends upon detection and treatment of cases, contact tracing and serologic testing of pregnant women. Possible cross-reactions between *T. pallidum* and the species causing yaws and pinta must be noted.

GENUS *Leptospira*

Two species: *L. interrogans* and *L. biflexa*; the former is parasitic, the latter contains free-living species. Within the species *interrogans* there are several different serogroups and serovars responsible for disease in humans and animals.

Leptospira interrogans

Characteristics	Finely coiled spirochetes with hooked ends. Cells 0.1–0.2 µm in diameter, up to 20 µm in length. Not visible by direct light microscopy unless stained by silver impregnation or immunofluorescent methods. Dark ground microscopy reveals rotational and directional motility by means of periplasmic flagella.
Laboratory identification	Direct microscopy of blood and urine possible, but difficult to interpret. Leptospira can be grown, with difficulty, in special serum-containing media. Serologic diagnosis is usual.
Diseases	Leptospirosis or Weil's disease in humans and animals.
Transmission	Leptospirosis in humans is a zoonosis, usual hosts being rodents, bats, cattle, sheep, goats and other domestic animals. Leptospires excreted in urine contaminate food and water. Infection occurs by contact either through occupation [e.g. sewer workers, farmers, abbatoir

workers) or recreation (e.g. canoeing, windsurfing) on inland waters]. Organisms may penetrate unabraded skin and conjunctiva.

Pathogenesis	After initial invasion there is hematogenous spread before the organisms localize in various organs including the liver and kidney. Subclinical infection common in endemic areas.
Treatment and prevention	Penicillin; tetracycline or erythromycin in penicillin-allergic patients. Disease may be prevented after exposure by penicillin or doxycycline.

GENUS *Borrelia*

Two species of *Borrelia* of importance in humans. *B. recurrentis* causes relapsing fever (now rare). *B. burgdorferi* causes of Lyme disease.

Characteristics	Less finely coiled than the leptospires. Cells 0.2–0.5 μm in diameter; stain readily, so are visible by light microscopy.
Laboratory identification	*B. recurrentis* demonstrated in blood smears by staining with Giemsa or acridine orange. *B. burgdorferi* much more difficult to visualize. Culture from biopsy material possible, but difficult; diagnosis usually by serology.
Diseases	In relapsing fever the relapsing element may be due to antigen switching. Lyme disease slowly progressive rather than relapsing. Characteristic skin lesion 'erythema chronicum migrans' occurs in approximately 50% of cases. Joint pains and fatigue common and later, in untreated cases, neurologic and cardiac manifestations.
Transmission	*B. recurrentis* spread from person to person by lice. Lyme disease is a zoonosis transmitted to humans by hard ticks (*Ixodes* spp.) associated with deer. Ticks are found on bracken and undergrowth and attach to exposed skin. Tick bite is often unnoticed, but less than a minute is required for the organisms to enter the host.
Pathogenesis	Little known about pathogenesis of either disease. Antigen switching in *B. recurrentis* presumably allows evasion of host's antibody response.
Treatment and prevention	Tetracycline; but erythromycin and penicillin have both been used successfully. Prevention depends upon avoiding contact with vectors (e.g. protective clothing for walkers and forestry workers).

OTHER BACTERIA

MYCOPLASMAS

Characteristics	Distinguished from other prokaryotes and placed in the class Mollicutes because they lack a true cell wall and consequent rigidity. This is a stable characteristic exhibited by the genera *Mycoplasma*, *Ureaplasma* and *Acholeplasma* and is distinct from cell wall-deficient and L-forms of other species. The outer membrane, the outermost layer, functions as the major antigenic interface. It is a flexible triple-layered structure of proteins and lipids. Many species also contain cholesterol in the membrane, which is absent from other bacterial cells. The important species is *M. pneumoniae*, but *M. hominis* and *U. urealyticum* may cause genital tract infections.
Laboratory identification	Many species are fastidious, and complex media and soft agar may be required for satisfactory culture. Cultures incubated for at least seven days although some species (e.g. *M. hominis*) grow readily on moist blood agar plates within 48 h. Cells very variable in size (up to 100 μm) and morphology; cannot be stained by Gram's stain (no cell wall), but impressions of colonies can be stained with Dienes' or Romanowsky's stains. Diagnosis of infection based on serology due to difficulties of culture.
Diseases	*M. pneumoniae* is an important cause of 'atypical pneumonia'. Mycoplasmas also associated with genital infections (e.g. non-gonococcal urethritis) and with joint and other inflammatory infections. Other mycoplasmas are important pathogens of animals and birds.

Transmission	Transmission of *M. pneumoniae* from person to person by airborne route. Other mycoplasmas and ureaplasmas can be transmitted by sexual contact.
Pathogenesis	Surface protein adhesin binds *M. pneumoniae* to sialogycolipids on respiratory epithelium of host. Other virulence factors are not yet clearly understood.
Treatment and prevention	Tetracycline or erythromycin (note that the lack of cell wall target means lack of susceptibility to beta-lactams). No vaccine currently available. Prevention by interruption of spread is difficult.

RICKETTSIAE

Characteristics	These organisms have requirement for coenzyme A, NAD and ATP, which they cannot supply themselves, and are therefore obligate intracellular parasites; with rare exceptions need to be grown in cell cultures or experimental animals.
Laboratory identification	Small (0.7–2 μm diameter), Gram-negative bacteria. Isolation in laboratory is difficult for the reasons outlined above (and may carry a high risk of laboratory-acquired infection); therefore rarely attempted outside specialized facilities. Diagnosis of infection based on serology.
Diseases	Typhus; Rocky Mountain, Mediterranean and other spotted fevers; Q fever.
Transmission	*Coxiella burnetii* survives drying and is transmitted in aerosols from animals or materials contaminated by infected animals and inhaled. All other rickettsiae maintained in animal reservoirs and transmitted by bites of ticks, fleas, mites and lice.
Pathogenesis	Mechanisms unclear, but organisms have a predilection for endothelial cells, giving rise to characteristic primary skin lesion (in spotted fevers) and vasculitis. The intracellular habitat is important to the organism's survival in the face of host defences.
Treatment and prevention	Tetracycline, erythromycin, chloramphenicol. The newer fluoroquinolones may be useful in treatment. Beta-lactams ineffective. Infection prevented by avoiding contact with vectors. Vaccines available for at-risk groups (e.g. veterinarians, farm workers).

CHLAMYDIAE

Characteristics	Obligate intracellular parasites with distinct life cycle involving elementary bodies and reticulate bodies. Small cells with genome approximately 25% of that of *E. coli*. Important species are *C. trachomatis*, *C. psittaci* and *C. pneumoniae*.
Laboratory identification	Chlamydiae must be grown in cell culture, so cultural techniques limited to specialized laboratories. In cell cultures, *C. trachomatis* forms characteristic, glycogen-containing inclusion bodies, which can be stained with iodine. Both *C. psittaci* and *C. trachomatis* contain specific surface antigens that allow detection by immunofluorescent antibody techniques. *C. pneumoniae* currently detectable only by serology.
Diseases	*C. trachomatis* causes trachoma (eye infection), urethritis and other infections of the genital tract, and pneumonitis in newborns, acquired during birth from infected mothers. *C. pneumoniae*, described more recently, now recognized as important cause of atypical pneumonia. *C. psittaci* causes the atypical pneumonia, psittacosis.
Transmission	*C. pneumoniae* and *C. psittaci* acquired by inhalation, the latter from infected birds or contaminated bird litter. *C. trachomatis* spread by direct contact and is sexually transmitted.
Pathogenesis	Virulence factors remain unclear, but the intracellular habitat and different life cycle forms help organisms to evade host defences. Uptake into cells may be by parasite-encoded mechanisms.
Treatment and prevention	Tetracyclines and erythromycin (tetracyline should not be used in children). The new fluoroquinolones may be useful. Vaccines not available and are unlikely to be useful because of the immunopathologic element of the infections.

FUNGI

SUPERFICIAL MYCOSES

DERMATOPHYTES

General term for species invading superficial layers of skin. Of the many species involved, those belonging to *Epidermophyton*, *Microsporum* and *Trichophyton* are of greatest importance.

Characteristics	Filamentous fungi invading surface keratinized structures – skin, hair, nails. Hyphae penetrate between cells.
Laboratory identification	Examination of KOH-treated skin scrapings for hyphae; fluorescence under Wood's lamp. Culture on media useful in identifying species. Both Sabouraud dextrose agar (SDA) and dermatophyte test medium (DTM) can be used.
Diseases	Tinea, ringworm, athlete's foot.
Transmission	By fungal material on skin scales.
Pathogenesis	Skin inflammation, pruritus – sometimes localized hypersensitivity reactions.
Treatment and prevention	Topical antifungal agents. Improved skin care and hygiene.

Sporothrix schenckii

Characteristics	Dimorphic fungus (capable of growing as both single-celled yeast and multicelled hyphae). Occurs in external environment. Invades subcutaneous tissues.
Laboratory identification	Budding cells in inflammatory exudate from lesions. Culture on SDA.
Diseases	Sporotrichosis.
Transmission	Direct fungal contamination of wounds in skin (e.g. those made by thorns).
Pathogenesis	Ulceration or abcess formation in draining lymphatics.
Treatment and prevention	Potassium iodide, ketoconazole. Protection of skin.

DEEP MYCOSES

ASPERGILLUS

A. fumigatus is the most important of three common species, the others being *A. flavus* and *A. niger*.

Characteristics	Filamentous fungi causing opportunistic infections in immunocompromised patients. Occur widely in external environment. Invade lungs and blood vessels.
Laboratory identification	Presence of hyphae in tissues. Culture on SDA. Serology.
Diseases	Aspergillosis.
Transmission	Inhalation of airborne stages (conidia).
Pathogenesis	Causes thrombosis and infarction when blood vessels invaded. Partial blockage of airways from fungal mass. Allergic bronchopulmonary reactions.

Treatment and prevention	Amphotericin B.

Blastomyces dermatitidis

Characteristics	Dimorphic fungus. Invades through lungs, can become widely disseminated in body.
Laboratory identification	Yeast cells in sputum or skin lesions. Culture on SDA.
Diseases	Blastomycosis.
Transmission	Inhalation of airborne spores.
Pathogenesis abscesses.	Fungal infection in lungs. Presentation may be confused with tuberculosis. Can produce
Treatment and prevention	Ketoconazole.

Candida albicans

Characteristics	Dimorphic fungus, occurring as yeast on mucosal surfaces as component of normal flora, but forms hyphae when invasive. Produces opportunistic infections in stressed, suppressed and antibiotic-treated individuals. *Paracoccidioides brasiliensis* in central and South America has many similarities.
Laboratory identification	Fungal stages in tissues. Culture on SDA.
Diseases	Candidiasis, thrush.
Transmission	Part of normal flora of skin, mouth and intestine.
Pathogenesis	Localized mucocutaneous lesions; invasion of all major organs in the disseminated condition.
Treatment and prevention	Oral and topical antifungals (e.g. nystatin, miconazole). Ketoconazole, amphotericin B and flucytosine for disseminated disease.

Coccidioides immitis

Characteristics	Dimorphic fungus, growing as hyphae in soils, but as yeast-like endospores within capsules (spherules) in tissues. Invasion through lungs; can become widely disseminated in body.
Laboratory identification	In sputum or tissues. Culture on SDA. Serology.
Diseases	Coccidioimycosis. Indigenous to the Americas.
Transmission	Inhalation of airborne stages (arthroconidia).
Pathogenesis	Lung infections give mild, influenza-like condition, but serious illness may follow dissemination.
Treatment and prevention	Amphotericin B, ketoconazole.

CRYPTOCOCCUS NEOFORMANS

Characteristics	Encapsulated yeast-like fungus common in soils where there are bird droppings. Invades through lungs; can spread to CNS.

Laboratory identification	Encapsulated yeast cells in sputum or cerebrospinal fluid. Culture on SDA. Serology.
Diseases	Cryptococcosis.
Transmission	Inhalation of airborne cells.
Pathogenesis	Lung infection may result in influenza-like condition or pneumonia. In immunocompromised patients, CNS involvment leads to meningitis.
Treatment and prevention	Amphotericin B and flucytosine.

Histoplasma capsulatum

Characteristics	Dimorphic fungus, growing as hyphae in soil where there are bird droppings. Invades through lungs and grows as yeast cells, which can survive intracellularly after phagocytosis. Can become widely disseminated in body.
Laboratory identification	Yeast cells in sputum or tissues. Culture on SDA. Serology.
Diseases	Histoplasmosis.
Transmission	Inhalation of airborne spores.
Pathogenesis	Can produce acute and chronic pulmonary disease. Serious illness results from dissemination into other organs.
Treatment and prevention	Amphotericin B, ketoconazole.

Pneumocystis carinii

Characteristics	Respiratory organism previously classed as a sporozoan protozoan, now classified as a fungus. Lives extracellularly within alveoli.
Laboratory identification	Histologic identification of organism in tissues.
Diseases	Pneumonia-like condition, severe in immunocompromised patients. Worldwide distribution.
Transmission	Assumed to be by droplets.
Pathogenesis	Inflammation in lung.
Treatment and prevention	Trimethoprim plus sulfamethoxazole or pentamidine.

PROTOZOA

Cryptosporidium parvum

Characteristics	Intestinal sporozoan, invades and reproduces in epithelial cells of small intestine. Forms oocysts, which are passed in feces.
Laboratory identification	Small (5 μm) oocysts in feces, detected by flotation and acid-fast staining.

Diseases	Cryptosporidiosis. Worldwide distribution.
Transmission	Fecal–oral. Swallowing infective oocysts, usually in contaminated water. Animal reservoirs of infection.
Pathogenesis	Invasion of epithelial cells causes diarrhea; can be profuse in immunocompromised patients.
Treatment and prevention	No routine treatment available; spiramycin can be used in immunocompromised. Improved sanitation.

Entamoeba histolytica

Characteristics	Intestinal ameba, lives in intestine as trophozoite; produces resistant cysts, which are passed in feces.
Laboratory identification	Motile trophozoites or four-nucleate cysts in feces, detected in fresh or fixed-stained smears.
Diseases	Amebic dysentery, liver abscess. Worldwide distribution, commonest in tropical and subtropical countries.
Transmission	Fecal–oral. Swallowing cysts in contaminated water or food.
Pathogenesis	Invasion of large bowel mucosa causes ulceration and diarrhea, often bloody. Spread to liver causes formation of sterile abscess.
Treatment and prevention	Metronidazole, tinidazole. Hygiene and sanitation.

Giardia lamblia

Characteristics	Intestinal flagellate; lives on mucosa of small bowel. Produces cysts, which are passed in feces.
Laboratory identification	Four-nucleate cysts in feces, detected in fixed stained smears. Direct recovery of binucleate trophozoites from bowel.
Diseases	Giardiasis. Wordwide distribution.
Transmission	Fecal–oral. Swallowing cysts, usually in contaminated water. Animal reservoirs of infection.
Pathogenesis	Large numbers of trophozoites can cause severe diarrhea and impaired absorption. Most severe in immunocompromised patients.
Treatment and prevention	Metronidazole, tinidazole. Improved sanitation, water treatment.

GENUS *Leishmania*

Genus contains several species, of which *L. brasiliensis*, *L. donovani* and *L. tropica* cause major disease.

Characteristics	Sporozoa living intracellularly in macrophages as amastigote stage. Transmitted by phlebotomine sandflies.
Laboratory identification	Clinical signs, presence of amastigotes in stained biopsy material, *in vitro* culture of tissue specimens to obtain promastigotes.
Diseases	Visceral *(donovani)*, cutaneous *(tropica)* and mucocutaneous *(brasiliensis)* leishmaniasis. Disease also known by many local names (e.g. kala-azar, Oriental sore, espundia). Commonest in tropical and subtropical countries.

Transmission	By bite of infected sandfly.
Pathogenesis	Visceral: hepatosplenomegaly from invasion of macrophages in liver and spleen; allergic reactions after treatment causing dermal nodules. Cutaneous: localized ulcers, which resolve. Mucocutaneous: progressive invasion of mucocutaneous tissues in nose and mouth.
Treatment and prevention	Antimonials, pentamidine. Avoidance of vectors.

GENUS *Plasmodium*

Genus contains four species causing disease: *P. falciparum, P. malariae, P. ovale* and *P. vivax. P. falciparum* and *vivax* are commonest.

Characteristics	Sporozoa living intracellularly in liver and primarily in red blood cells.
Laboratory identification	Parasites in red blood cells in stained blood smear.
Diseases	Malaria. Commonest in tropical and subtropical countries.
Transmission	By bite of infected anopheline mosquito.
Pathogenesis	Bursting of infected red cells causes periodic fevers. In *falciparum* malaria, sequestration of infected cells in brain capillaries can cause fatal cerebral malaria; this infection is sometimes associated with intravascular hemolysis. Infection with *P. malariae* can lead to nephritis due to immune complex deposition.
Treatment and prevention	Many antimalarial drugs, but parasites show considerable drug resistance. Avoidance of vectors. Mosquito control.

Toxoplasma gondii

Characteristics	Sporozoan living intracellularly, forming large tissue cysts. Natural host is cat, where parasite has enteric cycle, producing oocysts in feces. In humans organisms can invade many tissues.
Laboratory identification	Serology; need repeated tests to establish current infection.
Diseases	Toxoplasmosis. Worldwide distribution.
Transmission	Swallowing oocysts passed by cats; ingestion of tissue cysts in raw or undercooked meat; transplacental.
Pathogenesis	In adults causes mild influenza-like disease; lymph nodes may be enlarged. Symptoms more severe in immunocompromised patients. Congenital infections can damage eye or brain and prove fatal.
Treatment and prevention	Pyrimethamine, sulfadiazine. Hygiene, cooking of meat.

Trichomonas vaginalis

Characteristics	Flagellate living in urogenital system of females and, occasionally, males. Trophozoite form only, no cyst.
Laboratory identification	Identification of trophozoites in stained material from vaginal smears.
Diseases	Trichomoniasis. Worldwide distribution.

Transmission	Venereal.
Pathogenesis	Mild in males; causes vaginitis with discharge in females.
Treatment and prevention	Metronidazole, tinidazole. Use of condoms.

GENUS *Trypanosoma*

Genus contains three species that cause disease: *T. gambiense, T. rhodesiense* (African trypanosomiasis) and *T. cruzi* (American trypanosomiasis).

Characteristics	Flagellates living in blood and tissues. *T. cruzi* has intracellular stages.
Laboratory identification	Organisms in blood or cerebrospinal fluid (African) or blood, biopsy or culture (American). Serology.
Diseases	African trypanosomiasis (sleeping sickness): subSaharan Africa. American trypanosomiais (Chagas' disease): South America.
Transmission	By bite of infected insect vector: tsetse fly (African) or reduviid bug (American).
Pathogenesis	African: infection of CNS causing meningoencephalitis. American: destruction of infected cells, especially neurones, megacolon, megaesophagus, cardiac failure.
Treatment and prevention	Arsenicals. Avoidance of vectors. Vector control.

HELMINTHS

TAPEWORMS

Diphyllobothrium latum

Characteristics	Large adult tapeworm in intestine. Scolex with sucking grooves not suckers. Eggs released and passed in feces.
Laboratory identification	Fecal smears, fresh or stained. Eggs in feces have characteristic operculum (lid).
Diseases	Diphyllobothriasis (fish tapeworm). Worldwide distribution. Commonest where fish eaten raw.
Transmission	Larval stages in fish. Adult worm acquired when infected fish eaten raw or undercooked.
Pathogenesis	Usually harmless; may be associated with vitamin B_{12} deficiency.
Treatment and prevention	Niclosamide, praziquantel. Cooking of fish. Sanitation.

Echinococcus granulosus

Characteristics	Large fluid-filled (hydatid) cysts, in abdomen, liver, lungs, CNS.

Laboratory identification	Scans, serology.
Diseases	Hydatidosis, hydatid disease. Worldwide distribution, commonest in sheep-rearing countries.
Transmission	Swallowing eggs released from adult tapeworms in dogs. Natural cycle is adult (dog), larval cysts (sheep).
Pathogenesis	Cysts exert pressure on internal organs. Release of cyst fluid can cause anaphylaxis.
Treatment and prevention	Mebendazole. Surgical removal of cysts. Prevention of dogs eating infected viscera from sheep. Hygiene after handling dogs.

Hymenolepis nana

Characteristics	Small (2–4 cm) adult tapeworms in intestine. Scolex with suckers and hooks. Eggs passed in feces. Life cycle can be direct or via insect intermediate host.
Laboratory identification	Fecal smears, fresh or stained. Thin-shelled eggs in feces.
Diseases	Hymenolepiasis (dwarf tapeworm). Worldwide distribution.
Transmission	Swallowing eggs. Accidental ingestion of larvae in insects.
Pathogenesis	Usually harmless. Numbers of worms can build up by autoinfection (direct hatching of eggs from adult worms in intestine) and enteritis may result.
Treatment and prevention	Niclosamide, praziquantel. Hygiene and sanitation.

GENUS *Taenia*

Two species of this genus infect humans, *T. saginata* and *T. solium*.

Characteristics	Large (meters) adult tapeworms in intestine. Scolices with suckers (*saginata*) or suckers and hooks (*saginata* and *solium*). Proglottids (segments) passed in feces. Small cysts (larval stages of solium) in muscles, CNS and eyes.
Laboratory identification	Proglottids in feces. Species identifiable on basis of number of branches to uterus (*T. saginata* 15–20; *T. solium* 5–10).
Diseases	Taeniasis (beef and pork tapeworms). Cysticercosis (*T. solium* only). Worldwide distribution.
Transmission	Adult worms acquired by eating raw or undercooked meat (beef, *saginata*; pork *solium*) from animals infected with larval stages. *T. solium* eggs can hatch in humans, allowing cysts to develop.
Pathogenesis	Adult worms essentially harmless. In cysticercosis, cysts in brain can result in neurologic symptoms.
Treatment and prevention	Niclosamide, praziquantel. Adequate cooking of meat. Prevention of human feces contaminating grazing and feeding areas of cattle and pigs.

FLUKES

Clonorchis sinensis

Characteristics	Liver fluke. Narrow elongated worms in bile ducts.

Laboratory identification	Fecal smears, fresh or stained. Eggs in feces.
Diseases	Clonorchiasis (Asia).
Transmission	Larval stages in fish; adult flukes acquired when infected fish eaten raw or undercooked.
Pathogenesis	Damage to liver, inflammation of bile ducts.
Treatment and prevention	Praziquantel. Cooking of fish. Sanitation.

Paragonimus westermanii

Characteristics	Lung fluke. Thick fleshy worms living as pairs in cysts.
Laboratory identification	Eggs in sputum or feces.
Diseases	Paragonimiasis (Asia).
Transmission	Larval stages in crabs; adult flukes acquired when infected crab meat eaten raw or undercooked.
Pathogenesis§	Inflammation of lungs, secondary bacterial infections.
Treatment and prevention	Praziquantel. Cooking of crab meat. Sanitation.

GENUS *Schistosoma*

Genus contains several species able to infect humans. Three are of major importance *S. haematobium, S. japonicum* and *S. mansoni.*

Characteristics	Blood flukes; adult worms in blood vessels around intestine *(S. japonicum, S. mansoni)* or bladder *(S. haematobium).* Eggs in tissues.
Laboratory identification	Fecal smears, fresh or stained. Spined eggs in feces (*S. japonicum* – small lateral spine; *S. mansoni* – large lateral spine). Eggs in urine (*S. haematobium* – terminal spine).
Diseases	Schistosomiasis. Widely distributed in tropical/subtropical countries (*S. mansoni,* Africa, S America; *S. haematobium,* Africa, Middle East; *S. japonicum,* Asia).
Transmission	Larvae released from eggs infect aquatic snails. These release infective cercariae larvae, which actively penetrate human skin.
Pathogenesis	Hypersensitivity responses to eggs cause inflammation, granuloma formation, fibrosis and obstructive disease in intestine, bladder and liver.
Treatment and prevention	Praziquantel. Avoidance of infected waters. Removal of snails. Sanitation.

NEMATODES

Ascaris lumbricoides

Characteristics	Large (up to 30 cm) intestinal roundworm; migratory stages pass through liver and lungs.

Laboratory identification	Fecal smears, fresh or stained. Thick-shelled eggs in feces; worms also passed occasionally.
Diseases	Ascariasis. Worldwide distribution. Commonest in tropical and subtropical countries.
Transmission	Swallowing infective eggs in contaminated soil, food or water.
Pathogenesis	Migrating larvae cause pneumonia-like symptoms. Adults can obstruct intestine, interfere with digestion and absorption of food, migrate in bile duct. Allergic symptoms common.
Treatment and prevention	Mebendazole, pyrantel, piperazine. Hygiene and sanitation.

Enterobius vermicularis

Characteristics	Small (1 cm) roundworm in large bowel. Worms emerge from anus at night to lay eggs.
Laboratory identification	Eggs recovered from perinal skin; adult worms in feces.
Diseases	Enterobiasis, pinworm. Worldwide distribution. Commonest in children.
Transmission	Swallowing eggs, which can be carried on fingers and in dust. Eggs infective when laid, so direct reinfection is common.
Pathogenesis	Perianal pruritus.
Treatment and prevention	Mebendazole, pyrantel, piperazine. Hygiene.

FILARIAL NEMATODES

Large group. Most important species living in lymphatic tissues *(Wuchereria bancrofti, Brugia malayi)* or in skin *(Onchocerca volvulus).*

Characteristics	Adults very long, thin worms, living in lymphatics with microfilariae larvae in blood *(Wuchereria, Brugia)* or in subcutaneous nodules with microfilariae in skin *(Onchocerca).*
Laboratory identification	Detection of microfilariae in stained blood smear or fresh skin snip.
Diseases	Lymphatic filariasis *(Wuchereria, Brugia).* Onchocerciasis or river blindness *(Onchocerca).*
Transmission	Microfilariae taken up by blood-feeding insects (mosquitoes, *Wuchereria, Brugia*; *Simulium* blackflies, *Onchocerca*), develop to infective stage and reintroduced into humans at the next blood meal. Widely distributed in tropical and subtropical countries.
Pathogenesis	In lymphatic filariasis, adult worms cause inflammation of lymph nodes and blockage of lymphatics, sometimes causing elephantiasis (big leg). In onchocerciasis, hypersensitivity to microfilariae larvae leads to skin and eye lesions.
Treatment and prevention	Diethyl carbamazine (lymphatic) and ivermectin (onchocerciasis). Avoidance of vectors. Vector control.

HOOKWORMS

General term for intestinal bloodsucking worms. Two major species *Ancylostoma duodenale* and *Necator americanus.*

Characteristics	Small (1 cm) intestinal roundworms; migratory stages pass through skin and lungs. Adult worms have expanded mouths for attachment to intestinal mucosa.
Laboratory identification	Fecal smears, fresh or stained. Thin-shelled eggs in feces. Culture of feces, eggs hatching after 24 h to release larvae.
Diseases	Hookworm disease (ancylostomiasis, necatoriasis). Widespread in tropical and subtropical countries.
Transmission	Infective larvae penetrate skin (both species) or mucous membranes after ingestion (*Ancylostoma*).
Pathogenesis	Bloodsucking of worms can lead to anemia and protein loss. Larval penetration associated with dermatitis.
Treatment and prevention	Mebendazole, pyrantel. Hygiene and sanitation.

Strongyloides stercoralis

Characteristics	Minute (2 mm) intestinal roundworm, living in humans only as larvae and parthenogenetic females. Migratory stages pass through skin and (possibly) lungs. Eggs hatch in intestine, larvae in feces may become infective directly or initiate a free-living generation in soil, from which infective larvae develop.
Laboratory identification	Larvae in fresh fecal specimens.
Diseases	Strongyloidiasis. Widespread in tropical and subtropical countries.
Transmission	Infective larvae penetrate skin.
Pathogenesis	In immunocompromised patients, repeated autoinfection (development of larvae released from females in the intestine) can lead to hyperinfection (disseminated strongyloidiasis), with larvae invading all body tissues. Hyperinfection can be fatal. Diarrhea and malabsorption accompany heavy intestinal infections.
Treatment and prevention	Thiabendazole. Hygiene and sanitation.

Toxocara canis

Characteristics	Invasion of larvae of roundworm species normally maturing in intestine of dogs.
Laboratory identification	Serology.
Diseases	Toxocariasis, visceral larva migrans. Worldwide distribution.
Transmission	Swallowing infective eggs passed by dogs in contaminated soil, food or water.
Pathogenesis	Invasion of body tissues causing granulomatous inflammatory responses. Larvae in CNS may cause epilepsy-like condition; in the eye granulomas may cause blindness.
Treatment and prevention	Thiabendazole. Hygiene. Routine deworming of puppies and pregnant bitches.

Trichinella spiralis

Characteristics	Minute (2–3 mm) roundworms, living as adults in the intestine. Coiled larvae in muscles. Low host specificity; infects and matures in wide variety of mammals.
Laboratory identification	Clinical signs, serology, muscle biopsy.
Diseases	Trichinellosis (trichinosis). Worldwide distribution.
Transmission	Acquired by eating raw or undercooked meat (usually pork) containing infective larvae.
Pathogenesis	Diarrhea during intestinal phase. Allergic symptoms, muscle pain, cardiac effects during muscle invasion; latter phase can be fatal.
Treatment and prevention	Mebendazole. Cooking of meat.

Trichuris trichiura

Characteristics	Medium size (0.75 cm) roundworms in large bowel. Body of characteristic 'whipworm' form, with long thin anterior and short thicker posterior.
Laboratory identification	Fecal smears, fresh or stained. Eggs in feces have characteristic shape, oval with plug at each pole. Endoscopy.
Diseases	Trichuriasis. Worldwide distribution. Commonest in tropical and subtropical countries.
Transmission	Swallowing infective eggs in contaminated soil, food or water.
Pathogenesis	Diarrhea, intestinal inflammation, occasionally rectal prolapse.
Treatment and prevention	Mebendazole. Hygiene and sanitation.

APPENDIX II: PROTOCOLS FOR SPECIMEN PROCESSING

Subsequent sections of this appendix are devoted to the basic protocols used in the diagnostic laboratory for processing specimens. These protocols describe the processing of specimens for isolation of bacteria, and pathogenic fungi where relevant. Isolation of viruses from clinical specimens as a method of diagnosis is generally slower, more difficult and costly and viral infections are usually diagnosed by antigen detection or serologic methods (see Chapter 14). The following types of specimens are considered:

Urine

Feces

Genital tract specimens

Skin and soft tissue specimens

Respiratory tract specimens (including nose, throat, eye and ear swabs, and sputum)

Cerebrospinal fluid

Pus

Other fluids such as pleural, pericardial fluids and joint aspirates

Blood

Bone marrow

Biopsy samples

Autopsy samples

Forensic samples

Abbreviations

Culture media

BA	Blood agar (different species of blood may be specified)
DCA	Deoxycholate citrate agar
Mac	MacConkey agar
CLED	Cysteine lactose electrolyte deficient agar
EMB	Eosin methylene blue agar
TM	Thayer–Martin agar
WC	Wilkins Chalgren agar
CA	Chocolate agar
TCBS	Thiosulfate citrate bit salts sucrose agar
SDA	Sabouraud agar

Incubation conditions

CO_2	Air enriched with 7–10% carbon dioxide.
AnO2	Anaerobic environment; one in which oxygen has been removed and replaced by nitrogen and hydrogen. These conditions can be achieved in 'gas jars' with commercially available gas-generating sachets.

Duration and temperature of incubation are also stated.

Other abbreviations

RBC	Red blood cells
WBC	White blood cells
NaOH	Sodium hydroxide
KOH	Potassium hydroxide
NCL	Hydrogen chloride

URINE

Specimen type	Mid-stream urine (MSU). Catheter urine (CSU). Suprapubic aspirate (SPA). Early morning urine (EMU).
Examination of specimens	Macroscopically: note appearance (e.g. cloudy, bloodstained). Microscopically: examine drop of urine (wet preparation; unstained). Note presence and numbers of WBC (normal <10–50/cm^3). Note presence of RBCs, epithelial cells (a poorly-collected specimen), bacteria, crystals. Commercial test kits available to detect WBCs and RBCs.
Culture	Numbers of bacteria important so quantitative and semiquantitive methods used. Media: BA, Mac or CLED. Incubation: air for 18 h at 35–37°C.
Likely pathogens (basic method)	*Escherichia coli, Proteus, Staphylococcus saprophyticus, Enterococcus, Klebsiella, Pseudomonas, Salmonella, Candida* (note that growth of yeasts is improved on SDA). Growth significant if over 10^5 organisms/ml isolated from an MSU; presence of any number of bacteria in CSU or SPA specimens may be significant; any number of mycobacteria in EMU specimens may be significant.
Important pathogens (not isolated by above technique)	Mycobacteria: • EMU specimens best for isolation of mycobacteria; before culture, decontaminate with NaOH or HCl, centrifuge, neutralize deposit. • Microscopy: not recommended; other non-pathologic mycobacteria from water or environment may be detected. • Culture: inoculate centrifuged deposit on to Löwenstein-Jensen or Middlebrook agar (in screw-capped bottles to prevent desiccation and reduce hazard). • Incubation: air for 4–12 weeks at 35–37°C *Leptospira*: • Can be demonstrated in urine in weeks 2–3 of infection by dark ground microscopy; urine must be very fresh (<15 minutes); culture possible, but difficult; diagnosis usually serologic. *Schistosoma*: • Ova of *S. haematobium* can be seen by microscopy; urine usually contains RBCs.

FECES

Specimen type	Samples of feces preferable to rectal swabs; swabs from soiled diapers acceptable; because of random distribution of organisms in sample, take three sequential samples.
Examination of specimens	Macroscopically: note appearance, gross blood, mucus parasites. Microscopically: note WBCs and RBCs in wet preparation; ova, cysts and parasites in concentrated suspension. Electron microscopy can be useful for rapid detection of some viruses.
Culture	Media/inoculum: Mac or EMB/lightly for discrete colonies. DCA/heavy*. Bismuth sulphite agar/heavy*. Selenite F broth/>1 g feces (subculture to DCA after 18 h incubation). Incubation: air for 18–48 h at 35–37°C. *Because these selective media inhibit pathogens, but to a lesser extent than commensals.
Likely pathogens (basic method)	*Salmonella* spp., *Shigella* spp., *Escherichia coli* (see below for verotoxin-producers).

Important pathogens (not isolated by above technique)	History and presentation of patient dictates culture type.

| **Pathogens demonstrated by special culture techniques** | *Campylobacter*:
• Medium: Columbia BA (rich BA) made selective by addition of antibiotic cocktail.
• Incubation: microaerophilic (10% O_2) for 24–48 h at 43°C (for *C. jejuni*; lower temperature for other species). |

Verotoxin producing *E. coli* (EHEC)
• Medium: sorbitol Mac (verotoxin producers do not usually ferment sorbitol; other *E. coli* do).
• Incubation: as basic method above.

Yersinia enterocolitica:
• Medium: CIN (cefsulodin, irgasan, novobiocin) agar.
• Incubation: air for 48–96 h at 30°C.

Clostridium perfringens:
• Medium: Robertson's cooked meat medium (×2); heat one at 80°C for 10 min before incubation.
• Incubation: air (anaerobic conditions provided in depths of medium) for 18 h at 35–37°C.
• Subculture to medium: neomycin BA (note that hemolysis differs on horse and sheep blood); incubation: AnO_2 for 18 h at 35–37°C.

Vibrio cholerae:
• Medium: TCBS.
• Incubation: air for 18 h at 35°C.
• Medium for enrichment: alkaline peptone water (pH 9).
• Incubation: air for 3–6 h at 35°C.
• Subculture to TCBS and incubate as above.

Pathogens demonstrated microscopically:
• Ova.
• Cysts.
• Helminth parasites.
• *Entamoeba histolytica* (mobile form visible if specimen examined early on).
• *Giardia lamblia* trophozoites (acute diarrhea) or cysts.
• Rotaviruses (and certain other viruses) visible by electron microscopy.

GENITAL TRACT SPECIMENS

Specimen type	Swabs transported in buffered medium essential due to fastidiousness and multiplicity of species causing genital infections.

| **Examination of specimens** | Microscopically:
• Wet preparation (for *Trichomonas vaginalis*, *Candida*).
• Acridine orange stain: view by fluorescence microscopy *(T. vaginalis)*; obviates need for expensive time-consuming culture.
• Gram's stain: note WBCs, Gram-negative intracellular diplococci (*Neisseria gonorrhoeae*); presence of WBCs in absence of any of above species, consider *Chlamydia trachomatis*; clue cells characteristic of bacterial vaginosis. |

Culture	Media: BA, TM (or other medium selective for gonococci), Mac, WC, SDA, human BA if diagnosis of vaginal discharge or pelvic inflammatory disease.
	Incubation: BA (CO_2) for 18–72 h at 35–37°C.
	TM (CO_2) for 18–72 h at 35–37°C.
	Mac (air) for 18–72 h at 35–37°C.
	WC (AnO_2) for 18–72 h at 35–37°C.
	Human BA (AnO_2) for 18–72 h at 35–37°C.
	SDA (air) for 18–48 h at 30°C.
Likely pathogens (basic method)	*N. gonorrhoeae*, *Candida albicans*, *Streptococcus agalactiae* (group B streptococcus), *Bacteroides* spp., *Gardnerella vaginalis* (enhanced growth on human blood agar), *Mycoplasma* and *Ureaplasma* spp., *Listeria monocytogenes*.
Important pathogens (not isolated by above technique)	*Chlamydia trachomatis:* • Culture: inoculate specimen onto monolayer of irradiated McCoy cells; examine after 48 h for characteristic inclusions. • Alternatively direct examination of specimen by immunofluorescent staining techniques. *Haemophilus ducreyi:* • Medium: culture on CA + isovitalex 1%. • Incubation: CO2 for 2–9 days at 30–34°C. *Treponema pallidum:* • Cannot be cultured *in vitro*. • Demonstrated in primary and secondary lesions by dark ground microscopy of exudate; otherwise diagnosis depends upon serology.

SKIN AND SOFT TISSUE SPECIMENS

Specimen type	Sampling of skin lesions problematic; of doubtful value in absence of obvious lesion; serum-coated swabs or swabs soaked in broth or peptone helpful in sampling and conserving skin flora; sellotape effective for sampling skin for carriage; skin scrapings, required to establish dermatophyte fungal infections, must include apparently uninfected tissue from periphery of lesion. Soft tissue lesions (e.g. bites, traumatic injuries) often polymicrobial and anaerobes must be sought. Viral infections: electron microscopy of vesicle fluid and/or culture, but superficial bacterial contamination of open lesions presents serious interpretation problems.
Examination of specimens	Microscopically (skin scrapings): treat portion of scrapings with KOH (24 h) to dissolve keratin; examine in wet preparation for fungal hyphae.
Culture	Use untreated portion of sample. Medium: SDA. Incubation: air for 1–10 days at ambient temp (approximately 25°C).
Likely pathogens (basic method)	*Trichophyton*, *Epidermophyton* and *Microsporum* spp., *Candida* spp., and other skin yeasts (important in immunocompromised, e.g. *Trichosporon beigelii*, *Cryptococcus neoformans*; also *Sporothrix schenkii*).
Examination of specimens	Microscopically: Gram's stain (note that this is of limited value except for grossly infected open lesions).
Culture	Media: BA, WC. Incubation: air (BA) or AnO_2 (WC) for 18–48 h at 35–37°C.

Likely pathogens (basic method)	Frequent: *Staphylococcus aureus*, *Streptococcus pyogenes*, *Propionibacterium acnes*, enterobacteria and pseudomonads (in warmer climates or after exposure to detergents), *Candida*. Infrequent: *Corynebacterium diphtheriae* (from cutaneous diphtheria), *Corynebacterium ulcerans*, *Erysipelothrix rhusiopathiae*, *Bacillus anthracis*.
Important pathogens (not isolated by above technique)	*Mycobacterium* spp., particularly *M. marinum* (see section on sputum for technique, p. 551). *Treponema pallidum*: cannot be cultivated *in vitro*; examine fluid from primary and secondary lesions by dark ground microscopy. Pathogens demonstrated microscopically: • *Leishmania tropica*, *L. mexicana* (amastigotes in smear from skin lesion). • *Dracunculus medinensis* (adult, or in fluid from vesicle). • *Onchocerca volvulus* (microfilariae in skin snips from nodule). • *Sarcoptes scabiei* (mites in skin scrapings or hooked out from burrow).

RESPIRATORY TRACT SAMPLES

The upper respiratory tract flora is liable to alter as a result of environmental conditions (e.g. moist atmospheres encourage Gram-negative rods).

Specimen type	**Throat swabs**
Examination of specimens	Microscopy of no value, unless Ludwig's angina (a mixed infection caused by a spirochete and a Gram-negative anaerobic fusiform) suspected.
Culture	Media: BA, CA, tellurite BA (if *Corynebacterium diphtheriae* suspected).
Incubation:	• BA (AnO$_2$) – better for streptococcal hemolysis. • CA (CO$_2$) for 18–48 h at 35–37°C.
Likely pathogens (basic method)	*Streptococcus pyogenes* (also beta-hemolytic streptococci of groups C and G), *C. diphtheriae*, *Candida* (important in immunocompromised).
Specimen type	**Nasal swabs (usually to detect carriage of pathogens and not to sample site of infection)**
Culture	As for throat swabs with addition of Mac.
Likely pathogens (basic method)	*Staphylococcus aureus*, *Strep. pyogenes*, *Neisseria meningitidis*, *C. diphtheriae*.
Specimen type	**Pernasal swabs (can be used to sample the nasopharynx)**
Culture	Bordet–Gengou, or charcoal BA for *Bordetella pertussis*. BA or CA to detect carriage of *N. meningitidis*.
Specimen type	**Outer ear swabs**
Culture	As for throat swabs with addition of Mac agar
Likely pathogens (basic method)	*Strep. pneumoniae*, *Haemophilus influenzae*, *Staph. aureus*, Gram-negative rods, especially *Pseudomonas aeruginosa*.

Specimen type	**Eye swabs**
Examination of specimens	Microscopically: Gram-stained smears: note WBCs and bacteria Direct immunofluorescence (DFA; direct fluorescent antibody stain) for *Chlamydiatrachomatis* if clinical history suggestive.
Culture	Media: BA, CA. Incubation: $CO2$ for 18–48 h at 35–37°C.
Likely pathogens (basic method)	*Strep. pneumoniae, Staph. aureus, H. influenzae, Acinetobacter lwoffi, N. gonorrhoeae.*
Important pathogens (special techniques)	*C. trachomatis* (for methods see Genital Tract Specimens, p. 548).

Specimen type	**Sputum**
Examination of specimens	Macroscopically: note appearance (purulent, mucoid, salivary), volume. Microscopically: Gram's stain – note polymorphs, bacteria (numbers, different types, predominant morphotype), epithelial cells (contamination with mouth flora).
Culture	Media: BA, CA. Incubation: CO_2 for 24–48 h at 35–37°C.
Likely pathogens (basic method)	*Strep. pneumoniae, H. influenzae, Staph. aureus, Klebsiella pneumoniae, Pseudomonas* spp., *Branhamella catarrhalis, Candida* spp., *Aspergillus* spp.
Important pathogens (not isolated by above technique)	(Note that laboratory needs to be warned if these pathogens are suspected.) Anaerobes: • If lung abscess suspected, follow basic method and inoculate additional BA and incubate anaerobically for 48 h. *Legionella pneumophila:* • Medium: blood charcoal yeast agar supplemented with cysteine. • Incubation: CO_2 for 3–7 days at 35–37°C. Mycobacteria: • If mycobacteria suspected, handle sputum in safety cabinet. • Before culture: decontaminate sputum with an equal volume of 4% NaOH to kill other bacteria. Neutralize with HCl or dilute. • Microscopy: Ziehl-Neelsen or auramine stain; observe for acid-fast rods. • Culture Löwenstein–Jensen or Middlebrook agar (in screw capped bottles to prevent desiccation). • Incubation: air* for up to 12 weeks at 35°C for *M. tuberculosis*, 25, 35 and 43°C for *M. avium-intracellulare*. (*For mycobacteria other than tuberculosis (MOTT) incubation in dark and in continuous light may reveal pigments.) • Alternatively use radiometric growth detection system. Add sputum homogenate and antibiotic cocktail to suppress other respiratory organisms to commercial medium containing radioisotope. Incubation: air for 2–12 days at 35°C. Growth detected by automated detection of radiolabelled CO_2.

| **Other important pathogens** | Viruses such as respiratory syncytial virus and influenza virus detected by immunofluorescence imaging of nasopharyngeal washings; *Pneumocystis carinii* (sputum); *Paragonimus westermanii* (eggs in sputum). |

CEREBROSPINAL FLUID

| **Specimen type** | This specimen is irreplaceable and must be processed as soon as possible after collection, with utmost care. |

| **Examination of specimens** | Macroscopically: |

- Note volume, color (presence of xanthochromia); presence of clot (will invalidate attempts at accurate cell count).

Macroscopically:
- Wet preparations (in counting chambers) for accurate counts of WBCs and RBCs.
- Gram's stain.
- Cytologic stain (aids recognition of eosinophils indistinguishable in Gram-stained smears).
- Ziehl–Neelsen or auramine stain for acid-fast rods (when indicated by history).

Chemically:
- Analysis of protein and sugar content.
- Antigen detection techniques may aid rapid diagnosis.

Culture:
- Media: BA (×2); fluid enrichment medium (e.g. thioglycollate); SDA (if *Cryptococcus* suspected from microscopy or history); Löwenstein–Jensen, Middlebrook or other suitable for mycobacteria (if suspected from microscopy or history); radiometric growth detection systems incorporating Middlebrook medium.
- Incubation: BA (CO_2) for 18–48 h at 35–37°C; CA (CO_2) for 18–48 h at 35–37°C; BA (AnO_2) for 18–48 h at 35–37°C; SDA (air) for 18–48 h at 30°C; fluid enrichment medium: subculture to BA (×2) after 48 h and incubate as for BA above; Löwenstein–Jensen (or equivalent): air for up to six weeks at 37°C.

| **Likely pathogens (not isolated by above technique)** | *Leptospira interrogans*; viruses – cell culture to isolate enteroviruses, mumps virus, herpes simplex virus; *Naegleria* (amebae plus WBCs and RBCs may be visible). |

PUS

| **Specimen type** | Pus, rather than a swab dipped in the exudate, should be sent for culture whenever possible. Bacteria survive less well on swabs and because recovery in culture depends among other things, upon the number of organisms present in the sample, the larger the volume the better. |

| **Examination of specimens** | Microscopically: |

- Gram's stain: note WBCs (polymorphs), bacteria and fungi (numbers, different types, predominant type).
- If mycobacteria are suspected, Ziehl–Neelsen or auramine stain.
- If actinomycetes are suspected, examine pus for sulphur granules.
- If anaerobes are suspected, examine pus directly by gas-liquid chromatography for volatile fatty acid end-products of metabolism.

| **Culture** | Media: BA, WC, CA, Mac, fluid enrichment medium. |

Incubation:
- BA (air) 35–37°C for 1–5 days.
- Mac (air) 35–37°C for 1–5 days.
- Fluid enrichment 35–37°C for 1–5 days.
- CA (CO_2) 35–37°C for 1–5 days.
- WC (or equivalent) (AnO_2) 35–37°C for 1–5 days.

Note that many fastidious anaerobes are particularly susceptible to oxygen in early stages of colony formation, so one set of anaerobic plates should be incubated undisturbed for 48 h unless examined in an anaerobic cabinet.

Likely pathogens (basic method)	*Staphylococcus aureus, Streptococcus pyogenes,* enterococci, peptococci, *Listeria, Pasteurella* spp., *Yersinia* spp, *Neisseria* spp., enterobacteria and pseudomonads, anaerobes including *Clostridium* spp., *Bacteroides* spp., and *Fusobacterium* spp., *Nocardia* spp., and *Actinomyces* spp. (the last two may require more than 48 h incubation).
Important pathogens (not isolated by above technique)	*Mycobacerium* spp.: • Pus from which no organisms are recovered should be examined microscopically and cultured for mycobacteria (using methods for sputum above); from some lesions (e.g. injection abscesses) mycobacteria other than *M. tuberculosis* may be isolated and significant.

OTHER FLUIDS

Specimen type	Examples are pleural, pericardial, ascitic and joint fluids. In health, amount of fluid is small, but large volumes may accumulate in disease; transudates result from stasis or obstruction; exudates from inflammation; specimens should be collected aseptically by aspiration into two sterile containers, one of which contains anticoagulant.
Examination of specimens	Macroscopically: note appearance and volume. Centrifuge fluid and examine deposit (use supernatant for serology and chemical analysis). Microscopically: Gram's stain: note polymorphs, lymphocytes (if present, suspect mycobacteria), bacteria (numbers, different types, predominant type). Cytologic stain.
Culture	Use deposit. Media: BA, WC or BA (with additions suitable for anaerobes), fluid enrichment medium (e.g. thioglycollate).
Likely pathogens (basic method)	Wide range of pathogens may be found; any isolate from specimen collected aseptically considered significant.
Important pathogens (not isolated by above technique)	Examine microscopically and culture for mycobacteria if indicated (see Sputum above, p. 551).

BLOOD

Specimen type	Volume of blood collected, ratio of blood to culture medium and presence of antibiotics all affect this important diagnostic process; scrupulous adherence to aseptic collection of samples is essential; inoculate blood directly into culture medium at bedside; use two bottles of culture medium: one contains a good broth medium, the other a broth medium formulated to support growth of anaerobes; dilute at least one part blood to 15 parts culture medium; distribute at least 20 ml of blood between the two culture bottles. Some blood culture systems include a third bottle with broth medium containing liquid (sodium polyanethol sulfonate, 0.05%), which helps to neutralize antibiotics and antibacterial activity of blood; some commercial systems do not require subculture, but use automated techniques to detect bacterial growth.
Examination of species	Transport blood cultures rapidly to the laboratory, incubate at 37°C, and examine 6, 24 and 48 h after collection; prolonged incubation (up to 21 days) may be required for growth of some organisms (e.g. *Brucella* spp.). Detection of positive cultures: unless alternative commercial systems used, bacterial and fungal growth detected microscopically.

Gram's stain: note bacteria (Gram-negative organisms may be difficult to see as RBCs and protein debris also stain pink).

Culture	Media: BA, WC or BA (with additions suitable for anaerobes), Mac (if Gram-negative rods seen by microscopy).

Incubation:
- BA (CO_2) for 24–48 h at 35–37°C.
- Mac (air) for 24–48 h at 35–37°C.
- WC (AnO_2) for 24–48 h at 35–37°C.

Likely pathogens (basic method)	Any isolate from more than one blood culture considered significant; blood culture system can support growth of any bacterial species that can grow *in vitro* without specific growth requirements; polymicrobial infections may be found and isolation of one species does not preclude possibility of a second; normal skin commensals such as coagulase-negative staphylococci are common contaminants.

BONE MARROW

Specimen type	Usually only available for microbiologic evaluation when collected for hematologic reasons; if collected and manipulated aseptically, bone marrow can be processed as for blood culture.
Likely pathogens (basic method)	*Salmonella typhi*, *Brucella* spp., mycobacteria, *Leishmania donovani* can be demonstrated in stained smears.

BIOPSY SAMPLES

As with cerebrospinal fluid, process biopsy samples with care as these are irreplaceable; processing protocol dictated by patient history; divide sample into three parts for histology, bacteriology and virology (note that specimens for bacteriology and virology must not be placed in histologic fixatives). Lymph nodes and other tissues may require maceration; this process may produce aerosols and should be carried out with appropriate precautions.

AUTOPSY SAMPLES

Collection of samples requires collaborative effort; superficial contaminants may be eliminated by searing outer surface with hot iron before cutting or by washing the sample several times in sterile broth or saline.

FORENSIC SAMPLES

All samples must be retained for legal purposes, precluding any destructive processing; it is imperative that all samples and slides are clearly labelled; staff should sign for custody of samples.

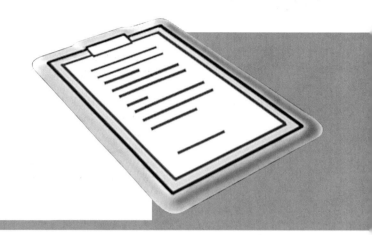

answers

Chapter 15

Upper respiratory tract infections

1. Diagnosis

Acute otitis media.

2. Most likely pathogens

Haemophilus influenzae and *Streptococcus pneumoniae* are the most common pathogens. Less commonly *Moraxella catarrhalis*, Group A β-hemolytic streptococci, and *Staphylococcus aureus* are implicated. Acute otitis media often follows a viral upper respiratory tract infection. Congestion of the eustachian tubes results in fluid stasis within the middle ear and secondary bacterial infection. The pressure building up within the anatomic constraints of the middle ear causes pain, and may lead to perforation of the tympanic membrane, with a discharge of pus.

3. Treatment

Treatment should involve antibiotics, usually oral unless the child is vomiting. Options include amoxycillin either alone or in combination with a beta-lactamase inhibitor such as clavulanic acid to cover the increasing proportion of *H. influenzae* that are beta-lactamase positive. Alternatives include orally-active second and third generation cephalosporins. Penicillin-allergic patients should be given cotrimoxazole or a new macrolide with increased activity against *H. influenzae*.

4. Possible complications

Complications include acute mastoiditis, which is rare since the advent of antibiotic therapy, and recurrent infections leading to chronic exudative otitis media (glue ear), which is a much more common problem.

Chapter 16

Infections of the eye

1. Infections associated with a choroidoretinitis

Cytomegalovirus (CMV), *Toxoplasma gondii*, *Toxocara* (*canis* or *catis*), *Mycobacterium tuberculosis*, or acute retinal necrosis, which is thought to be associated with varicella–zoster virus.

2. How would you make the diagnosis?

The diagnosis is almost invariably clinical and is made with the assistance of an ophthalmologist. In such a patient it can sometimes be difficult to differentiate between *Toxoplasma* and CMV. CMV retinitis sometimes has a classical appearance referred to as tomato ketchup and cottage cheese! Serology may be helpful in the diagnosis of *Toxoplasma* infection. In addition, in certain centers vitreous fluid from the affected eye can be collected. Detection of CMV DNA in this sample can be performed using a nested polymerase chain reaction approach involving two sets of primers, one set internal to the other, which increases the sensitivity of the test.

3. Treatment for CMV retinitis

Commence with a treatment course of intravenous ganciclovir while monitoring the hemoglobin, white cell count, and platelet count because this antiviral drug is myelosup-

pressive. If bone marrow suppression occurs, an alternative drug is foscarnet (which is nephrotoxic). It is best to site permanent intravenous access as this patient will need maintenance therapy with either of these drugs together with regular ophthalmologic follow-up to detect and prevent reactivation.

Chapter 17

Lower respiratory tract infections

1. Differential diagnosis

This case is suggestive of an atypical pneumonia. Causes are:

- Chlamydial infections such as *Chlamydia pneumoniae* (also referred to as TWAR) and *Chlamydia psittaci*.
- *Mycoplasma pneumoniae*.
- *Legionella pneumophila*.
- *Coxiella burnetii* (Q fever).

2. Other questions particularly relevant to the differential diagnosis to ask

- What is your occupation?
- Have you traveled recently?
- Do you have any pets at home or any hobbies?

These questions are always an important part of the history, but may be especially relevant with regard to *C. psittaci* (contact with infected birds), *L. pneumophila* (air conditioning systems) and *C. burnetii* (Q fever, contact with infected sheep/cattle).

3. Further investigations

Serology

- To detect *Mycoplasma pneumoniae* – particle agglutination test (IgM and IgG) and complement fixation test (CFT) on paired acute and convalescent sera collected 10–14 days apart, or test the acute serum specimen taken at least ten days after the illness. The hematology laboratory should also test for the presence of cold agglutinins.
- To detect chlamydiae – microimmunofluorescence for type-specific IgM/IgG or enzyme-linked immunosorbent assay (ELISA), and CFT on paired acute and convalescent sera collected 10–14 days apart, or test the acute serum taken at least ten days after the illness. The CFT uses the chlamydial group-specific antigen.
- To detect *L. pneumophila* – rapid microagglutination test (RMAT) to detect the presence of antibody.
- To detect *C. burnetii* – CFT of paired acute and convalescent sera collected 10–14 days apart, or test the acute serum specimen taken at least ten days after the illness. Phase 1 antibody is detected in chronic Q fever infection. Phase 2 antibody is detected in acute and chronic Q fever infection.

Culture for chlamydiae, mycoplasma, and *Legionella* may be attempted, depending upon available laboratory facilities.

4. Diagnosis

Mycoplasma pneumoniae infection on the basis of a fourfold rise in CFT, a positive agglutination test titer having diluted the serum 1 in 1024, and positive cold agglutinins.

5. Treatment

The antibiotics of choice are erythromycin or tetracycline.

Chapter 18

Urinary tract infections

1. Significance of bacterial count
This patient's urine specimen shows a bacterial count ($>10^5$ per ml of urine).

2. Why urine is screened for infection in pregnancy
Pregnant women have an increased risk of developing a urinary tract infection because the ureters dilate under the action of progesterone. This allows the urine to remain static and infection to ascend from the bladder. In the early stages of infection the patient may be asymptomatic, hence the need to screen the urine for the presence of infection. The risk of pyelonephritis is greater in the pregnant woman with a positive urine culture. Both urinary tract infection and pyelonephritis may cause septicemia, which may result in premature labour. It is therefore necessary to identify and treat urinary tract infections in pregnancy promptly.

3. The three most likely causes of this patient's infection
In the light of the culture result showing 'coliforms' the most likely causes are *Escherichia coli* followed by *Proteus mirabilis*. Other Gram-negative rods such as *Klebsiella* or *Pseudomonas* would be very unlikely unless the patient had a history of recurrent infection or previous instrumentation of the urinary tract.

4. Antimicrobials suitable for treating this infection in pregnancy
It may be possible to treat a simple urinary tract infection with a urinary sterilizing agent such as nitrofurantoin. Ampicillin is a suitable first-line antibiotic in areas where there is a low prevalence of resistant *Escherichia coli*. Where the prevalence of resistance is high, it may be necessary to use an oral cephalosporin. If the patient is unwell and requires parenteral antibiotics, an injectable cephalosporin can be given.

Chapter 19

Sexually transmitted diseases

1. Most likely diagnosis
Pneumocystis carinii pneumonia (PCP) in a person with HIV1 infection.

2. Further investigations
- Arterial blood gas analysis.
- Induced sputum or bronchoscopy and bronchoalveolar lavage for PCP examination.
- HIV1 and HIV2 antibody screening assay: this is positive and therefore a further confirmatory test is performed and demonstrates the presence of antibody to HIV1. In addition, *Pneumocystis* cysts are seen on cytology.

3. Management
The diagnosis should be discussed sensitively with the patient and a further serum specimen collected to confirm the diagnosis. A second specimen should always be retested to ensure that no errors in the collection, labeling of the specimen, dispatch, or handling of the specimen in the laboratory have occurred. The laboratory should have tested both the serum from the original specimen and repeat the test on any remaining serum in the original tube containing the blood clot.

First-line treatment for PCP, which would have already been started on clinical suspicion, generally comprises oxygen and cotrimoxazole, and in severe cases methylprednisolone. If the patient develops an allergy to the sulfa-containing drugs such as cotrimoxazole, intravenous pentamidine treatment should be instituted. Clinicians will be guided by the clinical signs and symptoms as well as the results of the blood gas analysis.

4. Prognosis and follow-up
This patient has an AIDS-defining diagnosis (i.e. PCP) and her prognosis in terms of survival duration is variable. Baseline CD4 counts and a p24 antigen test would be performed as would a syphilis and viral hepatitis screen.

Regular PCP prophylaxis with cotrimoxazole should be instituted and she should be followed-up regularly. She should be monitored clinically, and CD4 counts should be repeated at regular intervals. A decision about whether to start antiretroviral treatment should be discussed.

Other issues include a discussion regarding her partner and HIV testing, safe sex, and whether she has or is planning to have children. Counseling about the wider aspects and implications of her diagnosis with a health advisor should be arranged.

Chapter 20

a. Gastrointestinal tract infections

1. Most likely diagnosis and differential diagnosis
The most likely diagnosis is acute hepatitis B infection (HBV). The differential diagnosis includes hepatitis A, hepatitis C, delta hepatitis (as a hepatitis B coinfection/superinfection), (cytomegalovirus (CMV) infection, and Epstein–Barr virus (EBV) infection.

2. Investigations
- Collect a clotted blood specimen for hepatitis B surface antigen (HBsAg) testing and markers of HBV infection (see below).
- HBsAg testing: using enzyme-linked immunosorbent assay (ELISA) and the reverse passive hemagglutination (RPHA) test. The RPHA test allows an estimation of the HBsAg titer. The potential pitfall of the ELISA monoclonal antibody-based assay is that it is extremely specific and may not detect any of the rare HBV escape mutants with mutations in the region to which that monoclonal antibody has been made. The RPHA is a polyclonal-based test and should detect these mutants:
- Anti-HB core IgM.
- Anti-HB core (total IgM and IgG).
- HBeAg.

The results of these investigations are as follows: HBsAg enzyme immunoassay (EIA) positive (confirmed by specific neutralization with immune serum containing antibody to the HBsAg); HBsAg RPHA titer 1:1280; anti-HB core IgM positive; anti-HB core (total IgM and IgG) positive; HBeAg positive.

These results are consistent with an acute HBV infection.

If the sample is HBsAg negative, test for HAV IgM and HCV antibody. HCV antibody would not be detected at this early stage by EIA because anti-HCV seroconversion may be delayed for several months after an acute HCV infection. The test is usually repeated two months later if clinically indicated.

3. Management

- Repeat the HBV serology in one, three and six months to see whether the infection resolves. If HBsAg is still present after six months this man is a hepatitis B carrier and should be followed-up regularly because he may develop complications of chronic HBV infection (i.e. chronic active hepatitis, chronic persistent hepatitis, hepatocellular carcinoma). In addition, some individuals switch from being HBeAg positive to anti-HBe positive and some lose their HBsAg and become anti-HBs positive.

- Advise the patient to avoid alcohol and strenuous exercise.

- This man is also at risk of other infectious diseases because of his intravenous drug abuse and this should be discussed with him in the general context of health counseling.

4. Control of infection

HBV infection is a notifiable disease in the UK. Sexual partners or individuals with whom this man has shared needles should be followed-up, counseled and tested to see whether they have serologic evidence of a past hepatitis B infection as a matter of urgency. If there is no evidence of past HBV infection these individuals should be offered a course of hepatitis B immunization together with an injection of hepatitis B hyperimmuneglobulin (HBIG) to attenuate, modify or prevent HBV infection.

b. Gastrointestinal tract infections

1. Source of infection

Bacteria are well-preserved in ice cream and can multiply extensively before the product is frozen. Probable source was an asymptomatically infected worker in the factory, who could have acquired it from poultry, eggs, or meat.

2. Treatment

Treatment is by oral rehydration, and antibiotics are not usually necessary. If the infection is severe or invasive, ciprofloxacin or trimethoprim can be used.

3. Management

Screen factory workers for *Salmonella enteridis* in feces. Careful re-examination and enforcement of personal hygiene program.

c. Gastrointestinal tract infections

1. Immediate management.

- Admit to a source isolation room in the ward.
- Collect blood for urea and electrolyte determination.
- Rehydrate orally unless she is vomiting, in which case intravenous fluids are needed.
- Send a stool sample to bacteriology and virology for analysis.

2. Most likely viral causes of the diarrhea

Viral gastroenteritis can be divided into sporadic infantile gastroenteritis and epidemic viral gastroenteritis. The most common cause of sporadic infantile gastroenteritis is a rotavirus infection. Adenovirus infections are the second most common cause.

3. Diagnosis of a viral infection

- Electron microscopy (using phosphotungstic acid as a negative stain) is the method of choice because in this setting it is a 'catch-all' method that allows detection of a variety of viruses for which there are no generally available specific tests for detecting viral antigen or antibody to that antigen.

- There is a particle agglutination test that is specific for rotavirus infection. This is widely used, but may miss some rotavirus infections.

- In specialised laboratories enzyme-linked immunosorbent assays (ELISAs), radioimmunoassays (RIAs), or nucleic acid detection methods are available for some of the viruses associated with gastroenteritis.

Wheel-like particles which are 65nm diameter, are demonstrated by electron microscopy and rotaviral infection is diagnosed.

4. Natural course of the infection

If the child is dehydrated, fluid replacement therapy is needed. There is no specific treatment for any of the viral causes of diarrhea, and rotaviral excretion should decrease within a week. Avoid lactose-based fluids as the loss of the distal parts of the intestinal villi due to viral infection results in a disaccharidase deficiency and therefore lactose intolerance/malabsorption.

The most important measures to prevent nosocomial infection are to place the child in source isolation and maintain high standards of hygiene, in particular thorough hand-washing after contact with the child by any member of staff.

Chapter 21

Obstetric and perinatal infections

1. Likely diagnosis and likely pathogens

The baby is septicemic. The most likely pathogens responsible for septicemia in the newborn are organisms acquired from the mother's genital tract. Group B streptococci are the most common, but *Escherichia coli* and *Listeria monocytogenes* are also important pathogens in this age group.

2. Investigation

The baby should have a septic screen. In particular, this involves a blood culture and cerebrospinal fluid (CSF) sample. Deep ear swabs and a gastric aspirate may help to identify the pathogen responsible. A maternal vaginal swab should also be taken. Antimicrobial therapy should be started before the results of cultures are known and there are many different regimens which may be used. Common combinations are cefotaxime and benzylpenicillin, or ampicillin and gentamicin. The use of aminoglycosides requires careful monitoring of pre and post-dose serum levels to minimize toxicity. Once the pathogen has been identified, the antibiotic regimen can be tailored accordingly.

Group B streptococci were isolated from this baby's blood culture and he was treated with intravenous benzylpenicillin and gentamicin.

3. Risk factors in the mother's history

The maternal history that points to an increased risk of neonatal infection include the following:

- Early rupture of membranes
- Maternal pyrexia
- A long and difficult labour

Chapter 22

Central nervous system infections

1. Urgent investigations

A computerized tomographic (CT) scan of the patient's head followed by a lumbar puncture if the CT scan does not demonstrate raised intracranial pressure.

2. Diagnoses

It is important to rule out a subarachnoid hemorrhage, a subdural hemorrhage (both are unlikely in the absence of red blood cells and xanthochromic appearance in the CSF), a cranial space-occupying lesion including a cerebral abscess, metabolic causes of seizures, and meningitis.

The presentation and findings are more consistent with an encephalitic process and the most common causes of a viral encephalitis include herpes simplex (HSV), mumps, and enteroviruses. More detailed clinical examination revealed the presence of genital ulcers.

3. Management and treatment

There is enough evidence to implicate HSV infection as the cause of the encephalitis and so intravenous aciclovir should be started immediately together with other general supportive measures. It is important that this patient is treated with aciclovir for at least two weeks to prevent a relapse. Finding diffuse slow wave activity on an electroencephalogram (EEG) would further assist in making a diagnosis. A genital swab should be collected for viral isolation and cerebrospinal fluid (CSF) should be cultured, although it is extremely unusual to isolate HSV from CSF. Finally, it is possible to detect HSV DNA in CSF specimens using the polymerase chain reaction technology (PCR) and this service may be available in some laboratories.

Chapter 23

a. Infections of the skin, muscle, joints, bone and hemopoietic system

1. Likely diagnosis

The most likely diagnosis is an acute osteomyelitis. In children of this age, it may be accompanied with a history of minor trauma. It can be difficult to diagnose, particularly if vomiting is a major part of the illness.

2. Investigations

Investigations that should be performed are:
- Full blood count.
- Blood cultures.
- Radiographs of the affected area.

In acute osteomyelitis, radiographic changes usually lag behind the clinical picture. The most common pathogen in such cases is *Staphylococcus aureus*.

3. Treatment

Treatment should be commenced using intravenous flucloxacillin and oral fusidic acid (or other equivalent anti-staphylococcal treatment) while the results of cultures are awaited. Intravenous fluids and nasogastric aspiration should also be started. The limb should be immobilized by splinting, and traction will reduce the pain. Pain relief and antipyretics should also be given as appropriate. If the patient's temperature does not settle, it may be necessary to drain any collection of pus operatively. Any pus should be sent to microbiology for culture. How would you treat this condition?

b. Infections of the skin, muscle, joints, bone and hemopoietic system

1. Differential diagnosis

- Roseola infantum (also called exanthema subitum) due to human herpes virus 6 (HHV 6).
- Enteroviral infections (i.e. due to echoviruses, coxsackieviruses).
- Fifth disease due to parvovirus B19, which is unlikely because the classical presentation is red, slapped cheeks together with a fine rash.
- Measles and rubella, which are unlikely because of the clinical findings and she is up to date with her immunization schedule.

2. Investigations

- Collect a throat swab and stool specimen for viral isolation, in particular for the enteroviruses.
- Collect a serum specimen for the following tests: HHV 6 IgM (reference laboratory test), parvovirus B19 IgM, measles-specific IgM, rubella-specific IgM, and enterovirus specific IgM.

Her fever subsided over three days and HHV 6 specific IgM was detected in the serum specimen.

c. Infections of the skin, muscle, joints, bone and hemopoietic system

1. Most common infectious causes of an acute monoarthritis

Single joints can become infected as a result of a direct penetrating injury, or as a result of hematogenous spread. The large joints are usually affected by a hematogenous spread, especially the knee and hip. Disseminated *Neisseria gonorrhoeae* infection is renowned for its ability to produce a monoarthropathy. Other organisms can spread to joints, most common is *Staph. aureus* (60%), but other organisms such as non group A beta hemolytic streptococci (15%) and *Streptococcus pneumoniae* (3%) may be implicated.

2. Other points which may be helpful in the history

In an arthritis due to *N. gonorrhoeae*, there is usually a history of urethral discharge in a man. Where other organisms are involved, there is usually a source of the infecting organism, e.g. an infected skin wound. These points should be sought in the history.

3. Diagnosis

The most effective way of diagnosing an infected joint is to take a sample of joint fluid for analysis. In the presence of infection, there will be numerous polymorphonuclear white cells. In this case, microscopic examination of the knee fluid revealed more than 2000 white cells indicative of an inflammatory process within the joint. There may be organisms seen on the Gram stain which will give an initial guide to therapy. Culture of the fluid, including suitable media for the isolation of gonococci will demonstrate the pathogen.

4. Treatment

Treatment should involve antimicrobials to eradicate the infecting organism. Gonococci involved in joint infections are usually sensitive to penicillin although penicillin-resistant strains are being increasingly reported. Ceftriaxone is being used to treat gonococcal infections in many parts of the USA. Staphylococcal infection should be treated with flucloxacillin, depending on the antibiotic sensitivity pattern, in combination with another agent such as oral fusidic acid (or other equivalent anti-staphylococcal treatment).

Chapter 24

Worldwide virus infections

1. Differential diagnosis

Epstein–Barr virus (EBV) infection (also known as infectious mononucleosis or glandular fever) or cytomegalovirus (CMV) infection.

2. Investigation for EBV infection

Paul–Bunnell test or monospot for heterophile antibody. The heterophile antibody is an IgM antibody that reacts with an antigen unrelated to the host that produced the antibody. The test entails using guinea pig kidney (GPK) cells to adsorb out Forssman antibodies, which can cause a false positive test result and ox cell stroma (OCS) cells, which adsorb out the heterophile antibody. The serum specimen is pipetted in three places onto a test card:

- Nothing is added to the first (unadsorbed) serum.
- GPK cells are added to the second serum.
- OCS cells are added to the third.

Finally the indicator horse red blood cells are added to all three specimens and the cards are gently shaken. Agglutination should occur in only two of the three tests as the OCS cells absorb the heterophile antibody and no agglutination occurs.

In order to confirm the result the specimen should be tested for viral capsid antigen (VCA)-IgM and IgG and early antigen (EA)-IgG. A positive VCA-IgM and high titer EA-IgG indicate an acute EBV infection.

3. Interpretation of the results

The results are consistent with the presence of heterophile antibody and an acute EBV infection.

4. Common complications

- Hepatitis and hepatomegaly in 15–20%.
- Splenomegaly in up to 50–60%.
- Jaundice in 5–10%.
- Secondary bacterial infections (i.e. beta-hemolytic streptococci) in 25%.
- Occasional neurologic and hematologic complications.

5. Advice

- Rest.
- Avoid contact sports until symptoms improve.
- No alcohol until hepatitis resolves.

Chapter 25

Vector-borne infections

1. Differential diagnosis

Malaria, viral hemorrhagic fever and typhoid fever.

If someone has a history of travel to an area such as Sierra Leone (West Africa) and develops this clinical picture within three weeks of their return, then the risk of having a viral hemorrhagic fever must be considered. This is important as these patients are placed in a category of suspicion of illness risk, which is graded as minimal, moderate or strong. The type of hospital isolation unit to which the patient is admitted depends upon this risk assessment. This patient was graded as a medium risk and was admitted to a high security unit in which he could be investigated and treated. In addition, any individuals in close contact with him should be contacted as they may be at risk.

2. Immediate investigations

After the patient is transferred to the high security isolation unit, which contains its own laboratory, a full blood count including a differential cell count and thick and thin films, blood urea, electrolytes and glucose, an electrocardiogram, a midstream urine (MSU) specimen and stool and blood cultures should be collected.

A picture of a hemolytic anemia, leukopenia and a slightly lowered platelet count was seen in this case. The thin film revealed normal size, multiple infected red blood cells and approximately 10% of the red blood cells contained flimsy ring forms (malarial trophozoites). A diagnosis of falciparum malaria was made.

A serum sample should be sent for arboviral serology as individuals from endemic areas can present with dual infections.

3. Management

Management comprises full supportive care and treatment with intravenous quinine. Hematologic and biochemical parameters should be monitored, and in particular the level of parasitemia in response to treatment, blood glucose and renal function.

This patient made an uneventful recovery and was found to have had chloroquine-resistant falciparum malaria.

Chapter 26

Multisystem zoonoses

1. Questions to ask to help make the diagnosis

Asking about an individual's occupation is always important. This man is a sailor who has traveled to the Far East as well as Africa. Questions should be asked about:

- His lifestyle.
- Contact with any cases of infectious disease, pets or animals.
- Whether he has been bitten by any insects.
- Whether he has had any unpasteurized milk or cream or eaten any goats' cheese.

These questions may be critical in determining the cause of a PUO. In fact, this patient had drunk some milk in Africa directly after milking a few cows.

2. Most likely diagnosis
Brucellosis is the most likely diagnosis.
3. Further investigation
- Collect blood cultures and use a special biphasic (solid/liquid) medium called Casteñeda's medium, which should be incubated in carbon dioxide for up to six weeks.
- Test serum using the standard tube agglutination test for *Brucella* agglutinins and *Brucella* complement fixation test (CFT). A single serum tested by CFT had a titer of 2048.
4. Management
Treatment with doxycycline and rifampicin for six weeks, but relapses occur.

Chapter 27

Pyrexia of unknown origin
1. Probable diagnosis and critical further investigations
It is probable that this patient has infectious endocarditis. She has an artificial aortic valve, which makes this diagnosis highly likely given the presence of a fever and a murmur. In these circumstances it is important to take blood cultures to identify the pathogen responsible. At least three sets of cultures should be taken on three separate occasions to ensure the highest chances of isolating the organism. An echocardiogram, which is most sensitive if performed by a transesophageal approach should be performed. The presence of vegetations on echocardiography are diagnostic, although their absence does not exclude the diagnosis.
2. Most common pathogen
Streptococci, usually of the viridans type and found as part of the normal flora of the mouth are the most common organisms responsible for endocarditis. However, with the increasing use of cardiac surgery to replace damaged valves, staphylococci, both *Staphylococcus aureus* and coagulase-negative staphylococci (CNS) are important. CNS are especially implicated in prosthetic valvular endocarditis. Many other organisms have been implicated as the cause of endocarditis, including some fastidious Gram-negative rods, and more unusually, fungi.

The majority of cases of endocarditis used to be due to rheumatic valve disease as a consequence of rheumatic fever. An increasing number of cases are associated with prosthetic valves, and staphylococci are the most prominent organisms found in this group of patients. Infection can be acquired at the time of surgery, when it will present within the first few months postoperatively and usually manifests within a few weeks. Alternatively it may present later, as in this case, when it is the result of organisms settling on the valve during a bacteremia. The classic signs of endocarditis may not be present in this group of patients and the presentation may be more acute.

This patient's blood cultures revealed *Staphylococcus aureus* in all three sets.
3. Crucial components of management
It is essential that a physician, a surgeon, and a microbiologist are involved at an early stage. It may be necessary to remove an infected valve surgically if there is no response to antimicrobial therapy. A multidisciplinary team is best placed to make such a decision for each individual case.

4. Possible complications
The most serious complications include abscess formation within the valve and endocardium. Infected tissue embolizing from an infected valve on the left side of the heart may result in cerebral, renal, or more unusually, bone abscesses.
5. Guidelines to reduce the risk of this disease occurring
In the UK, guidelines are available from the British Heart Foundation in conjunction with the British Society for Antimicrobial Agents and Chemotherapy on the use of antimicrobial prophylaxis before dentistry. Prophylactic and therapeutic guidelines are available in most countries.

Although there is little evidence that the majority of cases of endocarditis are due to dental manipulation, litigation has ensued where a dentist has failed to give prophylaxis to patients known to be at risk of endocarditis.

Chapter 28

Infections in the compromised host
1. Most likely diagnosis and diagnostic tests
The most likely diagnosis is *Cryptococcus neoformans* (fungal) infection. The serum can be immediately tested for cryptococcal antigen and an Indian ink or nigrosin stain performed on the cerebrospinal fluid (CSF) deposit. Rapid detection of cryptococcal antigen in CSF and serum may be performed using a latex particle agglutination test.
2. Other confirmatory investigations
Culture of *C. neoformans* together with antifungal sensitivity tests, which are usually performed in reference laboratories.

Cryptococcal antigen was detected in both the serum and the CSF and capsulated yeasts were seen in the CSF.
3. Management
- Treat with antiemetics, analgesics, and intravenous amphotericin B (with or without 5 flucytosine) or fluconazole depending upon the clinical picture.
- Continue fluconazole maintenance therapy to prevent recurrences after recovery.
- Consider that this patient now has two AIDS-defining diagnoses and this has prognostic implications.
- Repeat the cryptococcal antigen tests monthly for six months or if the patient is symptomatic. Lumbar punctures may be repeated at one and six months to monitor recovery.

Chapter 34

Hospital infection, sterilization and disinfection
1. Common causes of postoperative infections in patients and steps to reduce these problems
The most common cause of a postoperative pyrexia is a wound infection. Other causes of pyrexia include chest and urinary infections. Chest infections are particularly common after abdominal surgery because the patient is in pain and finds coughing difficult. Urinary infections are often a result of catheterization. Non-infectious causes of postoperative pyrexia include deep venous thrombosis.

Surgical wound infections are substantially reduced by giving prophylactic antibiotics, which should be effective against the most common pathogens responsible for infection in the type of surgery being used.

2. Investigations

It is important that the wound dressing is removed so that the wound can be examined and a swab is taken. Sputum culture and urine culture should also be sent. A chest radiograph is needed if there is clinical evidence of a chest infection.

This man's wound is red and discharging small amounts of pus at the lower end and a wound swab grows *Staphylococcus aureus*.

3. Treatment

Initially this patient would be treated with flucloxacillin. The laboratory will have the results of antibiotic sensitivity testing the following day. Methicillin is used in the laboratory to detect flucloxacillin resistance. The organism is resistant to flucloxacillin and is referred to as a 'methicillin-resistant *Staphylococcus aureus*' or MRSA strain.

The patient should be source isolated in a side room and staff should be made aware of the risks of carrying the organism on their hands. *Staph. aureus* is carried on a variety of sites on the body, including the nose, hair, axillae, wrists and hands, and the perineum. Swabs should be collected from these sites in this patient to check for carriage.

The carriage rate is higher in hospitals than in the community. MRSA ward outbreaks may occur, especially as the organism survives in dry environments. In this case, the most likely source of the MRSA is the patient's skin or nose.

The following measures should be taken to reduce the chance of the MRSA spreading: these include isolating the patient and careful wound dressing technique and good handwashing technique by any member of staff attending him. In addition, he should be treated with a glycopeptide antibiotic, either vancomycin or teicoplanin. If vancomycin is used, the serum concentration must be monitored.

Index